Textbook of
NEUROANATOMY

Textbook of
NEUROANATOMY

ALVIN M. BURT, Ph.D.
Professor of Cell Biology
Division of Anatomy
Department of Cell Biology
Vanderbilt University
School of Medicine
Nashville, Tennessee

W. B. SAUNDERS COMPANY
Harcourt Brace Jovanovich, Inc.
Philadelphia   London   Toronto   Montreal   Sydney   Tokyo

W. B. SAUNDERS COMPANY
Harcourt Brace Jovanovich, Inc.

The Curtis Center
Independence Square West
Philadelphia, Pennsylvania 19106

Library of Congress Cataloging-in-Publication Data

Burt, Alvin M.
    Textbook of neuroanatomy / Alvin M. Burt. — 1st ed.
        p.   cm.
    ISBN 0-7216-2199-6
    1. Neuroanatomy.   I. Title.
    [DNLM: 1. Nervous System — anatomy and histology.   2. Nervous System —
physiology.   WL   101 B973t]
QM451.B885   1992
612.8 — dc20
DNLM/DLC   91-35154

Textbook of Neuroanatomy   ISBN 0-7216-2199-6
                                International Edition   ISBN 0-7216-4899-1

Printed in the United States of America.

Last digit is the print number: 9   8   7   6   5   4   3   2   1

This book is dedicated to the memory
of the late Dr. Jack Davies
anatomist, scholar, teacher, and friend (1919–1991)

Preface

Exciting interdisciplinary research has led to new and rapid advances in the field of neurobiology. Technical advances, in such diverse fields as molecular biology and solid state physics, have made these studies possible. And now neurobiologists, in the once separate disciplines of neuroanatomy, neurophysiology, neurochemistry, neuropharmacology, and clinical neurology, are working together on the frontier of this rapidly expanding science.

Consequently, many of today's introductory courses, in what traditionally has been neuroanatomy, contain basic elements of morphology, chemistry, physiology, and neurology. This is as it should be—for the clinical neurologist now has tools available that were unheard of 20 years ago.

Computed axial tomography and magnetic resonance imaging provide *in situ* views of the living brain in serial section. In the near future, positron emission tomography will find wider application in the *in situ* study of focal changes in metabolism, amino acid incorporation, and the synthesis and uptake of specific neurochemical transmitters in the human brain. Patients with chronic pain now obtain relief from the neurosurgical implantation of self-stimulating electrodes, and the condition of many patients with Parkinson's disease is alleviated with L-dopa therapy. These are but a few examples of how traditional boundaries between disciplines have disappeared in neurobiology.

Along with these changes is the need for a change in the composition of the introductory textbook, one that integrates the subdisciplines of neurobiology. *Textbook of Neuroanatomy* was written on the premise that gross morphology and molecular structure are at opposite ends of a continuum, a continuum that forms the foundation for physiological function.

Within the field of neurobiology, the body of knowledge is vast and well beyond the scope of a single textbook. *Textbook of Neuroanatomy* is an introductory text and not a reference. The material selected for inclusion is fundamental to an understanding of the organization and function of the human nervous system. With the rapid developments in the field of neurobiology, no text can be current with the latest discovery. In the selection of new material, the objective was to achieve a balance between what is "state of the art" and what will stand the test of time while, at the same time, providing a broad introduction to the field.

The student is introduced to the general organization of the adult nervous system through its embryonic and fetal development in Part I, *Organization and Development of the Nervous System.* Neuroembryology is an excellent medium in which to (1) introduce the student to the organization of the nervous system and (2) lay the ground plan, or anlage, for subsequent material. In my experience, the intricate relationships of the adult nervous system are more comprehensible when the student has followed its development from the simple to the complex.

Basic cell biology, the structure and function of the fundamental units of nervous activity, is presented in Part II, *Cellular Elements.* This part contains the basic histology and fine structure of the nervous system as well as the fundamentals of cellular neurophysiology and the biochemistry of neurotransmission, neuromodulation, and molecular plasticity.

Part III, *Morphology of the Adult Nervous System,* is an overview of the anatomy of the adult central nervous system. This part provides the foundation for the study of functional systems. Included in these chapters are photomicrographs of a large number of Weigert-stained sections of the brain stem and a detailed description of the vascular system, the ventricular system, and the meninges.

Part IV, *Sensory Systems,* covers the neuroanatomical pathways of the sensory systems, from receptor to cerebral cortex. This material is correlated with our knowledge of the physiology and the neurochemistry to provide a more comprehensive picture of each system. More attention is devoted to information processing in some systems than in others—a reflection of our understanding of those systems. However, many of the basic principles that apply to information processing in one system are applicable to others. The vestibular system has been included in this section, rather than in the section on motor systems, because this presentation is sensory in its orientation. The role of the vestibular system in motor function is discussed in Part V.

Part V, *Motor Systems,* deals with the neuroanatomy of motor pathways and forms the framework for the physiological and the neurochemical bases of motor function. The first four chapters deal with the different levels of organization and function of the somatic motor system: the spinal cord and brain stem, the motor cortical areas, the basal ganglia, and the cerebellum. The final chapter in this part discusses the visceral motor system (autonomic nervous system) and the hypothalamus.

Part VI, *Cranial Nerves,* includes a comprehensive discussion of the cranial nerves. Although the motor and the sensory components are covered in the preceding chapters, a working knowledge of the individual cranial nerves is essential for the neurological examination in clinical practice. Cranial nerves of special sense (olfactory, optic, and vestibulocochlear) are discussed separately in Part IV.

Part VII, *Higher Integrative Centers,* begins with the organization of the thalamus, and the principles of thalamocortical organization. This chapter is followed by a discussion of the neuroanatomical and functional organization of the neocortex in the human brain. The final chapter discusses the limbic system. This chapter includes the cortical components of the limbic lobe and the many subcortical structures that together compose the limbic system.

Because this textbook is written by a single author, it provides the reader with both continuity in subject matter and consistency in writing style. *Textbook of Neuroanatomy* is an introduction to the anatomy of the human nervous system, integrating morphological, physiological, and clinical material. This introduction is intended to be comprehensive but not overwhelming.

Throughout the text, clinical examples are utilized as aids to understanding the basic systems or mechanisms under discussion. Selected readings are provided after each chapter in order that students may pursue topics of interest in greater depth.

Although *Textbook of Neuroanatomy* was written as an introductory text for students in health-related sciences, the nature and organization of the material is appropriate for basic courses in neuroanatomy and neurobiology at both the graduate and advanced undergraduate levels as well.

Acknowledgments

The writing and illustrating of *Textbook of Neuroanatomy* would not have been possible without the encouragement and help of many colleagues and friends. I am indebted to those who critically reviewed individual chapters or sections of this textbook: Lucille Aulsebrook, Vivien A. Casagrande, Michael Conley, William L. R. Cruce, James D. Fix, Paula C. Hoos, Jon H. Kaas, Theodore J. Voneida, and the late Jack Davies. I am especially indebted to Duane E. Haines who kindly reviewed, critically and constructively, the manuscript for over half of this textbook.

A general note of thanks to those many colleagues who granted me permission to use illustrative material. The list is too long to mention here, but specific acknowledgements are made in the legend of each figure. However, special thanks are due those who provided original illustrative material: Vivien A. Casagrande, Michael Conley, Duane E. Haines, and C. Leon Partain.

A good, accessible, medical library collection is a *sine qua non* when writing a book of this nature. Thanks are due Mark Hodges, Director of the Vanderbilt University Medical Center Library, and his staff, especially Gayle Grantham and Susan Dow, for their excellent cooperation and assistance during the preparation of the textbook.

My editors and their staff at W. B. Saunders Company have done an outstanding job, especially Marty Wonsiewicz and Linda Mills. Through their encouragement, guidance, and understanding, *Textbook of Neuroanatomy* has become a reality. Thanks are also due the many individuals at W. B. Saunders Company who had a role in converting my manuscript into a finished product.

I am especially grateful for the patience and understanding of my lovely wife Judy. Her gentle but firm reminders that I had a job to complete kept me going when I'd rather be fishing. Her encouragement and hours of work at my side on the seemingly endless stream of galley proofs, illustration dummies, and page proofs made the final stages of this book a joy.

Contents

Chapter 13

Taste and Olfactory Pathways 282

Part V

MOTOR SYSTEMS 301

Chapter 14

Spinal Cord and Brain Stem Control of Motor Function 303

Chapter 15

Motor Cortex and Descending Motor Pathways 322

Chapter 16

Basal Ganglia and Related Nuclei 335

Chapter 22

Limbic System   479

Part

I

ORGANIZATION AND DEVELOPMENT OF THE NERVOUS SYSTEM

Chapter

1

Organization and Development of the Nervous System

The vertebrate nervous system receives information from the external and internal environments and regulates somatic and visceral motor functions. In humans, the central nervous system has an extraordinary capacity to store and retrieve bits of information as memory, to initiate thought processes, and to regulate emotions and behavior. These capacities arose parallel to an extensive development of the cerebral cortex.

Anatomically, this complex system can be divided into the *central nervous system (CNS)* — the brain and spinal cord — and the *peripheral nervous system (PNS)* — the receptors and effectors of the body, the peripheral ganglia, and the nerve processes connecting these structures with the CNS. Although many nerve fibers in the PNS have cell bodies in the CNS, and vice versa, this division is not arbitrary. Important morphological and physiological differences exist between the PNS and CNS, differences that are functionally significant in such areas as neuropharmacology.

The functional unit of the nervous system is a highly specialized, excitable cell, the *neuron*. Neurons are capable of receiving information from other neurons and from specialized receptors, integrating this information, and sending a message to other neurons or effectors. Typical neurons have many small *dendrites*, extensions of the cell specialized for the reception of information, and a single *axon*, a long slender process specialized for the transmission of information as an electrical impulse or *action potential*. Interneuronal communication takes place at a *synapse* or a *synaptic junction,* the specialized coupling between the terminal of an axon of one neuron and the dendrite of another. When an action potential reaches the axon terminal, it triggers the release of a chemical message or a *neurotransmit-*

3

ter. The chemical message is "read" by a specialized receptor molecule on the recipient neuron and triggers an appropriate response.

Estimates of the number of neurons in the human brain range from 10 to 100 billion, with up to 60 or 70% of these in the cerebral cortex alone. Most neurons are present at birth or shortly thereafter. As the brain continues to grow during the postnatal period, the number and the complexity of these interneuronal connections increase.

The nervous system originates as a simple epithelial disc that rapidly rolls into a tube. After bending and ballooning, thinning and thickening, this tube differentiates into the very complex adult organ. In the adult brain, many of the anatomical relationships are difficult to understand initially. However, by examining the brain's development, from the simple to the complex, the adult nervous system is more readily understood. The objective of this chapter is not to examine the subject of neuroembryology comprehensively but to examine a few of the primary developmental changes leading to the formation of the complex adult brain.

Early Neural Tube

NEURULATION

The CNS develops from the embryonic *neural plate.* The PNS develops from a specialized strip of ectoderm lateral to the neural plate, known as the *neural crest,* and from portions of the *neural plate.*

Toward the end of the 3rd week of embryonic development, the dorsal ectoderm in the head process area of the embryonic disc thickens to form the *neural plate* (Fig. 1–1). This thickening is most apparent at the rostral end of the embryonic disc. This process proceeds in a caudal direction, following Hensen's node and the primitive streak. After the initial thickening, the neural plate folds longitudinally, forming the primitive neural tube. During this process of *neurulation,* the lateral margins of the neural plate become elevated and the central portion, immediately overlying the primitive notochord, becomes depressed, forming the *neural groove* (Fig. 1–2). At the same time, the mesoderm, lateral to the notochord, becomes segmented into somites. During neurulation, the lateral margins of the neural plate make initial contact in the region of the fourth somite. This initial closure of

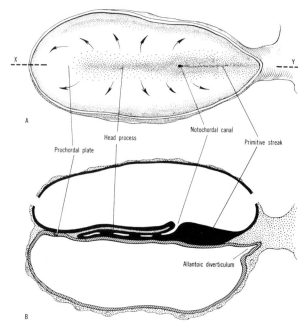

FIGURE 1–1

An early embryonic disc viewed from the dorsal surface *(A)* and in sagittal section *(B)* along the plane XY. The head process extends forward from the primitive knot as a rod of cells between the ectoderm and endoderm. The head process shows a discontinuous lumen or notochordal canal that opens caudally into the amniotic cavity at the primitive knot (later, the neurenteric canal).

The ectoderm and endoderm are in firm contact at two places: the prochordal plate and primitive streak. The directions of spread of the intraembryonic mesoderm from the head process, the primitive knot, and the primitive streak are indicated by arrows in *A.* The head process is the presumptive neural plate. (Reproduced with permission from J. Davies, *Human Developmental Anatomy,* Ronald Press, 1963.)

the neural tube is at the level of what ultimately will be the upper cervical spinal cord.

At this early stage, the more rostral portion (presumptive brain) is already larger than the spinal portion (Fig. 1–3). Commencing at the initial point of contact, neural tube formation proceeds in both rostral and caudal directions (Fig. 1–3). While the neural tube is closing, in a zipper-like fashion, the embryo is elongating in the caudal direction. By the 14-somite stage (Fig. 1–4), the brain region has enlarged greatly and the anterior and posterior *neuropores* mark the rostral and the caudal boundaries of the neural tube, respectively. Because neural tube formation proceeds caudally as the embryo elongates, the rostral portions of the neural tube are more advanced in development than the caudal portions.

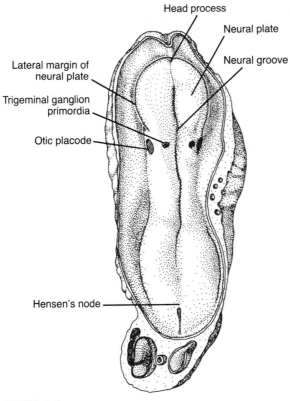

FIGURE 1-2

Dorsal view of the reconstruction of an early presomite human embryo showing the open neural groove. In the region of the future rhombencephalon, the otic placode and the trigeminal (fifth) ganglion appear as dark, rounded areas. (Redrawn from N. W. Ingalls, Contrib. Embryol., 11: 61–90, 1920.)

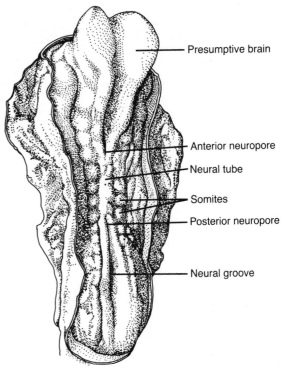

FIGURE 1-3

Dorsal view of the reconstruction of a seven-somite human embryo showing the early neural tube closure and the partial segmentation of paraxial mesoderm into somites. (Redrawn from F. Payne, Contrib. Embryol., 16: 117–124, 1925.)

Figure 1–5 is a schematic representation of early neural tube formation. During this process, a specialized portion of the neural plate separates from both the neural tube and the overlying ectoderm, the *neural crest*. In later development, this will form the neurons of the peripheral ganglia and other components of the PNS.

Neural Tube Histogenesis

MATRIX LAYER AND NEUROBLASTIC PROLIFERATION

The early neural tube consists of a pseudostratified columnar epithelium in which the cells extend from the primitive neural canal to the external surface of the neural tube. These germinal or *matrix cells* proliferate rapidly during early devel-

opment and at later stages produce neuroblasts and finally glioblasts.

Figure 1–6 represents the well-ordered mitotic cycle of the matrix cell. During the first phase of mitosis (t_s) the nuclei in the outer or S zone of the neural tube rapidly synthesize DNA. When synthesis is complete, the nuclei migrate toward the neural canal (t_2) and the matrix cells round up at the luminal surface and divide (t_m) in the M zone. The daughter cells elongate and reach the outer surface of the neural tube. The nuclei once again migrate out to the S zone during t_1 and repeat the cycle. The symbol t_g represents one generation or cycle. All DNA synthesis takes place in the outer or S zone, but the actual cell division takes place in the M zone.

At a predetermined time, daughter cells leave the matrix or germinal layer and migrate laterally to form the mantle layer. These are the early neuroblasts. Once they leave the matrix layer, they lose their capacity to undergo cell division. Experimental studies have shown that neuroblasts

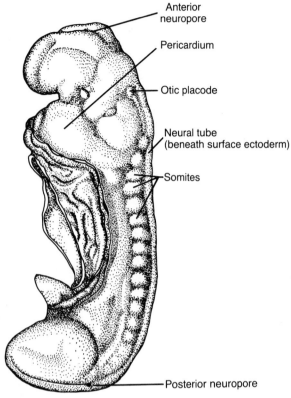

Anterior
neuropore

Pericardium

Otic placode

Neural tube
(beneath surface ectoderm)

Somites

Posterior neuropore

FIGURE 1-4

Lateral view of the reconstruction of a 14-somite human embryo. Note the enlargement of the head region and the development of visceral (branchial) arches. (Redrawn from C. H. Heuser, Contrib. Embryol., 22: 135–154, 1930.)

destined to form functionally related neurons are produced at approximately the same time during embryogenesis.

MANTLE LAYER AND EARLY NEURONAL DIFFERENTIATION

Neuroblasts leave the matrix layer and migrate peripherally to form the *mantle layer*. Here, they grow rapidly and differentiate into functional neurons (Fig. 1–7). The migrating neuroblast, although an undifferentiated bipolar cell, is already programmed to differentiate into a specific type of neuron and become part of a specific nuclear group. The matrix layer produces more neuroblasts than required. Cell death is an important feature in the later differentiation and patterning of neuronal groups (nuclei). Many factors contribute to this attrition, including the lack of functional synaptic connections and the size of the peripheral field innervated. During cellular differentiation, neuroblasts gradually acquire the morphological properties of adult neurons (see Chapter 2).

GLIAL PROLIFERATION AND DIFFERENTIATION

Once the production of neuroblasts is complete, the matrix cells produce *glioblasts*—cells that will differentiate into *astrocytes, oligodendrocytes,* and *ependymal cells*. The ependymal cells, lining the ventricular cavities of the CNS, and the astrocytes differentiate first. Later, in association with the vascularization of the nervous tissue, many astrocytes develop vascular end-feet. This ensheathment of the blood vessels may represent the onset of their regulation of electrolyte balance and metabolism in the surrounding neurons.

Also coincident with vascularization is the differentiation of *microglia* from glioblasts. These small glial elements respond to injury and become active phagocytes. In later development, glioblasts will form oligodendrocytes, marking the beginning of CNS myelination.

Glioblasts and glia, in contrast to neurons, retain the ability to undergo cell division. In general, the production of neuroblasts is complete in a given segment of the nervous system before the formation of glioblasts. With the rostrocaudal gradient in neural tube differentiation, at a given stage of development, glioblasts can be found in the anterior portions of the nervous system while neuroblasts are still being produced in the more posterior segments.

NEURAL CREST DEVELOPMENT

During neurulation, a portion of the neuroectoderm known as the *neural crest* is pinched off and remains separated from the neural tube and the overlying surface ectoderm. Neural crest cells differentiate into the sensory neurons of the *dorsal root* and *cranial nerve ganglia* and into the *sympathetic* and *parasympathetic* motor neurons of the *autonomic ganglia* (see Figs. 1–5 and 1–7).

At spinal levels, dorsal root ganglia differentiate from clusters of neural crest cells arranged segmentally in a manner reflecting early somite formation. Other neural crest cells migrate ventrally to a position adjacent to the developing vertebral column, forming the *paravertebral sympathetic ganglia* (see Fig. 1–7), and others migrate farther, forming the *prevertebral* (*celiac* and *mesenteric*)

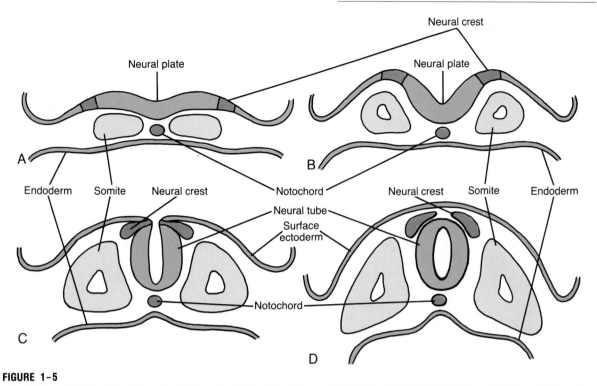

FIGURE 1-5

Stages of early neural tube formation illustrated in cross section. *A*, Thickening of the neural plate; *B*, formation of the neural folds and the neural groove; *C*, opposition of the lateral margins of the neural plate; and *D*, fusion of the neural plate to form the neural tube and associated neural crest tissue.

FIGURE 1-6

Mitotic cycle diagram of the matrix cell in the early neural tube. The matrix, or germinal layer, is divided into three zones: S, I, and M. The generation time (t_g) is divided into four periods: t_s, t_2, t_m, and t_1. See text for discussion. (Redrawn with permission from S. Fujita, J. Comp. Neurol., 122: 311–328, 1964.)

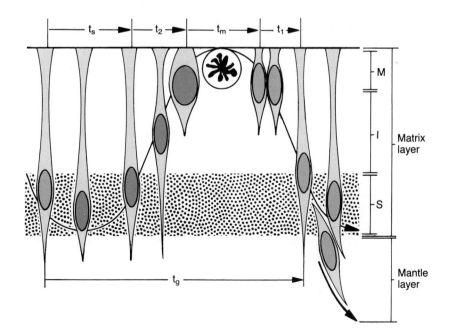

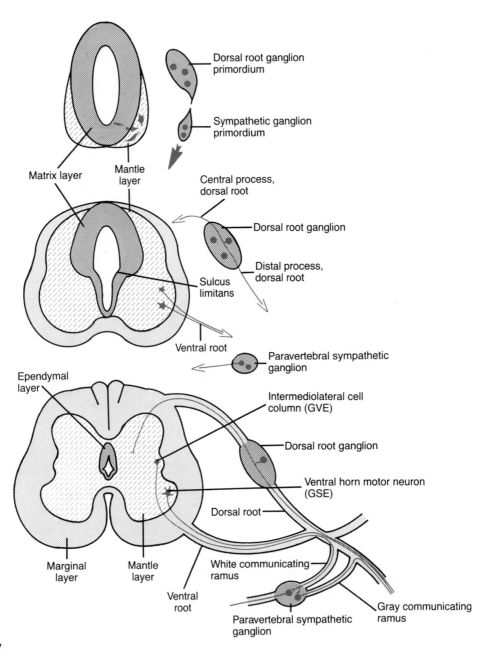

FIGURE 1–7

Stages in spinal cord development.

   A, Neuroblasts from the matrix layer of the basal plate migrate to the mantle layer, and neural crest cells form the primordia of dorsal root ganglia and paravertebral sympathetic ganglia.

   B, Neuroblasts of the mantle layer differentiate, and the marginal layer appears. Axons of motor neurons grow from the neural tube, forming the ventral roots. Proximal and distal processes of the dorsal root ganglion cells appear. Axons from developing sympathetic ganglion cells grow toward visceral targets.

   C, Dorsal and ventral roots merge to form a mixed (sensory and motor) spinal nerve. The sympathetic ganglion receives preganglionic motor fibers from the spinal cord via the white ramus and sends postganglionic fibers to join the spinal nerve via the gray ramus. (GVE, general visceral efferent; GSE, general somatic efferent.)

ganglia. Some of these cells invade developing visceral organs and form the *parasympathetic* and *enteric ganglia* or the *chromaffin cells* of the adrenal medulla.

At cranial levels, neural crest cells form the sensory ganglia of cranial nerves (V, VII, IX, and X) and the parasympathetic ganglia (ciliary, otic, sphenopalatine, and submandibular ganglia).

The *Schwann sheath cells* and the *satellite cells* of the dorsal root ganglia also develop from neural crest cells. The Schwann cells ensheath and myelinate the peripheral nerve fibers, and the satellite cells encapsulate the neuronal cell bodies in the dorsal root ganglia. Although most Schwann cells are of neural crest origin, substantial numbers migrate from the ventral or basal portion of the neural tube in association with the outgrowth of peripheral nerve processes.

MYELINATION

Myelination in the CNS begins during the 4th month when the fetus is approximately 100 mm in length and is not complete until the 2nd or 3rd year of postnatal life. A wide variation exists in the pattern of myelination; but, in general, the oldest pathways—phylogenetically—are myelinated first and the newest pathways, last. Neurons function long before myelination; but, with the completion of myelination, the conduction of action potentials becomes more rapid and efficient.

In the spinal cord, the cervical segments myelinate first. The first fibers myelinated are the intrasegmental fibers to motor neurons. In spinal nerves, ventral or motor roots myelinate before dorsal or sensory roots. Dorsal columns become myelinated during the 6th fetal month. Myelination of the corticospinal tract begins near term but is not completed until the 2nd year of postnatal life.

DEVELOPMENT OF MENINGES AND CHOROID PLEXUS

By the time the embryo is 6 to 8 mm in length, a rich capillary plexus has developed in the loose connective tissue surrounding the neural tube. This vascular mesodermal tissue forms the *meninx primitiva* or primitive meninges. The thin ependymal roof of the forebrain and hindbrain is soon invaded by these capillaries, forming the *choroid plexus.* The choroid plexus is responsible for the formation of cerebrospinal fluid (see Chapter 9). The vascularized ependymal roof of the ventricles is the *tela choroidea.*

The meninx primitiva rapidly separates, forming a thick protective outer layer, the *dura mater,* a highly vascular inner layer, the *pia mater,* and an avascular middle layer, the *arachnoid.* The arachnoid remains in close contact with the inner surface of the dura. However, with cerebrospinal fluid formation, the contact between the arachnoid and the pia is reduced to a fine reticulated network of fibers, which bridges the fluid-filled space between the two layers, the *subarachnoid space.*

During the 3rd month of development, an opening appears in the midline of the roof of the fourth ventricle, the *medial foramen of Magendie* and, later, an opening appears in each lateral recess of the fourth ventricle, the *lateral foramen of Luschka.* These openings permit the free flow of cerebrospinal fluid from its source, i.e., the choroid plexus of the ventricles, into the subarachnoid space, surrounding the brain and spinal cord.

Spinal Cord Development

SPINAL CORD GROWTH

The anterior neuropore closes by the end of the 1st month of fetal development. The posterior neuropore, however, does not close until the 2nd month, after the formation of new mesoderm from the primitive streak is complete. All later growth of the spinal cord is interstitial, from the proliferation and growth of the cells within the neural tube. At this time, the caudal end of the neural tube is adjacent to the caudal end of the notochord. A few coccygeal nerves develop, but these disappear when the rudimentary tail of the embryo atrophies.

The caudal end of the developing spinal cord is opposite the first coccygeal vertebra in the 30-mm fetus. During later development, growth of the vertebral column is more rapid than the interstitial growth of the spinal cord and, in the 221-mm fetus, the caudal end of the cord is opposite the third lumbar vertebra (Fig. 1–8). Both spinal cord and vertebral column continue to grow differentially during postnatal life until, in the adult, the caudal end of the cord is oppo-

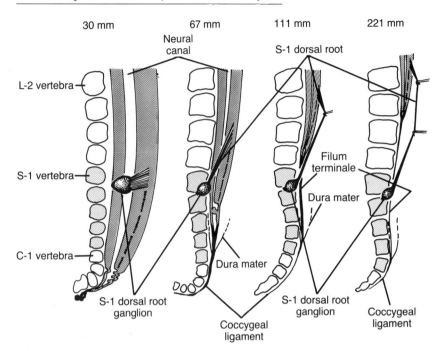

30 mm	67 mm	111 mm	221 mm

Neural canal

S-1 dorsal root

L-2 vertebra

S-1 vertebra

C-1 vertebra

Filum terminale

Dura mater

Dura mater

S-1 dorsal root ganglion

S-1 dorsal root ganglion

Coccygeal ligament

Coccygeal ligament

FIGURE 1–8

The caudal end of the spinal cord in the human fetus from the eighth to 25th week of development. These diagrams illustrate the rate and extent of caudal displacement of the vertebral canal relative to the spinal cord. In each case, the dorsal root of only the first sacral nerve is drawn. See text for discussion. (Redrawn from G. L. Streeter, Am. J. Anat., 25: 1–11, 1919. Copyright © 1919 Wiley-Liss, reprinted by permission of Wiley-Liss, a Division of John Wiley and Sons Inc.)

site the intervertebral disc between the first and second lumbar vertebrae. Throughout this period, the upper cervical segments retain their original position, relative to the vertebrae. The caudal end of the spinal cord maintains a slender, fibrous connection with the base of the vertebral canal, the *filum terminale* (see Fig. 1–8). The dural sac surrounding the spinal cord grows at nearly the same rate as the vertebral canal and, in the adult, this sac extends to the third sacral vertebra.

As a result of the "relative shortening" of the cord, spinal nerves in the upper cervical region exit from the vertebral canal at right angles to the cord, and those at lower levels travel increasing distances before exiting. Roots of the first sacral nerve exit the spinal cord immediately opposite the first and second sacral vertebrae in early development. At the 221-mm stage, the roots of the first sacral nerve are opposite the first lumbar vertebra (see Fig. 1–8). These roots descend in the dural sac, within the vertebral canal, to the original point of exit in the sacrum. The dorsal root ganglia remain associated with the intervertebral foramen in which they first developed. The fluid-filled dural sac, from the caudal end of the spinal cord to the third sacral vertebra, contains only dorsal and ventral nerve roots and the filum terminale, collectively called the *cauda equina*. Clinically, this area is important for the with-

drawal of cerebrospinal fluid (spinal tap) and the administration of spinal anesthetics. A large needle can be inserted into this fluid-filled, subarachnoid space with little damage to the nerve roots.

DIFFERENTIATION OF SPINAL CORD

As neuroblasts accumulate in the mantle layer, a longitudinal sulcus or groove appears in the lateral wall of the neural canal, the *sulcus limitans*. This groove separates the spinal cord into alar (dorsal) and basal (ventral) plates. Usually, neurons of basal plate origin are motor in function and those of the alar plate are sensory (Fig. 1–9).

Axonal processes of motor neurons exit the neural tube in the *ventrolateral sulcus* and grow toward the somite adjacent to their point of exit. This attraction of rootlets to the nearest somite produces a segmental pattern for peripheral spinal nerves, a pattern retained in the adult.

At the same time, neural crest cells, in the differentiating dorsal root ganglia, form primary sensory neurons. The peripheral processes of these neurons grow into the surrounding tissue and contact specialized receptors. The central processes form the dorsal roots and enter the spinal cord at the *dorsolateral sulcus* (see Fig. 1–7). Some processes ascend to the brain stem in

FIGURE 1-9

Differentiation of alar and basal plates in the spinal cord. In early development, the cord is divided into alar and basal plates at the sulcus limitans *(A)*. With later differentiation, the motor and sensory columns appear *(B)*. (GSA, general somatic afferent; GVA, general visceral afferent; GSE, general somatic efferent.)

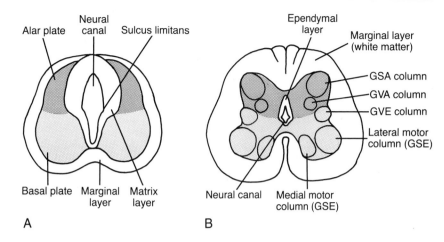

the dorsal columns of the marginal layer. Others make synaptic connections with interneurons in the alar (dorsal) half of the cord and establish reflex connections with motor neurons of the basal plate.

Ventral and dorsal roots merge as they exit the vertebral canal to form a mixed (sensory and motor) segmental spinal nerve. In the adult, the cutaneous innervation is segmental (dermatomal), a pattern that reflects the differentiation of the dermatome from the original somite. The motor component of the spinal nerve innervates striated muscle formed from the myotome of the same somite.

In addition to somatic motor and somatic sensory fibers, most spinal nerves have visceral motor and visceral sensory components. Thoracic and upper lumbar nerves contain sympathetic preganglionic motor (visceral efferent) fibers and sacral levels contain parasympathetic preganglionic motor (visceral efferent) fibers. Some of the sensory neurons in the dorsal root ganglia innervate visceral structures and are, therefore, visceral afferent fibers.

Most spinal nerves contain all four functional components: general somatic efferent (*GSE*), general visceral efferent (*GVE*), general somatic afferent (*GSA*), and general visceral afferent (*GVA*) (see Fig. 1–9). GSE fibers innervate skeletal or striated muscle of somite origin. GSA fibers provide sensory innervation to muscles and dermatomal structures of somite origin. GVE fibers innervate visceral structures of endodermal or mesodermal origin, usually containing smooth muscle. GVA fibers provide sensory innervation to these visceral structures. These four basic functional components (GSE, GSA, GVE, and GVA) are present in the cranial nerves along with three additional special functional components (see following discussion).

INFLUENCE OF PERIPHERAL FIELD

The excessive production of neuroblasts and selective cell death are important factors in determining the final cell pattern in the CNS. Limb buds arise in the lower cervical and lumbosacral segments with the eventual formation of the upper and lower extremities. The spinal organization of GSE neurons reflects this increase in the peripheral field. In spinal segments innervating the extremities, the ventral (anterior) horns are large and contain prominent *lateral motor columns*. The smaller *medial motor columns* that innervate the axial musculature are present throughout the length of the spinal cord.

GVE columns are present in thoracic and upper lumbar segments of the spinal cord as the *intermediolateral cell column*. However, the GVE columns are absent from cervical levels. Although not as distinct, a GVE column for the parasympathetic innervation of visceral structures is present in sacral levels.

Differentiation of the alar plate has a similar dependence on the peripheral field. Dorsal (posterior) horns—"receiving stations" for afferent information—are larger in lower cervical and lumbosacral levels and are a reflection of the increased sensory information entering the cord from the extremities. Similarly, dorsal root ganglia innervating the extremities are larger and

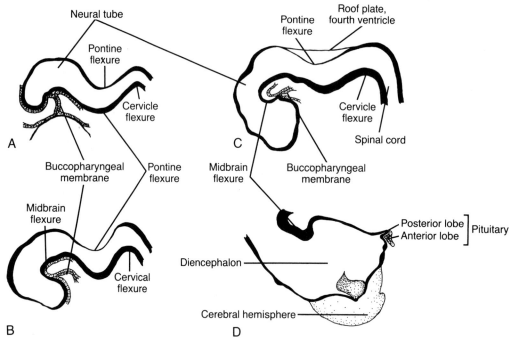

FIGURE 1-10

Primary brain flexures and the formation of the anterior pituitary from Rathke's pouch.

A, This represents an early stage in brain flexion. Note the extensive overgrowth of the anterior portion of the neural tube and the relative displacement of the buccopharyngeal membrane to a position under the developing forebrain.

B and *C*, These represent successive stages in the overgrowth of the forebrain and the gradual formation of Rathke's pouch from the ectoderm of the nasopharynx.

D, This represents a later stage in forebrain development. Rathke's pouch (anlage of the anterior pituitary) has separated from the nasopharynx. (*A* and *B* redrawn with permission from J. Davies, *Human Developmental Anatomy*, Ronald Press, 1963; *C* and *D* modified with permission, from G. L. Streeter, Contrib. Embryol., 31: 27–63, 1945, and 32: 133–203, 1948.)

contain more sensory neurons than do upper cervical and thoracic ganglia.

Primary Brain Flexures and Early Regional Differentiation

PRIMARY BRAIN FLEXURES

Before closure of the anterior neuropore, the rostral end of the neural tube grows much faster than the surrounding tissues of the head. The early prochordal plate of Figure 1–1 becomes tucked under the rapidly growing forebrain and forms the buccopharyngeal membrane (Fig. 1–10). During this period, the neural tube flexes, or bends, at three principal locations. The *midbrain* and *cervical flexures*, both with concavities toward the ventral surface, are present in the 6-mm embryo (Fig. 1–11). By the 12-mm stage,

the *pontine flexure*, with its dorsal concavity, is visible (Fig. 1–12). The result is a neural tube that is folded like an accordion, occupying half the space it would if fully extended (Fig. 1–13).

PRIMARY BRAIN DIVISIONS

The primary divisions of the brain are readily identified after the primary flexures appear (Figs. 1–12, 1–13, and Table 1–1). At the rostral end of the neural tube is the *prosencephalon*, or *forebrain*, which is further subdivided into *telencephalon* and *diencephalon*. Immediately behind the prosencephalon and "capping" the midbrain flexure, is the *mesencephalon*, or *midbrain*. The *rhombencephalon*, or *hindbrain*, extends from the mesencephalon to the spinal cord and is subdivided into a rostral *metencephalon* (*pons* and *cerebellum*) and a caudal *myelencephalon* (me-

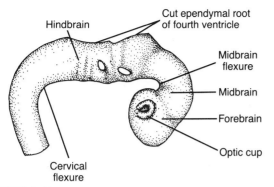

FIGURE 1-11

Lateral view of a model of the brain from a 6-mm human embryo. Note the presence of well-developed midbrain and cervical flexures and the appearance of the optic cup at the base of the diencephalon. (Redrawn from F. Hochstetter, Beitrage zur Entwicklungsgeschichte des menschlichen Gehirns, Bd. II, F. Deuticke, Wien und Leipzig, 1929.)

dulla oblongata, or *medulla*) by the pontine flexure.

Matrix cell proliferation and neuroblast migration into the mantle layer are similar to those described for the spinal cord, except for the cerebral hemispheres and the cerebellum (see subsequent discussion). The differentiation of specific nuclear groups is due, largely, to regional variations in the patterns of proliferation and migration and the selective attrition of neuroblasts.

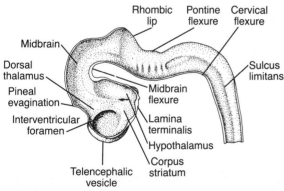

FIGURE 1-12

Midsagittal view of a model of the brain from an 11.8-mm human embryo. Note the formation of the telencephalic vesicle and the presence of three primary flexures. (Redrawn from M. Hines, J. Comp. Neurol., 34: 73-169, 1924. Copyright © 1919 Wiley-Liss, reprinted by permission of Wiley-Liss, a Division of John Wiley and Sons Inc.)

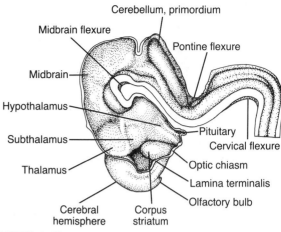

FIGURE 1-13

Midsagittal view of a model of the brain from a 16.8-mm human embryo. Note the presence of three well-defined brain flexures. (Redrawn from G. L. Streeter, Contrib. Embryol., 32: 133-203, 1948.)

Hindbrain and Midbrain Development

FORMATION OF FOURTH VENTRICLE

The hindbrain of the 6-mm embryo has begun to open, like a book, and the roof plate has become a thin ependymal layer. With formation of the pontine flexure, the roof plate is stretched farther

TABLE 1-1

Primary Divisions of the Embryonic Brain

PRIMARY DIVISION	SUBDIVISION	ADULT STRUCTURES
Prosencephalon (Forebrain)	Telencephalon	Cerebral Cortex Basal Ganglia
	Diencephalon	Dorsal Thalamus Hypothalamus Epithalamus Ventral Thalamus (Subthalamus)
Mesencephalon (Midbrain)	Mesencephalon (Midbrain)	Tectum Tegmentum Cerebral Peduncles
Rhombencephalon (Hindbrain)	Metencephalon	Pons Cerebellum
	Myelencephalon	Medulla Oblongata

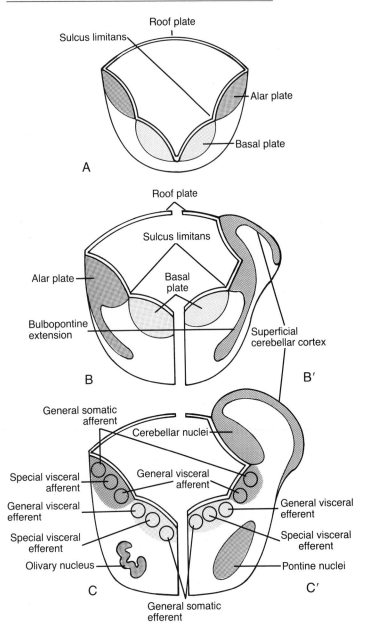

FIGURE 1-14

Alar and basal plate differentiation in the rhombencephalon. *A*, This represents an early stage of development. *B* and *C* represent successive stages in the differentiation of the myelencephalon, and *B'* and *C'* represent successive stages in the differentiation of the metencephalon. (Redrawn with permission from W. J. Hamilton and H. W. Mossman, *Human Embryology*, 4th Edition. Williams & Wilkins, Baltimore, 1972.)

and the "book" opened wider (Fig. 1–14*A*). The spreading or flaring of the neural tube is widest at the flexure. This enlarged neural canal becomes the *fourth ventricle*, bounded above by the ependymal roof and below by the alar and basal plates of the neural tube (see Fig. 1–14*A*). The floor of the fourth ventricle, shaped like a diamond or rhombus when viewed from above, is the *rhomboid fossa*. With later growth, the ependymal roof forms a small diverticulum on each side, at the widest point of the ventricle, the *lateral recess*. The cerebellum develops from the *rhombic lip*, a portion of the alar plate forming the lateral margin of the rostral half of the ventricle (Figs. 1–13 and 1–14*B'*). Capillaries from the meninx primitiva invade the ependymal roof to form the choroid plexus and tela choroidea of the fourth ventricle.

DIFFERENTIATION OF MYELENCEPHALON

The portion of the rhombencephalon caudal to the pontine flexure is the myelencephalon, *medulla oblongata*, or simply *medulla*. The caudal end of the medulla is similar in basic structure to the upper cervical spinal cord. As one ascends in the medulla, the neural tube spreads laterally, the roof plate expands, and the fourth ventricle widens.

During medullary differentiation, alar and basal plates give rise to the nuclei of cranial nerves VIII (*vestibulocochlear*), IX (*glossopharyngeal*), X (*vagus*), XI (*spinal accessory*), and XII (*hypoglossal*), and to portions of a nucleus of cranial nerve V (*trigeminal*). Concurrently, a ventral migration of neuroblasts from the alar plate forms the *inferior olivary nuclei*, which are cerebellar relay nuclei (Fig. 1–14*A*, *B*, and *C*). At later stages of development, the appearance of ascending and descending fiber pathways and the migration of specific nuclei further alter the organization of the medulla.

DIFFERENTIATION OF METENCEPHALON

The metencephalon (*pons* and *cerebellum*) is that portion of the rhombencephalon rostral to the pontine flexure. During differentiation, alar and basal plates give rise to nuclei of cranial nerves VI (*abducens*) and VII (*facial*) and the remainder of the nuclei of cranial nerve V (*trigeminal*). These nuclei become located in the *pontine tegmentum* (see Fig. 1–14).

Two features characterize the differentiation of the metencephalon, and both involve cells of alar plate origin. A large number of alar plate neuroblasts migrate ventrad, forming the *pontine nuclei*, or *basal pons*, part of a large corticopontocerebellar relay complex. In addition, other alar plate neurons enter the rhombic lip and form the cerebellum (see Fig. 1–14).

FORMATION OF CEREBELLUM

In the initial phase, alar plate neurons proliferate rapidly, causing the rhombic lip to enlarge and protrude into the fourth ventricle (Figs. 1–13, 1–15*A*, and 1–16). As development proceeds, a population of neuroblasts migrates toward the surface (marginal layer), forming the anlage of the *cerebellar cortex* (Fig. 1–15*B*). This outer layer grows rapidly, throwing the cortex of the cerebellum into a series of transverse folds or *folia* (Fig. 1–15*C*). During this period, the two

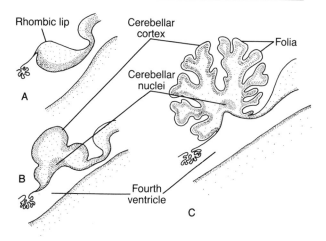

FIGURE 1–15

Successive stages in the development of the cerebellum as seen in sagittal section. *A*, An early stage in the enlargement of the rhombic lip. *B*, At a later stage, neuroblasts migrate into the marginal layer and form the early cerebellar cortex. *C*, By the 140- to 160-mm stage, rapid cortical growth has thrown the cerebellum into a series of transverse folds or folia.

halves of the cerebellum fuse in the midline. The entire structure grows back over the roof of the fourth ventricle, trapping much of the tela choroidea beneath it. At the same time, several clusters of neuroblasts remain in the mantle layer to form the *cerebellar nuclei* (see Fig. 1–15).

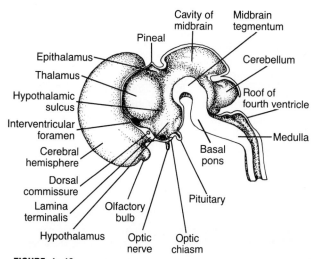

FIGURE 1–16

Midsagittal view of a model of the brain from a 43-mm human embryo. (Redrawn from M. Hines, J. Comp. Neurol., 34: 73–169, 1924. Copyright © 1924 Wiley-Liss, reprinted by permission of Wiley-Liss, a Division of John Wiley and Sons Inc.)

Later in development, fibers grow from the cerebral cortex to the pontine nuclei as part of a massive *corticopontocerebellar* pathway. Axons from the pontine neurons enter the cerebellar cortex, forming the large *middle cerebellar peduncle* or *brachium pontis*. Similarly, ascending *spinocerebellar* fibers, along with *olivocerebellar* and *vestibulocerebellar* fibers, form the *inferior cerebellar peduncle*, composed of the *restiform body* and the *juxtarestiform body*. Information leaves the cerebellum by way of the cerebellar nuclei, forming the *superior cerebellar peduncle*, or *brachium conjunctivum*.

DIFFERENTIATION OF MESENCEPHALON

The mesencephalon, or midbrain, is immediately rostral to the pons and caps the midbrain flexure (see Figs. 1–12, 1–13, and 1–16). The motor nuclei of cranial nerves III (*oculomotor*) and IV (*trochlear*) and much of the *midbrain tegmentum* differentiate from the basal plate. In comparison, the alar plate, becomes the *tectum*, the *superior* and *inferior colliculi* that contain reflex centers for the visual and auditory systems, respectively. Two large nuclei, the *red nucleus* and the *substantia nigra*, develop in the ventral portion of the tegmentum. It is not clear whether they arise from the neuroblasts of the alar plate or basal plate.

The neural canal remains large during early midbrain development, but as the tectum and tegmentum grow and as the ascending fibers from the cerebellum (superior cerebellar peduncle) pass through the tegmentum, the neural canal becomes restricted, forming the narrow *cerebral aqueduct* (*aqueduct of Sylvius*). This is an ependymal lined channel connecting the fourth ventricle of the rhombencephalon with the third ventricle of the more rostral diencephalon.

Later, development of the very prominent *cerebral peduncles* further alters the ventral surface of the midbrain. These structures carry descending fibers from the cerebral cortex, principally corticopontine and corticospinal fibers.

Forebrain Development

EARLY DEVELOPMENT OF THE EYE

Soon after closure of the anterior neuropore, a pair of vesicles sprout from the anteroventral portion of the lateral walls of the forebrain, the *optic vesicles*. These hollow processes arise from an area that will become part of the *diencephalon*. The optic vesicle grows toward the surface ectoderm, which subsequently thickens, invaginates, and pinches off to form the *lens vesicle*. At the same time, the optic vesicle becomes depressed, forming the *optic cup* (see Fig. 1–11). The optic cup, lens vesicle, and surrounding mesoderm will form the eye (see Chapter 11).

Initially, the connection between the optic vesicle and the diencephalon, the *optic stalk*, has a lumen, continuous with the central cavity of the forebrain (*third ventricle*). This lumen gradually becomes obliterated and, as the *retina* differentiates, fibers forming the *optic nerve* grow through the optic stalk to reach the diencephalon. Although traditionally considered a nerve, the optic nerve (*cranial nerve II*) is actually a pathway within the CNS. The optic cup and stalk are part of the diencephalon, and the retinal ganglion cells differentiate from the neuroblasts of the optic cup.

EARLY DIFFERENTIATION OF TELENCEPHALON

During the 5th week of development, two massive *telencephalic vesicles* grow out from the dorsolateral portion of the forebrain. These vesicles are the anlagen of the *cerebral hemispheres* and the *basal ganglia* (see Fig. 1–12). Together the hemispheres and the basal ganglia make up the *telencephalon*. The remainder of the forebrain becomes the *diencephalon*.

The ependymal roof plate of the third ventricle grows laterally as part of the telencephalic vesicle. Hence, the early cerebral hemispheres have an ependymal roof that is continuous with the roof of the third ventricle (Fig. 1–17A). The two vesicular cavities become the *lateral ventricles* and are in continuity with the third ventricle through the *interventricular foramina of Monro* (Figs. 1–16 and 1–18). The foramen is bounded anteriorly by the lamina terminalis, superiorly by the ependymal roof of the diencephalon, posteriorly by the thalamus, and inferiorly by the hypothalamus.

During the period of rapid telencephalic growth, large numbers of neuroblasts migrate through the mantle layer to the outer or marginal layer and form the *cerebral cortex* or *pallium*. At the base of the telencephalic vesicle, however, vast numbers of neuroblasts accumulate in the mantle layer, forming the *basal ganglia*.

FIGURE 1-17

The dorsal surface of the fore-brain showing how the ependymal roof plate of the diencephalon (shaded) is carried out on the dorsomedial surface of the cerebral hemispheres (A) and is finally carried into the temporal lobes as a result of the C-shaped growth pattern of the hemispheres (B).

Angioblastic mesoderm (meninx primitiva) is trapped between the hemispheres and the wall of the diencephalon, forming the velum interpositum (see lower arrows). (Reproduced with permission from J. Davies, *Human Developmental Anatomy*, Ronald Press, 1963.)

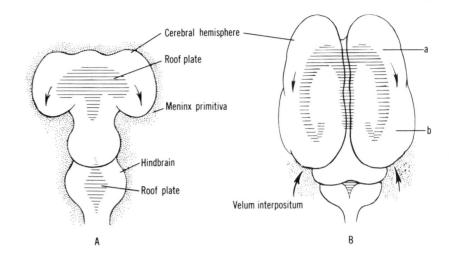

A   B

FORMATION OF CEREBRAL HEMISPHERES AND BASAL GANGLIA

During the 3rd and 4th months of fetal development, the entire telencephalon grows much more rapidly than the rest of the brain. In the developing *pallium*, or *cerebral cortex*, the walls remain very thin. The extensive growth rapidly increases the surface area of the telencephalic vesicle, especially the lateral and dorsal surfaces (Fig. 1–19). In the ventral telencephalon, most of the growth is associated with the *basal ganglia*. The cortical

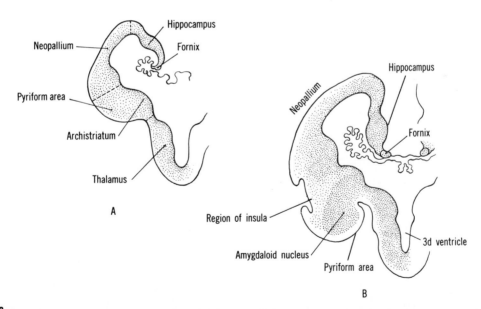

A

B

FIGURE 1-18

Coronal sections through the interventricular foramen of the human forebrain at two stages in its development.

A, The neopallium occupies a restricted area in the lateral surface of the hemisphere between the hippocampus and the piriform area. Associated deeply with the piriform area is the amygdaloid nucleus of the basal ganglia.

B, The neopallial cortex has expanded greatly, displacing the hippocampus onto the medial surface close to the ependymal roof of the diencephalon and the piriform area onto the medioventral surface. The insula, attached to the underlying basal ganglia, is overgrown by the opercula of the neopallial cortex and is submerged in the depths of the lateral fissure (fissure of Sylvius). (After J. E. Frazer, *Manual of Human Embryology*. Bailliere, Tindall & Cox, Ltd., London, 1940.)

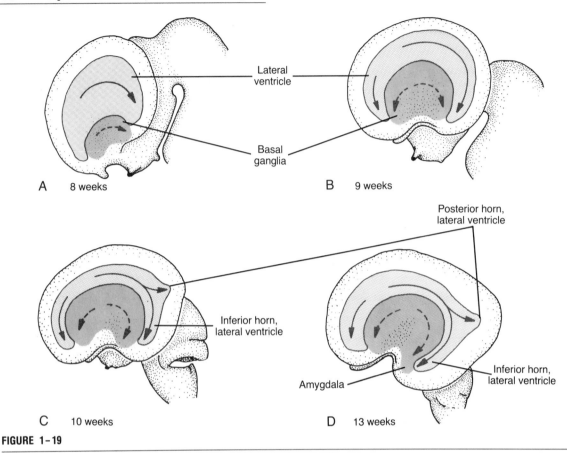

FIGURE 1-19

Development of the telencephalon from the eighth *(A)* to the 13th *(D)* week of gestation. In the development of the pallium (black), note the fixed position of the insula (black stipple over basal ganglia) and the growth of the cortex around this fixed point. Development of the underlying ventricle and basal ganglia are in red. Dashed arrows show relative directions of growth in the basal ganglia. Solid red arrows indicate change in the lateral ventricles. These changes correspond to growth patterns in the developing pallium. Note the relative position of the olfactory bulb, as the lateral olfactory stria grows toward the amygdala in *C* and *D*. (Adapted from F. Hochstetter, Beitrage zur Entwicklungsgeschichte des menschlichen Gehirns, Bd. II, F. Deuticke, Wien und Leipzig, 1929.)

component of the ventral telencephalon is small, has no ventricular cavity beneath it, and becomes the cortex of the *insula* in the adult (see Fig. 1–18). The *growth pattern of the pallium is planar*, growing rapidly as an expanding two-dimensional sheet of tissue. In contrast, the *growth pattern of the basal ganglia is three-dimensional*, growing rapidly as a spheroidal mass, deep to the cortical tissue and the ventricles. By comparison, the ependymal roof grows at a much slower rate than do the pallium and the basal ganglia and is drawn out along the dorsomedial surface of the developing hemispheres (see Fig. 1–17).

As a result of the differential growth patterns, the pallium expands like the shell of a balloon (the cavity being the lateral ventricle). At the same time, the rapidly growing basal ganglia push into the balloon like an expanding fist. As a result of the combination of these growth patterns, the basal ganglia expand into the ventricle from the ventromedial side and the pallium balloons outward, forward, and to the rear. These differential growth patterns result in the ventricle and hemisphere curving or bending around the basal portion of the telencephalon, in a C shape, much like the curved horns of a ram (see Fig. 1–19). However, the original ventral portion of the pallium (the presumptive insula) is attached firmly to the underlying basal ganglia and does not balloon. As the pallium balloons around this portion of the telencephalon, it carries the lateral ventricle with it, forming the *inferior horn* of the *lateral ventricle*. Concurrently, the basal ganglia grow rapidly and protrude into the lateral ventri-

FIGURE 1-20

Drawing of the lateral surface of a 6-month human fetal brain. Note the development of neopallial opercula and the "burying" of the insula in the depths of the lateral fissure.

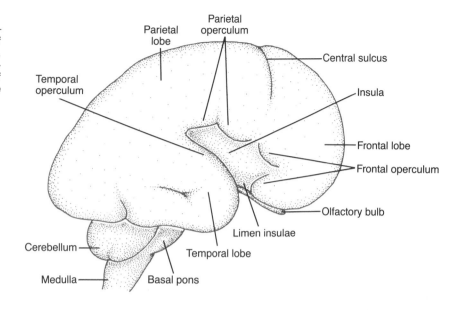

cle, forming the inner margin of the C (see Fig. 1–19).

At this stage, the pallium can be divided tentatively into the *frontal, parietal, occipital,* and *temporal lobes* and the *insula (island of Reil).* Definitive identification requires the later formation of fissures and sulci. During the remainder of development, the surface area of the pallium continues to increase rapidly. Portions of the neopallium roll over the surface of the insula, burying the insula beneath cortical *opercula,* or lids (Fig. 1–20). Eventually, the opercula meet, but do not fuse. The resultant cleft between the *frontal* and *parietal opercula* above and the *temporal operculum* below becomes the *lateral* or *Sylvian fissure.* The insula lies in the depths of this fissure (see Fig. 1–20).

FORMATION OF CHOROID FISSURE

As the pallium enlarges, the slower growing ependyma is drawn out into a slender C-shaped strip (Fig. 1–17B). At the same time, it is displaced to the medial surface of the hemisphere by the more rapidly growing pallium, forming part of the medial wall of the lateral ventricle. The ependyma now extends from the interventricular foramen, where it is continuous with the ependyma of the third ventricle, around the inner curvature of the lateral ventricle to the rostral end of the inferior horn. The *choroid fissure* forms when capillaries from the meninx primitiva invade this C-shaped

strip of ependyma to form the choroid plexus of the lateral ventricle. Thus, the choroid fissure is not a true fissure or cleft, but the delicate choroid plexus forming a portion of the medial wall of the lateral ventricle.

DEVELOPMENT OF ARCHIPALLIUM, PALEOPALLIUM, AND NEOPALLIUM

The cerebral cortex can be divided into the *archipallium (hippocampal formation), paleopallium (piriform and entorhinal cortex),* and *neopallium,* based on anatomical and phylogenetic criteria (see Chapter 21). The archipallium is the oldest and the neopallium the newest. The neopallium accounts for over 90% of the cortical area in humans. The older portions of the cortex develop first and are disproportionately large during the early stages. The archipallium develops from the medial surface of the telencephalic vesicle, adjacent to the ependyma, and the paleopallium develops from the ventral surface (Fig. 1–18A). As development proceeds, the neopallium grows at a much faster rate and both the hippocampus and the piriform cortex are displaced to more medial positions (Fig. 1–18B). Extensive neopallial growth in frontal and lateral areas further displaces the hippocampus caudad, around the convexity of the C and onto the medial wall of the temporal lobe, adjacent to the choroid fissure and the inferior horn of the lateral ventricle. The piriform and entorhinal cortex is displaced to the

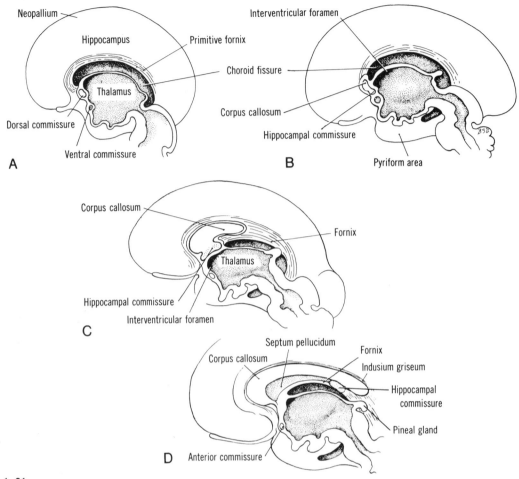

FIGURE 1–21

Four sagittal sections of the human fetal brain showing successive stages in the formation of the corpus callosum and the hippocampal commissure.

A, The corpus callosum arises by the massing of commissural fibers of neopallial origin dorsal to the dorsal commissure in the lamina terminalis.

B, The callosal fibers extend caudad breaking up the fornix fibers, which lie in their path.

C and *D,* As the callosal fibers extend caudad, fornix fibers are split into a dorsal component (the vestigial indusium griseum and longitudinal striae) and a ventral component (the columns of the fornix). The fornix columns pass across the midline in the dorsal commissure, *(A)* and *(B),* which now becomes the hippocampal commissure and is displaced out of the lamina terminalis by the caudal growth of the corpus callosum. A portion of the lamina terminalis is stretched and incorporated into the septum pellucidum.

The choroid fissure lies entirely within the concavity of the fornix. (Reproduced with permission from J. Davies, *Human Developmental Anatomy*, Ronald Press, 1963.)

medial and inferior surfaces of the temporal lobe, adjacent to the hippocampus.

GROWTH OF COMMISSURAL FIBERS

The cerebral hemispheres develop extensive connections with the hemisphere of the opposite side. However, the nerve fibers are not able to grow across the single-cell layer of the ependyma.

Because the ependymal roof of the third ventricle is continuous with the choroid fissure of the hemisphere, the lamina terminalis (the anterior end of the original neural tube) provides the only available path.

The first commissural fibers to develop are those from the oldest part of the cortex, the hippocampus. Fibers leave the hippocampus as the *fornix* and travel anteriorly, between the hip-

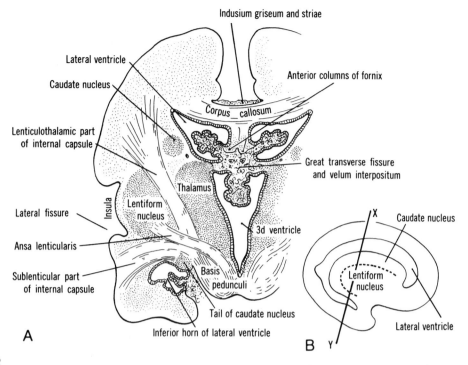

FIGURE 1-22

A, Transverse section of the cerebral hemisphere and the diencephalon after the formation of the corpus callosum. Note that the latter, along with the columns of the fornix, forms a false roof for the diencephalon, the true roof being the tela choroidea of the third ventricle. Between the false roof and the true roof are the great transverse cerebral fissure and the entrapped velum interpositum.

The internal capsule (dashed line in *B*), formed by neopallial fibers, breaks through the corpus striatum along a C-shaped line, which again reflects the C-shaped growth pattern of the hemisphere. The corpus striatum external to the internal capsule forms the caudate nucleus; that internal to the capsule forms the lentiform nucleus. These developmental features help to explain the complex anatomical relationships of the ventricle, internal capsule, and caudate nucleus as shown in *A*. (Reproduced with permission from J. Davies, *Human Developmental Anatomy*, Ronald Press, 1963.)

pocampus and the choroid fissure, to the lamina terminalis (Figs. 1–18 and 1–21*A*). Fibers of the fornix cross to the opposite side as the *dorsal commissure*. These fibers become the *hippocampal commissure*.

As differentiation proceeds, neopallial fibers descend on the lamina terminalis, crossing in the area of the dorsal commissure. With the addition of these fibers, the dorsal commissure separates into the *corpus callosum* (neopallial fibers) and the *hippocampal commissure* (archipallial fibers) (Fig. 1–21*B*). With the extensive growth of the neopallium, the corpus callosum cannot be contained in the lamina terminalis and it grows caudad, forcing its way between fibers of the fornix (Fig. 1–21). During the same period, the hippocampus is displaced to the medial wall of the temporal lobe (see previous discussion). With this posterior growth of neocortical commissural fibers, the fornix and the hippocampal commis-

sure assume a position ventral to the corpus callosum. The displacement is not complete, and some rudiments of the hippocampus and fornix are trapped dorsal to the corpus callosum. These become the *indusium griseum* and the *medial* and *lateral longitudinal striae* (*striae of Lancisi*) (see Fig. 1–21).

Additional hippocampal fibers join the fornix but grow toward the hypothalamus and the areas of the ventral forebrain. With the continued growth of the corpus callosum, the hippocampal commissure is displaced caudad and the fornix, rostral to the hippocampal commissure, consists principally of fibers to forebrain areas. Gradually, the fornix separates from the corpus callosum, suspended by the *septum pellucidum*. Cells from the lamina terminalis form the septum, and this bilaminar structure becomes part of the medial wall of the lateral ventricle (Figs. 1–21*D* and 1–22).

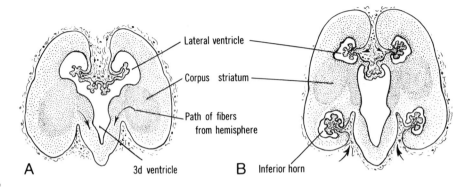

FIGURE 1–23

Two coronal sections of the hemispheres: plane A through the interventricular foramen and plane B posterior to this foramen. Note that the basal ganglia and the thalamus are in contact from the beginning and that this connection is the natural pathway for fibers (shown by arrows, *A*) passing from the hemispheres to the lower centers. These fibers later form the internal capsule. The arrows in *B* indicate the site of invagination of the velum interpositum into the lateral ventricle. (Reproduced with permission from J. Davies, *Human Developmental Anatomy*, Ronald Press, 1963.)

As the corpus callosum grows posteriorly, part of the meninx primitiva is trapped between the corpus callosum and the tela choroidea of the third ventricle. This trapped tissue, the *velum interpositum*, fills the space between the roof of the third ventricle and the corpus callosum and between the pallium and the diencephalon. This space becomes the *great transverse cerebral fissure* (see Fig. 1–22).

DEVELOPMENT OF THE INTERNAL CAPSULE

Many neurons of the neopallium project to lower levels of the CNS and, in turn, receive extensive projections from the diencephalon, particularly the thalamus. In order to reach the diencephalon and lower levels, these fibers pass through the basal ganglia and between the basal ganglia and the thalamus, forming the *internal capsule* (Figs. 1–22*A* and 1–23*A*). The internal capsule, following the C curvature of the basal ganglia and the pallium, divides the basal ganglia into the *lentiform nucleus* (*globus pallidus* and *putamen*), lateral and within the C, and the *caudate nucleus,* medial and along the outer convexity of the C (see Fig. 1–22).

Fibers from the anterior portions of the frontal lobe pass between the *head of the caudate nucleus* and the lentiform nucleus to form the *anterior limb* of the internal capsule. Those from the posterior frontal lobe and parietal lobe first pass between the lentiform nucleus and the *body of the caudate nucleus* and then between the lentiform nucleus and the thalamus to form the *lenticulothalamic* portion of the internal capsule.

Fibers from the occipital lobe pass behind the lentiform nucleus, forming the *retrolenticular* portion of the internal capsule. Those from the temporal lobe pass beneath the lentiform nucleus, forming the *sublenticular* portion of the internal capsule (see Fig. 1–22).

DEVELOPMENT OF OLFACTORY SYSTEM

In the 16.8-mm human embryo, a small protrusion, the *olfactory bulb*, grows from the antero-inferior surface of each telencephalic vesicle and makes contact with the specialized epithelium of the *olfactory placode* in the nasopharynx (see Figs. 1–13 and 1–19). These epithelial cells form the specialized chemoreceptors and the several hundred *olfactory nerves* (*cranial nerve I.*) Olfactory nerves pass through the surrounding connective tissue and enter the developing olfactory bulb. In the adult, this connective tissue becomes the bony *cribriform plate* of the skull. Fibers from the olfactory bulb grow into the neck of the olfactory bulb and along the base of the frontal cortex, forming the *olfactory tract*. At the base of the telencephalon, the olfactory tract splits to form the *lateral, medial,* and *intermediate olfactory striae* (see Fig. 1–19). The lateral olfactory stria swings across the anteroinferior margin of the insula to end in the temporal lobe, near the piriform cortex and the *amygdaloid nucleus,* a division of the basal ganglia situated in the tip of the temporal lobe (see Fig. 1–19). The medial olfactory stria ends in the inferomedial portion of the frontal lobe, just rostral to the lamina terminalis. The intermediate olfactory stria ends at the

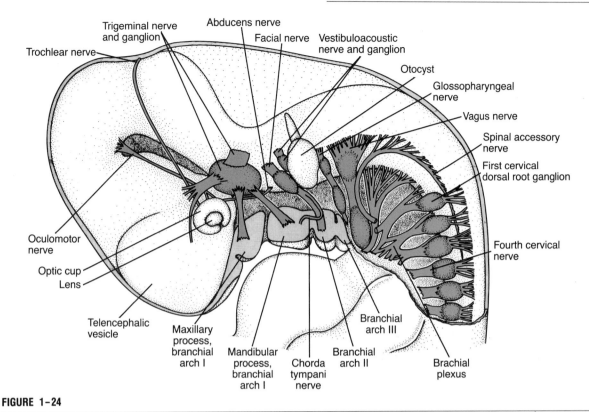

Trigeminal nerve and ganglion
Abducens nerve
Facial nerve
Vestibuloacoustic nerve and ganglion
Trochlear nerve
Otocyst
Glossopharyngeal nerve
Vagus nerve
Spinal accessory nerve
First cervical dorsal root ganglion
Fourth cervical nerve
Oculomotor nerve
Optic cup
Lens
Telencephalic vesicle
Maxillary process, branchial arch I
Mandibular process, branchial arch I
Chorda tympani nerve
Branchial arch II
Branchial arch III
Brachial plexus

FIGURE 1-24

Lateral view of a reconstruction of a 10-mm human embryo showing the origin and distribution of the cranial and upper cervical nerves (in red). (Redrawn with modification from G. L. Streeter, Am. J. Anat., 8: 285–301, 1908.)

base of the forebrain, in an area known as the *olfactory tubercle* in the adult. These pathways are considered further in Chapter 13.

DIFFERENTIATION OF DIENCEPHALON

In the 11.8-mm human embryo, swellings in the ventricular wall of the diencephalon mark the early appearance of the four subdivisions of the diencephalon, the *thalamus (dorsal thalamus), subthalamus, hypothalamus,* and *epithalamus.* Characteristic of this differentiation are the appearance of local areas of rapid proliferation and focal aggregations of differentiating neuroblasts in the lateral walls of the third ventricle. This growth, more apparent in the 16.8-mm embryo, reduces the third ventricle to a thin cavity. Of the diencephalic subdivisions, the thalamus grows most rapidly, and by 43 mm, it is the most prominent structure bordering the third ventricle. The rapid growth and development of the thalamus parallels that of the neopallium, with which it has extensive reciprocal connections (see Figs. 1–12, 1–13, and 1–16).

Cranial Nerves

EARLY CRANIAL NERVE FORMATION

As early as the 10-mm human embryo, the cranial nerves have formed and their peripheral pattern of innervation is straightforward (Fig. 1–24). The complexity observed in the adult is due to the later differentiation and migration of tissues innervated by these nerves. The cranial nerves are considered in detail in Chapter 19.

FUNCTIONAL COMPONENTS OF CRANIAL NERVES

Besides the four general components (*GSA, GVA, GSE,* and *GVE*) characteristic of spinal nerves, cranial nerves have three additional "special" components: special somatic afferent (*SSA*) is a sensory component for special senses of somatic origin (auditory, vestibular, and visual); special visceral afferent (*SVA*) is a sensory component for special senses considered visceral (taste and olfaction); and special visceral efferent (*SVE*) is a motor component for innervation of striated

TABLE 1-2

Functional Components of the Cranial Nerves*

CRANIAL NERVE (NO.)	COMPONENT	BRAIN STEM NUCLEUS
Oculomotor nerve (III)	GSE	Oculomotor nucleus
	GVE	Edinger-Westphal nucleus
Trochlear nerve (IV)	GSE	Trochlear nucleus
Trigeminal nerve (V)	SVE	Motor nucleus of V
	GSA	Main sensory and spinal nuclei of V
Abducens nerve (VI)	GSE	Abducens nucleus
Facial nerve (VII)	SVE	Facial nucleus
	GVE	Superior salivary nucleus
	GVA	Solitary nucleus
	SVA	Solitary nucleus
	GSA	Spinal nucleus of V
Glossopharyngeal nerve (IX)	SVE	Nucleus ambiguus
	GVE	Inferior salivary nucleus
	GVA	Solitary nucleus
	SVA	Solitary nucleus
	GSA	Spinal nucleus of V
Vagus nerve (X)	SVE	Nucleus ambiguus
	GVE	Motor nucleus of X
	GVA	Solitary nucleus
	SVA	Solitary nucleus
	GSA	Spinal nucleus of V
Spinal accessory nerve (XI)	SVE†	Nucleus ambiguus and accessory nucleus
Hypoglossal nerve (XII)	GSE	Hypoglossal nucleus

* Excluding the nerves of special sense: olfactory nerve (I), optic nerve (II), and vestibulocochlear nerve (VIII). These are discussed in Chapters 13, 11, and 12, respectively.
† Some consider the spinal accessory nerve as GSE (see Chapter 19).
Cranial nerves VII, IX, and X have the same five functional components and use many of the same brain stem nuclei.

muscle of visceral (branchial) arch origin. SVE is often called *branchial efferent,* or *branchiomotor.*

The functional components of the brain stem form columns. However, unlike the spinal cord, the columns are not continuous. In addition, whereas most spinal nerves have four components (GSA, GVA, GVE, and GSE), cranial nerves may have as many as five or as few as one (Table 1-2).

In the basal plate of the early embryo, the position of the functional components (medial to lateral) is as follows: GSE, SVE, and GVE. The sequence (medial to lateral) in the alar plate is GVA, SVA, GSA, and, when present, SSA (see Fig. 1-14). In the adult, except for SVE, these columns maintain the same relative position.

SVE nuclei migrate to a ventrolateral position in the brain stem. The best example of this is the facial nucleus (Fig. 1-25). The motor nucleus of V, the nucleus ambiguus, and the accessory nucleus have a similar developmental history. In Figure 1-25A, motor fibers from both facial and abducens nuclei begin to grow (see black arrows) and cell bodies of the facial neurons migrate dorsomedially, over the abducens nucleus (see red arrow). As development proceeds (Fig. 1-25B), the nucleus of the facial nerve, now medial to the abducens nucleus, migrates ventrolaterally (see red arrow) with the nerve fibers trailing. In Figure 1-25C, the facial nucleus assumes the adult position in the ventrolateral portion of the pontine tegmentum. Axons forming the facial nerve course in a dorsomedial direction, "hook over" the abducens nucleus, and exit in a ventrolateral direction. Motor fibers from all SVE nuclei have a similar intramedullary course, although not as pronounced as that of the facial nerve—fibers course dorsomedially, make a 180-degree bend, and exit ventrolaterally.

Developmental Abnormalities

A variety of factors (single gene mutations, chromosomal abnormalities, environmental agents, diseases, drugs, and toxins) can lead to congenital malformations. Nervous system development is a complex process, a fine-tuned orchestration of differential growth rates, cell migrations, and focal proliferations along with selected cell attri-

FIGURE 1-25

Diagram of the sequence of events in the migration of the motor nucleus of the facial nerve (special visceral efferent, SVE). (See text for discussion.)

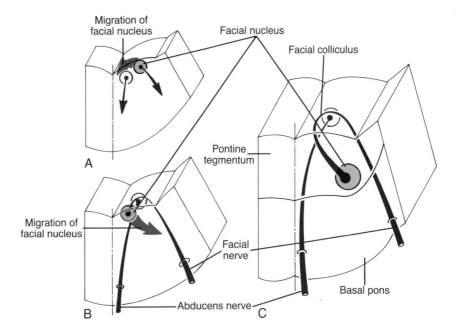

tion. The sequence of events is precisely timed and coordinated. Anything that can interfere with or retard one of the many steps may "de-synchronize" the events and produce a developmental defect.

Some congenital malformations are massive and incompatible with life; others are minor and asymptomatic. The following discussion includes a few examples of what can go wrong during development. It is not an all-inclusive list but illustrates some of the types of deficits that can and do occur. About 1% of all births have some form of congenital malformation of the CNS.

NEURAL TUBE DEFECTS

The most common group of congenital malformations of the nervous system are *neural tube defects*. These represent developmental abnormalities of the neuroectoderm and/or the surrounding mesoderm. Usually, skeletal (skull or vertebral column) defects occur along with a malformation of the underlying brain or spinal cord. The last results from an improper closure of the neural tube during neurulation.

Some vocabulary review will be helpful. The suffix *-schisis* means *opening*, or cleft; hence, *cranioschisis* is an opening, or a cleft, in the skull. *Rachischisis* is a cleft in the dorsal spine of the vertebra, from the Greek word *rachis*, meaning spine. Often, long compound words are combinations of basic word elements, usually Greek,

and these compound words are "translated" with a working knowledge of these basic word elements. For example, *-cele* means *cavity*; *encephalo-* means *brain*; *meningo-* means *meninges* or *membrane,* and *myelo-* literally means *marrow* but more often signifies *spinal cord*. If we put these together, a *meningoencephalocele* (meninges-brain-cavity) is a cavity containing meninges and brain tissues and *myeloschisis* is a cleft spinal cord or one that failed to close during neurulation.

Spina bifida is the most common of the spinal cord malformations. Characteristic of these neural tube defects is a lack of fusion of the vertebral arches (Fig. 1–26). In *spina bifida occulta*, lack of fusion of the vertebral arches is the principal defect. The underlying neural and meningeal tissues are rarely damaged, and the individual usually remains asymptomatic (Fig. 1–26A). In more severe cases of spina bifida, portions of the underlying meninges and/or neural tissue protrude from the opening in the vertebral canal. In *spina bifida with meningocele*, the meninges protrude through the defect and the spinal cord remains within the vertebral canal (Fig. 1–26B). In more severe defects, *spinal bifida with meningomyelocele*, both the spinal cord tissue and the meninges protrude into the sac (Fig. 1–26C). In the most severe form, *spina bifida with myeloschisis*, the neural tube fails to close (Fig. 1–26D). In the last case, the neural tube is spread out and often the tissue is difficult to recognize as neural tissue, because of its expo-

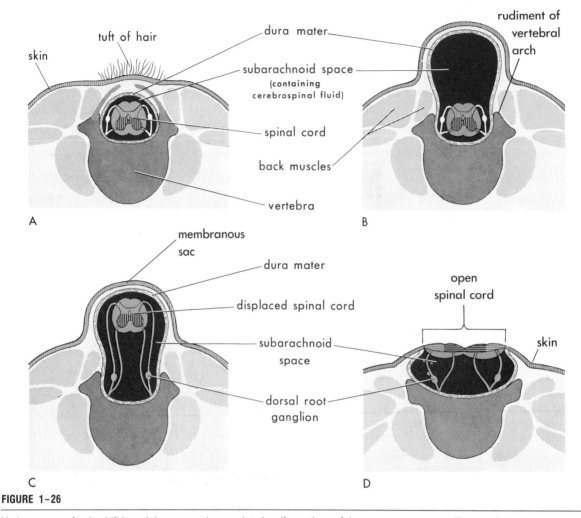

FIGURE 1-26

Various types of *spina bifida* and the commonly associated malformations of the nervous system are illustrated.

A, Spina bifida occulta. About 10% of people have this vertebral defect in L-5, S-1, or both. It usually causes no back problems.

B, Spina bifida with meningocele.

C, Spina bifida with meningomyelocele.

D, Spina bifida with myeloschisis. The types illustrated in *B* to *D* are often referred to collectively as *spina bifida cystica* because of the cyst-like sac that is associated with them. (Reproduced with permission from K. L. Moore, *The Developing Human: Clinically Oriented Embryology*, 4th Edition, W. B. Saunders Co., Philadelphia, p. 375, 1988.)

sure to the amniotic fluid and the trauma of the birth process. Most forms of spina bifida occur at vertebral level L-5 or S-1.

With spina bifida occulta and spina bifida with meningocele in which there are no neurological deficits, the prognosis is very good. However, usually with a meningocele, the spinal cord does sustain some damage, even though it does not protrude through the skeletal defect. Severe neurological deficits invariably accompany spinal bi-

fida with meningomyelocele or with myeloschisis. The extent of the deficit varies and reflects both the total amount of neural tissue damaged and the spinal level involved.

When the bony defect is in the skull, the general classification is *cranium bifidum* (Fig. 1-27). The defect usually occurs in the midline at the level of the posterior fontanelle or near the foramen magnum (Fig. 1-27A). As with spinal bifidum, several categories of cranium bifidum

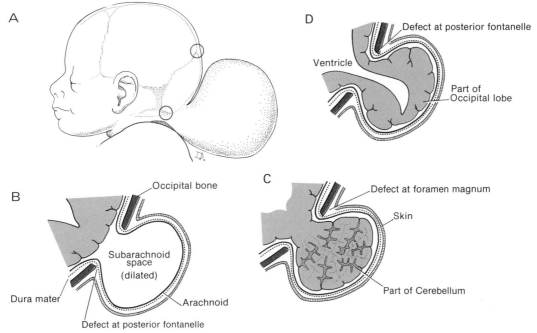

FIGURE 1-27

Cranium bifidum (bony defect in the cranium) and various types of herniation of the brain and/or meninges are illustrated.

A, The head of a newborn infant with a large protrusion from the occipital region of the skull. The upper circle indicates a cranial defect at the posterior fontanelle, and the lower circle indicates a cranial defect near the foramen magnum.

B, Meningocele consisting of a protrusion of the cranial meninges that is filled with cerebrospinal fluid.

C, Meningoencephalocele consisting of a protrusion of part of the cerebellum that is covered by meninges and skin.

D, Meningohydroencephalocele consisting of a protrusion of part of the occipital lobe that contains part of the posterior horn of a lateral ventricle. (Reproduced with permission from K. L. Moore, *The Developing Human: Clinically Oriented Embryology*, 4th Edition, W. B. Saunders Co., p. 391, 1988.)

are based on the tissues involved. *Cranium bifidum with meningocele* is a protrusion of meninges (Fig. 1-27*B*); *cranium bifidum with meningoencephalocele* is a protrusion of both the brain and meninges (Fig. 1-27*C*); and *cranium bifidum with meningohydroencephalocele* is a protrusion of the brain, ventricle, and meninges (Fig. 1-27*D*). Wide variation exists in the degree of permanent damage. The viability of the newborn therefore depends on the amount and nature of the damage to the neural tissue.

The most severe example of a neural tube defect is complete *anencephaly*, an absence of the brain and the overlying cranial vault, i.e., complete *cranioschisis with encephaloschisis*. Usually, the facial features are present, but the cranial vault and brain are absent, except for a hemorrhagic mass of tissue representing the remains of the brain, the *area cerebrovasculosa*. Often this defect is accompanied by *rachischisis with mye-* *loschisis*, the probable result of either absence of neurulation or faulty closure of the entire neural tube. These conditions are not compatible with life.

DEFECTS IN THE ANTERIOR TELENCEPHALIC WALL

When the anterior neuropore closes, the *lamina terminalis* forms. This portion of the anterior wall provides the principal route for the commissural fibers of the corpus callosum in their growth from one side of the telencephalon to the other. A defect in the dorsal portion of the lamina terminalis, in the area of the dorsal commissure (see Fig. 1-16), prevents the formation of the corpus callosum, a condition known as *agenesis of the corpus callosum*. An absence of the cingulate gyrus often accompanies this deficit. Although agenesis of the corpus callosum can occur alone, it often is a component of more extensive malformations involving other structures associated with the anterior wall and forebrain area.

The telencephalic vesicles normally arise from the dorsolateral portion of the forebrain, separated anteromedially by the lamina terminalis. If, during the outgrowth process, the vesicles do not remain separated but fuse anteromedially in the midline, they will not develop into a pair of hemispheres. Instead, they will grow out as a single, large vesicle from the forebrain or prosencephalon, a condition known as *holoprosencephaly*. This large, single prosencephalic vesicle will grow back over the diencephalon, without the separation of the longitudinal cerebral fissure and without the corpus callosum. Holoprosencephaly represents the extreme example of a group of anterior wall defects. In *lobar holoprosencephaly*, for example, the two hemispheres are nearly separate, except for the anterior portion.

If the anterior wall defect also involves the more rostral prochordal mesoderm, formation of the facial features will be abnormal. The most extreme example is *cyclopia*, in which the bony orbits are fused and contain either two eyeballs or a single fused eyeball, with a single optic nerve. The nose is present as a small rudimentary protuberance immediately above the single orbit. Often the basal ganglia and dorsal thalami are fused in the midline as well. The combination of holoprosencephaly and severe facial abnormalities usually suggests a chromosomal disorder. Holoprosencephaly without prochordal mesodermal involvement (facial features) suggests some teratological agent.

GENERALIZED DISTURBANCES OF GROWTH

The adult human brain has a weight of approximately 1400 gm. Although the rules for "normal" and "abnormal" size are not clear-cut, if the brain weighs less than 900 gm, it is considered *microencephalic*. Microencephaly is commonly associated with mental retardation and is often accompanied with seizures and motor disorders. However, a mass of less than 900 gm has been reported for the brains of apparently "normal" individuals. *Megaloencephaly*, an abnormally large brain of greater than 1400 or 1600 gm, also is associated with mental retardation. However, this condition has been found in some individuals with higher than normal intelligence.

SUGGESTED READING

Gottlieb, G. (Editor). *Studies on the Development of Behavior and the Nervous System.* Academic Press, New York. (Volume 1 (1973). *Behavioral Embryology.* Volume 2 (1974). *Aspects of Neurogenesis.* Volume 3 (1976). *Neural Behavior and Specificity.* Volume 4 (1978). *Early Influences.*)

A four-volume series dealing with experimental studies of nervous system development, with special emphasis on the development of behavior.

Jacobson, M. (1978). *Developmental Neurobiology,* 2nd Edition. Plenum Press, New York.

An in-depth coverage of experimental embryology, with special emphasis on mechanisms of development.

Ludwin, S. K. and M. G. Norman (1985). Congenital malformations of the nervous system. In *Textbook of Neuropathology*, R. L. Davis and D. M. Robertson (Editors). Williams & Wilkins, Baltimore, pp. 176–242.

A comprehensive and systematic survey of congenital malformations of the human nervous system.

Moore, K. L. (1988). *The Developing Human: Clinically Oriented Embryology,* 4th Edition. W. B. Saunders Co., Philadelphia.

A good, basic textbook covering all aspects of human embryology, including the nervous system. Congenital malformations and other developmental problems are correlated with normal development throughout the text.

Part
II

CELLULAR ELEMENTS

Chapter

2

Histology and Fine Structure of Nervous Tissue

NEURONS
NEUROGLIA
EPENDYMA AND CHOROID PLEXUS
PERIPHERAL NERVOUS SYSTEM
DAMAGE AND REPAIR

To early neurobiologists, the central nervous system (CNS) was a complex syncytium in which all neurons were structurally continuous. However, by the late 1800's, this view was challenged by proponents of the *neuron doctrine*. According to this doctrine, the nervous system was made up of individual cells, each a distinct genetic, anatomical, and functional unit. The concept was not immediately accepted, however, and the issue remained controversial during the first half of the 20th century.

Electron microscopical studies provided the definitive evidence for the neuron doctrine. In these studies, a small, distinct separation always was found between neurons at the point of apparent contact. These points of "near contact" were called *synapses* as early as the turn of the century, even though the extremely narrow space, the *synaptic cleft*, could not be seen with the light microscope.

In addition to the neuronal elements, the CNS contains *neuroglial cells*. Generally regarded as the "connective tissue" of the CNS, neuroglial cells far outnumber neurons yet account for only half the brain's mass. Unlike neurons, neuroglial cells retain the capacity to proliferate. Most brain tumors, benign and malignant, are of neuroglial origin. When the CNS is injured, glial cells mobilize, clean up the debris, and seal off the local area, leaving behind a "glial scar." This scar is partially responsible for the lack of neuronal regeneration in the mammalian CNS (see subsequent discussion).

Neurons

COMPONENTS

The three principal components of a neuron are the *soma*, the *dendrites*, and the *axon*. These are illustrated for a *multipolar neuron* in Figure 2–1*A*. The soma contains the *nucleus* and its surrounding cytoplasm, the *perikaryon*. The dendrites arise as multiple branches from the soma. Collectively, all the dendrites and their branches form the *dendritic tree*. Neurons have a single *axon*, originating from the soma at the *axon hillock* and ending in a terminal arborization, the *telodendron*. Each terminal branch of the telo-

31

A

Dendrites

Soma

Nucleus

Mitochondria

Recurrent axon
collateral

Axon

Ribosome
rosettes

Telodendron

Synaptic terminals

B

Base of dendrite

Neurofilaments

Golgi
apparatus

Rough
endoplasmic
reticulum

Nuclear
membrane

Nucleolus

Barr body

Axon hillock

Initial segment

Myelin sheath

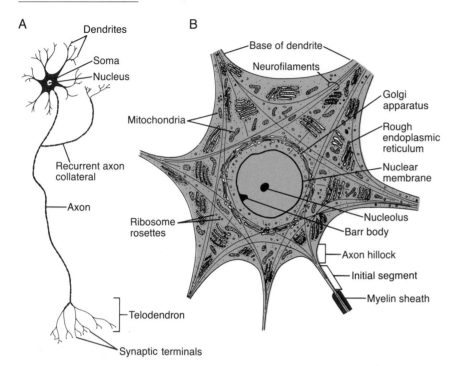

FIGURE 2-1

Multipolar neuron *(A)* illustrates the major components, and a higher magnification of the soma *(B)* illustrates a number of cell organelles. The axon hillock area is devoid of rough endoplasmic reticulum, ribosome rosettes (polysomes), and free ribosomes. However, these organelles extend for varying distances into the base of the dendrites. Neurofilaments and microtubules (not illustrated) pass through the perikaryon and into the axonal and dendritic processes.

dendron has an enlarged, bulbous ending, the *synaptic terminal* (*bouton terminaux* or *synaptic button*). The surface membrane of the soma and dendritic tree is specialized for the reception and integration of information, whereas that of the axon is specialized for the transmission of information in the form of an *action potential* or a *nerve impulse*.

In the CNS, functionally related neurons grouped together are known as *nuclei*. Within such a *nucleus*,* and between the neuronal cell bodies, is an area called the *neuropil*. The neuropil, packed with dendrites, axonal branches, and glia, contains a very high concentration of synapses.

Incoming nerve impulses produce focal changes in the *resting membrane potential* of the neuron, changes that spread passively along the membrane of the dendrites and soma. The level of excitability of a neuron at any point in time is determined by the temporal and spatial summation of all excitatory and inhibitory signals received. An *action potential* is generated at the *initial segment* of the axon when the resting membrane potential of this "trigger zone"

reaches a threshold level. Once triggered, the self-propagating action potential travels rapidly along the entire length of the axon, ending with the depolarization of the synaptic terminal (see Chapters 3 and 4).

TYPES AND CLASSIFICATION

Adult neurons have a wide variety of shapes and degrees of morphological complexity, to the extent that each neuron has a unique identity. Nevertheless, certain similarities in structure occur between groups of neurons. These similarities are the bases for classification into broad categories.

Multipolar neurons have many processes, a single axon, and more than one dendrite, and account for most of the neurons in the vertebrate nervous system (Fig. 2–2*A*, *B*, and *C*). *Bipolar neurons* have two processes and, most commonly, are associated with pathways of special sense, such as visual, auditory, and vestibular systems (Fig. 2–2*E*). *Pseudounipolar neurons*, located principally in sensory ganglia of cranial and spinal nerves, have only one process leaving the cell body (Fig. 2–2*D*). Embryonically, pseudounipolar neurons develop from bipolar neuroblasts and the two neuronal processes fuse during later development, hence the prefix *pseudo-*.

An additional classification of multipolar neurons is based on the length of the axon relative to

---

* In neuroanatomy, the term *nucleus* is used in two ways: (1) to refer to the cell organelle and (2) to refer to a population of functionally and/or anatomically related neurons.

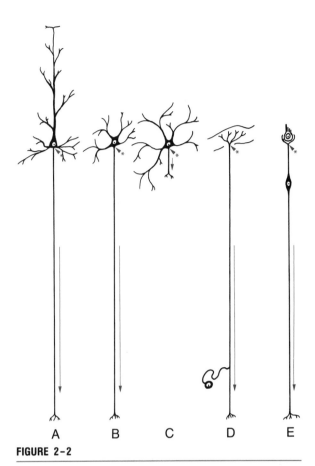

FIGURE 2-2

Five different types of neurons illustrate the principle of dynamic polarization. *A*, Cortical pyramidal neuron; *B*, Golgi type I multipolar neuron; *C*, Golgi type II multipolar neuron; *D*, pseudounipolar sensory neuron; and *E*, bipolar neuron from the vestibular ganglion. Arrowheads with asterisks identify the "trigger zone" for the action potential. The long arrows indicate the direction of impulse conduction. (See text for discussion.)

the dendritic tree. *Golgi type I* neurons have an axon that extends beyond the limits of the dendritic tree. These usually function as *relay neurons*, i.e., they send information to another area of the CNS or to peripheral effectors in the case of motor neurons (Fig. 2–2*B*). *Golgi type II* neurons have an axon that terminates in the immediate area of the cell body and does not extend beyond the limits of the dendritic tree. These neurons usually function as *associational neurons,* or *interneurons* (Fig. 2–2*C*).

A few examples of other classifications, based on general morphology, are illustrated in the drawings and photomicrographs of Golgi-stained neurons in Figures 2–3 and 2–4. The heavy-metal Golgi stains impregnate a select population of neurons producing a solid black, three-

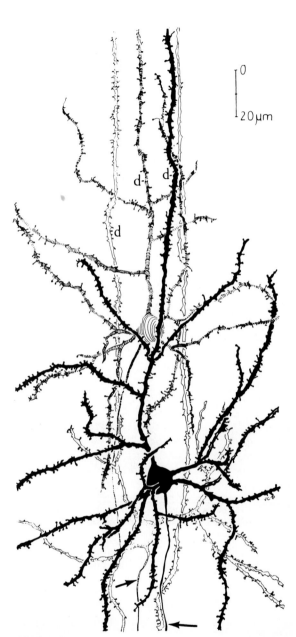

FIGURE 2-3

Camera lucida drawing of three small, cortical pyramidal neurons from an adult *Macaca.* Cells give rise to apical and basal dendrites (d) of varying caliber, which display numerous spiny appendages of diverse shapes and sizes. A thin axon (arrows) springs from each cell body and descends to deeper layers. Rapid Golgi preparation. (Reproduced with permission from S. L. Palay and V. Chan-Palay, General morphology of neurons and glia. *In* E. R. Kandel (Editor), *Handbook of Physiology*, Section 1, Volume I, p. 7, 1977.)

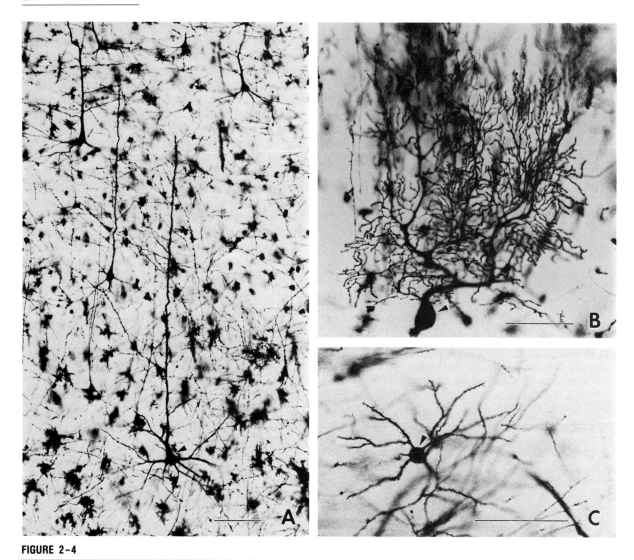

FIGURE 2-4

A, Medium-sized pyramidal neuron from the human cerebral cortex; B, human cerebellar Purkinje cell; and C, a small stellate neuron from the cerebral cortex of the cat. Golgi-Cox stain. Arrows point to the soma of the neuron. The bars represent 100 μm.

dimensional silhouette of the entire cell. This totally obscures the intracellular structures. Camillio Golgi first described these stains over 100 years ago, yet the chemical basis of the reaction and why so few neurons stain at one time remain unknown.

The *Purkinje cells* of the cerebellar cortex have an elaborate dendritic tree and a single axon projecting to the nuclei of the cerebellum (Fig. 2-4B). In the cerebral cortex, the apical dendrites of the *pyramidal cells* radiate toward the cortical surface and a single axon leaves the soma to terminate in another cortical area or in a lower center (see Figs. 2-3 and 2-4A). Small *stellate cells* of the cerebral cortex have short axons that

terminate in the immediate vicinity of the perikaryon (Figs. 2-2C and 2-4C). By definition, a pyramidal cell and a Purkinje cell are also Golgi type I neurons as are lower motor neurons. However, the Golgi type I and Golgi type II nomenclature is usually used for neurons that do not have a more precise label. This is a "catchall" nomenclature, but one that still describes the general features of the multipolar neuron.

DYNAMIC POLARIZATION

The concept of *dynamic polarization* is helpful in the definition of the functional components of the neuron. The location of the "trigger zone" defines the origin of the axon. Receptor surfaces of the neuron passively integrate incoming information. When the trigger zone is depolarized to a threshold level, an action potential is generated.

For each neuron in Figure 2–2, the direction of the action potential conduction is indicated with an arrow and the trigger zone, with an arrowhead and asterisk. A cortical pyramidal neuron is represented in *A*, a Golgi type I neuron in *B*, and a Golgi type II neuron in *C*. All three are multipolar neurons. The trigger zone of the axon is adjacent to the soma.

Dorsal root ganglion cells (pseudounipolar neurons) (see Fig. 2–2D) carry sensory information from the periphery to the spinal cord via a long axon. The single neuronal process attached to the soma bifurcates, with a peripheral arm extending to the sensory receptor and a central arm extending to the CNS. Sensory stimulation alters the resting potential of the peripherally located dendritic tree. When the trigger zone reaches threshold, an action potential is generated. In this type of neuron, the soma is some distance from the

axon and is not involved directly in the generation or conduction of the action potential.

In the case of *bipolar neurons*, such as those of the vestibular ganglion (see Fig. 2–2E), the soma is in the middle of the axon. One segment of the axon extends from the receptor to the soma and the other from the soma to the brain stem. As with dorsal root neurons, the trigger zone defines the beginning of the axon. The action potential passes from the trigger zone, across the membrane of the soma, and into the brain stem via the central process of the neuron.

SOMA

The cell body or *soma* contains the nucleus and the surrounding cytoplasm, or *perikaryon* (see Fig. 2–1). In large neurons, the perikaryon is extensive; in small neurons, it is limited. The soma is the trophic center of the neuron and provides a constant supply of organelles and macromolecules for axonal and dendritic processes. Accordingly, the soma is well equipped for

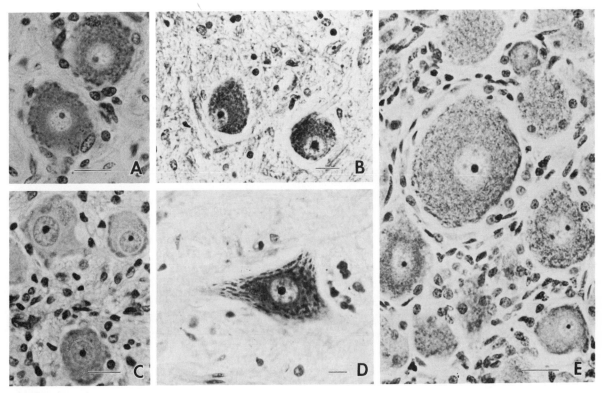

FIGURE 2–5

A, Nissl-stained neurons from the celiac ganglion; *B*, Clarke's column of the thoracic spinal cord; *C*, sympathetic ganglion; *D*, sympathetic preganglionic motor neuron from the thoracic spinal cord; and *E*, a dorsal root ganglion. Human tissue; bars represent 20 μm.

the synthesis of proteins, phospholipids, and other macromolecules. In multipolar neurons, the unit membrane of the soma is important in the reception and integration of synaptic information.

The *nucleus* of a neuron is usually large, spherical, and centrally located; an exception is the eccentric location of the nucleus in neurons from the nucleus dorsalis (Clarke's column) (Fig. 2–5B). Within the nucleus, the chromatin is dispersed and stains lightly with a web-like pattern, whereas the one or more very prominent nucleoli stain intensely (Figs. 2–5 and 2–6).

A characteristic feature of the perikaryon in large neurons is an abundance of ribonucleoprotein associated with the rough endoplasmic reticulum, polysomes, and free ribosomes. In light microscopic preparations with nucleic acid stains, this feature appears as large dense-staining clumps, or *Nissl bodies*. The pattern of clumping is characteristic of different types of neurons and serves as a means of identification. For example, Nissl bodies in lower motor neurons stain with a pattern of large clumps, whereas those in dorsal root ganglion cells stain with a fine granular pattern (compare Fig. 2–5D with Fig. 2–5E). With the electron microscope, we can see that these clumps are actually small stacks of rough endoplasmic reticulum (Fig. 2–7).

In most neurons, the very prominent *Golgi apparatus* is present as a loose net surrounding the nucleus and, in smaller neurons, extends into the base of dendrites (see Figs. 2–1 and 2–7).

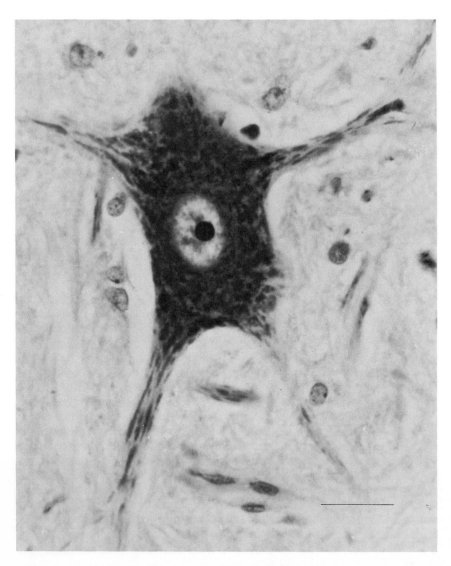

FIGURE 2–6

Nissl-stained anterior horn cell from the human lumbar spinal cord. Cresyl fast violet stain; bar represents 20 μm.

FIGURE 2-7

The nuclear envelope, Nissl
bodies, and Golgi apparatus. The
electron micrograph shows part
of the nucleus and perikaryon of
an anterior horn cell. In the cytoplasm are small Nissl bodies and
parts of the Golgi apparatus in
different section planes. The fen-
estrations in the cisternae of the
Golgi apparatus can be seen in
the surface view near the center
and in the transverse section
near the right edge. Lysosomes
(Ly) of diverse sizes and shapes
are collected near the nucleus.

The nucleus is bounded by a
double-layered envelope, which
arches across the lower third of
the micrograph. The inner membrane of the envelope is smooth.
The outer membrane undulates
irregularly. Periodically, both
membranes come together to
form the walls of pores (arrows),
each bridged by a diaphragm
(see insets).

Notice that ribosomes are only
rarely attached to the outer cytoplasmic surface of the nuclear
envelope and that the chromatin
does not approach very close to
its inner aspect. Spinal cord of
adult rat; ×34,000.

The insets at the lower edge of
the micrograph are enlargements
of the left half of the nuclear
envelope. The thin fibrous lamina (triangles) adherent to the inner surface of the envelope, the
nuclear pores with their dia-
phragms, and the crown-like
array of threads (ct) are shown
(×91,000). (Reproduced with
permission from A. Peters, S. L.
Palay, and H. DeF. Webster, *The
Fine Structure of the Nervous
System*, 2nd Edition, W. B.
Saunders Co., Philadelphia, p. 51,
1976.)

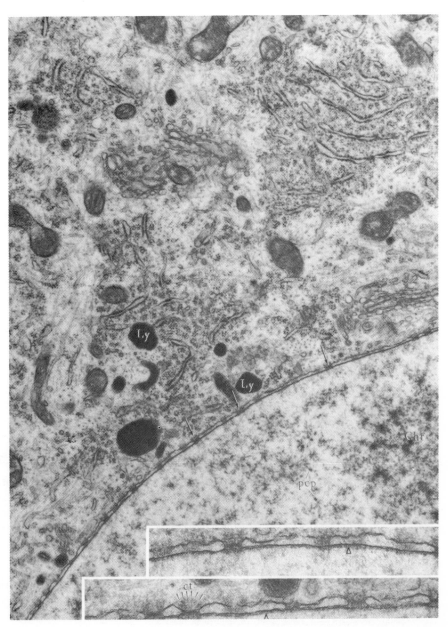

Functions of the Golgi apparatus include the post-translational modification of proteins, such as glycosylation, and the packaging of macromolecules for transport to nerve terminals. Numerous *mitochondria* reside in the perikaryon, axon, and dendrites, consistent with a cell that maintains a high rate of oxidative metabolism.

Neurofibrils are another distinctive feature of neurons, and these can be visualized in light microscopic preparations with reduced silver stains (Fig. 2–8). These fibrils extend through the perikaryon and into the dendritic and axonal processes.

Comparable structures cannot be identified with the electron microscope, and the neurofibrils are believed to be clumps or bundles of submicroscopic *neurofilaments* (100 Å in diameter). In addition to neurofilaments, the perikaryon and nerve processes contain large numbers of *microtubules*, approximately 250 Å in diameter and visible with the electron microscope (Fig. 2–9).

The soma also contains many dense lysosomes and, occasionally, a yellowish pigmented substance in the form of *lipofuscin granules*. The last, more prevalent in older neurons, probably represent the residue of old lysosomes. *Melanin* pigment is found within lysosome-like structures of some neurons, such as those in the substantia nigra of the midbrain.

DENDRITES

The dendritic tree is the primary receiving station for synaptic information. In multipolar neurons, the soma also receives synapses, but the surface area and the number of synapses are small compared with those of the dendrites. The dendritic surface of many neurons is modified by the presence of *dendritic spines*. These small protuberances (up to 1.0 μm in length and 0.2 to 2.0 μm in diameter), which further increase the synaptic surface area, are visible with Golgi-stained preparations for the light microscope (Figs. 2–3 and 2–10*A*) but are more visible with the electron microscope (see Fig. 2–13).

Dendrites have an abundance of microtubules and neurofilaments, regularly arranged and parallel to the long axis of the nerve process (see Fig. 2–9). Secondary dendritic branches are smaller in diameter and contain proportionally fewer neurofilaments and microtubules. The rough endoplasmic reticulum of the soma may extend into the base of the dendrite. Free ribosomes and polysomes are found throughout the dendritic tree, although the concentration is less in secondary and tertiary branches. Mitochondria are found throughout the dendrite (see Fig. 2–9).

AXON

In multipolar neurons, the axon arises from the soma in an area devoid of Nissl substance, the *axon hillock* (see Fig. 2–1). The *initial segment*, the narrowest part of the axon, is the site of action potential generation, the trigger zone. The diameter of the axon increases slightly after the initial segment. Unlike the gradually tapering dendrite, the diameter of the axon remains constant from the initial segment to the terminal arborization. In some neurons, an axon may arise from the base of a dendrite instead of the soma.

In *myelinated axons*, a myelin sheath extends from the initial segment to the telodendron (see Fig. 2–1). Many axons have collateral branches, some at or near the soma (*recurrent collaterals*). Others are at various locations throughout the course of the axon. Some axons terminate in a rather restricted area, whereas others branch profusely and terminate in many different areas of the CNS.

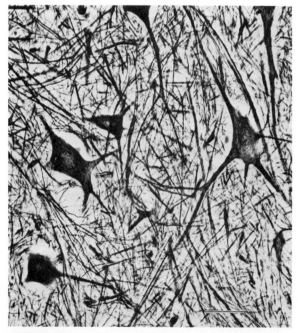

FIGURE 2–8

Neurofibrils of anterior horn cells from the human lumbar spinal cord. Pyridine-silver stain; bar represents 40 μm.

FIGURE 2-9

Dendrites in longitudinal and transverse section. In this electron micrograph of the neuropil of the anterior horn are two dendrites (Den$_1$ and Den$_2$) sectioned longitudinally and a third (Den$_3$) sectioned transversely. In the upper dendrite (Den$_1$) some extent of the individual microtubules (m) and neurofilaments (nf) may be seen. These structures have regular outlines, which contrast with the more varicose outlines of the tubules of the smooth endoplasmic reticulum (SR), with which clusters of free ribosomes (r) are often associated, Such large numbers of neurofilaments in groups are characteristic of the dendrites arising from large anterior horn neurons and are not seen in dendrites generally.

With the exception of ribosomes, the same organelles are also present in the transversely sectioned dendrite (Den$_3$). This smaller dendrite has two axon terminals synapsing upon its surface. In the upper terminal, the synaptic vesicles are spherical, whereas in the lower one they are mostly ellipsoidal. Extending around the axon terminals and the postsynaptic dendrite is an astrocytic sheath (As). Spinal cord of adult rat; ×44,000. (Reproduced with permission from A. Peters, S. L. Palay, and H. DeF. Webster, *The Fine Structure of the Nervous System*, 2nd Edition, W. B. Saunders Co., Philadelphia, p. 75, 1976.)

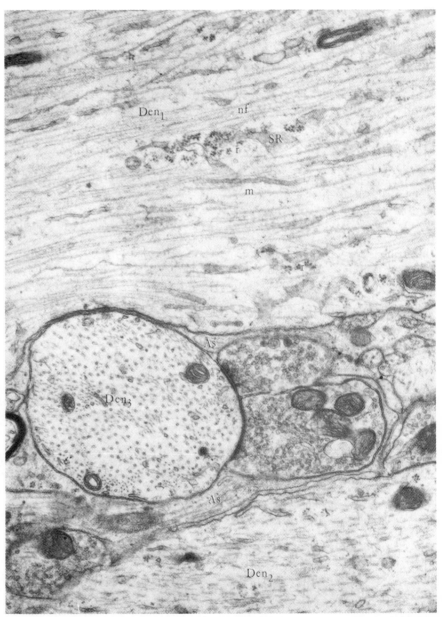

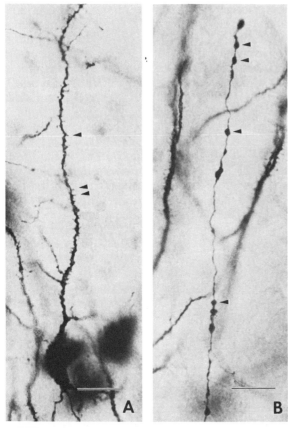

FIGURE 2-10

A, Portion of the apical dendrite of a pyramidal neuron illustrating the dendritic spines. *B,* A segment of an axon illustrates axonal varicosities or boutons en passant. Golgi-Cox stain, human cerebral cortex; bars represent 20 μm.

SYNAPTIC TERMINALS AND SYNAPSES

The *synaptic terminal* (*bouton terminaux* or *synaptic button*) is specialized for the transmission of a chemical message in response to the arrival of an action potential. The *synapse* is the junctional complex between the *presynaptic terminal* of an axon and a *postsynaptic membrane* or receptor surface. The prefixes *pre-* and *post-* refer to the direction of synaptic transmission: *presynaptic* referring to the transmitting side (usually axonal) and *postsynaptic* to the receiving side (usually dendritic or somal but sometimes axonal).

At a CNS synapse, the presynaptic and postsynaptic membranes are separated by a space of 200 to 300 Å, the *synaptic cleft.* Electron-dense material on the inner surfaces of the two membranes forms the *presynaptic* and *postsynaptic densities* (Fig. 2-11). The presynaptic density

usually has a series of conical projections protruding into the presynaptic terminal. The postsynaptic density is of uniform thickness. When the postsynaptic density is thicker than the presynaptic, the synapse is an *asymmetrical synapse.* When the thickness is nearly the same, it is a *symmetrical synapse* (see Fig. 2-11). In general, asymmetrical synapses are excitatory and symmetrical synapses inhibitory.

Presynaptic terminals contain a large number of membrane-bound vesicles, *synaptic vesicles.* These range in size from 400 to 1000 Å in diameter and contain the neurotransmitter. The vesicles of asymmetrical, excitatory synapses are always spherical, whereas the vesicles of symmetrical, inhibitory synapses can be either spherical or ellipsoidal. Presynaptic terminals also contain mitochondria, components of the smooth endoplasmic reticulum, some microtubules, and a few neurofilaments (Figs. 2-11, 2-12, and 2-13).

Synapses are classified by their location on the postsynaptic neuron (Fig. 2-14): *axospinous* synapses are axon terminals synapsing on a dendritic spine; *axodendritic* synapses are axon terminals on the shaft of a dendrite; and *axosomatic* synapses are axon terminals on the soma. The *initial segment synapse* is an axon terminal synapsing on the initial segment of an axon, and the *axoaxonal* synapse is an axon terminal synapsing on another axon terminal. A *chain synapse* is the special case of an axoaxonal synapse in which both axon terminals also synapse on the same postsynaptic receptor surface (see Fig. 2-14). Not illustrated are *dendrodendritic* synapses, junctions between two dendritic processes.

The axons of some neurons, especially those with catecholamines as primary neurotransmitters, have specialized swellings along their courses. The swellings of these varicose or "beaded" axons contain synaptic vesicles and release neurotransmitter in response to an action potential. These swellings, known as *boutons en passant,* form *nondirected synapses* (Figs. 2-10*B* and 2-14). A postsynaptic specialization is lacking, and the released transmitter may diffuse to receptors on distant neurons, up to several millimeters away from the bouton.

Although rare in the vertebrate nervous system, there also are direct, fused connections between neurons. The presynaptic and postsynaptic membranes of these *electrical synapses* or *gap junctions* are partially fused. Action potentials cross from the membrane of one neuron to the next without attenuation and without neurotransmitter intervention. These synapses often lack the

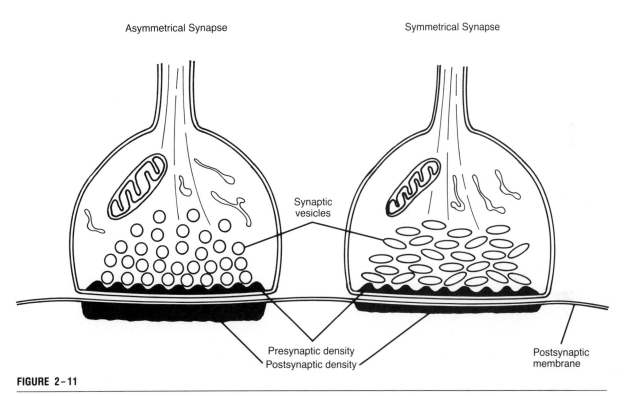

Asymmetrical Synapse   Symmetrical Synapse

Synaptic
vesicles

Presynaptic density
Postsynaptic density

Postsynaptic
membrane

FIGURE 2-11

An asymmetrical synapse and a symmetrical synapse. The classification is based on the relative thickness of the postsynaptic density.

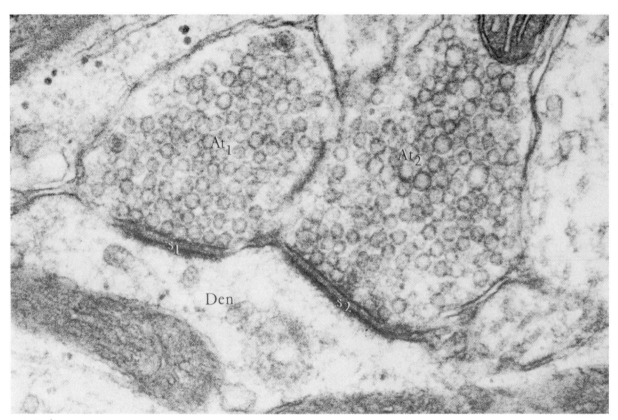

FIGURE 2–12

Two asymmetrical synapses (S_1 and S_2) between two axon terminals (At_1 and At_2) and the smooth dendrite (Den) of a stellate cell. At the synaptic junctions the presynaptic and postsynaptic membranes are separated by a cleft that contains intercellular material. The postsynaptic membrane has a prominent coating of dense material on its cytoplasmic face. Rat auditory cortex; ×100,000. (Reproduced with permission from A. Peters, S. L. Palay, and H. DeF. Webster, *The Fine Structure of the Nervous System*, 2nd Edition, W. B. Saunders Co., Philadelphia, p. 131, 1976.)

FIGURE 2-13

A large spine or protrusion (center of field) from the perikaryon of a neuron. Surrounding this structure is a variety of axon terminals. Two of the terminals (At_1 and At_2) contain small, spherical synaptic vesicles. The spherical vesicles in two other terminals (At_3 and At_4) are somewhat larger. The other axon terminals (At_5 to At_9) contain some elongate synaptic vesicles.

The synaptic junctions in which these various axon terminals participate all seem to be symmetrical. The junction formed by At_5 is noteworthy because of the regular array of presynaptic densities (arrows). At the other synaptic junctions, only one or two of these densities (arrows) are apparent. Ventral cochlear nucleus of adult rat; ×44,000. (Reproduced with permission from A. Peters, S. L. Palay, and H. DeF. Webster, *The Fine Structure of the Nervous System*, 2nd Edition, W. B. Saunders Co., Philadelphia, p. 161, 1976.)

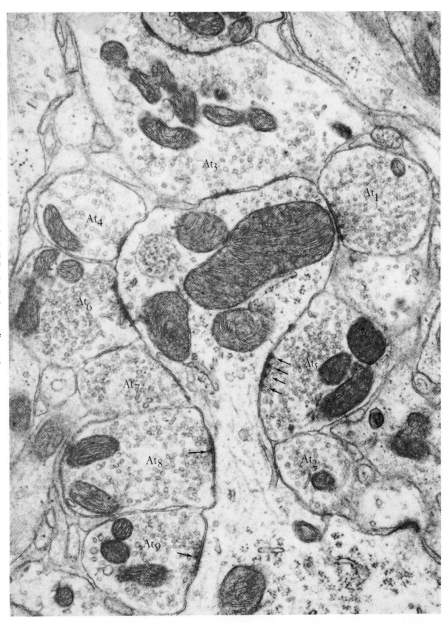

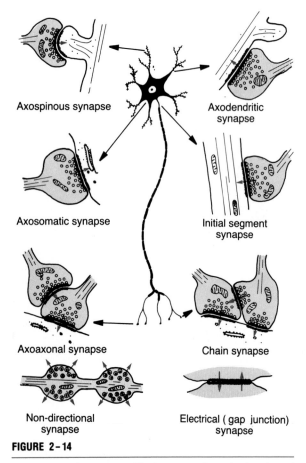

Axospinous synapse

Axodendritic synapse

Axosomatic synapse

Initial segment synapse

Axoaxonal synapse

Chain synapse

Non-directional synapse

Electrical (gap junction) synapse

FIGURE 2–14

Eight types of synapses. Black arrows show the location of the synapse. Red arrows show the direction of the synaptic transmission.

directional specificity of chemical synapses and may transmit an impulse in either direction (see Fig. 2–14).

Neuroglia

ASTROCYTES

Morphologically, astrocytes are divided into three categories: *fibrous astrocytes, protoplasmic astrocytes,* and *velate protoplasmic astrocytes.* All are variations of the same basic cell type; examples typical of each can be found. However, many astrocytes are not easily classified as one type or another. Fibrous astrocytes reside predominantly in white matter and have long slender processes with few branches; protoplasmic astrocytes reside predominantly in gray matter and have shorter, stouter processes with many short branches; and

the velate protoplasmic astrocytes have short, thin, veil-like processes (Figs. 2–15A, 2–15B, and 2–16).

The nuclei of astrocytes are large (6 to 10 μm) and ovoid, with a granular, vesiculated chromatin pattern. The indented oval nucleus rarely has a nucleolus.

One of the most characteristic features of astrocytes is the presence of a large number of *glial filaments.* Similar in structure to neurofilaments, glial filaments are much more abundant (Fig. 2–17). The perinuclear cytoplasm of the astrocyte contains few organelles: however, a prominent Golgi apparatus is always present.

Although astrocytes are present in large numbers, their function is largely unknown. Most brain capillaries are completely surrounded by astrocytic vascular end-feet and a dense *glial limitans* (see Figs. 2–15 and 2–17). At one time, this glial membrane was thought to be the morphological basis for the "blood-brain barrier." However, the barrier to macromolecules actually resides in the tight junctions between the nonfenestrated endothelial cells of brain capillaries. Processes, similar to vascular end-feet, form a glial membrane beneath the external surface of the brain, just under the pia mater. This membrane is not a macromolecular barrier. Gaps between end-feet provide an avenue of communication between the cerebrospinal fluid–filled, subarachnoid space and the intercellular spaces within the brain.

The close association of astrocytes and brain capillaries suggests a role in the regulation of brain metabolism, both in the uptake of nutrients and essential compounds and in the elimination of metabolic waste and toxic substances. Large quantities of K$^+$ are absorbed by astrocytes when surrounding neurons are stimulated repeatedly, apparently regulating the ion balance of the neuronal milieu. Astrocytes envelop neurons and neuronal processes in areas devoid of myelin sheaths, possibly insulating them from surrounding electrical "noise" as well as forming a structural matrix for the nervous system. However, most of the proposed functions for these abundant small cells are based on indirect evidence.

OLIGODENDROGLIA

Oligodendroglia, or *oligodendrocytes,* are smaller than astrocytes and their nuclei are irregular and more densely staining (see Fig. 2–17). The cytoplasm is more electron dense and there are more cellular organelles, especially free and attached

FIGURE 2-15

A, Fibrous astrocytes with multiple vascular end-feet. Silver carbonate stain; white matter of the cat cerebral cortex. B, Velate protoplasmic astrocyte. Silver carbonate stain, gray matter of the cat cerebral cortex. C, Microglial cell from the cerebral cortex of the rabbit. Silver-gold stain; all bars indicate 20 μm.

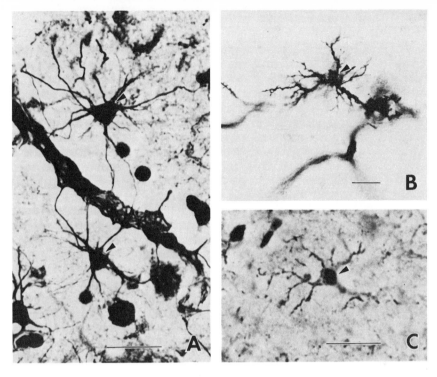

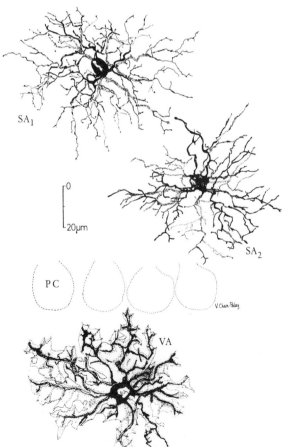

FIGURE 2-16

Smooth protoplasmic astrocytes and the velate protoplasmic astrocyte. Two protoplasmic astrocytes are shown in the molecular layer of the adult rat cerebellar cortex (SA₁ and SA₂). Both cells have radiating processes that are slender, branched, and contorted.

The smooth astrocyte is to be contrasted with the velate protoplasmic astrocyte (VA) of the granular layer with its laminar, veil-like processes extending in umbrella-like fashion from the cell body. The Purkinje cell (PC) layer is indicated. Golgi-Kopsch modification of the Rio-Hortega method. (Reproduced with permission from S. L. Palay and V. Chan-Palay, *Cerebellar Cortex, Cytology and Organization*, Springer-Verlag, New York, p. 317, 1974.)

45

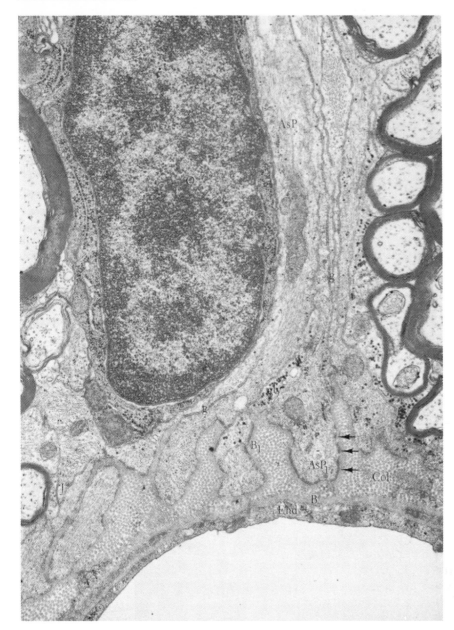

FIGURE 2-17

The perivascular glia limitans. The lower portion of the electron micrograph is occupied by part of a large capillary. The endothelial cells (End) are bounded by a basal lamina (B). Streaming toward the capillary are processes (AsP) of fibrous astrocytes, with cytoplasm that contains fibrils and dense glycogen granules (gly). These processes terminate in end-feet (AsP$_1$), which form a complete layer around the capillary. They are bounded by their own basal lamina (B$_1$), which is separated from that of the endothelial cells by a space containing collagen fibers (Col).

   Note that where the plasma membrane of an end-foot is covered by the basal lamina, localized cytoplasmic densities occur (arrows). These densities resemble hemidesmosomes and probably serve as attachment sites between the end-feet and the basal lamina (B$_1$). The dark cell lying in the middle of the field is an interfascicular oligodendrocyte (O). Optic nerve from adult rat; $\times$40,000. (Reproduced with permission from A. Peters, S. L. Palay, and H. DeF. Webster, *The Fine Structure of the Nervous System*, 2nd Edition, W. B. Saunders Co., Philadelphia, p. 245, 1976.)

ribosomes, an extensive Golgi apparatus, and many mitochondria. A distinguishing feature is the large number of microtubules, within both the perikaryon and the oligodendroglial processes.

Based on their location within the CNS, oligodendroglia are identified as *intrafascicular oligodendroglia* (between the fascicles of axonal processes, especially in the white matter) and *perineuronal satellite oligodendroglia* (surrounding the individual neurons and their dendrites, especially in the neuropil) (Fig. 2–18). The last

location suggests a role in insulation or in regulation of cell metabolism. However, convincing evidence to support this hypothesis is lacking.

One established function of oligodendroglia is axonal *myelination*. Processes of oligodendroglia envelope axons and form a sheath-like covering, a complex fusion of oligodendroglial cell membranes (Figs. 2–19, 2–20, and 2–21). Formation of this sheath is similar, in principle, to that of Schwann cells in peripheral nerves (see Peripheral Nervous System). Myelin sheaths extend from the

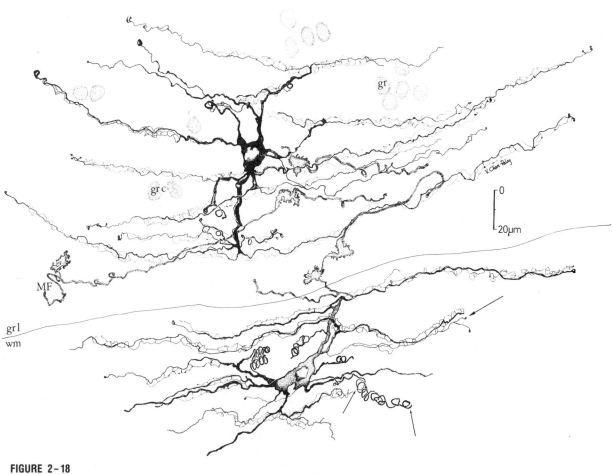

FIGURE 2-18

Camera lucida drawings of oligodendroglia in the white matter and the granular layer of the rat cerebellum. The cell in the lower half lies entirely within the white matter. Here the myelinated fibers are plaited in regular groups that crisscross at right angles to one another.

The long, coiled processes extending from the oligodendroglia are the continuous cytoplasmic ribbons in the myelin sheaths. The limits of the granular layer (grl) and white matter (wm) are indicated. Several mossy fibers (MF) with rosettes are present in the field among a few granule cells (grc). Golgi-Kopsch modification of the Rio Hortega method. (Reproduced with permission from S. L. Palay and V. Chan-Palay, *Cerebellar Cortex, Cytology and Organization*, Springer-Verlag, New York, p. 318, 1974.)

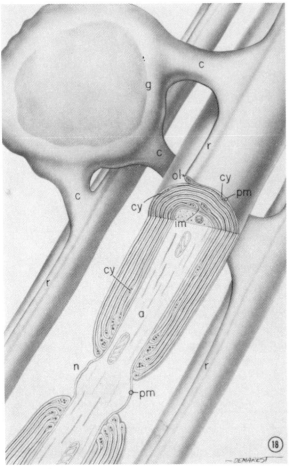

FIGURE 2-19

Three-dimensional reconstruction of an oligodendroglia forming internodes with three adjacent axons: r, outer tongue; n, node of Ranvier; pm, plasma membrane; a, axon; im, inner mesaxon; cy, cytoplasm; ol, outer lip; and g, oligodendroglia. (Reproduced with permission from M. B. Bunge, R. P. Bunge, and H. Ris, J. Biophys. Biochem. Cytol., 10: 79, 1961.)

initial segment of axons to their terminal branches. The segments of myelin formed by individual oligodendroglial processes are *internodes*, or *internodal segments;* the periodic gaps between the internodes are *nodes of Ranvier* (see Figs. 2-19 and 2-20). A single oligodendroglial cell has many processes and may form 40 or 50 internodes.

During the formation of the myelin sheath, a process from the oligodendroglial cell wraps around the axon and, after one full turn, the external surface of the glial membrane makes contact with itself, forming the *inner mesaxon*

(see Fig. 2-21). As the process from the oligodendroglia continues to spiral around the axon, the external surfaces fuse to form the first *interperiod line*. At the same time, cytoplasm is "squeezed" from the intracellular space (like toothpaste from a tube), and the cytoplasmic surfaces fuse to form the first *dense line*. Spiraling continues until the axon is invested with a predetermined number of wrappings. The alternate fusion of both the cytoplasmic and external surfaces of the membrane results in an interdigitated double spiral, one of *interperiod lines* (fused external surfaces) and one of *dense lines* (fused cytoplasmic surfaces). The dense line terminates when the membrane surfaces separate to enclose the cytoplasm at the surface of the sheath (the *tongue*) and the interperiod line terminates as the tongue turns away from the sheath (see Fig. 2-21).

Nodes of Ranvier are naked segments of axon between the internodal segments of myelin (see Fig. 2-20). This region of high membrane capacitance and low electrical resistance contains a high concentration of voltage-gated sodium channels, essential for the *saltatory conduction* of the action potential. During saltatory conduction in the myelinated axons, the action potential literally "leaps" from one node to the next, with little evidence of membrane depolarization in the internodal region.

As the myelin sheath approaches the nodal region, an additional ring of cytoplasm separates the cytoplasmic surfaces of the cell membrane. These "tongues" make contact with the *axolemma*, or surface membrane of the axon, in the paranodal region (see Fig. 2-20). Whenever axons branch to form collaterals, they do so at a node of Ranvier.

In the human brain, oligodendroglia begin to form myelin as early as the 14th week of prenatal development. This process accelerates during the last trimester and is completed only after several years of postnatal development. Once an axon is myelinated, internodes are not added during later growth. Instead, existing internodes increase in length with the growing axon.

MICROGLIA

Phagocytosis is the primary function of *microglia* (see Fig. 2-15). These cells, probably an undifferentiated form of glial stem cells, become activated in response to injury. In normal, nonpathological CNS tissue, distinguishing microglia from

FIGURE 2-20

Node of Ranvier in the central nervous system. At the node, the axon is bare. In the cytoplasm beneath the axolemma (Al) is a dense undercoating (D). On each side of the node are the terminal, or paranodal, portions of the two adjacent segments of myelin. The sheath becomes thinner as successive lamellae terminate to enclose pockets (P) of paranodal cytoplasm, which contain microtubules (m_1).

The pockets indent the surface of the axon and their enclosing plasma membranes become closely apposed to the axolemma. In this uranyl acetate–stained block preparation, the intermittent densities of the outer leaflet of the axolemma are not very apparent. Although the pockets of cytoplasm are regularly arranged in the paranodal region of the upper length of myelin, in the lower paranode they are piled up so that not all of them reach the axolemma.

The axoplasm of this longitudinally sectioned axon contains microtubules (m) and neurofilaments (nf) and some profiles of the smooth endoplasmic reticulum (SR). Basal ganglia of adult rat; $\times$60,000.

Inset shows part of the paranode from a myelinated axon. This material was not stained in the block with uranyl acetate. Hence, the intermittent densities (arrows) associated with the outer leaflet of the axolemma are apparent. Optic nerve of adult rat; $\times$100,000. (Reproduced with permission from A. Peters, S. L. Palay and H. DeF. Webster, *The Fine Structure of the Nervous System*, 2nd Edition, W. B. Saunders Co., Philadelphia, p. 215, 1976.)

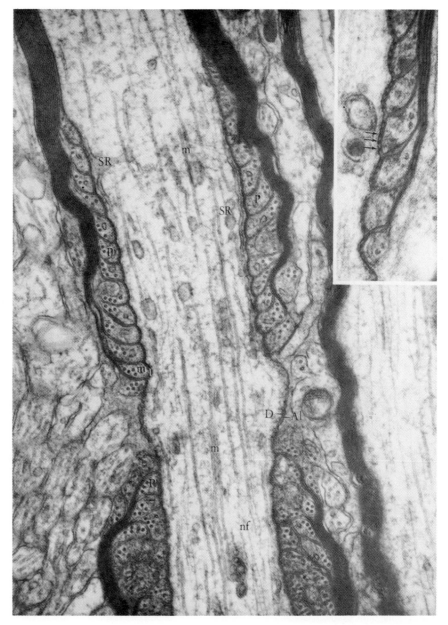

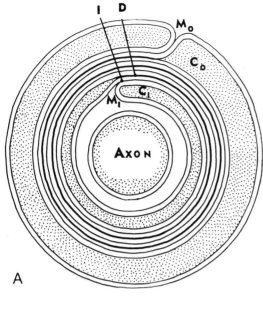

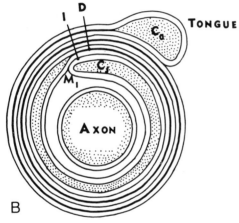

FIGURE 2-21

Diagrams to show the structure of the peripheral myelin *(A)* and the central myelin *(B)*. Cytoplasm of the axon, Schwann cell *(A)* and oligodendroglia *(B)* is stippled. In both, the inner cytoplasmic process, C_i, surrounds the axon and its membranes come together to form the inner mesaxon, M_i, in which the first intraperiod line, I, arises.

The first dense line, D, is formed by the apposition of the cytoplasmic surfaces of the same membrane. These lines continue in a spiral and terminate at the outside of the sheath. In the peripheral nerve, the intraperiod line terminates in the outer mesaxon, Mo. The dense line terminates by a separation of the cytoplasmic surfaces to enclose the cytoplasm of the outer process, Co, of the Schwann cell.

In the central sheath *(B)*, the dense line terminates as the membranes separate to enclose the cytoplasm, Co, of the tongue. The intraperiod line ends as the tongue membrane turns away from the outside of the sheath. (Reproduced with permission from A. Peters, J. Biophys. Biochem. Cytol., 7: 123, 1960.)

small astrocytes and oligodendrocytes is difficult. If the glial limitans is damaged, small *pericytes* (mesodermal cells associated with small blood vessels and outside the brain tissue) invade the damaged area. Originally, these mesodermal cells were believed to be the source of microglia. However, because microglia are present in the CNS in the absence of damage to the glial limitans, microglia now are considered to be neuroectodermal. When active as phagocytes, the microglia swell and are called *gitter cells*.

Ependyma and Choroid Plexus

EPENDYMA

Ependymal cells form a simple cuboidal epithelium, lining the ventricular cavities of the brain and the remnants of the central canal in the spinal cord. These cells differentiate from the germinal or matrix cells of the embryonic neural tube following the formation of neuroblasts and glioblasts. Characterized by an abundance of microvilli and one or more cilia on the apical or ventricular surface, these cells line the entire ventricular cavity (Figs. 2-22 and 2-23).

Ependymal cell nuclei stain lightly, and the chromatin material is fine and evenly dispersed. The cytoplasm has the usual complement of organelles: many small mitochondria, a Golgi apparatus, but a minimum of rough endoplasmic reticulum (see Fig. 2-22). Tight junctions, or zonulae adherens, hold the apical or luminal edges of adjacent ependymal cells together. These junctions do not completely circumscribe the ependymal cells, and large molecules move freely between the cerebrospinal fluid and the subependymal space.

CHOROID PLEXUS

During development, the ependymal layer comes in contact with the highly vascularized meninges, forming the *tela choroidea*, in the roof of the third and fourth ventricles and along the choroid fissure of the lateral ventricles. These cells of the ependymal layer differentiate into a secretory epithelium which, in combination with the meningeal blood vessels, forms the *choroid plexus*.

Fine microvilli cover the ventricular surface of these epithelial cells. The lateral margins are thrown into a complex series of interdigitating folds, and the inferior surface rests on a basal

FIGURE 2–22

Ependymal cells have rather light nuclei (Nuc) in which the chromatin is evenly dispersed. Sometimes, a filamentous inclusion (f) is present. The cytoplasm is also light and contains mitochondria (mit) and a Golgi apparatus (G). At their apical ends, the cells show rather short and uneven microvilli (mv) as well as tufts of cilia (cil). In the subependymal layer are both astrocytic (As) and microglial (M) processes. Some of the profiles at the apical surfaces of these cells appear to be axons (Ax). Rat lateral ventricle; ×12,000. (Reproduced with permission from A. Peters, S. L. Palay, and H. DeF. Webster, *The Fine Structure of the Nervous System*, 2nd Edition, W. B. Saunders Co., Philadelphia, p. 267, 1976.)

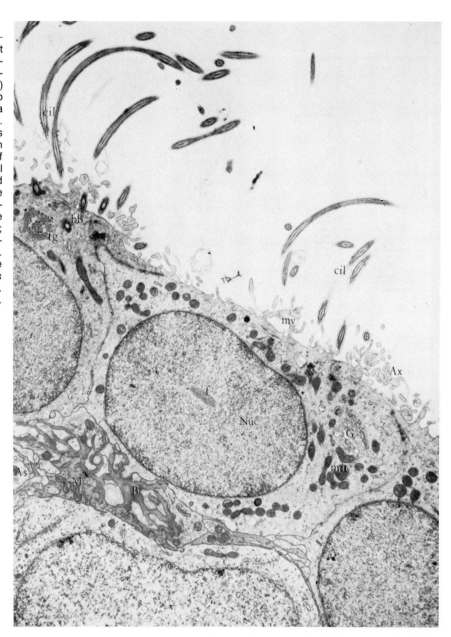

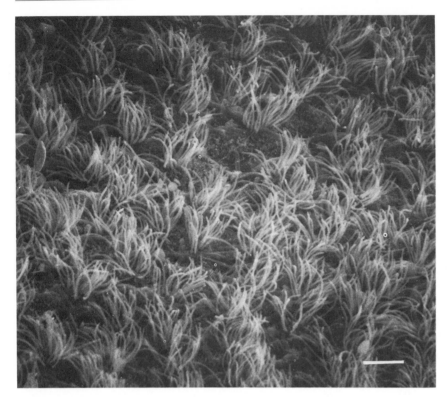

FIGURE 2-23

Scanning electron micrograph showing the ciliated surface of the lateral ventricle in a *Macaca* monkey. Bar represents 5 μm.

lamina. Beneath this complex are capillaries with fenestrated endothelial cells (Fig. 2-24). The macromolecular components of blood plasma pass freely into the subepithelial space; however, they cannot pass directly into the cerebrospinal fluid because of the elaborate interdigitations along the lateral margins of these cells and the tight junctions around their apical margins.

Production of cerebrospinal fluid is an active, energy-dependent process and, to provide the energy, the epithelial cells contain many mitochondria. Also consistent with the secretory function is the presence of clear vesicles and a well-developed Golgi apparatus in the apical portion of the cell (see Fig. 2-24).

Peripheral Nervous System

The peripheral nervous system contains all neuronal elements outside, or peripheral to, the brain and spinal cord, including the sensory neurons with their receptors, the axons of lower motor neurons extending from the brain stem and spinal cord to the striated muscle, and the peripheral components of the autonomic or visceral motor system.

SCHWANN CELLS

Individual nerve fibers of the peripheral nervous system are ensheathed by *Schwann cells*, or *neurolemmal cells*. In myelinated fibers, individual Schwann cells wrap around the axon, forming a myelin sheath analogous to that of the oligodendroglia of the CNS (Figs. 2-21 and 2-25). With nonmyelinated fibers, a single Schwann cell envelops many axons (Fig. 2-26). Although both Schwann cells and oligodendroglia are neuroectodermal in origin, there are two important differences. First, a single Schwann cell forms only one internodal segment of myelin, whereas a single oligodendroglia may form 40 to 50 (see Fig. 2-19). Second, unmyelinated fibers in the periphery are embedded in Schwann cells, whereas those of the CNS are not ensheathed by oligodendroglia but may have an investment of astrocytic processes (see Fig. 2-26).

STRUCTURE OF PERIPHERAL NERVES

Besides Schwann cells, peripheral nerves have three additional investments: the *epineurium*, the *perineurium*, and the *endoneurium* (Fig. 2-27). The epineurium is a thick connective tissue

FIGURE 2-24

Choroid plexus. Microvilli (mv) project from the ventricular surfaces of the choroid cells. The basal ends of the cells rest on the basal lamina (B), beneath which is a thin layer of attenuated cell processes (x). Deeper still are endothelial cells (End) making up the walls of a fenestrated capillary (Cap).

The choroidal cells have pale nuclei (Nuc), and the mitochondria (mit) are concentrated at their apical ends. The Golgi apparatus (G) is represented by small stacks of cisternae. Also conspicuous in the cytoplasm are short cisternae of the granular endoplasmic reticulum (ER) and many clear vesicles (v). The cell on the left contains two lysosomes (Ly). The intercellular junction (J) displays many complex infoldings (arrow) at its basal end. The lateral ventricle of adult rat; ×12,000. (Reproduced with permission from A. Peters, S. L. Palay, and H. DeF. Webster, *The Fine Structure of the Nervous System*, 2nd Edition, W. B. Saunders Co., Philadelphia, p. 283, 1976.)

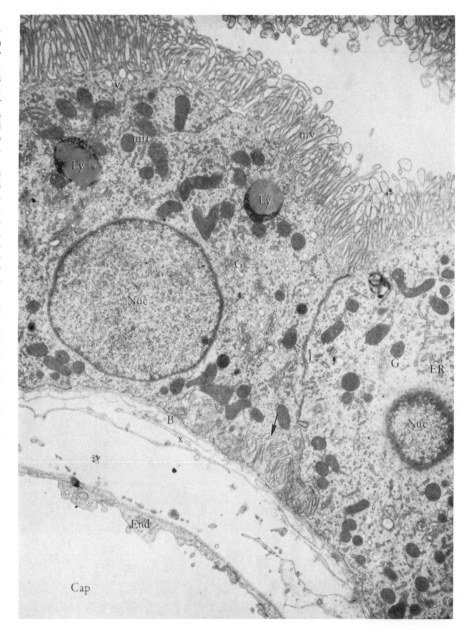

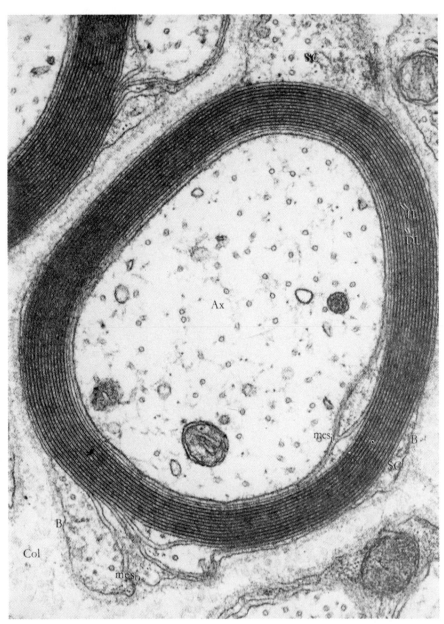

FIGURE 2-25

Myelinated axon, adult peripheral nerve. An electron micrograph of a transversely sectioned axon (Ax) is surrounded by a myelin sheath composed of lamellae formed from the spiralled plasma membrane of a Schwann cell. In the myelin sheath, the alternating major dense lines (DL) and the intraperiod lines (IL) are visible.

Surrounding the myelin is a thin rim of Schwann cell cytoplasm (SC). Outside the Schwann cell is a basal lamina (B) and beyond this the collagen fibers (Col) of the endoneurium. Adult rat sciatic nerve; ×100,000. (Reproduced with permission from A. Peters, S. L. Palay, and H. DeF. Webster, *The Fine Structure of the Nervous System*, 2nd Edition, W. B. Saunders Co., Philadelphia, p. 193, 1976.)

FIGURE 2-26

Unmyelinated axons, adult peripheral nerve. In the electron micrograph, above the center of the field, is a myelinated axon (Ax_1) sectioned transversely through the paranodal region.

The other axons in the field are unmyelinated, and a number of them are separately embedded within each Schwann cell. Although most axons are completely surrounded by their Schwann cells, others (e.g., Ax_2) are only partially enclosed. In such cases, part of the axon is covered only by the basal lamina (B) that surrounds the Schwann cell (SC).

Another unmyelinated axon (Ax_3), although apparently embedded within this Schwann cell, is surrounded by a completely separate process, which is probably an extension of the next Schwann cell in the series.

Note the microtubular and neurofilamentous components of the axons. Between the Schwann cells is the collagen (Col) of the endoneurium. Sciatic nerve from adult rat; ×48,000. (Reproduced with permission from A. Peters, S. L. Palay, and H. DeF. Webster, *The Fine Structure of the Nervous System*, 2nd Edition, W. B. Saunders Co., Philadelphia, p. 189, 1976.)

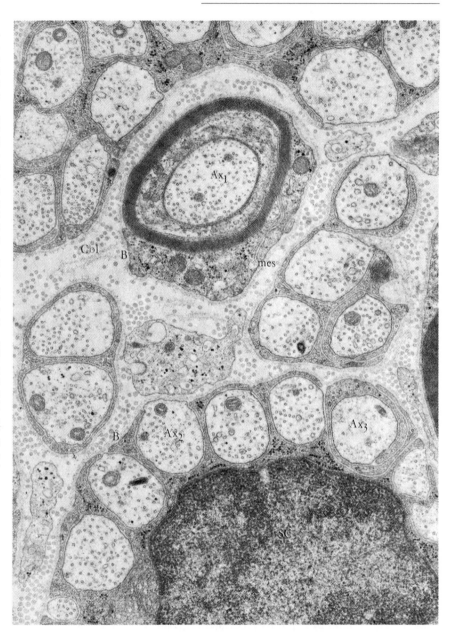

sheath, rich in collagen fibers, that covers the entire nerve. Within the nerve, additional connective tissue elements, i.e., the perineurium, segregate fibers into fascicles. The endoneurium is a loose organization of connective tissue elements (fibroblasts, collagen fibers, and small blood vessels) surrounding individual axons and their associated Schwann cells (see Fig. 2-27).

PERIPHERAL GANGLIA

Neuronal cell bodies in sensory ganglia are surrounded by modified Schwann cells known as *satellite*, *perineuronal*, or *capsular cells*. These cells encapsulate the soma of the sensory neuron and are continuous with the layer of Schwann cells surrounding the ganglion cell process. Con-

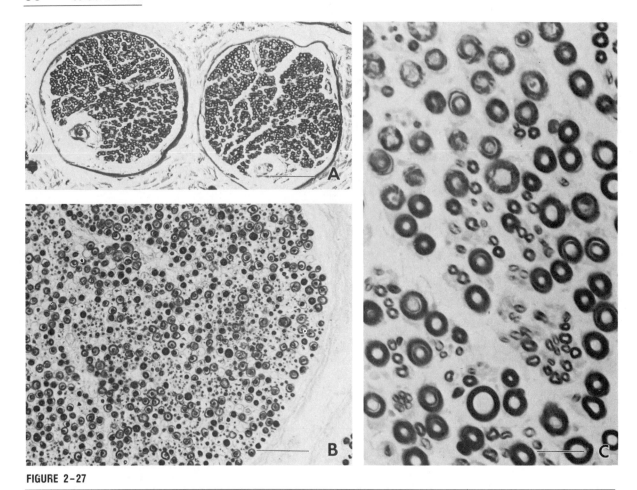

FIGURE 2-27

A, Low-power magnification of two fascicles of the vagus nerve embedded within the dense epineurium. *B*, A portion of a large fascicle of a mixed, motor and sensory, nerve. Note the wide range in fiber size. *C*, A higher magnification of *B*. Bars in *A* and *B* represent 100 μm; the bar in *C* represents 20 μm. Human tissue stained with osmic acid.

nective tissue elements, comparable to the endoneurium, perineurium, and epineurium of the peripheral nerve, invest the entire sensory ganglion. Neurons of the autonomic ganglia are similarly invested, although the layer of satellite cells is not as complete as that in sensory ganglia. The nuclei of satellite cells can be seen in Nissl-stained preparations of autonomic and sensory ganglia (see Fig. 2–5*A*, *C*, and *E*).

Damage and Repair

Trauma often produces irreversible damage to nervous tissue. Unlike the cells of many organ systems, neurons have lost the ability to proliferate. When the damage leads to degeneration of the entire neuron, the cell is lost, never to be replaced.

The entire neuron responds to damage or trauma, a coordinated effort aimed at survival and restoration of function. Damaged and severed processes *degenerate*. The cell body undergoes *chromatolysis*, a swelling of the perikaryon and a dispersion of the Nissl bodies. All these are changes related to the synthetic requirements of *repair* and *regeneration*.

Some of the changes begin immediately, others several days or weeks later. Secondary changes may not occur for months or even years. Changes occurring distal to the damaged area are *anterograde changes*; those occurring in the neuron cell body and proximal portion of the axon are *retrograde changes*. *Local changes* take place in the immediate vicinity of the lesion.

Neuronal degeneration is an essential feature of normal CNS development. If a developing neuron fails to establish adequate connections, it degenerates. Adult neurons retain this property, and their survival requires appropriate interactions with other neurons. If an intact neuron loses either an adequate source of stimulation or an adequate target, it will atrophy and may ultimately die, i.e., *transneuronal degeneration*.

In addition to synaptic transmission, neurons communicate through biochemical signals collectively called *trophic factors*. Through a combination of trophic and synaptic signals, neurons can "sense" the quality and integrity of synaptic contacts and the status of other neurons in a pathway.

Damage to a peripheral nerve along with the associated changes in the lower motor neuron is a good example of a neuron's response to trauma. Local anterograde and retrograde changes all occur simultaneously. Although they are considered separately, Figure 2–28 summarizes the temporal relationship. In the CNS, many of the

FIGURE 2-28

The principal events in peripheral nerve degeneration and regeneration.

A, Intact lower motor neuron with neuromuscular synapses on striated muscle.

B, Early responses to injury include phagocytosis of debris in the area of trauma by invading macrophages, swelling and initial degeneration of axon terminals, and early chromatolytic changes in the soma.

C, Growth processes arise from the proximal axon, and Schwann cells span the gap in the local trauma area. Completion of axon terminal degeneration, initiation of distal axon degeneration (wallerian degeneration), continued phagocytosis by macrophages, and peak chromatolytic changes in the soma are noted.

D, Growth processes, guided by Schwann cells, enter the connective tissue matrix of the distal nerve. Completion of axonal degeneration and degeneration of aberrant growth processes take place.

E, Growth processes reach the target and form new neuromuscular synapses. Aberrant processes degenerate.

F, Regeneration is complete. The new axon has a smaller diameter and a slower conduction velocity but forms functional neuromuscular synapses. Internodal segments of the myelin sheath are shorter than those of the original axon. Completion of the functional synapse is the signal to reverse the chromatolytic changes in the neuron. Swelling is reduced, and Nissl bodies reform.

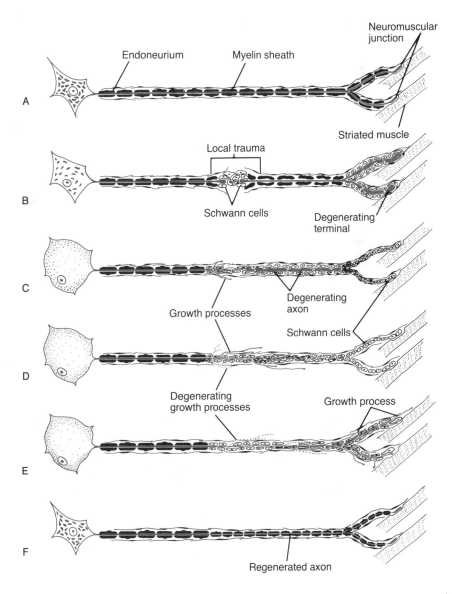

responses to trauma are quite different. These differences are indicated in the discussion of the peripheral nerve.

LOCAL CHANGES

When an axon is severed, the cut ends immediately retract several millimeters. The axonal membrane fuses at the cut surface, isolating the axoplasm from the surrounding extracellular material. Axoplasmic flow continues for some time in both directions and, because of this, each cut end begins to swell. Macrophages migrate into the trauma area and phagocytize the damaged tissue debris in the local area (Fig. 2–28*A* and *B*).

In the CNS, astrocytes and microglia invade the area phagocytizing the debris. At the same time, fibrous astrocytes rapidly form a *glial scar* around the damaged area, isolating it from the surrounding nervous tissue. If the blood vessels or the surface of the CNS is damaged, macrophages also invade the area of trauma. However, the glial scar restricts the macrophages to the local area. Later, this glial scar becomes a barrier to axonal regeneration in the CNS. Peripheral nerves, however, will regenerate if the cut ends are opposed and if scarring is kept to a minimum.

ANTEROGRADE CHANGES

Axon terminals immediately swell; neurofilaments increase in number; mitochondria rupture; and, within several days, an electron-dense debris fills the axon terminal (Fig. 2–28*B*). In 5 to 7 days, the synaptic terminals detach from the postsynaptic membrane and Schwann cells invade the area of synaptic contact. The Schwann cells proliferate and rapidly phagocytize the remnants of the degenerating axon terminal (Fig. 2–28*C*).

Within 1 to 2 weeks, the remainder of the distal segment of the axon begins to degenerate. The myelin sheath separates from the axon and breaks down, the axon swells and disintegrates into a number of beaded fragments, and the proliferating Schwann cells phagocytize the debris. The slower anterograde degeneration of the distal segment of the axon is also called *wallerian degeneration* (Fig. 2–28*C* and *D*). Wallerian degeneration occurs in the CNS as well, with glial cells functioning in the same capacity as Schwann cells.

The connective tissue matrix of the damaged peripheral nerve remains intact. Once the remnants of the old axon and its myelin sheath have

been removed, Schwann cells remain in the channel to guide the regenerating axon (Fig. 2–28*D* and *E*). In the CNS, however, there is no connective tissue matrix and glial cells fill the area, forming an additional barrier to later regeneration.

RETROGRADE CHANGES

Few retrograde degenerative changes occur in the axon. During the first 2 to 3 days after the lesion, a short segment of the proximal stump of the axon and its associated myelin sheath degenerate. The distance varies from the length of several internodes to several centimeters, often stopping at the point of origin of the next axon collateral.

During the same period, the soma of the injured neuron begins to swell. Nissl bodies disperse with small fragments of the Nissl substance moving toward the periphery of the swollen cell body (Figs. 2–28*A* to *C* and 2–29). These changes in the soma, collectively called *chromatolysis*, may last for several weeks or a month, or until the regenerating axon re-establishes synaptic contact. During chromatolysis, the number of free polysomes and the rate of synthesis of RNA, protein, and other macromolecules essential for the repair and regeneration increase. When a regenerating axon establishes functional connections, the chromatolytic neuron returns to nor-

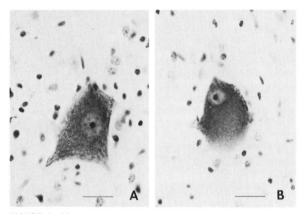

FIGURE 2–29

Chromatolysis in motor neurons of the spinal cord. Nissl-stained neurons from the lateral motor columns of the human lumbar spinal cord.

A, Early chromatolysis demonstrating initial swelling of the soma, and the initial stages of Nissl substance dispersion.

B, Advanced chromatolysis, characterized by extensive swelling of the soma and dispersion of the Nissl substance are noted. (See text for discussion.) Cresyl fast violet stain; bars represent 20 μm.

mal (Fig. 2–28*E* and *F*). If functional contact is not made, which is the usual case in the CNS, the neuron will undergo atrophy. The number of axon collaterals remaining intact determines the degree of atrophy. If this number is insufficient to maintain the viability of the neuron, it degenerates.

During chromatolysis, glial cells surround the soma of the injured neuron and send processes into the clefts of the synapses on the soma and proximal dendrites, literally "lifting" the synaptic terminal from the surface of the chromatolytic neuron. This effect reduces the stimulation of the injured neuron, now actively engaged in the synthetic tasks associated with regeneration. Once the axon has regenerated, these glial processes retract and the synapses re-form.

The severity of the chromatolytic changes reflects the location of the damage to the axon. Chromatolytic changes are more severe when the damage is closer to the cell body. The farther the injury is from the cell body, the more collateral axonal branches remain intact and the greater the probability of a succesful regeneration of the damaged axon.

REGENERATION

In most neurons, chromatolysis is a prerequisite for regeneration. During this period, a large number of "sprouts" emerge from the proximal stump of the axon, each with a growth cone, resembling that of a developing neuron (see Fig. 2–28*C*). A single axon may send out as many as 20 to 30 sprouts, each seeking a viable path toward the target.

The growth processes soon span the gap between the proximal stump of the axon and the connective tissue matrix of the distal nerve sheath. Schwann cells bridge the gap and guide the growth processes into the distal nerve sheath, now nearly devoid of the remnants of the degenerating distal axon (see Fig. 2–28*D*). As the growth processes enter the distal sheath, Schwann cells continue to act as guides, lining the channels within the connective tissue matrix of the peripheral nerve stump. During this period, several growth processes may occupy a single nerve channel. However, only one reaches the target and establishes a functional connection; the others degenerate (see Fig. 2–28*D* to *F*). Under normal conditions, an axon regenerates as much as 3 to 4 mm per day, or about 1 ft in 100 days.

Regeneration stimulates the synthesis of a number of specific *growth-associated proteins*, or *GAPs*. These proteins appear during development and again during regeneration. However, they are absent or undetectable in the normal, mature neuron. The precise role of GAPs in nerve growth is still unknown.

In the CNS, except for short axonal projections within the neuropil, axons usually do not regenerate. Part of the explanation has been the physical barrier of the glial scar. Some evidence suggests that Schwann cells actively facilitate the regeneration of peripheral nerves. Experiments have shown that CNS neurons can regenerate in a matrix containing Schwann cells and that peripheral nerves do not regenerate in the presence of glial cells. It is not known whether glial cells lack some growth promoting factor present in Schwann cells or whether they contain a growth inhibitory factor.

TRANSNEURONAL CHANGES

When a neuron degenerates, the loss can have a cascade effect. If the target neurons no longer receive sufficient synaptic signals, those target neurons will atrophy, or worse, degenerate. This process is *anterograde transneuronal degeneration*, and the time required for these changes is much longer than that required for the primary neuronal degeneration (Fig. 2–30). Similarly, if degeneration results in the loss of targets for other neurons, those neurons not directly injured but projecting to the degenerated neurons will no longer have an adequate target. They too will atrophy or even degenerate. This process is *retrograde transneuronal degeneration* (Fig. 2–30). Unless the primary damage is extensive, transneuronal degenerative changes are not very common. Usually, there are sufficient collateral branches and terminals from other neurons and, at most, there may be some atrophy but not degeneration.

Specific sensory pathways, in which there is a high degree of point-to-point projection and very few collateral branches, are an exception. The visual pathways provide good examples of both anterograde and retrograde transneuronal degeneration. If the optic nerve is cut, anterograde transneuronal degeneration of neurons in the lateral geniculate nucleus occurs. Several months later, a loss of neurons in the visual cortex (the target of lateral geniculate neurons) is noted. If there is damage to the lateral geniculate nucleus, anterograde transneuronal degeneration is observed in the visual cortex. Retrograde transneuronal degeneration occurs in the retinal ganglion

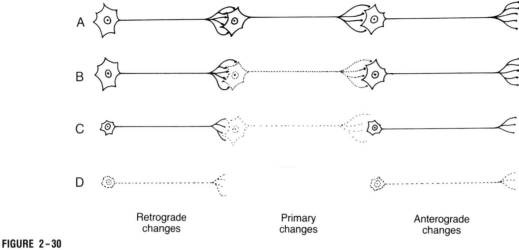

Retrograde   Primary   Anterograde
changes   changes   changes

FIGURE 2-30

The anterograde and retrograde transneuronal degenerative changes in response to the degeneration of an injured neuron. The degeneration of a neuron is represented in the center. Anterograde transneuronal changes are on the right and retrograde transneuronal changes on the left. Following degeneration of the damaged neuron *(B)*, the transneuronal changes are initially atrophy *(C)* and then degeneration *(D)*. (See text for discussion.)

cells, cells with axons that normally project to the lateral geniculate nucleus.

INJURY AND PLASTICITY

In some areas of the CNS, new synaptic connections are made in response to the loss of the original connections through degeneration. In the hippocampal formation, for example, if a particular afferent pathway is cut, those synaptic terminals in the hippocampal formation degenerate. However, other axons normally terminating on adjacent sites of the same hippocampal neuron actively "sprout" collateral branches and form new synapses on the old sites, thus preserving the synaptic sites on the recipient neuron. If, however, the original afferents are able to regenerate, they will reestablish their original connections, displacing the collateral branches that had temporarily occupied the site. We do not know how widespread this phenomenon is or if this is only an isolated example. It does not occur in the visual pathway. For example, a partial removal of the optic nerve does not stimulate collateral "sprouting" in the lateral geniculate nucleus. The one generality that can be made is that different pathways or systems in the CNS respond to trauma in different ways.

SUGGESTED READING

Jones, E. G. and W. M. Cowan (1983). The nervous tissue. In *Histology, Cell and Tissue Biology,* 5th Edition, L. Weiss (Editor). Elsevier Biomedical Publishers, New York, pp. 282–370.

This chapter, in a major histology textbook, provides an overview of the light and electron microscopic anatomy of central and peripheral nervous tissues including the sensory receptors and motor effectors.

Palay, S. L. and V. Chan-Palay (1977). General morphology of neurons and neuroglia. In *Handbook of Physiology,* Section 1, *The Nervous System,* Volume I, *Cellular Biology of Neurons,* Part 1, E. R. Kandel (Editor). American Physiological Society, Bethesda, MD, pp. 5–37.

An overview of the light and electron microscopic anatomy of neurons and glia of the central nervous system, including an extensive discussion of synaptic structure.

Peters, A., S. L. Palay, and H. DeF. Webster (1976). *The Fine Structure of the Nervous System,* 2nd Edition. W. B. Saunders Co., Philadelphia.

A systematic survey of the electron microscopic anatomy of central and peripheral nervous tissues.

Chapter

3

Excitable Membranes

RESTING POTENTIALS
PASSIVE MEMBRANE PROPERTIES
ACTION POTENTIALS

The *transmission, receipt,* and *integration* of *electrical signals* are fundamental to information processing within the central nervous system (CNS)—be it a simple reflex arc or a more complex, higher integrative activity, such as decision making or memory storage.

Neurons, like many other cell types, maintain a *membrane potential* in which the inside of the cell is electrically negative with respect to the extracellular fluid. Because of their unique structural and molecular specializations, nerve cells are able to utilize this membrane potential for intercellular communication in the form of electrical signals.

In the "unstimulated" neuron, or the neuron "at rest," the *membrane potential* is called a *resting potential.* Although some variation exists from neuron to neuron, this potential usually ranges from -70 to -90 millivolts (mV). When a neuron is stimulated, the resting potential is altered. Excitatory stimuli *depolarize* the cell membrane (decrease the internal negativity of the resting membrane potential), and inhibitory stimuli *hyperpolarize* the cell membrane (increase the internal negativity of the resting membrane potential).

The electrical excitability of a neuron is due in large measure to *voltage-sensitive ion channels* or *ionophores.* These are large protein complexes that span the unit membrane of the neuron and form hydrophilic channels through which specific ions can move. These *ion channels* are highly selective. They allow the controlled movement of only selected ions along electrochemical gradients, producing *ion currents.*

When excitatory stimuli depolarize the *initial segment* of an axon to a threshold level, an *action potential* is generated. The *action potential*—a rapidly moving, self-propagating wave of membrane depolarization—travels the length of the axon and enables the neuron to transmit signals rapidly and over relatively long distances (Fig. 3–1).

Upon reaching the *synaptic bouton*, the *action potential* triggers a sequence of molecular events, culminating in the release of chemical *neurotransmitters.* These transmitters, in turn, diffuse across the *synaptic cleft* and bind to specific *receptor molecules* on the recipient cell, be it the *postsynaptic membrane* of another neuron or the *motor endplate* of a muscle cell.

Neurotransmitter-receptor interactions produce focal alterations in the resting potential of the postsynaptic membrane with the generation of either an *excitatory postsynaptic potential (EPSP)* or an *inhibitory postsynaptic potential (IPSP).* The nature of the postsynaptic response is a property of the receptor molecule involved.

61

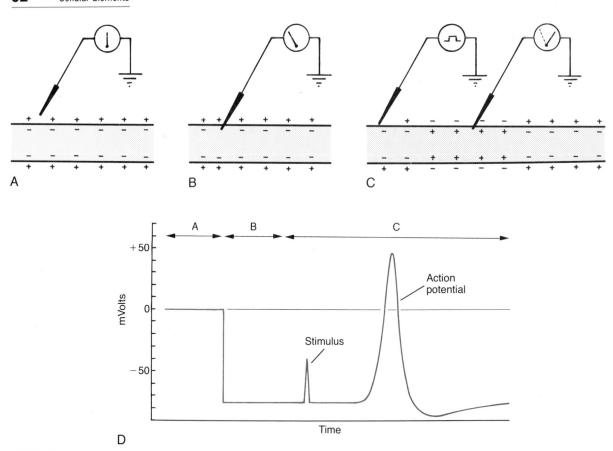

FIGURE 3-1

Measurement of electrical activity in a nerve axon with microelectrodes. Positions of recording and stimulating electrodes are illustrated in *A*, *B*, and *C*, with the corresponding measurements of membrane potential in *D*.

A, The recording electrode is extracellular. *B*, The electrode has penetrated the cell membrane, and the recording electrode is intracellular.

C, The stimulating electrode (left) has delivered a brief depolarizing pulse triggering the generation of an action potential measured at the recording electrode (right). (See text for discussion.)

Often, the magnitude of this response is modulated by the physiological state of the recipient cell.

This chapter considers the *membrane or resting potential,* and those factors contributing to the maintenance of this potential. The *action potential* and the mechanism of propagation of the action potential are also discussed.

Chapter 4 reviews the physiology and cell biology of *synaptic transmission,* the communication between neurons and that between neurons and their targets. Chapter 5 focuses on the biochemistry of *synaptic transmission* and *neuronal modulation.*

Much of our understanding of the physiological properties of individual neurons—membrane po-

tentials, conduction velocities, and ionic currents—has come from studies utilizing intracellular microelectrodes. These electrolyte-filled glass electrodes with tips of less than a micron in diameter record changes in membrane potential and stimulate neurons electrically or through the application of specific drugs or chemicals by a process known as *ionophoresis.*

Micromanipulators position the recording microelectrodes on the surface of the neuron for *extracellular* measurements, or they penetrate the cell membrane for *intracellular* measurements (see Fig. 3–1). As the tip of the electrode penetrates the neuron, the cell membrane seals tightly around the electrode, electrically isolating the tip from the extracellular space.

When one electrode stimulates a neuron, a second electrode can record the response, as illustrated in Figure 3–1*C* and *D*. When an electrical stimulus is of sufficient magnitude to generate an action potential, this self-propagating wave of depolarization sweeps along the neuronal membrane and can be recorded with the second electrode positioned at some distance from the first. The time elapsed between the application of the stimulus and the recording of the action potential (measured in milliseconds, msec) can be utilized to calculate the conduction velocity. This is the speed at which the action potential moves from its point of origin—the stimulating electrode—to its point of measurement—the recording electrode.

Resting Potentials

The *resting potential* of a neuron is the electrical potential maintained by the unit membrane of the neuron at times when it is not being altered by EPSPs and IPSPs (dendrites and soma) or when it is not propagating an action potential (axon). In theory, the resting potential represents a basal or resting level; however, this state is transient because most neurons continually receive EPSPs and IPSPs and generate action potentials.

Neurons expend metabolic energy to maintain the resting membrane potential. Without this expenditure, the membrane potential would gradually dissipate. The term steady-state potential is a more apt description; however, *resting potential* is the accepted term.

ESSENTIAL NEURONAL MEMBRANE PROPERTIES

Three properties of the neuronal membrane are essential for the establishment and maintenance of the resting potential: the *lipid bilayer* of the unit membrane, *ion channels*, and *electrogenic ion pumps* (Fig. 3–2).

LIPID BILAYER AS A CAPACITOR

Because the hydrophobic *lipid bilayer* of the unit membrane is relatively impermeable to charged particles, such as ions, it functions as an *electrical capacitor*. At rest, the lipid bilayer acts as a dielectric, separating the negative charges, which line the inner surface of the membrane, from the positive charges on the outer surface.

ION CHANNELS OR IONOPHORES

The other property of the neuronal membrane is the presence of complex proteins known as *ion channels* or *ionophores,* which span the lipid bilayer and form hydrophilic channels or gaps in the dielectric membrane. These *ion channels* are highly selective and allow the controlled passage of specific ions along their electrochemical gradients, producing *ion currents*.

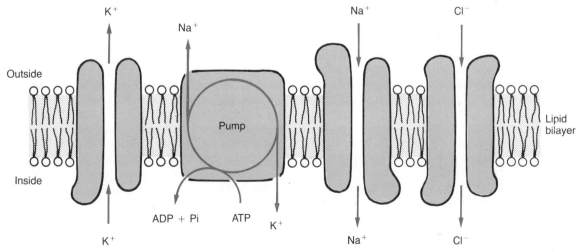

FIGURE 3-2

Three components of a neuronal membrane essential for the establishment and maintenance of the resting potential are (1) the *lipid bilayer,* (2) the *ion channels* for Na+, K+, and Cl−, and (3) the Na+/K+–*electrogenic pump.*

Many ion channels open and close in response to small changes in the membrane potential, a property fundamental to the processes of impulse conduction and neuronal signaling. Ion channels with voltage-sensitive properties are often referred to as *gated* or *voltage-sensitive channels.* At rest, these ion channels are closed, permitting the passage of few, if any, ions. However, in the "resting" state of a neuron, a small, net movement of ions across the cell membrane takes place. It is not clear whether this movement represents a separate subpopulation of ion channels or whether some voltage-sensitive channels "leak."

The principal ion channels associated with the maintenance of the resting potential and the propagation of the action potential are the *sodium channel* and the *potassium channel.* In addition, the *calcium channel* is of major importance at the axon terminal for synaptic transmission.

All of the voltage-sensitive ion channels share a similar basic molecular organization for their large, α-subunit. Greater diversity, however, is found in the one or more smaller β-subunits associated with them. As an example, the organization of the α-subunit of the sodium channel is illustrated in Figure 3–3. Common to the sodium channel, and other cation channels, are four homologous domains (I, II, III, and IV), each with six membrane-spanning segments in the form of α-helices (S1 to S6). The S-segment peptides of one domain are similar to but not identical with the corresponding segments in the other three domains. When seen from the surface, the four domains are arranged symmetrically around a central pore or canal, believed to be the ion channel per se (Fig. 3–3B).

Of the membrane-spanning segments, S4 (labeled with a +), contains positively charged amino acids arranged in regular intervals. In one working model, a small change in membrane potential causes the S4 α-helix to rotate approximately 60 degress, like a corkscrew, resulting in a net outward movement of positive charges. If this net outward movement of charges were of sufficient magnitude to generate the required gating current, it could account for the voltage-sensitive changes in ion conductance observed for these channels.

Although the similarities between ion channels suggest a common molecular mechanism for voltage gating, the differences in structure between ion channels are of equal importance and are responsible for the *ion selectivity* (i.e., sodium

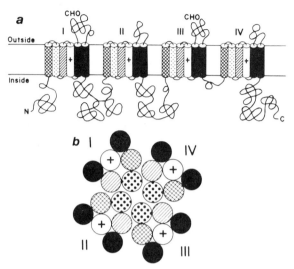

FIGURE 3–3

Organization of the sodium channel. *a,* Proposed transmembrane topology of the sodium channels; *b,* proposed arrangement of the transmembrane segments viewed perpendicular to the membrane.

In *a,* the four units of homology spanning the membrane are displayed linearly. Segments S1-S6 in each repeat (I-IV) are indicated by cylinders as follows: S-1, crosshatched; S-2, stippled; S-3, hatched; S-4, indicated by a plus sign; S-5 and S-6, solid.

Putative sites of *N*-glycosylation (CHO) are indicated. In *b,* the ionic channel is represented as a central pore surrounded by the four units of homology. Segments S1-S6 in each repeat (I-IV) are represented by circles indicated as in *a.* (Reproduced with permission from M. Noda, T. Ikeda, T. Kayano, et al.: Nature, 230:191, 1986. Copyright © 1986 Macmillan Journals Limited.)

channels for sodium ions and potassium channels for potassium ions) and for the *unique gating properties* of these different channels.

All channels for a given ion are not identical but appear to represent a "family" of ion channels, each member with slightly different amino acid sequences and with correspondingly different physiological properties. For example, although we usually refer to the sodium channels as if they were of identical structure, a number of different sodium channels with slightly different physiological properties exist, imparting subtle variations in function to different neurons or to different areas of the same neuron. This finding is true for the other ion channels as well.

Furthermore, the physiological state of a cell can lead to the modification or *modulation* of existing ion channels through a number of biochemical processes, including phosphorylation. The capacity to be modulated may be an intrinsic property of most, if not all membrane ion channels. Mechanisms of modulation are discussed in Chapter 5.

Sodium channels have three essential properties setting them apart from the other channels: (1) a *selectivity* for sodium ions, (2) a very rapid *voltage-sensitive activation* or opening, and (3) a *voltage-sensitive inactivation* or closing of the channel (Fig. 3–4).

The last two properties are central to the generation of the action potential. At rest, the sodium channel is closed, but a small depolariza-

tion of the membrane will activate it rapidly. *Activation* (opening) results in an immediate *inward surge of sodium ions,* which further depolarizes the membrane. During this extremely brief and transient period of activation, sodium ions move through the channel at a rate in excess of 10^7 ions/sec, a value approaching the rate of movement of sodium in free solution. Following the activation, an immediate inactivation of the sodium channel and the consequent cessation of the sodium current occur. In the inactive state,

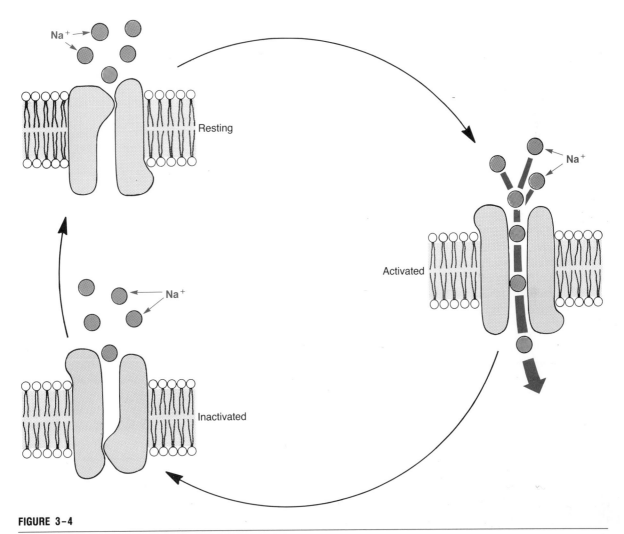

FIGURE 3–4

Voltage-sensitive sodium channel. The sodium channel exists in one of three states: *resting*, *activated*, and *inactivated*. When the membrane potential is near the resting potential, the channel is in a *resting* or closed state.

Depolarization of the surrounding membrane (e.g., an action potential or an excitatory postsynaptic potential) *transiently activates* or opens the channel, and sodium ions rapidly enter the cell, flowing down their concentration gradient. Within a fraction of a millisecond, the activated sodium channel is *inactivated* and the ion flow ceases. In the inactivated state, the channel remains closed and will not respond to voltage changes. Following repolarization of the membrane, the inactivated sodium channel returns to the resting state.

the channel cannot respond to voltage changes and remains refractory until the membrane potential has returned to the resting state (see Fig. 3–4).

Sodium channels make up less than 1% of the total membrane protein; hence, the excitability of the neuron is dependent on the efficient operation of strategically located channels. Certain toxins bind selectively to the sodium channel with a high affinity, a property that has been used to map the distribution of sodium channels on the neuronal cell membrane (Table 3–1). The region of the initial segment of the axon and the nodal regions of the myelinated axons have relatively high concentrations of sodium channels. These areas are essential for action potential generation and saltatory conduction, whereas the neuronal membrane of the soma and dendrites has relatively few sodium channels.

Potassium channels are among the most heterogeneous of the ion channels. Members of this large family of ion channels are either resting (closed) or activated (open) (Fig. 3–5). When the voltage-sensitive channels are activated, an *outward flow of potassium current* occurs. However, unlike sodium channels, potassium channels remain open as long as the membrane is depolarized. Because the outward flow of potassium ions increases the internal negativity of the cell, potassium currents work toward the repolarization of the membrane. As repolarization occurs, the potassium channels return to the resting state.

In addition to voltage sensitivity, many forms of the potassium channel are activated directly by intracellular calcium. The calcium is released from the internal stores via the second messenger systems or enters the neuron through voltage-sensitive calcium channels. The activation mechanisms of calcium concentration and the membrane potential, although not strictly additive, appear to work together. When calcium concentrations are low, a relatively large depolarization is required to activate potassium channels. When free calcium levels are elevated, however, the potassium channels are activated with a much smaller change in membrane potential.

Some potassium channels, known as "BK" channels or "maxi-K" channels, have very high conductances (200 to 300 pS/channel, where S = Siemens, reciprocal ohms). They are characterized by very large potassium currents when activated, a marked contrast to the "SK" channels, which have very low conductances (10 to 14 pS). These two categories of potassium channels have different voltage and calcium sensitivities and can be differentiated further by specific channel blocking agents. However, both are essential for the repolarization of the neuron following an action potential. A number of potassium channels do not fit into either category. These channels cover a broad span of conductance ranges and activation properties.

Although the general structure is similar for all potassium channels, the differences in physiological properties have been attributed to α-subunit proteins with slightly different amino acid sequences, or to different β-subunits.

SODIUM/POTASSIUM PUMP— NA$^+$/K$^+$-ATPase

The third property of the neuronal membrane essential for the establishment and maintenance of the resting potential is the presence of *electro-*

TABLE 3–1

Sodium Channel Distribution and Density in a "Typical" Mammalian Neuron

CELL COMPARTMENT	SODIUM CHANNEL DENSITY (NUMBER/MICRON^2)	METHOD OF LOCALIZATION
Cell body	50 to 75	Saxitoxin binding
Axon initial segment	350 to 500	Scorpion toxin autoradiography
Unmyelinated axon	110	Saxitoxin binding
Myelinated axon		
Node of Ranvier	2000 to 12000	Electrophysiology and saxitoxin binding
Internode	<25	Electrophysiology, saxitoxin binding, and immunocytochemistry
Nerve terminals	20 to 75	Saxitoxin binding and scorpion toxin binding

Reproduced with permission from W. A. Catterall. Science, 223: 653–661, 1984. Copyright 1984 by AAAS.

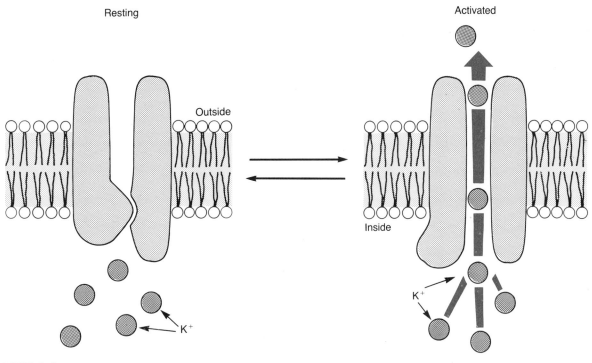

Resting   Activated

Outside

Inside

K⁺   K⁺

FIGURE 3–5

Voltage-sensitive potassium channel. The potassium channel exists in one of two states: *resting* or *activated*. When the membrane potential is near the resting potential, the channel is in the *resting* or closed state. Depolarization of the membrane (e.g., an action potential or an excitatory postsynaptic potential) activates or opens the channel, and potassium ions exit the cell, flowing down their concentration gradient. Most voltage-sensitive potassium channels remain open as long as the membrane is depolarized, returning to the resting state as the membrane becomes repolarized.

genic ion pumps. These are catalytic membrane proteins capable of pumping ions across the membrane against a concentration gradient. The principal pump is the *sodium/potassium pump* or *Na^+/K^+ – ATPase.*

Without this energy-dependent pump, ionic concentration gradients would "leak" to equilibrium and the resting potential would disappear. Up to 70% of the ATP generated from intermediary metabolism in the brain is utilized by the pump, but the K_m for ATP is relatively low (0.1 to 0.6 mM). The level of this substrate rarely becomes rate limiting. Under conditions of anoxia or metabolic poisoning, however, ATP does become rate limiting and the resting potential is rapidly lost.

Na^+/K^+-ATPase utilizes the energy of ATP to translocate Na^+ and K^+ ions against their respective concentration gradients, pumping three Na^+ ions out of the cell for every two K^+ ions pumped into the cell. Although not directly involved in the generation of action potentials and synaptic transmission, the electrogenic pump maintains the ionic gradients necessary for these processes, thereby maintaining the cell in a state of "excitability" (Fig. 3–6).

This large, membrane-spanning protein, with a molecular weight of approximately 170 kiloDaltons (kDa), consists of a major α-subunit and a minor β-subunit. The α-subunit contains the catalytic sites, the Na^+ and K^+ binding sites, and the phosphorylation site (see Fig. 3–6). Most of the β-subunit, a peptide of 40 to 60 kDa, is on the external surface of the membrane and contains a number of glycosyl groups.

Both subunits are highly conserved between species, with homologies as high as 95% in the amino acid sequences reported for the α-subunit and 60% for the β-subunit. All of the catalytic sites are located on the α-subunit, and the precise function of the β-subunit is unknown.

At least five genes code for the catalytic subunit, with two of these found in nervous tissue. The two brain isoenzymes can be differentiated

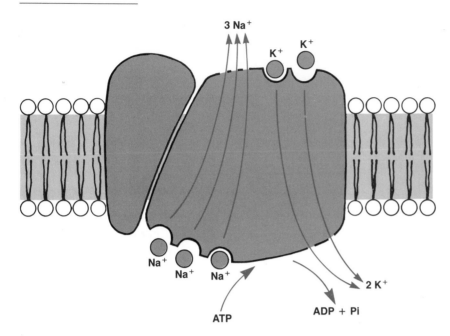

FIGURE 3-6

The Na^+/K^+-ATPase, an electro-genic ion pump, is essential for establishing and maintaining the ionic gradients responsible for the resting membrane potential. This large, ATP-dependent membrane protein catalyzes the coupled translocation of sodium and potassium ions: three sodium ions are pumped out of the cell for every two potassium ions pumped into the cell.

by their relative sensitivities to inhibition by the cardiac glycoside, ouabain.

Cells regulate pump activity in two ways: (1) by adjusting the capacity of existing pumps and (2) by increasing or decreasing the number of pumps per unit of membrane. Intracellular concentrations of sodium are a major regulator of pump activity, with very small elevations increasing the activity of existing pumps. The concentration of potassium has little effect on pump activity. In addition, changes in the intracellular sodium concentration over time will alter the number of pumps per unit area of membrane. As with other large membrane proteins, the activity of the pump can be modulated via a number of second messenger systems.

IONIC CONCENTRATION GRADIENTS

The electrical basis for the *resting potential* is the unequal distribution of specific ions between the intracellular and extracellular compartments. The principal *ion potentials* contributing to the *resting potential* are those for *Na+*, *K+*, and *Cl−*. Na+ and Cl− concentrations are considerably higher outside the neuron, and K+ concentration is higher inside the cell (Table 3–2).

NERNST EQUATION

When the concentration of an ion on one side of a semipermeable membrane is greater than the concentration on the other side, an electrical potential and a chemical concentration gradient exist for that ion, which tend to drive it toward equilibrium.

This potential, *E*, can be expressed by the *Nernst equation:*

$$E_{ion} = \frac{RT}{zF} \ln \frac{[ion]_o}{[ion]_i} \qquad [3-1]$$

where E_{ion} is equal to the electrical potential for the ion, R is the gas constant (8.3143 joules/°K/mole); T is the absolute temperature (310.15°K); z is the charge of the ion, and F is the Faraday constant (96,500 coulombs/mole). The $[ion]_o$ is

TABLE 3-2

Intracellular and Extracellular Concentrations of Selected Ions in a Typical Mammalian Nerve Cell

IONS	EXTRACELLULAR (mM)	INTRACELLULAR (mM)	RELATIVE PERMEABILITY*
Na+	140	15	1.0
K+	4.7	138	66.7
Ca++	4.0	1.5†	
H+	4×10^{-5} (pH 7.4)	4×10^{-5} (pH 7.4)	
Cl−	110	6.6	133

* When the membrane is "at rest."
† Most of the intracellular Ca++ is bound; less than .0001 mM is free.

the concentration of the ion outside the cell, and [ion]$_i$ the concentration inside the cell.

Using these constants, converting ln to log_{10}, and expressing the potential in millivolts (1 joule/coulomb = 10^3 millivolts, mV), the equation, for univalent cations, becomes as follows:

$$E_{ion} (mV) = 61.5 \cdot log_{10} \frac{[ion]_o}{[ion]_i} \qquad [3-2]$$

In other words, a concentration difference across a semipermeable membrane for an ion is accompanied by an electrical potential that is proportional to the log of the concentration gradient.

Using the values from Table 3–2 and assuming the membrane were permeable only to K$^+$, the Nernst potential for K$^+$ would be as follows:

$$E_K = 61.5 \cdot log_{10} \frac{[4.7]}{[138]} = -90 \text{ mV}$$

Similarly, if the membrane were permeable only to Na$^+$, the Na$^+$ potential would be as follows:

$$E_{Na} = 61.5 \cdot log_{10} \frac{[140]}{[15]} = +60 \text{ mV}$$

And likewise, if the membrane were permeable only to Cl$^-$:

$$E_{Cl} = -61.5 \cdot log_{10} \frac{[110]}{[6.6]} = -75 \text{ mV}$$

Since chloride is a monovalent *anion*, z in Equation 3–1 is −1, and the constant in Equation 3–2 becomes −61.5.

GOLDMAN CONSTANT FIELD EQUATION

In the resting state, the membrane has a finite permeability to all three ions: hence, the *resting potential* (E$_M$) is a function of the individual ion gradients and the relative permeability (P) of each ion. This relationship is expressed by the *Goldman constant field equation,* sometimes referred to as the Goldman-Hodgkin-Katz equation, as follows:

This equation predicts that, if the permeability of one ion becomes much greater than that of the other ions, the membrane potential, E$_M$, will approach the potential for that ion as defined by the Nernst equation.

For example, in Equation 3–3, if P$_{Na}$ >>> P$_K$ and P$_{Cl}$, those terms with K$^+$ and Cl$^-$ become small relative to those with Na$^+$, and the membrane potential, E$_M$, approaches the Nernst potential for Na$^+$, E$_{Na}$.

ION FLOW IN RESTING MEMBRANE

Assume (1) a nerve cell at "rest," (2) an unequal distribution of ions as illustrated in Table 3–2, and (3) a cell membrane permeable *only* to K$^+$. Under these conditions, both P$_{Na}$ and P$_{Cl}$ will equal 0, and Equation 3–3 becomes the Nernst equation for the K$^+$. Thus, the resting potential will equal the Nernst potential for K$^+$, E$_M$ = E$_{K^+}$ = −90 mV.

If we now insert Na$^+$ channels, the membrane will become permeable to Na$^+$ in addition to K$^+$, and there will be a net flow of Na$^+$ ions into the cell. The Na$^+$ flow into the cell is driven by the chemical gradient (140 mM outside vs. 15 mM inside) and by the electrical potential (+60 mV Nernst potential for Na$^+$ is 150 mV away from the −90 mV resting potential).

Although relatively powerful electrical and chemical forces are present to drive Na$^+$ ions into the cell, the resting membrane is much more permeable to K$^+$ than to Na$^+$. The K$^+$ chemical gradient (138 mM inside vs. 4.7 mM outside) tends to drive K$^+$ ions out of the cell. Although the electrical potential favors the movement of K$^+$ ions into the cell, the force of the chemical concentration gradient is greater and there is a net flow of K$^+$ out of the cell. This net efflux of K$^+$ counters much of the effect of incoming Na$^+$ ions on the membrane potential, and a "new" resting potential is established. Because both Na$^+$ and K$^+$ are moving down concentration gradients, the new steady-state or resting potential must lie between the Nernst potentials for K$^+$ (−90 mV) and Na$^+$ (+60 mV) but closer to the K$^+$ potential, as the membrane at rest is much more permeable to K$^+$, in this example, E$_M$ = −75 mV.

Thus, in the "resting" state, Na$^+$ ions flow constantly into the cell and K$^+$ ions flow con-

$$E_M = 61.5 \cdot log_{10} \frac{(P_K \cdot [K^+]_o + P_{Na} \cdot [Na^+]_o + P_{Cl} \cdot [Cl^-]_i)}{(P_K \cdot [K^+]_i + P_{Na} \cdot [Na^+]_i + P_{Cl} \cdot [Cl^-]_o)} \qquad [3-3]$$

stantly out of the cell. Once chemical concentration gradients are established and maintained, the actual value for the resting potential becomes a function of the relative permeability of the two ions. Any change in the relative concentration of the two ions and/or any change in ion permeability (the ease with which an ion moves through its ionophore) will alter the steady state and, hence, change the value of the resting membrane potential, E_M. In nerve cells, as discussed subsequently, the permeabilities of ions are subject to change, thereby altering the membrane potential and providing a principal mechanism for neuronal signaling.

The resting potential cannot be maintained indefinitely, because both K^+ and Na^+ are flowing along concentration gradients. In time, the chemical gradients would dissipate and the membrane potential would be gone, much like a battery running down. However, the Na^+/K^+ pump functions as a "battery charger," maintaining the chemical gradients and, hence, the resting potential. Because the pump extrudes three Na^+ ions for every two K^+ ions it moves into the cell, when the neuron is at "rest," there must be a passive efflux of two K^+ ions for every three Na^+ ions that enter to maintain the steady state.

Chloride is the third principal ion associated with the membrane potential. The membrane normally is very permeable to Cl^-, and the ions are not actively pumped in or out of the neuron. Thus, Cl^- is free to diffuse, subject only to passive forces—the internal negativity of the membrane favoring movement of the ion out of the cell and the outside concentration favoring diffusion of the ion into the cell. The final concentration of Cl^- reflects an equilibrium between the inward and outward movements of the ion. Under these conditions, there is no net flux of Cl^- and $E_M = E_{Cl} = -75$ mV.

Other ions, such as Mg^{++} and Ca^{++}, behave in a manner similar to Na^+ and K^+. However, the concentrations and permeabilities of these ions are very small, and they do not contribute significantly to the *resting membrane potential, E_M.*

OHM'S LAW

In electrical circuits, the total current flow, in this case I_M, is equal to the sum of the component currents as follows:

$$I_M = I_{Na} + I_K + I_{Cl} \qquad [3-4]$$

where I_{Na} represents the Na^+ current, I_K the K^+ current, and I_{Cl} the Cl^- current.

A fundamental law of physics, *Ohm's law,* defines current in terms of electromotive force (E) and resistance (R):

$$I = \frac{E}{R} \qquad [3-5]$$

where I is the current in amperes, E is the electromotive force in volts, and R is the resistance in ohms.

Conductance is the reciprocal of the resistance and Equation 3–5 can be rewritten as follows:

$$I = g \cdot E \qquad [3-6]$$

where g is the *conductance* measured in reciprocal ohms or Siemens (S), and 1 S = 1/ohm.

The current for each ion can be expressed with a similar equation:

$$I_{Na} = g_{Na} \cdot (E_M - E_{Na})$$

$$I_K = g_K \cdot (E_M - E_K)$$

and

$$I_{Cl} = g_{Cl} \cdot (E_M - E_{Cl})$$

Note that E of Equation 3–6 is the resting membrane potential (E_M) less the Nernst "battery" potential for each ion, i.e., the *total* electromotive driving force for that particular ionic current.

At the resting membrane potential, by definition E_M does not change ($dE/dt = 0$); hence, $I_M = 0$. Therefore, substituting in Equation 3–4 as follows:

$$0 = I_M = I_{Na} + I_K + I_{Cl}$$

or with further substitution:

$$0 = g_{Na} \cdot (E_M - E_{Na}) + g_K \cdot (E_M - E_K) + g_{Cl} \cdot (E_M - E_{Cl})$$

At the resting potential, E_{Cl} is equal to E_M; hence, $g_{Cl} \cdot (E_M - E_{Cl}) = 0$. Therefore, when the previous equation is solved for E_M:

$$E_M = \frac{(g_{Na} \cdot E_{Na}) + (g_K \cdot E_K)}{g_{Na} + g_K} \qquad [3-7]$$

This relationship is fundamental to understanding the behavior of the neuronal membrane, especially as it relates to action potentials (see subsequent discussion). If the conductance of Na^+, for example, increases greatly relative to that of K^+, the value for the membrane potential,

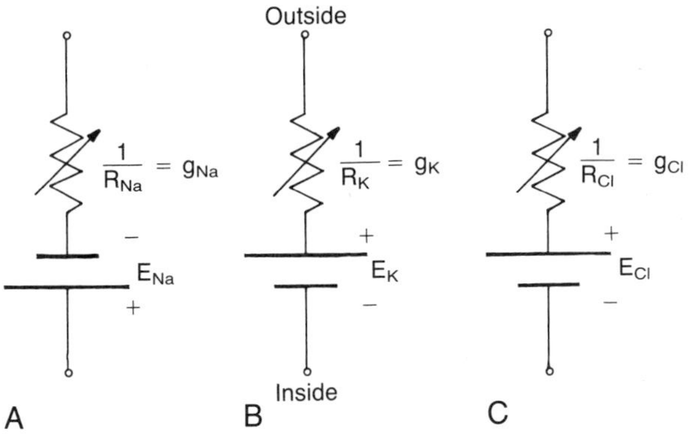

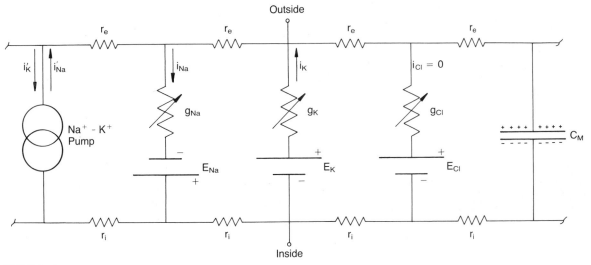

FIGURE 3-7

Equivalent electrical circuits for Na$^+$ (A), K$^+$ (B), and Cl$^-$ (C). Ionic currents are a function of both the electromotive force, E, and the conductance, g. Conductance will vary with the physiological state of the ionophore.

E_M, will approach that for E_{Na}. Similarly, if the K$^+$ conductance becomes large relative to that of Na$^+$, E_M will approach E_K.

Equation 3-7 can be rewritten in a more general form to apply to those situations in which the chloride ion is not distributed passively and E_M does not equal E_{Cl}:

$$E_M = \frac{(g_{Na} \cdot E_{Na}) + (g_K \cdot E_K) + (g_{Cl} \cdot E_{Cl})}{g_{Na} + g_K + g_{Cl}} \quad [3-8]$$

Similarly, conductances and potentials for other ions could be added to this same equation.

However, in most cases, their concentrations and/or conductances are so small, relative to those of Na$^+$, K$^+$ and Cl$^-$, that they have no significant effect on the calculation of the membrane potential.

Although a neuron maintains a "resting" potential, this is not a passive process. A small inward Na$^+$ current and a small outward K$^+$ current are always present. At the same time, equal but opposite currents are generated by the Na$^+$/K$^+$ pump, maintaining the steady state of the resting membrane potential.

EQUIVALENT CIRCUIT MODEL OF MEMBRANE

It is helpful to think of the nerve membrane, with its ion gradients and currents, in terms of an equivalent electrical circuit.

The Nernst potential for each ion is equivalent to an *ionic battery*. Because ion flow or *current* is a function of both the conductance of the ion channel and the electromotive force or electrical potential, an equivalent electrical circuit can be drawn for each ionic component (Fig. 3-7).

Similarly, the individual ion circuits can be combined with other components of the membrane to create an equivalent electrical circuit diagram for the membrane (Fig. 3-8). To complete the circuit diagram, several more elements have been inserted: the Na$^+$/K$^+$ pump (Na$^+$/K$^+$-ATPase); the capacitance of the lipid bilayer, C_M;

FIGURE 3-8

An equivalent electrical circuit for the neuronal membrane at rest. Ionic current components represent both the ionophore and the concentration gradient for the respective ions. The Na$^+$/K$^+$ pump is the ATP-dependent electrogenic pump. Membrane capacitance (C_M) is an inherent property of the lipid bilayer. At rest, $i_{Cl} = 0$ (see text. Note the symbol for ion current is i in figure and I in text). The symbols r_i and r_e represent the electrical resistance of the intracellular and extracellular fluid media, respectively.

and the resistance of the intracellular (r_i) and extracellular (r_e) fluids.

Passive Membrane Properties

Neuronal electrical signaling can be classified as either passive or active. *Passive signals (electrotonus)* are subject to attenuation, highly localized, and generally confined to the dendrites and soma of the neuron. *Active signals (action potentials)* are self-propagating, can travel relatively long distances, and are generally axonal.

The most common examples of *passive signals* are *postsynaptic potentials* (EPSPs and IPSPs) and *receptor potentials.* The last are covered with sensory systems. These are important short-distance signals in intraneuronal communication, especially for the temporal-spatial integration of synaptic signals.

ELECTROTONIC CURRENT SPREAD

Assume a small, localized increase in the membrane conductance for sodium—from some focal stimulus to the membrane. This increase generates a small, inward sodium current leading to a 2-mV depolarization of the membrane, a depolarization that is not sufficient to activate voltage-sensitive ion channels. Equation 3–7 predicts that a small increase in g_{Na} will produce a small shift in the membrane potential E_M in the positive direction, i.e., toward the sodium equilibrium potential, E_{Na}.

An electrical current always follows the path of least resistance. In this case, the current spreads radially from the point of origin, creating a local area of depolarization. The extent of the radial spread depends on two factors: the internal resistance (r_i) and the transmembrane resistance (R_M). R_M represents the total membrane resistance (the lipid bilayer and the reciprocal of the ion channel conductances), and r_i represents the resistance of the intracellular fluid. Because R_M is much greater than r_i, the current will spread for some distance. *The greater the membrane resistance relative to the internal resistance, the greater the passive spread.*

When a drop of water strikes the surface of a puddle, the impact produces a series of ripples, with each ripple attenuating rapidly as it spreads radially from the point of impact. The electrotonic spread of a small membrane depolarization is like a single ripple. The height of the ripple is analogous to the magnitude of the depolarization, and the trailing edge of the ripple represents a return of the membrane potential to the resting state.

Two properties characterize the electrotonic spread: the *length* or *space constant* (λ) and the *time constant* (τ). The first is a measure of the attenuation of the potential as it spreads passively along the membrane, and the second is a measure of the speed with which the potential spreads over the membrane.

LENGTH OR SPACE CONSTANT

Figure 3–9 illustrates the passive spread of current following a small focal depolarization. In *A*, the current spreads laterally, in both directions (red arrows) from the focal depolarization in the center. In *B*, the lateral spread of the depolarization is represented as a percent of the maximum, E_M. The *length* or *space constant* (λ) is defined as the distance from the point of stimulus to the point where the E_M has attenuated to 37% of the original value. Alternately, using our example of 2 mV, it is the distance away from the point of stimulation, where the maximum change in membrane potential is 0.74 mV (0.37 × 2 mV). For most neurons, this value ranges from 0.1 to 1.0 mm. To return to the analogy of a ripple, the length constant is that distance from the point of impact to the point where the height of the ripple has attenuated to 37% of the maximum.

TIME CONSTANT

The second property, the *time constant* (τ), is a measure of the speed with which the membrane responds to the stimulus and is defined as the time required for the change in membrane potential to reach 63% of its maximum value. This property is a function of both the membrane resistance and capacitance. For most neurons, the time constant will be from 1 to 20 msec. If the time constant is relatively large, the passive depolarization will have a relatively long rise time and a correspondingly long period of repolarization to the resting value. Small time constants indicate relatively short-lived passive potentials.

SUBTHRESHOLD STIMULI

Single EPSPs are usually *subthreshold stimuli.* The individual stimuli are not sufficient to trigger an action potential, and the change in membrane potential spreads passively (Figs. 3–10 and 3–11). To trigger an action potential, the passive depolarization must reach a *threshold level of intensity* at a location with an *adequate density of*

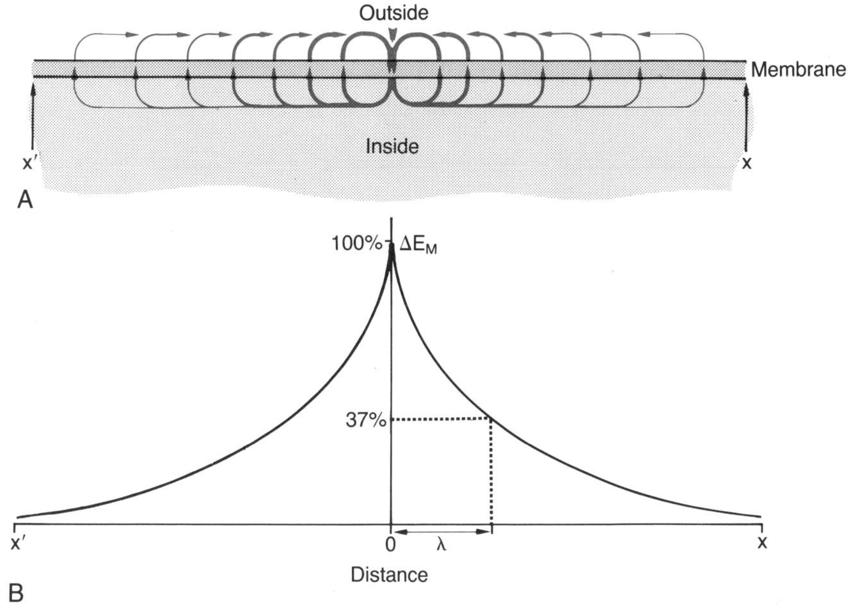

FIGURE 3-9

Passive spread of membrane current. A focal change in E_M will passively spread across the membrane of the soma or a dendrite in all directions. The characteristics of this spread depend on the conductance properties of the intracellular compartment relative to the membrane. The membrane has a relatively high resistance (low conductance). The greater this resistance is, relative to the intracellular resistance, the farther the change in membrane potential will spread before it is dissipated.

The distance from the origin of the focal change in potential (E_M) to the point where the change is 37% of the maximum is defined as the length constant. This type of passive spread is characteristic of most excitatory postsynaptic potentials and inhibitory postsynaptic potentials.

voltage-sensitive sodium channels (the axon or the initial segment of the axon, see Table 3–1). Depolarizations of the soma and dendrites generally spread passively because the density of voltage-sensitive sodium channels is sparse.

Again, the ripple analogy applies: if the ripple is of sufficient magnitude when it reaches the initial segment of the axon it will trigger an action potential. Figure 3–10 illustrates the simplest mechanism whereby an excitatory stimulus can trigger an action potential. If the excitatory stimulus is of sufficient magnitude to reach the threshold at the initial segment, an action potential will be triggered.

TEMPORAL SUMMATION

Another property of passive conduction is *temporal summation* (see Fig. 3–11). The small, single EPSP on the left is subthreshold and atten-

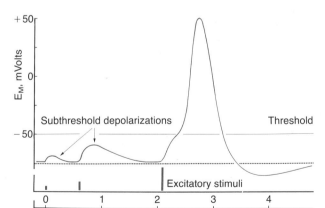

FIGURE 3-10

An elevation in the magnitude of an excitatory stimulus increases the degree of membrane depolarization. When a single stimulus is sufficient to raise the membrane potential to threshold, an action potential is triggered.

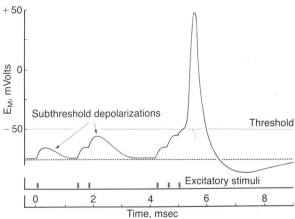

FIGURE 3-11

Temporal summation of excitatory postsynaptic potentials. A single excitatory stimulus (left bar) dissipates within 1.5 to 2.0 msec. Two similar stimuli within a brief time period (center bars) summate, but they still do not reach the threshold and, hence, do not trigger an action potential. Three such stimuli (right bars) summate, raising the membrane potential to threshold and triggering an action potential.

uates with time. Multiple subthreshold stimuli to the same location can be additive. In the second example, two subthreshold stimuli summate. However, the summated depolarization is still subthreshold and this too attenuates. If three such stimuli occur (on the right), the additive effect is sufficient to reach threshold and an action potential is triggered. This additive phenomenon depends on the time constant for the membrane. If the time constants given in Figure 3–11 had been shorter, the individual depolarizations would have attenuated before the next stimulus arrived, and there would not have been a *temporal summation* of the potentials. Similarly, if the time interval between stimuli had been longer, there would have been no summation.

SPATIAL SUMMATION

If more than one subthreshold depolarization occurs at the same time but at different sites on the neuron, the effects are also additive. This characteristic is known as *spatial summation*. If we again refer to the ripple analogy, when ripples that spread radially from two foci reach the initial segment at the same time, the effect will be additive—*spatial summation*.

TEMPORAL-SPATIAL SUMMATION

The two summation phenomena, *temporal summation* and *spatial summation,* act together. At any point in time, multiple depolarizations spread passively over the dendritic and somal membrane of the neuron. If the *spatial* and *temporal* parameters are suitable, there will be summation. In addition, if the summation depolarizes the initial segment of the axon to threshold, an action potential will be triggered.

IPSPs are processed in a similar manner— passive spread, time and length constants, and temporal and spatial summation. However, IPSPs have the reverse effect on the membrane potential—instead of decreasing the internal negativity (depolarization), an IPSP *increases* the internal negativity (*hyperpolarization*). Thus, the summative effect of a 2 mV EPSP and a 2 mV IPSP is zero. However, for an IPSP to reduce the effect of an EPSP on the initial segment, the IPSP must be generated at some geographic point between the EPSP and the initial segment of the axon. The integration of postsynaptic potentials is discussed in Chapter 4.

Action Potentials

ACTION POTENTIAL PROPERTIES

Neurons, when suitably stimulated, are able to convert a small portion of the energy stored as ionic potentials into a self-propagating electrical signal—the *action potential*. Under normal physiological conditions, an action potential is generated when the initial segment of the axon is depolarized to a threshold level. Once triggered, the action potential travels the entire length of the axon in an all-or-none fashion.

In Figure 3–1C, an action potential is triggered with a stimulating electrode. The event is recorded with a second electrode at some distance from the point of stimulation (see Fig. 3–1D). As the action potential passes the intracellular recording electrode, a sequence of rapid changes in the membrane potential is recorded. These changes are further illustrated in Figure 3–12.

The first phase, the *spike potential*, is a very rapid depolarization of the membrane, followed by an equally rapid repolarization. In this example, the membrane is depolarized from a resting potential of −75 mV through 0 to +45 or +50 mV in 0.5 msec or less. This effect is immediately followed by a rapid repolarization of the membrane to about −40 mV. The entire sequence takes place in a period of 1 msec or less.

A second phase of slower repolarization follows, the *negative after-potential*, in which the membrane returns to the original resting potential.

During the third and final phase, the *positive after-potential*, the repolarization process "overshoots" and then gradually returns to the original resting potential. The positive after-potential can last from a few milliseconds to several seconds and can vary in magnitude from a fraction of a mV to several mV (see Fig. 3–12).

The terms positive after-potential and negative after-potential are often confused, because the negative after-potential is more positive than the positive after-potential. However, they were first described from recordings made with *extracellular* electrodes, and under those conditions the polarity is reversed.

Once an action potential has been triggered, it is a self-propagating event. The magnitude of the depolarization and the speed of conduction are constant throughout the length of the axon.

Figure 3–13 illustrates a neuron with a stimulating electrode on the initial segment of the axon and three intracellular recording electrodes

FIGURE 3-12

The three components of an action potential are an initial *spike potential,* a negative *after-potential,* and a positive *after-potential.* The dotted line represents the resting membrane potential. E_{Na} and E_K represent the sodium and the potassium potentials, respectively.

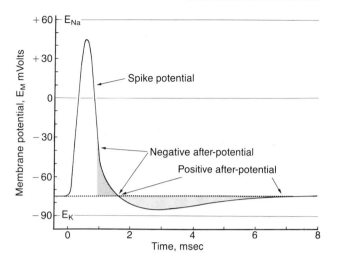

equally spaced along the axon at points a, b, and c. In the lower portion of the illustration, tracings A, B, and C represent recordings made from electrodes a, b, and c, respectively.

Two features are of special importance. First, the size and shape of the action potential is the same in all three tracings. Second, the action potential has a constant rate of propagation. The time elapsed between the stimulus and the recording of the action potential (the arrows under tracings A, B, and C) are directly proportional to

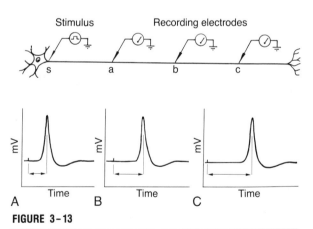

A   B   C

FIGURE 3-13

Time course for the movement of an action potential along an axon. A threshold stimulus is applied to the initial segment of an axon, point *s,* and recordings are made from points *a, b,* and *c* (top). The tracings in *A, B,* and *C* (lower portion) represent the recordings made at points *a, b,* and *c.* Note that the size and shape of the action potential are identical in all three tracings.

Arrows beneath the tracings in *A, B,* and *C* represent the time required for the action potential to travel from its origin (point of stimulus) to the recording electrode. The action potential moves at a constant velocity.

the distance between the recording electrode and the point of stimulation.

Although the size and shape of an action potential and its speed of conduction are not the same for all nerve fibers, once generated an action potential will retain the same properties throughout its course (the length of the axon).

MOLECULAR MECHANISM: VOLTAGE-SENSITIVE ION CHANNELS

Voltage-sensitive Na^+/K^+ channels are the keys to a neuron's ability to generate an action potential from the energy stored in the form of the resting potential.

Consider a hypothetical situation in which the membrane potential of an axon is abruptly increased from the resting negative value of -75 mV to a positive value of $+15$ mV for a period of 3 msec and is then returned to the resting value of -75 mV (Fig. 3–14). During this period, the conductance properties of both voltage-sensitive channels change in different but distinctive manners.

On the one hand, sodium conductance increases immediately, as the sodium channels go from the resting to the activated state. Within a fraction of a millisecond, the conductance abruptly decreases, as the channels rapidly change from the activated to the inactivated state (see Fig. 3–4).

The potassium conductance, on the other hand, increases at a much slower rate as the channels change from the resting to the activated state (see Fig. 3–5). The potassium conductance, however, remains high as long as the membrane is depolarized. The potassium ion channels re-

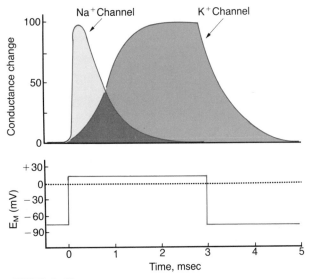

FIGURE 3-14

Changes in conductance of sodium and potassium ion channels when the membrane potential is suddenly increased from a resting value of −75 mV to a positive value of +15 mV for 3 msec. The sodium channels open (activate) and then close (inactivate) within 3 msec. In comparison, the potassium channels only open (activate) with the depolarization and do not begin to close until the the membrane potential returns to the resting level. (Adapted with permission from A. C. Guyton, Textbook of Medical Physiology, 7th Edition, W. B. Saunders Co., Philadelphia, 1986.)

main in the open or activated state. When the membrane potential returns to the resting state, the potassium conductance returns to the original level, as the ion channels return to the resting state (see Fig. 3–14).

CONDUCTANCE CHANGES ASSOCIATED WITH ACTION POTENTIAL

The pattern of membrane depolarization and repolarization observed for the action potential (see Fig. 3–12) can be related directly to changes in the conductances of the voltage-sensitive sodium and potassium channels (Fig. 3–15).

The density of voltage-sensitive sodium channels in the initial segment of the axon is seven times higher than that of the soma and dendrites (see Table 3–1). When a wave of membrane depolarization, spreading passively, reaches the relatively high concentration of sodium channels in the initial segment, a sufficient number of channels are activated, increasing their conductance 4000- to 6000-fold, to trigger an action potential.

The channel activation produces (1) an inward sodium current, (2) an immediate depolarization of the membrane of the initial segment, and (3) an ionic current that spreads laterally through the intracellular fluid and out through the membrane adjacent to the initial segment (see Fig. 3–9A).

The concentration of sodium channels is relatively high in the axon (see Table 3–1). This outward sodium current is sufficient to activate the sodium channels in the patch of membrane

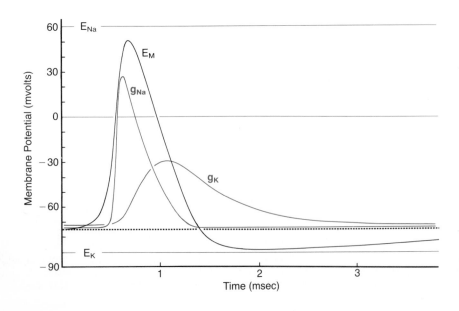

FIGURE 3-15

Time course of changes in sodium and potassium conductances (red), as they relate to the action potential (E_M, black). Note that sodium channels are characterized by the very rapid activation-inactivation sequence, whereas potassium channels are slower to respond (as in Fig. 3–14). (Adapted with permission from A. L. Hodgkin and A. F. Huxley, J. Physiol., 117: 500–544, 1952.)

immediately adjacent to the initial segment. This effect triggers a similar sequence of events—an inward sodium current through the newly activated sodium channels followed by an ionic current which spreads laterally and then out through the next adjacent patch or segment of membrane. This outward current activates more sodium channels and, in this manner, the action potential becomes a self-propagating wave of depolarization, spreading the entire length of the axon.

The self-propagating feature of the action potential is dependent on two factors: (1) the sufficient density of voltage-sensitive sodium channels and (2) the passive membrane properties compatible with the spread of enough current to activate additional voltage-sensitive sodium channels, in the immediately adjacent patch of membrane.

As we have reviewed in Figure 3–14, the activated sodium channel becomes inactivated within a fraction of a millisecond, blocking the further influx of sodium. However, within this brief period, the membrane potential has changed approximately 120 mV, moving from -75 mV to $+45$ mV, approaching the E_{Na} of $+60$ mV, a change predicted by Equation 3–7. As g_{Na} becomes greater than g_K, E_M approaches E_{Na}. At the same time, this membrane depolarization has activated slower responding, voltage-sensitive potassium channels. As these channels open, potassium ions flow out of the cell. The outward movement of potassium ions helps to restore the membrane potential to the original resting level. As the membrane potential returns to the resting level, potassium conductance returns to the original level (see Fig. 3–15).

When the sodium and potassium conductance changes are related to the action potential (see Fig. 3–15) the spike potential corresponds to (1) the activation-inactivation sequence of the sodium channels and (2) the initial activation of the slower responding potassium channels. Potassium conductance is maximal during the negative after-potential, with g_K returning to the resting level during the positive after-potential. In short, the depolarization is due to the rapid activation-inactivation sequence of the voltage-sensitive sodium channels and the repolarization to the activation of voltage-sensitive potassium channels.

IMPULSE PROPAGATION

In *nonmyelinated nerve fibers*, voltage-sensitive sodium channels are distributed uniformly over the surface of the axon. The action potential moves along the entire axonal membrane, spreading sequentially from one segment of axonal membrane to the segment immediately adjacent. The depolarization of one segment produces sufficient ionic current to activate the voltage-sensitive sodium channels in the adjacent segment of the membrane.

In *myelinated nerve fibers*, the action potential moves along the axon by a phenomenon known as *saltatory conduction*. The action potential literally leaps from one node of Ranvier to the next—a much more rapid means of impulse conduction. Two structural features are responsible: (1) an extremely high concentration of voltage-sensitive sodium channels at the nodes of Ranvier (see Table 3–1) and (2) a marked increase in the membrane resistance, R_M, in the internodal region due to the presence of the myelin sheath.

As a result, the node becomes a focal point of depolarization, generating a large, inward sodium current because a large number of voltage-sensitive sodium channels are activated. The high R_M of the internodal region means a greater lateral spread of the ionic current (current flow always follows the path of least resistance), through the intracellular fluid and then outward through the next node of Ranvier (Fig. 3–16). The outward current, in turn, activates the sodium channels at the node, resulting in an inward sodium current.

As long as the inward sodium current at one node produces sufficient ionic current to activate the voltage-sensitive sodium channels at the next node (up to 1 mm away) the action potential will leap rapidly from node to node as *saltatory conduction*.

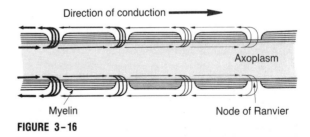

Direction of conduction ⟶

Axoplasm

Myelin   Node of Ranvier

FIGURE 3–16

Pattern of current flow during saltatory conduction in myelinated nerves. The combination of the increased membrane resistance from the myelin sheath, the very high concentration of voltage-sensitive sodium channels at the nodes of Ranvier, and the relatively low resistance in intracellular and extracellular fluids results in the ionic currents "leaping" from node to node. The end result is a much faster conduction velocity than that in nonmyelinated fibers.

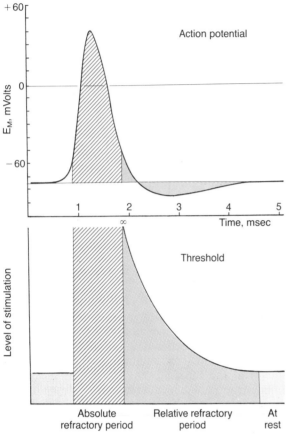

FIGURE 3-17

When an action potential is triggered, there is a finite period during which a second action potential cannot be evoked, regardless of the stimulus strength — the *absolute refractory period*. This is followed by the *relative refractory period*, a time during which the threshold for the generation of the action potential declines to the original level of the resting nerve. During the relative refractory period, an action potential can be generated provided the stimulus is sufficient to reach the threshold. However, the threshold is greater than normal.

When changes in the threshold (below) are compared with the action potential (above), the absolute refractory period corresponds to the spike potential — a period when the sodium channels are initially activated and subsequently inactivated. During the relative refractory period, coincident with the negative and positive after-potentials, an increasing number of sodium channels have moved from the inactivated to the resting state.

REFRACTORY PERIODS

Once an action potential has been triggered, a finite period occurs during which the axon cannot be stimulated, regardless of the strength of the stimulus (depolarization). This period, known as the *absolute refractory period,* coincides with the period of the spike potential (Fig. 3–17). During this period, the voltage-sensitive sodium channels have become inactivated and are unable to respond to a second stimulus until they return to the resting state. This period is followed by the *relative refractory period,* a period in which a second action potential can be triggered, if the stimulus is great enough. During this period, the membrane becomes repolarized and more and more of the inactive sodium channels return to the resting state. As the number of sodium channels in the resting state increases, the threshold for triggering another action potential decreases (see Fig. 3–17).

SUGGESTED READING

Catterall, W. A. (1988). Structure and function of voltage-sensitive ion channels. Science, 242: 50–61.

A excellent review of the molecular biology of the voltage-sensitive sodium, calcium, and potassium channels in excitable cells. This article reviews studies of the structure of the ion channels, including subunits, functional organization, and post-translational modification of proteins. Concepts from molecular biology, biophysics, and pharmacology are drawn together for the proposed structural models of channel function.

Kuffler, S. W., J. G. Nicholls, and A. R. Martin (1984). *From Neuron to Brain: A Cellular Approach to the Function of the Nervous System,* 2nd Edition. Sinauer Associates Inc., Sunderland, Massachusetts.

A basic text on neurobiology with special emphasis on neuronal physiology. This text contains an excellent, in-depth discussion of many of the points touched on briefly in this chapter. Part 2, Mechanisms of Neuronal Signaling, *is particularly relevant to the material in this chapter.*

Rossier, B. C., K. Geering, and J. P. Kraehenbuhl (1987). Regulation of the sodium pump: how and why? Trends Biochem. Sci., 12: 483–487.

A review of the Na⁺/K⁺-ATPase and the biochemistry of this membrane protein, an essential protein in the regulation of activity in excitable cells.

Chapter

4

Neuronal Communication

ELECTRICAL SYNAPSES
GENERAL FEATURES OF THE CHEMICAL SYNAPSE
NEUROCHEMICAL TRANSMISSION
SYNAPTIC INTEGRATION

Chapter 3 deals with membrane and action potentials, both properties of individual neurons. In this chapter, we discuss how neurons utilize these electrical properties for communication — both with each other and with effector organs.

The most direct form of communication is the *electrical synapse* or *gap junction*. In the electrical synapse, the presynaptic terminal of one neuron forms a very tight connection with the postsynaptic neuron. When an action potential reaches the presynaptic terminal, channel continuities between the presynaptic and postsynaptic elements permit the flow of the electrical signal, with little or no attenuation and little or no time delay. Although quite common in invertebrate nervous systems, neuronal electrical synapses are relatively rare in mammalian nervous systems. However, numerous gap junction–like connections exist between glial elements.

By far, the most common form of interneuronal communication in the mammalian nervous system is the *chemical synapse*. In the chemical synapse, the action potential depolarizes the presynaptic terminal leading to an influx of calcium ions with the resultant release of a chemical neurotransmitter. The neurotransmitter diffuses across the synaptic cleft and interacts with a specific receptor protein in the postsynaptic membrane. In the most straightforward case, the

neurotransmitter/receptor complex alters the conductance of an ion channel in the postsynaptic membrane. The ionic current then alters the postsynaptic resting potential, producing either an *excitatory postsynaptic potential (EPSP)* or *inhibitory postsynaptic potential (IPSP)*.

Neuroendocrinology — the study of the synthesis and release of neurotransmitters or neurohormones into the blood stream, either for short distances through the parvocellular neurosecretory cells or for systemic distribution through the magnocellular neurosecretory cells — is an important part of the understanding of neuronal communication. Neuroendocrinology is also discussed in Chapter 18. This chapter is limited to chemical and electrical synapses.

Electrical Synapses

Electrical synapses or gap junctions can be found in many types of non-neuronal, nonexcitable cells. Their function in these cells and their tissues is principally one of metabolic or chemical communication and not electrical signal transmission. In neurons, however, electrical synapses provide a direct electrical coupling between the presynaptic and postsynaptic elements. The electrical signal (usually an action potential) passes from one cell to the next, with little or no attenuation and without the "synaptic delay" so characteristic of chemical synapses.

The presynaptic and postsynaptic membranes of the *electrical synapse* are in close apposition, separated by a space of only 25 to 40 Å. Embedded within the presynaptic and postsynaptic membranes are protein complexes arranged in a pattern not unlike the ion channels described in Chapter 3. These proteins, referred to as *connexons*, consist of six subunits and form a protein-lined tube or canal through the unit membrane. Connexons of the presynaptic membrane are tightly paired with a similar connexon in the postsynaptic membrane, completing a channel of about 20 Å in diameter—an intercellular aqueous bridge—between the two cells (Fig. 4–1). These channels have a high conductance, relative to the voltage-sensitive ion channels (110 to 150 pS, 150×10^{-12} ohms^{-1}), and are large enough for the passage of small molecules from one cell to the next. Thus, the electrical current generated in the presynaptic terminal passes directly to the postsynaptic neuron with little attenuation and no time delay.

The area of contact between the presynaptic and postsynaptic elements in an *electrical synapse* varies from 0.1 to 10 μ^2, and the entire contact area is densely packed with connexons organized in a tight hexagonal array (see Fig. 4–1).

Functionally, the electrical synapse can be bidirectional, i.e., an electrical signal can pass in either direction, or the electrical synapse can be "rectified." If rectified, the synapse has a higher resistance (lower conductance) in one direction, making it effectively unidirectional in nature. Because of the lack of delay and attenuation, the synapse functions well for the synchronization of populations of neurons, especially those associated with stereotypical actions. Although the physiological properties of electrical synapses are less susceptible to alterations than those of their chemical counterparts, they can be modulated by the physiological state of the cell, the membrane potential, the intracellular calcium concentration, the pH, and by the phosphorylation through various second messenger systems.

In the mammalian brain stem, *electrical synapses* have been described between dendritic spines of adjacent neurons in the inferior olivary nucleus, between axon terminals and cell bodies in the lateral vestibular (Deiters') nucleus, and between cell bodies in the mesencephalic nucleus of V.

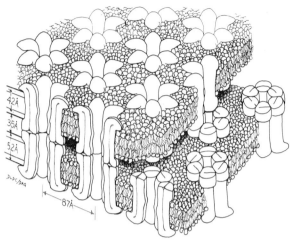

FIGURE 4-1

Structure of the gap junction or electrical synapse. The lipid bilayers of the presynaptic (upper) and postsynaptic (lower) membranes are separated by a finite cleft of 35 Å. Both membranes are studded with a dense concentration of channels or *connexons*, each composed of six protein subunits. Presynaptic connexons are tightly paired with postsynaptic connexons, forming protein-lined tubes or canals. The connexons provide direct intercellular continuity between the presynaptic and postsynaptic neurons. Small molecules pass freely from one cell to the next as do the ionic currents of the nerve signals.

The connexons are subject to modulation, through changes in membrane potential and second messenger systems, which activate/inactivate protein kinases, phosphatases, or both. (Reproduced from L. Makowski, D. L. D. Casper, W. C. Phillips, and D. A. Goodenough, *The Journal of Cell Biology*, 74: 629–645, 1977. By copyright permission of the Rockefeller University Press.)

General Features of the Chemical Synapse

MOLECULAR ARCHITECTURE

The basic fine structure of a chemical synapse is discussed in Chapter 2 (see Figs. 2–11 to 2–13). A number of the more important molecular components of the chemical synapse are represented in Figure 4–2. The presynaptic element, the *axon terminal* or *bouton terminaux*, is the termination of the axon proper and is bounded by an excitable membrane with voltage-sensitive sodium and potassium channels. In addition to these channels, the membrane of the axon terminal contains voltage-sensitive *calcium channels*,

FIGURE 4-2

The principal molecular components and events of a chemical synapse. *1, 2* and *3,* Voltage-sensitive ion channels in the presynaptic terminal for sodium, potassium, and calcium. *4,* Presynaptic receptor coupled to a second-message system. *5,* Presynaptic receptor coupled to an ion channel. *6,* Synaptic vesicle forming from the presynaptic membrane. *7,* Synthesis of neurotransmitter and storage in synaptic vesicles. *8,* Quantal release of neurotransmitter from synaptic vesicle by exocytosis. *9,* Postsynaptic receptor coupled to an ion channel. *10,* Postsynaptic receptor coupled to an ion channel through a second reaction such as a cyclic nucleotide–dependent phosphorylation. *11,* Postsynaptic receptor coupled to a second messenger system, which in turn modulates the postsynaptic neuron through the activation of a modulator protein or peptide.

Several neurotransmitters are represented by the different sized particles in the vesicles. Receptors selectively respond to one transmitter or the other. (See text for discussion.) All or some of the illustrated components may coexist at the same synaptic terminal.

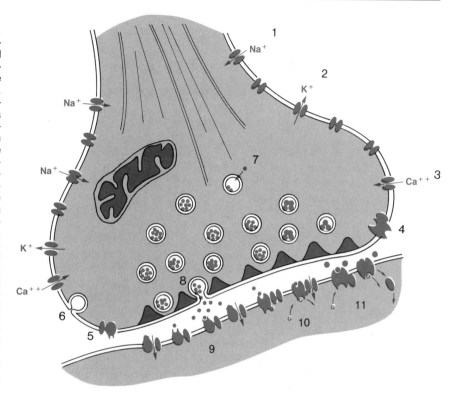

an essential ingredient for the release of the chemical neurotransmitter.

Both the presynaptic and postsynaptic membranes contain a variety of receptors for the neurotransmitter released by the axon terminal. Those on the postsynaptic membrane convert or translate the chemical message into an electrical signal, and those on the presynaptic membrane modulate the subsequent release of neurotransmitter.

TYPES

Physiologically, chemical synapses are either *excitatory* or *inhibitory*. Excitatory synapses produce focal *depolarizations* of the postsynaptic membrane (*EPSPs*), whereas inhibitory synapses produce focal *hyperpolarizations* of the postsynaptic membrane (*IPSPs*) (Fig. 4–3).

Morphologically, most chemical synapses can be classified as *asymmetrical* or *symmetrical synapses* (see Fig. 2–11). Asymmetrical synapses

characteristically have clear, round synaptic vesicles. Their postsynaptic density is thicker than their presynaptic density; hence, the term asymmetrical. These synapses are primarily excitatory in function. Alternately, symmetrical synapses usually have flattened vesicles. Presynaptic and postsynaptic densities are of similar thickness. Generally, symmetrical synapses are inhibitory.

Chemical synapses are further defined according to their anatomical location (Fig. 2–14). *Axospinous, axodendritic, axosomatic,* and *axoaxonal synapses* refer to axon terminals synapsing on dendritic spines, dendrites proper, neuronal soma, and other axon terminals, in that order. In addition to axonal synapses, some dendrites form chemical connections with other dendrites, i.e., *dendrodendritic synapses.* These are found in some areas of the neuropil and are important in the modulation and integration of incoming synaptic signals.

The foregoing classifications refer principally to synapses within the central nervous system

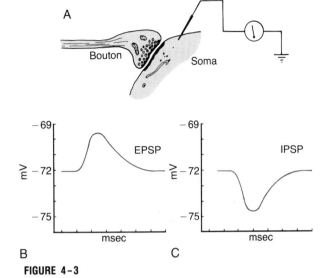

A

Bouton   Soma

EPSP

IPSP

B   C

FIGURE 4-3

Excitatory and inhibitory postsynaptic potentials (EPSPs and IPSPs). *A*, Axosomatic synapse with the recording electrode in the soma of the postsynaptic neuron.

B, If the synapse in *A* were excitatory, a single EPSP could depolarize the postsynaptic membrane from the resting potential of −72 mV to −69.5 mV as illustrated.

C, If the synapse were inhibitory, a single IPSP could hyperpolarize the postsynaptic neuron from the resting potential of −72 mV to −74.5 mV as illustrated. In either case, the change in membrane potential would spread passively over the soma.

(CNS). In the peripheral nervous system, there are several types of synaptic connections. In the ganglia of the autonomic nervous system, *preganglionic* fibers of the sympathetic and parasympathetic nervous system form both axodendritic and axosomatic synapses on the *postganglionic* neurons. These synapses are similar to those found in the CNS. In addition, motor neurons form synaptic connections with their target organs. In the case of somatic motor neurons, these would be the skeletal muscle fibers. These connections are *neuromuscular junctions* or *neuromuscular synapses*. They have a characteristic morphology, and the point of contact between the nerve and muscle is known as the *motor end plate*.

Chemical synapses are further classified according to the neurotransmitter: those in which acetylcholine (ACh) is the principal neurotransmitter are *cholinergic synapses*; those with glycine are *glycinergic*, and those with dopamine are *dopaminergic*. Because many synapses in the CNS utilize more than one neurotransmitter, which is probably the rule rather than the exception, this type of nomenclature must be em-

ployed with caution. A CNS neuron, however, will receive a multitude of different chemical messages, but *the effect of each chemical message on the resting membrane potential is dictated by the properties of the postsynaptic receptor.*

DALE'S PRINCIPLE

Chemical transmission, as a means of communication between neurons, was proposed in the mid 1930's but was not generally accepted until years later. With the acceptance of chemical transmission came another precept—*Dale's principle.* Named for a noted British neurophysiologist, Dale's principle proposed that the multitude of axon terminals arising from a single neuron utilized the same chemical message.

Today we know that some neurons may utilize as many as three different neurotransmitters at the same synaptic terminal, a concept unheard of at the time of Dale's proposal. However, the basis for Dale's principle was the biochemical and physiological unity of the individual neuron. Applying Dale's principle to the present understanding of neurotransmission, we can say that axon terminals arising from a single neuron utilize the same chemical message, be it either a single neurotransmitter or a *combination* of several neurotransmitters.

Although the narrow interpretation of Dale's principle—one neuron, one neurotransmitter—is now limited, the broader, more fundamental principle of the biochemical unity of the individual neuron remains valid.

Neurochemical Transmission

PRESYNAPTIC DEPOLARIZATION

The unit membrane of the *axon terminal* is continuous with the axon. The membrane contains both voltage-sensitive sodium and potassium channels and is depolarized, transiently, by the action potential. Unlike the electrical synapse, no physical continuity exists between the *presynaptic axon terminal* and the *postsynaptic membrane.* The two are separated by the *synaptic cleft*, a gap of from 150 to 200 Å. The electrical signal of the action potential must be converted to a chemical message.

A third population of voltage-sensitive ion channels, *calcium channels*, are present in the presynaptic membrane (see Fig. 4–2 (3)). When the presynaptic terminal is depolarized, the voltage-sensitive calcium channels are activated. A rapid influx of calcium ions into the presynaptic terminal takes place. For most chemical synapses, the influx of calcium is the trigger for the subsequent events leading to the release of neurotransmitter(s).

VOLTAGE-SENSITIVE CALCIUM CHANNELS

Voltage-sensitive calcium channels belong to the same "family" of ion channels as the voltage-sensitive sodium and potassium channels (see Chapter 3). The large, α_1-subunit of the calcium channel resembles the α-subunit of the sodium channel. Both have four homologous domains. Each one is composed of six membrane-spanning α-helices. The domains are arranged symmetrically around a central canal (see Fig. 3–3). These similarities are not unexpected, because both function as voltage-sensitive channels for cations. In addition, one might expect the same basic molecular mechanism to function in each case.

Calcium channels, however, represent a more diverse population of ion channels. In the presynaptic terminal, there are at least three types of channels based on activation-inactivation kinetics, voltage dependence, single-channel conductance, and on sensitivity to various pharmacologic antagonists. The best characterized are the *L-type*, with long-lasting calcium currents and sensitivity to inhibition by three classes of pharmacologic agents: dihydropyridines (nifedipine), phenylalkylamines (verapamil), and benzothiazepines (diltiazem).

Because the highest concentrations of L-type calcium channels are found in the transverse tubule systems of skeletal muscles, these muscle channels were used for much of the original molecular structure work. Subsequent research indicates the neuronal L-type channel is similar to, if not the same as, the muscle channel.

Associated with the α_1-subunit, is an α_2/δ-subunit complex and β- and γ-subunits (Fig. 4–4). The α_1-subunit contains the ion channel and external binding sites for the pharmacological antagonists and agonists. Phosphorylation of the L-type channel by a cAMP-dependent protein kinase shifts the channel from an inactive to active state. Both the α_1- and β- subunits contain phosphorylation sites for this kinase. In addition, these voltage-sensitive channels are inhibited by several of the G-proteins and other second messenger systems. A number of neurotransmitters, acting on the presynaptic terminal, can modulate

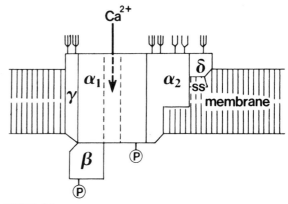

FIGURE 4-4

A proposed model for the voltage-sensitive calcium channel structure. The basic subunits ($\alpha_1, \alpha_2, \beta, \gamma,$ and δ) and the sites of cAMP-dependent phosphorylation (P) and glycosylation (Ψ and Ψ) are illustrated. (Reproduced with permission from M. Takahashi, M. J. Seagur, J. F. Jones, et al., Proc. Natl. Acad. Sci. USA, 84: 5478–5482, 1987.)

calcium channel activity directly or through second messenger systems. As discussed further, modulation of the presynaptic calcium channel is an important mechanism in the regulation of synaptic activity.

In the resting neuron, measurable calcium currents have been recorded with depolarizations as small as 20 mV (i.e., a shift in the resting membrane potential from −70 mV to −50 mV). Peak calcium currents are observed at membrane potentials near 0 mV, with half-maximum activation at −15 mV. The reversal potential for the calcium current is +40 mV.

RELEASE OF TRANSMITTER COUPLED TO INCREASED CALCIUM CONDUCTANCE

The inward surge of calcium triggers the release of the neurotransmitter from the presynaptic terminal. We know little of the actual molecular events. However, we know that these events occur rapidly, because synaptic delay is only 1 to 2 msec. During this period, voltage-sensitive calcium channels are activated. An inward surge of calcium ions and a binding of calcium to cytoplasmic sites and/or molecules occur. This signal triggers the exocytosis of synaptic vesicles with the release of the neurotransmitter into the synaptic cleft (see Fig. 4–2 (8)).

The transmitter release is quantal. Each synaptic vesicle contains one quantum of transmitter. For the neurotransmitter acetylcholine, 1 quantum, approximately 10,000 molecules, will produce an EPSP of about 0.4 mV at the neuromuscular synapse.

As synaptic vesicles fuse with the presynaptic membrane during the process of exocytosis, the membrane of the old vesicles becomes incorporated into the presynaptic membrane. At the same time, new vesicles are actively formed by pinocytosis from an adjacent surface of the presynaptic terminal (see Fig. 4–2 (6)). These vesicles are subsequently filled with newly synthesized or "recycled" neurotransmitter (see Chapter 5).

Because the time interval of synaptic delay is so brief, it is unlikely that the release of the neurotransmitter involves a cascade of enzymatic reactions, although one or two enzyme reactions could occur. Once the actual "trigger molecule" has been identified, the actual molecular mechanism can be described. Good evidence exists for some, yet to be defined, involvement of a calcium/calmodulin–dependent protein kinase, known to be present in nerve terminals, in the transmitter release mechanism.

Whatever the mechanism, calcium influx triggers an energy-dependent reaction culminating in the exocytotic release of the transmitter (see Fig. 4–2 (8)). The electrical signal of an action potential is thereby converted to a chemical message.

DIFFUSION OF TRANSMITTER AND BINDING TO RECEPTOR

Following release, the neurotransmitter diffuses, passively but rapidly, across the narrow 150 to 200 Å synaptic cleft. On reaching the postsynaptic membrane, the neurotransmitter is bound to a receptor molecule with specific recognition/binding sites for that particular transmitter (see Fig. 4–2 (9)). The binding of the ligand triggers a postsynaptic response specific for that receptor. *Note that the intrinsic properties of the postsynaptic receptor and not the neurotransmitter determine the nature of the postsynaptic response.*

POSTSYNAPTIC RECEPTORS

Receptors fall into two broad categories: *ion channel–coupled receptors*, in which the binding of the ligand to the receptor directly activates an ion channel, and *second messenger–coupled receptors*, in which the binding of the ligand activates one or more second messenger systems. Another name for *ion channel–coupled receptors* is *ligand-gated ion channels*. These ion channels are activated (gated) by the binding of a ligand (i.e., a neurotransmitter). This "family" of channels is large and includes many different neurotransmitter receptors coupled to the principal ion channels, Na^+, K^+, Ca^{++}, and Cl^-.

For example, the nicotinic acetylcholine receptor (nACh-R) is coupled to a sodium channel. Ligand activation of the receptor opens the sodium channel transiently, resulting in an inward surge of sodium current, a depolarization of the postsynaptic membrane, and the generation of an EPSP (see Fig. 4–3).

Two of the receptors for gamma-aminobutyric acid (GABA) and glycine are coupled to the chloride channel. Both GABA and glycine are inhibitory neurotransmitters. Ligand binding to these receptors produces an inward chloride current, a hyperpolarization of the postsynaptic membrane, and the generation of an IPSP (see Fig. 4–3).

Ion channel–coupled receptors have the fastest response time of the neurotransmitter receptors. Because channel activation occurs with the binding of the ligand to the receptor and does not require an additional chemical reaction, the changes in ion conductance occur almost instantaneously. Neurotransmitter receptors coupled to sodium or calcium channels are excitatory. Increased conductance of these ions leads to a depolarization of the postsynaptic membrane. However, receptors coupled to chloride or potassium channels hyperpolarize the membrane and are inhibitory.

Second messenger–coupled receptors are not linked directly to an ion channel, and accordingly their response time is somewhat longer than the ion channel–coupled receptors. Some, such as the norepinephrine β-receptors (i.e., β-adrenergic receptors) activate adenyl cyclase and a cAMP-dependent protein kinase. This activation leads to a phosphorylation of the receptor and an activation of the associated ion channel. Other transmitter receptors are coupled to G-proteins or other second messenger systems. Although the second messenger–coupled receptors are slower to respond, the duration of the response is greater.

Stimulation of any receptor that produces an EPSP may also indirectly activate a second messenger system. The membrane of the postsynaptic neuron contains voltage-gated calcium channels. Depolarization of the postsynaptic membrane by one or more EPSPs may activate adjacent voltage-sensitive calcium channels. When this occurs, there is an inward flow of calcium ions. This has the potential for activating of the calcium/calmodulin–dependent kinase system. This activation, in turn, can trigger a cascade of second messenger signals, in addition to the original EPSP.

Second messenger systems can modulate postsynaptic receptors and ion channels, and they can trigger the transcription of specific genes. The chemical synapse is part of a vast, highly adaptable communication system. It is no longer possible to consider a chemical synapse simply as an anatomical entity with a fixed set of physiological properties. Instead, it is a dynamic structure possessing a broad potential for modulation and adaptation to changing circumstances.

In summary, the principal responses to activation of the postsynaptic receptor are (1) the translation of the chemical message to an electrical signal (either an IPSP or an EPSP) and (2) the activation of second message systems that have the potential of activating and/or modulating ion channels, receptor responses (sensitivity), and transcription of specific mRNAs.

TERMINATION OF POSTSYNAPTIC RESPONSE

Unlike many hormones and growth factors, the chemical transmitter/receptor complex is not internalized by the postsynaptic neuron following the binding of the ligand to the receptor. Instead, neurotransmitters are removed by enzymatic inactivation, by re-uptake by the presynaptic neuron, or by a combination of the two.

The ACh system is a classic example of enzymatic inactivation. Acetylcholinesterase, present in the synaptic cleft and on the postsynaptic membrane, catalyzes the rapid hydrolysis of ACh to choline and acetate, both of which are neurochemically inactive. The choline is taken up by the presynaptic terminal via a high affinity uptake system and is recycled. Some neurotransmitters, such as the catecholamines, may be either inactivated by an enzyme-catalyzed O-methylation or taken up by the presynaptic terminal via some active mechanism. Other neurotransmitters, including some of the neuroactive peptides, are taken up by either the presynaptic neuron or the surrounding glial cells. In all cases, the removal of the active form of the neurotransmitter from the synaptic cleft is necessary for the termination of the action.

MULTIPLE NEUROTRANSMITTERS AND MODULATORS

Most of the discussion to this point deals with a single neurotransmitter. This is probably the exception rather than the rule, however. Most chemical synapses in the CNS appear to utilize two or more neurotransmitters. In some cases, the release of the second transmitter is dependent on the rate of firing of the presynaptic neuron. Often, the second transmitter has no effect by itself but modulates the action of the first transmitter—either presynaptically or postsynaptically. In the case of presynaptic modulation, the presynaptic terminal may contain receptors specific to the second neurotransmitter, and activation of this receptor can modify the release of the first transmitter (see Fig. 4–2 (4,5)). Postsynaptic modulation can involve an interaction of the second neurotransmitter with specific postsynaptic receptors. Through a second messenger system, these receptors can amplify the postsynaptic response of the first neurotransmitter. The combinations of interactions are vast and provide a mechanism for the dynamic "fine tuning" of synaptic sensitivity.

Synaptic Integration

SINGLE NEURONS

The CNS integrates neuronal signals at all levels of organization, from molecular modulation at the synapse to convergence and divergence of the multisynaptic neuronal pathways.

Rarely is a single EPSP of sufficient magnitude to generate an action potential in the postsynaptic neuron. EPSPs and IPSPs spread passively over the neuronal membrane and are summated both spatially and temporally. When the summated membrane potential at the initial segment of the axon reaches threshold, the neuron generates an action potential (see Figs. 3–10 and 3–11).

As a *postsynaptic potential (PSP)* spreads over the membrane of the dendritic tree and soma, it becomes attenuated and gradually dissipates. The more peripheral the origin of the PSP on the dendritic tree, the greater its attenuation when it reaches the soma.

If the receptive surfaces of the dendritic tree and soma are viewed as a chain of ten equal compartments (Fig. 4–5A), a theoretical pattern for an EPSP generated in each compartment and

FIGURE 4-5

A. Diagrammatic representation of the transformation of the soma and dendritic receptive surfaces of a neuron into a chain of ten equal compartments.

B. Graphs of computed excitatory postsynaptic potentials (EPSPs) occurring in compartment 1 obtained with this compartmental model. Synaptic currents generated in compartments 1, 4, and 8 provided the respective computed graphs for the EPSPs.

C, A plot of shape indices for computed EPSPs such as those in *B.* EPSPs generated in each compartment have characteristic features in shape when they reach the soma, compartment 1 (time to peak and duration of half-width value).

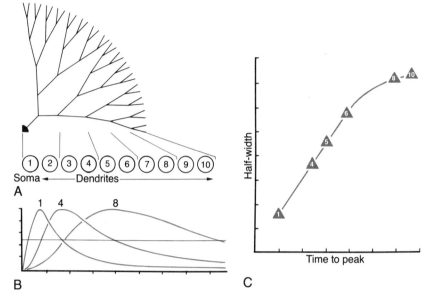

EPSPs generated closer to the soma have shorter times to peak and briefer half-width values than those generated farther out on the dendritic tree.

Note: Scales are in units of the dimensionless ratio, t/τ. (Adapted, with permission, from W. Rall, R. E. Burke, T. G. Smith, et al., J. Neurophysiol., 30: 1169–1193, 1967.)

measured at the soma can be calculated (Fig. 4–5*A* and *B*). Each compartment generates EPSPs with unique shape indices for *time-to-peak* (i.e., the time required for an EPSP to reach its peak) and *duration of half-width* (i.e., the duration of the EPSP measured between the points on the rising and falling phases which are one-half peak amplitude) (Fig. 4–5*B* and *C*). From the ratio of the shape indices, it is possible to predict the origin of EPSPs (see Fig. 4–5*C*).

Several generalizations can be made from this model. EPSPs generated in different compartments of the dendritic tree have different shape indices when they reach the soma. The closer a synapse is to the soma, the "faster" the shape indices of the PSP (i.e., a shorter time-to-peak and a shorter half-width). Conversely, the more distal the synapse, the "slower" the shape indices. A postsynaptic event in the distal part of the dentritic tree will therefore have a longer duration and lower amplitude than one closer to the initial segment of the axon.

STRATEGIC PLACEMENT OF INHIBITORY SYNAPSES

The magnitude of an IPSP will vary with the resting potential of the neuron. Most inhibitory synapses increase the conductance of either potassium or chloride. The Nernst potentials for potassium and chloride are close to the "normal" resting potentials (−90 mV and −75 mV, respectively, see Equation 3-2). If the membrane resting potential is more positive than the Nernst potential for that ion or if it is partially depolarized from EPSPs, the effect of the IPSP is greater. For example, at a resting potential of −70 mV, the increased chloride conductance cannot make the membrane potential more negative than −75 mV, or a maximum change of −5 mV. If, however, the resting potential were −60 mV, an increased chloride conductance could change the potential as much as −15 mV (from −60 mV to near −75 mV).

An IPSP-induced increase in the chloride conductance of an area of the membrane effectively "short-circuits" the passive spread of an EPSP across that area. However, if the inhibitory synapse is located more distally on the dendritic tree than the excitatory synapse, it will have little effect in inhibiting the excitation. To be effective, an inhibitory synapse must be located between the excitatory input it is designed to inhibit and the initial segment of the axon. Specific examples of the regional distribution of synaptic input to motor neurons are discussed in Chapter 14.

REPETITIVE FIRING

When the initial segment of the axon reaches threshold, a single action potential is generated and the neuron becomes refractory for 1 to 2 msec (Fig. 3–17). If, however, the EPSPs responsible for the depolarization are of long duration (i.e., those with ion conductance changes coupled to second messenger systems), they may persist for several seconds or longer. As soon as the initial segment is no longer in the absolute refractory state (1 to 2 msec), the persisting EPSP will trigger another action potential (see Fig. 3–17).

A prolonged EPSP translates into a volley of action potentials, each separated in time by milliseconds. This phenomenon of an EPSP persisting for a longer time than the refractory period of the neuron and then generating additional action potentials is often called *synaptic after-discharge.*

A large or prolonged depolarization of a neuron will never produce an increased action potential. An action potential can only approach and never exceed the Nernst potential for sodium. A large depolarization of a neuron produces a volley of action potentials fired in rapid succession. Therefore, neuronal communication is frequency modulated as opposed to amplitude modulated.

Many neurons have resting potentials at or near the threshold. These neurons may discharge repetitively, with little or no additional stimulus. Large numbers of neurons are transmitting impulses continuously in the brain, even during deep sleep and coma, unless the individual is "brain dead". For these neurons, a change in basal firing frequency often carries the significant message.

Theoretically, nearly every neuron in the CNS is directly or indirectly connected with every other neuron. Hence, inhibitory circuits within the nervous system are as important as excitatory pathways. If it were not for inhibition, a single sensory stimulus could trigger a cascade of firing involving every neuron. To a degree, this is what happens to regions of the brain during some forms of epileptic seizure. A jacksonian seizure starts with a focal cortical discharge, and the "excited" area spreads over the cortex in an uncontrolled fashion.

Another factor restraining uncontrolled neuronal discharge is fatigue. Maintaining a resting potential requires energy. Up to 70% of the brain's ATP is used to maintain this potential. With prolonged stimulation, ATP and neuro-transmitter stores are consumed at a rate faster than they are replaced. When this occurs, the neuronal firing rate will diminish.

PRESYNAPTIC MODULATION

In addition to "modulating" synaptic activity through intrinsic molecular mechanisms, the effectiveness of a synapse can be indirectly modified by "modulating" neurons forming axoaxonal synapses on the presynaptic axon terminal (Fig. 4–6). This presynaptic modulation can lead to either *inhibition* or *facilitation* of the excitatory presynaptic neuron as illustrated. The effect of the modulating neuron is determined by the nature of the receptors for its neurotransmitter.

In the illustration of *presynaptic inhibition* (Fig. 4–6, lower left), the axoaxonal synapse of the modulating neuron has reduced calcium channel conductance through a second messenger system, thus decreasing the magnitude of the inward calcium current produced by the action potential of the excitatory neuron. Calcium influx is the trigger for neurotransmitter release. Hence, as calcium influx is reduced, so too is the amount of transmitter released. The EPSP is also reduced—less transmitter released, fewer postsynaptic receptors activated (see Fig. 4–6).

Another mechanism of presynaptic inhibition operates through the activation of chloride channels. If chloride conductance is increased (refer to Equation 3-8), the degree of depolarization of the axon terminal by the action potential is reduced. Because the number of calcium channels activated is proportional to the change in membrane potential, a reduced change in potential activates fewer calcium channels and thereby reduces the influx of calcium.

In *presynaptic facilitation* (see Fig. 4–6, lower right), the axoaxonal synapse of the modulating neuron has blocked or inactivated potassium channels in the presynaptic terminal of the excitatory neuron through a second messenger system. Because potassium conductance is essential for the rapid repolarization of the membrane, blocking potassium channels prolongs the time required for the membrane to repolarize. Notice the longer, more attenuated action potential (see Fig. 4–6). The prolonged period of depolarization increases the calcium influx that, in turn, increases the amount of neurotransmitter released by the excitatory neuron; thereby, the EPSP increases.

In both examples, *presynaptic inhibition* and *presynaptic facilitation*, the modulating neuron

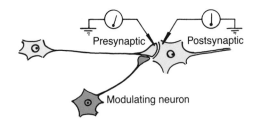

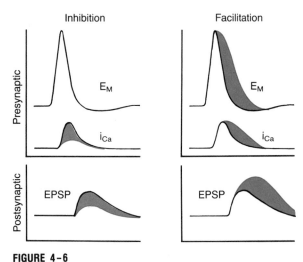

Inhibition   Facilitation

Presynaptic

Postsynaptic

FIGURE 4-6

Presynaptic inhibition and presynaptic facilitation. A modulating neuron forming an axoaxonal synapse can alter the effectiveness of an excitatory synapse. In cases in which this effect increases the performance of the synapse, it is *presynaptic facilitation*. When the effect hinders the performance, it is known as *presynaptic inhibition*.

In the illustration, electrodes record from both the excitatory presynaptic terminal and the postsynaptic neuron (top). If the modulating neuron is inhibitory, events illustrated in the lower left may be seen. The presynaptic action potential is unaltered, but the calcium current is markedly reduced. The reduction in calcium current leads to a corresponding reduction in the release of the neurotransmitter. The result is a diminished EPSP.

When the modulating neuron is facilitory, events illustrated in the lower right may be observed. The duration of the presynaptic action potential is prolonged, with a corresponding attenuation in the calcium current. The increased calcium influx triggers the release of an increased amount of neurotransmitter. The result is an increased EPSP.

Other examples of presynaptic modulation exist—these two serve only as illustrations. The message conveyed to a postsynaptic neuron at a synapse is not always the same—often it is modulated presynaptically by other neurons. (See text for further discussion.)

has no direct effect on the postsynaptic neuron (see Fig. 4-6). The effect is one of modulating the incoming excitatory signal, either by inhibiting or facilitating the release of neurotransmitter at that synapse.

NEURONAL CIRCUITS

The CNS is composed of many specific circuits or pathways. Information is transmitted by groups of neurons signaling in concert or in a particular temporal-spatial pattern. For example, the signal for the voluntary flexion of the lower extremity originates in the cerebral cortex and travels to the spinal cord via the corticospinal tract. Once in the spinal cord, the axons synapse with interneurons that excite motor neurons innervating the flexor muscles and synapse with other interneurons that inhibit motor neurons to the extensor muscles.

These neuronal signals have a specific spatial and temporal pattern. Another level of organization has been achieved, from the temporal and spatial summation of PSPs on individual neurons to the temporal and spatial discharge patterns produced by large numbers of neurons.

The synaptic connections between the neurons that compose a CNS pathway are very complex. The detailed circuitry is not well documented. However, it is helpful to visualize these very

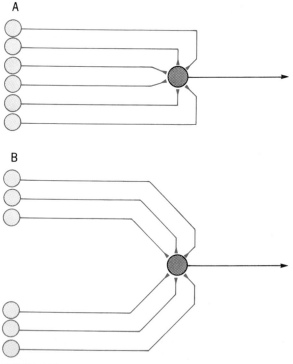

FIGURE 4-7

Convergence. *A*, A number of neurons from a single pathway or source (red) converge on a single neuron.

B, A number of neurons from more than one pathway or source (red) converge on a single neuron.

complex patterns in terms of basic and highly simplified models. These models and the concepts they convey are utilized in the discussion of specific pathways in this text.

CONVERGENCE

When a single neuron is the focused target of a number of neurons, it is called *convergence* (Fig. 4–7). The simplest example is illustrated in Figure 4–7*A* in which the axons of six neurons converge on a single neuron. Convergence can also occur when a single neuron forms multiple synapses with a single target neuron. The probability is greater of exciting a postsynaptic neuron when there is convergence. *Convergence* also describes neurons from several different pathways focusing on a single target, as in Figure 4–7*B*. The spinal motor neuron is a good example; it receives synaptic input from a number of pathways—corticospinal, vestibulospinal, and reticulospinal, to name a few, along with the interneurons of the spinal cord.

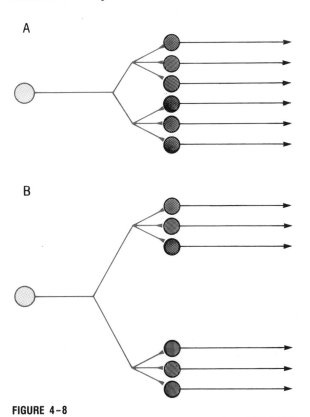

FIGURE 4–8

Divergence. *A,* A single neuron (red) projects to a number of other neurons within a single nucleus or locus.

B, A single neuron (red) projects to a number of other neurons in more than one nucleus or locus.

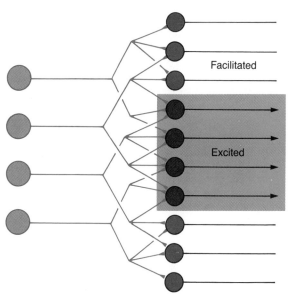

FIGURE 4–9

Multiple synaptic input can excite or facilitate neurons. When arriving at the same time, the synaptic input from the neurons (red) is sufficient to excite the neurons in the shaded area. Above and below the excited area, the neuronal input is insufficient to cause firing, but the excitatory postsynaptic potentials generated will raise the resting potentials closer to threshold values and, hence, facilitate them. The facilitation, however, is transient and will decay with time.

DIVERGENCE

When a group of neurons is innervated by a single neuron, the pattern is one of *divergence* (Fig. 4–8*A*). This pattern provides a mechanism for signal amplification. The signal from a single neuron of the corticospinal tract may excite as many as 100 interneurons. *Divergence* also describes the innervation of several groups of neurons by a single neuron (Fig. 4–8*B*). With the corticospinal tract used as an example, branches (collaterals) from axons of the corticospinal tract terminate in the cerebellar relay nuclei of the brain stem and on the interneurons of the spinal cord. The signal generated in the cerebral cortex has diverged to spinal and cerebellar targets.

EXCITATION AND FACILITATION

EPSPs depolarize the membrane. If the summated depolarization reaches threshold, an action potential is generated; if the summated depolarization remains subthreshold, the neuron is said to be *facilitated.* It will take less additional stimulation to trigger an action potential as long as the EPSP persists. In Figure 4–9, those neurons in the shaded area are sufficiently *excited* (three synapses, in this example) to generate action potentials. In contrast, those above and below are *facilitated,* having received one or two synapses they are depolarized but to subthreshold levels.

INHIBITORY CIRCUITS

Inhibition is as important to the processing of information in the CNS as excitation. Not only does inhibition prevent a massive, uncontrolled spread of neuronal excitation, it functions to "sharpen" the signals generated by excitatory neurons. Several inhibitory circuits are illustrated

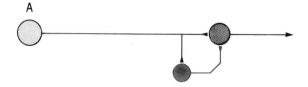

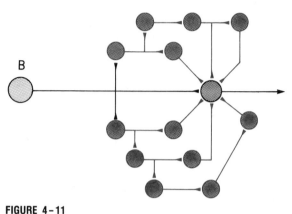

FIGURE 4 – 11

Signal amplification and prolongation. *A,* Stimulation of an excitatory interneuron (red) will provide a second excitatory input to the stimulated neuron, arriving by approximately 0.5 to 1.0 msec after the primary stimulation owing to the synaptic delay.

B, When more interneurons are involved, the signal amplification can be quite prolonged. In this example, the stimulated neuron would receive excitatory input for several milliseconds from the recruitment of a large number of excitatory interneurons (red). Thus, a single input can be amplified and prolonged from the recruitment of interneurons.

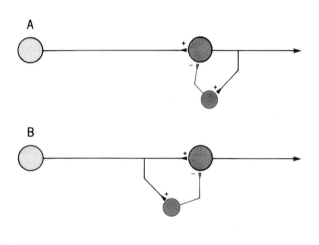

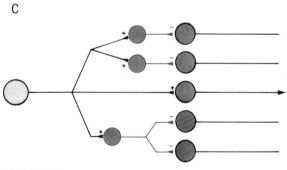

FIGURE 4 – 10

Inhibitory circuits. *A,* Feedback inhibition: a collateral from the stimulated neuron excites an inhibitory interneuron (red). This effect reduces the firing rate of highly stimulated neurons and is similar to the Renshaw cell inhibitory loop on the lower motor neurons.

B, The excitatory neuron also excites an inhibitory interneuron (red). Because of the synaptic delay, the inhibitory signal will arrive after the primary excitatory input.

C, Lateral inhibition. The excitatory neuron also stimulates one or more inhibitory interneurons (red). These inhibit the neurons surrounding the stimulated neuron. This is a feature of many projection pathways, and the effect is to increase the contrast of the projected signal.

in Figure 4 – 10. In *feedback inhibition,* an axon collateral from the excited postsynaptic neuron stimulates an inhibitory interneuron. This, in turn, inhibits the excitatory postsynaptic neuron.

A similar circuit exists in the spinal cord, with collaterals of lower motor neurons innervating small inhibitory interneurons, the Renshaw cells. The inhibition, arriving at the postsynaptic neuron after the initial volley of action potentials, turns off the excited neuron, blocks any synaptic after-discharge, and inhibits further stimulation for the duration of the IPSP (Fig. 4 – 10*A*). If the presynaptic excitatory neuron stimulates the inhibitory interneuron, the effect is similar but more rapid. Only one synaptic delay instead of two occurs (Fig. 4 – 10*B*).

Lateral inhibition occurs when an excitatory signal is relayed through a postsynaptic neuron and when collaterals from the presynaptic axon excite inhibitory interneurons. These, in turn,

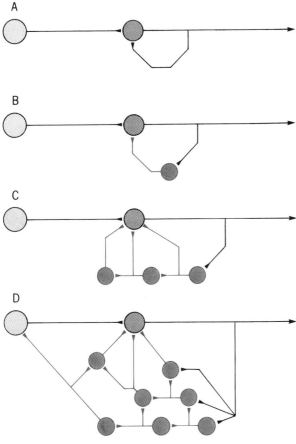

FIGURE 4-12

Feedback or reverberatory loops. *A*, The simplest form of feedback loop is a collateral from the stimulated neuron feeding back on itself.

B, *C*, and *D*, These represent feedback loops of increasing complexity and involve excitatory interneurons (red) feeding back on the stimulated neuron and in *D*, on the excitatory neuron as well. Such loops serve to prolong the firing and the level of excitation for extended periods.

inhibit adjacent postsynaptic neurons. This pattern is quite common in topographically organized ascending sensory pathways, with tight point-to-point representation. The inhibition of surrounding relay neurons serves to increase the "contrast" of the projected excitatory signal. A number of examples of this type of circuit in ascending sensory pathways are known.

AMPLIFICATION CIRCUITS

Signal amplification, in its simplest form, occurs when an excitatory interneuron excites the same

postsynaptic neuron (Fig. 4-11*A*). The end result is two excitatory stimuli separated temporally by the duration of one synaptic delay, 1 to 2 msec. If more than one interneuron is involved (Fig. 4-11*B*) the effect can be quite prolonged. The postsynaptic neuron receives a number of excitatory stimuli over a period of 4 to 5 msec.

Feedback or *reverberating loops* also prolong the period of excitation of a postsynaptic neuron. In theory, this could trigger the perpetual firing of a neuronal circuit. In the simplest form, an axon collateral from the postsynaptic neuron feeds back on itself (Fig. 4-12*A*). Feedback loops of increasing complexity are represented in Figure 4-12*B*, *C*, and *D*. With these reverberating loops, a single stimulus can initiate a very prolonged period of continuous firing and excitation of the postsynaptic neuron (dark gray).

SUGGESTED READING

Augustine, G. J., M. P. Charlton, and S. J. Smith (1987). Calcium action in synaptic transmitter release. Ann. Rev. Neurosci., 10: 633-693.

A good review of the literature and our understanding of the molecular processes involved in neurotransmitter release.

Catterall, W. A. (1988). Structure and function of voltage sensitive ion channels. Science, 242: 50-61.

A excellent review of the molecular biology of the voltage-sensitive sodium, calcium, and potassium channels in excitable cells. This article reviews studies of the structure of the ion channels, including the subunits, their functional organization, and the post-translational modifications of the channel proteins. Concepts from molecular biology, biophysics, and pharmacology are drawn together for the proposed structural models of channel function.

Guyton, A. C. (1986). *Textbook of Medical Physiology*, 7th Edition. W. B. Saunders Co., Philadelphia.

Chapters 46 and 47 of this basic medical physiology textbook contain excellent material pertinent to the subject matter in this chapter.

Rall, W. (1977). Core conductor theory and cable properties of neurons. In *Handbook of Physiology*, Section I, The Nervous System, Volume I, Cellular Biology of Neurons, Part 1. E. R. Kandel (Editor). American Physiological Society, Bethesda, MD, pp. 39-97.

An excellent but highly technical review of theoretical and experimental studies of postsynaptic potentials and their relation to the cable theory of the neuronal dendritic tree.

Trends in Neuroscience, Volume 11, No. 10, October, 1988. (Special Issue) Calcium and Neuronal Excitability.

This special issue of *Trends in Neuroscience* is devoted to a collection of review articles covering various aspects of the role of calcium in the neuron, especially as it relates to mechanisms of neurotransmitter release.

Chapter

5

Chemical Transmission

Reappraisal of Traditional Concepts of Chemical Synaptic Transmission

Until the late 1970's, it generally was accepted that each neuron utilized one and only one neurotransmitter. However, today, the concept of a single neuron having more than one chemical transmitter is well established. Multiple transmitters are more likely the rule rather than the exception.

At most synapses, a principal neurotransmitter activates an ion channel directly, or indirectly via a second messenger system, thereby producing an electrical event postsynaptically, i.e., an excitatory postsynaptic potential (EPSP) or an inhibitory postsynaptic potential (IPSP). The second or third neurotransmitter generally functions as a modulator of the activity of the primary neurotransmitter, from facilitating or inhibiting the presynaptic and postsynaptic effects of the primary neurotransmitter to initiating messenger ribonucleic acid (mRNA) transcription for the synthesis of specific peptide or protein molecules.

Central nervous system (CNS) neurons receive signals from thousands of synaptic terminals, representing input from many different neurons. Although a single neuron sends a specific message or combination of messages, it receives a variety of neurochemical signals. Hence, the receptive mechanisms of a single neuron must be as varied as the messages they receive.

Many neurons have *autoreceptors*, receptors on

the presynaptic membrane sensitive to one or more of the neurotransmitters released by that neuron. Autoreceptors generally function to inhibit the release of additional neurotransmitter. Sometimes, they facilitate release or raise the rate of synthesis of a neurotransmitter by altering the kinetic properties of rate-limiting enzymes or increasing the availability of substrate.

Neurotransmitter release may be regulated, in part, by *synapsin-I*. This protein associates with the synaptic vesicles and is the substrate for both cAMP-dependent and calcium-dependent protein kinases. Autoreceptor-coupled second messenger systems can activate both kinases.

Neurotransmitters are grouped into seven categories: (1) *acetylcholine;* (2) *catecholamines*, dopamine, norepinephrine and epinephrine; (3) *indole amines*, serotonin or 5-hydroxytryptamine; (4) *histamine;* (5) *inhibitory amino acids*, glycine and gamma aminobutyric acid (GABA); (6) *excitatory amino acids*, glutamate and aspartate; and (7) *peptides*, including the opioid peptides, substance-P, neurotensin, and thyrotropin-releasing hormone (TRH).

Neurotransmitter receptors are grouped into two classes: (1) *ion channel–coupled receptors* and (2) *second messenger–coupled receptors*. *Ion channel–coupled receptors* bind the ligand (neurotransmitter) and undergo an immediate conformational change, which opens the ion channel, generating an EPSP or IPSP. These receptors have a short latency (μsecs) and a short duration of response (1 to 2 msec). *Second messenger–coupled receptors* bind the ligand and activate a second messenger system, usually through a molecular transducer, a G-protein. These receptors have latencies of 100 to 250 msec and durations of response that can last from milliseconds to minutes or even longer.

Modulators, Signal Transducers, and Second Messengers

At the molecular level, the nervous system is very malleable and is continually "fine tuned" or *modulated*. Ion channels and chemical receptors are frequently modified, rendering them more sensitive or less sensitive in accord with the physiological state of the neuron. Second messenger systems initiate many of these biochemical changes and adapt the nervous system to conditions of the moment.

PROTEIN PHOSPHORYLATION

Reversible protein phosphorylation is a common mechanism of molecular modulation and produces conformational changes in membrane proteins, such as ion channels and receptor molecules. These changes often alter function. They modify a receptor's affinity for a ligand, the sensitivity of a voltage-gated ion channel, or the kinetic properties of an enzyme. Four ingredients are essential: (1) a *protein kinase* to catalyze the phosphorylation, (2) a source of *high energy phosphate* (ATP), (3) a *target protein*, and (4) a specific *protein phosphatase* to reverse the process.

We know less about the protein phosphatases. However, if phosphorylation turns a process on, a phosphatase must play an equal role in turning it off. Second messenger systems activate some protein phosphatases and *phosphatase inhibitors*. A good example of a phosphatase inhibitor is DARPP-32, a small protein from neurons with dopamine receptors coupled to the activation of adenyl cyclase. Phosphorylation of DARPP-32 by a cAMP-dependent protein kinase transforms an inactive protein into a potent phosphatase inhibitor. Thus, a second messenger system can activate a specific protein kinase and the protein kinase, in turn, activates a phosphatase inhibitor. The net effect is an amplification of the initial signal.

G-PROTEINS AS SIGNAL TRANSDUCERS

The guanyl nucleotide binding proteins, or *G-proteins*, link incoming messages (activated receptors) to effectors (second messenger systems). G-proteins probably function as signal transducers for all second messenger–coupled receptors. This mechanism provides an additional dimension to signal amplification at the molecular level, with one receptor coupled to as many as ten or 20 G-proteins.

G-proteins are heterotrimers, composed of three subunits (α, β, and γ). The 39-52 kD α-subunit is the specific signal transducer. This α-subunit contains the guanyl nucleotide binding sites, is activated by the neurotransmitter receptor, and in turn stimulates the second messenger system. The tightly linked β- and γ-subunits are similar in molecular structure from one G-protein to the next. The α-subunit is reversibly coupled to the β-subunit. The hydrophobic properties of the γ-subunit anchor the G-protein complex to the inner surface of the unit membrane (Fig. 5–1).

G-protein specificity for second messenger sys-

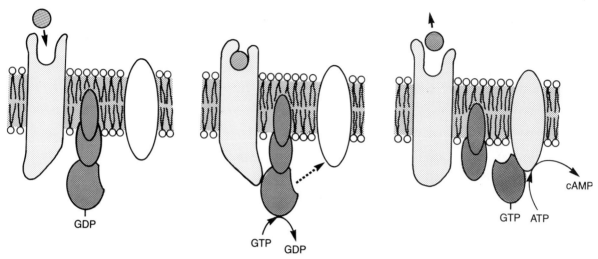

FIGURE 5-1

Guanyl nucleotide binding protein (G-protein) as a signal transducer. An example is illustrated of a G-protein linking an activated receptor to a second messenger system. Excitation of the receptor leads to the formation of cAMP. In the resting state (left), the G-protein (G$_S$) is situated between the membrane-spanning receptor and the adenyl cyclase (effector). The γ-subunit anchors the G-protein to the inner surface of the membrane, and guanosine diphosphate (GDP) is bound to the α-subunit.

The binding of the neurotransmitter to the receptor (center) activates the receptor, which in turn promotes the displacement of GDP with guanosine triphosphate (GTP). The GTP · G$_\alpha$ complex dissociates from the membrane-bound G$_{\beta-\gamma}$ complex and activates the adjacent adenyl cyclase (right). The activated adenyl cyclase catalyzes the formation of cAMP.

When the intrinsic GTPase activity of the G$_\alpha$-subunit hydrolyzes the GTP to GDP, the inactive GDP · G$_\alpha$ complex rapidly reassociates with the G$_{\beta-\gamma}$ complex and the system returns to the resting state (left).

tems resides in the α-subunit. For example, G$_S$-proteins activate adenyl cyclase activity and a cAMP-dependent protein kinase; G$_I$-proteins inhibit adenyl cyclase activity; and G$_P$-proteins activate phospholipase C and the phosphatidylinositol system. The G$_K$-proteins directly activate K$^+$ channels. The brain has a high level of another G-protein known as G$_O$ (for "other")—a molecular transducer with undefined receptors and effectors.

In the "resting" state, guanosine diphosphate (GDP) is bound to the α-subunit of the G-protein heterotrimer (GDP · G). Activation of the neurotransmitter receptor accelerates the displacement of GDP with GTP, forming an activated GTP · G$_\alpha$ complex. The GTP · G$_\alpha$ complex separates from the β-γ subunit and activates the effector. The intrinsic GTPase activity of the G$_\alpha$-subunit then hydrolyzes the GTP, deactivating the GTP · G$_\alpha$ complex, leading to the re-formation of the inactive GDP · G complex (see Fig. 5-1).

ADENYL CYCLASE AND cAMP-DEPENDENT PROTEIN KINASES

Adenyl cyclase, a transmembrane glycoprotein, catalyzes the synthesis of the active second mes-

senger, *cAMP* (adenosine-3',5'-monophosphate), from ATP. In the nervous system, cAMP functions exclusively to activate cAMP-dependent protein kinases. A cyclic nucleotide phosphodiesterase terminates the activity of cAMP by converting it to the inactive AMP (adenosine-5'-monophosphate). Activation of adenyl cyclase is a multistep process (see Fig. 5-1). For the β-adrenergic receptor, this process can amplify the signal 30-fold, because each receptor activates up to 30 G$_S$-proteins. In the brain, the calcium/calmodulin system can also activate adenyl cyclase.

The G$_I$-proteins inactivate adenyl cyclase in one of two ways. In one system, the GTP · G$_{I\alpha}$ complex inactivates the enzyme directly; in the other, the G$_{I\beta,\gamma}$ complex inhibits the activation of adenyl cyclase by competing for the previously activated GTP · G$_{S\alpha}$. This may explain why many receptors coupled to the inhibition of adenyl cyclase are more effective after another neurotransmitter system has activated the adenyl cyclase. G$_{I\alpha}$ is also a substrate for protein kinase C, and the phosphorylated G$_{I\alpha}$-subunit has less inhibitory activity.

The brain cyclic nucleotide phosphodiesterases represent a heterogeneous population of enzymes. The most abundant form is activated by a calcium/calmodulin–dependent protein kinase but is inhibited by a cAMP-dependent protein kinase. Activation of adenyl cyclase has a cascade effect. Activation of cAMP-dependent protein kinases can open ion channels, converting the post-synaptic chemical signal to an electrical event. The cAMP-dependent protein kinases also inhibit cyclic nucleotide phosphodiesterase activity. The half-life of cAMP is thus extended, and the initial event prolonged. Many neurotransmitters have receptors that can either activate or inhibit adenyl cyclase. The response is dependent on the specific receptor rather than on the neurotransmitter.

PHOSPHATIDYLINOSITOL TURNOVER

The phosphatidylinositols are an important source of second messengers for neurotransmitter systems. Of these, phosphatidylinositol-4,5-bisphosphate (PIP_2) is the most common (Fig. 5-2). These phospholipids have two long-chain fatty acids attached to a glycerol backbone, with phosphoinositol in the 3 position. In the brain, 80% contain the 18-carbon stearic acid and the 20-carbon arachidonic acid esterified to carbons 1 and 2 of the glycerol, respectively.

The metabolically active diacylglycerol (DG), specifically, 1-stearyl-2-arachidonyl-*sn*-glycerol, is attached to the inner leaflet of the cell membrane. After an ATP-dependent phosphorylation, DG becomes phosphatidic acid (PA). PA reacts with cytidine triphosphate (CTP) to form the cytidine nucleotide complex, CDP · PA. Inositol combines with CDP · PA to form phosphatidylinositol (PI). With a two-step phosphorylation of the inositol ring, PI becomes, sequentially, phosphatidylinositol-4-phosphate (PIP) and PIP_2 (Fig. 5-3).

Phospholipase C, activated by a G-protein, cleaves PIP_2 to DG and inositol-1,4,5-triphosphate (IP_3). Both DG and IP_3 act as second messengers. The soluble IP_3 mobilizes intracellular calcium stores and the membrane-bound DG activates protein kinase C (PKC), a potent regulator of neuronal activity. IP_3 may mobilize some of the calcium required for full activation of PKC. In addition, calcium mobilization may activate calcium/calmodulin-dependent protein kinases (see Fig. 5-3).

Phosphorylation of DG to PA inactivates DG. A 5'-inositol phosphatase inactivates IP_3, forming inositol-1,4-diphosphate (IP_2), which rapidly becomes inositol. Both the DG (now as PA) and inositol are used for the resynthesis of PIP_2. Diacylglycerol lipase can also inactivate DG, with the formation of 1-stearyl monoglyceride and arachidonic acid. This pathway provides a source of

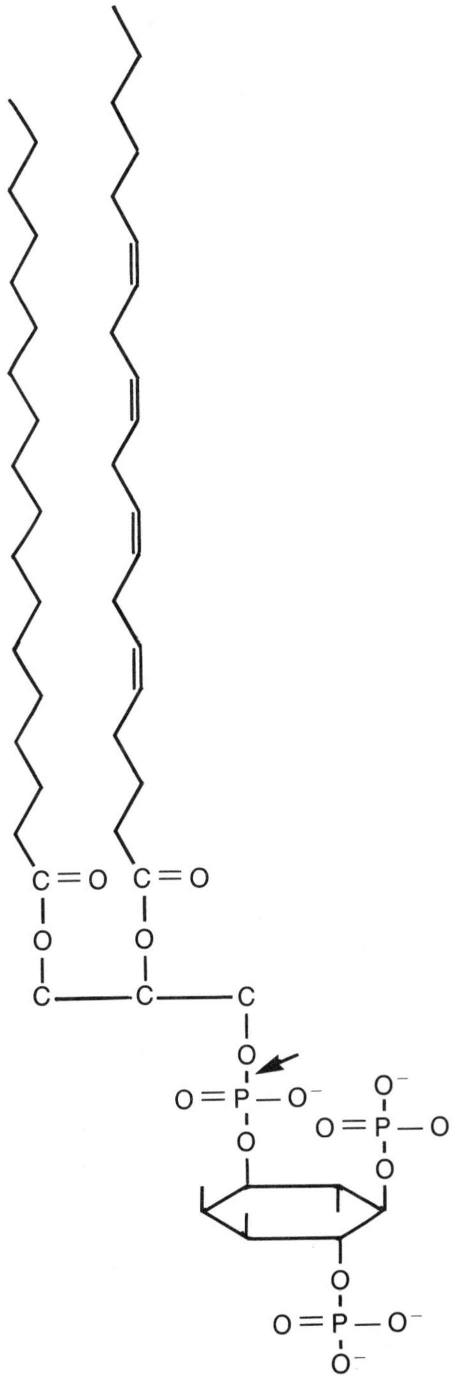

FIGURE 5-2

Structure of phosphatidylinositol-4,5-bisphosphate (PIP_2). PIP_2 is a phosphodiester of diacylglycerol and inositol-1,4,5-triphosphate. Esterified to the 1-position of the glycerol is the saturated, 18-carbon stearic acid and esterified to the 2-position is the unsaturated, 20-carbon arachidonic acid. This forms *sn*-1-stearyl-2-arachidonyl-glycerol-3-phosphoinositol-4,5-bisphosphate (PIP_2). The phosphatidylinositols are quite homogenous, with nearly 80% containing stearic and arachidonic acid esters as illustrated.

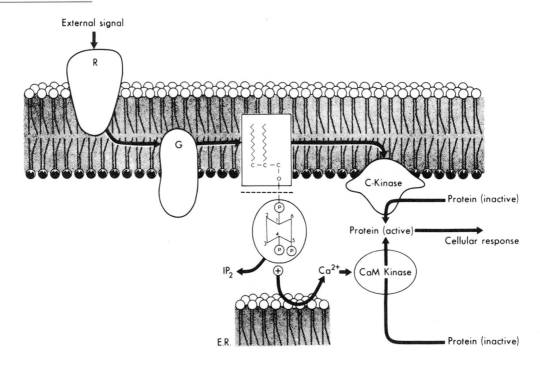

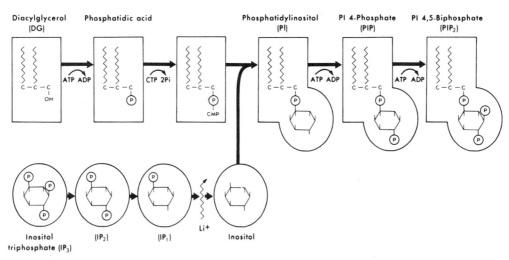

FIGURE 5-3

Proposed model for the role of phosphatidylinositol in receptor activation. Binding of a neurotransmitter to its receptor (R) activates a G-protein (G) that requires guanosine triphosphate (GTP). The G-protein then activates phospholipase C (not illustrated), which splits the phosphatidylinositol-4,5-bisphosphate (PIP$_2$) to inositol-1,4,5-triphosphate (IP$_3$) and diacylglycerol (DG) (site of cleavage indicated by ----------). IP$_3$ releases Ca^{2+} ions from internal membrane stores. The Ca^{2+} ions then combine with calmodulin (CaM) to activate protein kinases or participate in other intracellular events. DG activates protein kinase C (C-kinase), which can also activate proteins to produce further intracellular events.

Resynthesis of PIP$_2$ involves the merging of two cycles that are shown as enlargements of the DG area (rectangles) and the IP$_3$ area (circles). In the circle series, there is stepwise removal of the three phosphate groups to form first, inositol-1,4-diphosphate (IP$_2$), second, inositol-1-phosphate (IP$_1$), and finally, inositol. In the rectangle series, DG is converted to a phosphatidic acid by the addition of a phosphate group and then, by the addition of cytosine triphosphate, to the cytosine nucleotide complex CDP · DG.

The products of the two cycles, inositol and CDP · DG, combine to produce phosphatidylinositol (PI), which is phosphorylated to phosphatidylinositol-4-phosphate (PIP). Phosphorylation of PIP regenerates phosphatidylinositol-4,5-bisphosphate (PIP$_2$). (Reproduced with permission from P. L. McGeer, J. C. Eccles, and E. G. McGeer, *Molecular Neurobiology of the Mammalian Brain*, 2nd Edition, Plenum Press, New York, 1987.)

arachidonic acid, although most of the arachidonic acid generated in the brain is through the activation of phospholipase A_2, which cleaves the arachidonic acid group directly from PIP_2 or phosphatidylcholine.

Both PI and PIP can be split by phospholipase C, forming DG and either IP or IP_2. Neither IP nor IP_2 mobilizes calcium, and both are rapidly dephosphorylated to inositol. The DG formed activates *protein kinase C (PKC)* if sufficient free calcium is available. In some systems, photoreceptors for example, IP_3 exists in a cyclic form $(c1:2,4,5\text{-}IP_3)$. Inactivation is through the action of a phosphodiesterase. The importance of the cyclic inositol phosphates in bioregulatory functions is largely unknown.

PROTEIN KINASE C (PKC)

High concentrations of PKC exist in the CNS. This membrane-associated enzyme plays an important role in the modulation of neuronal activity, from the regulation of calcium, potassium, and chloride channels to the regulation of the amount of neurotransmitter released during synaptic transmission.

DG, produced from the phospholipase C–catalyzed cleavage of PIP_2, activates PKC. For full activation, PKC also requires phosphatidylserine, which is a major component of nerve cell membranes and not rate limiting, and calcium. The activated form of neuronal PKC remains in close association with the inner surface of the cell membrane, adjacent to ion channels and receptors, which are substrate proteins for this kinase (see Fig. 5 – 3).

CALCIUM/CALMODULIN-DEPENDENT PROTEIN KINASES

Nerve terminals and postsynaptic membrane areas are rich in a calcium-binding protein of 148 amino acids—*calmodulin*. When an action potential depolarizes the nerve terminal, there is an influx of calcium ions through voltage-gated calcium channels and calcium binds to calmodulin. Activation of one molecule of calmodulin requires four calcium ions. Once activated, the calcium/calmodulin complex can stimulate several specific calcium/calmodulin–dependent protein kinases, some membrane bound and others soluble.

Calcium/calmodulin–dependent protein kinases are important for the exocytotic release of neurotransmitter, the modulation of neurotransmitter synthesis, long-term potentiation, and other metabolic functions associated with in-creased activity and the need for additional metabolic energy sources.

MODULATION THROUGH GENE TRANSCRIPTION

Neurotransmitter systems, besides producing electrical changes (IPSPs and EPSPs) and altering specific proteins (receptors, ion channels, and enzymes) via second messenger systems, play an active role in the regulation of gene expression. Neurotransmitter-activated second messenger systems can initiate or enhance the transcription of mRNAs for the synthesis of specific receptors, enzymes, ion channels, and other molecules involved in neuronal communication. This is the third and most complex dimension of neuronal communication, but one of major importance in the regulation of the synthesis of protein precursors of neuroactive peptides and in complex processes, such as learning and memory.

Cholinergic Transmission

Acetylcholine (ACh) is the principal neurotransmitter at the neuromuscular junction, the peripheral ganglia of the autonomic nervous system, numerous autonomic effector organs, and many of the synapses in the CNS. The cholinergic system is unique for two reasons. First, large numbers of cholinergic terminals are located outside the CNS and, second, certain exotic fish have very high concentrations of cholinergic synapses (e.g., in the electric organ of *Torpedo californica*). Because of these unique features, some of the pioneering work in the field of neurotransmitter chemistry was done on the cholinergic system. As new techniques evolved, studies included the more complex and heterogeneous CNS, verifying and expanding many earlier conclusions.

SYNTHESIS, STORAGE, AND RELEASE

ACh is synthesized in the axon terminal from the substrates choline and acetyl-coenzyme A (acetyl-CoA). Catalyzed by the enzyme, *choline acetyltransferase (ChAT)*, the acyl transfer reaction has apparent Michaelis constants (K_ms) of 1.0 mM for choline and 10 μM for acetyl-CoA. The enzyme, although synthesized in the cell body, is transported to the nerve terminal. Acetyl-CoA comes principally from the metabolism of glucose and secondarily from phospholipids. Normally, the *in vivo* availability of the enzyme and the availability of acetyl-CoA are not rate limiting.

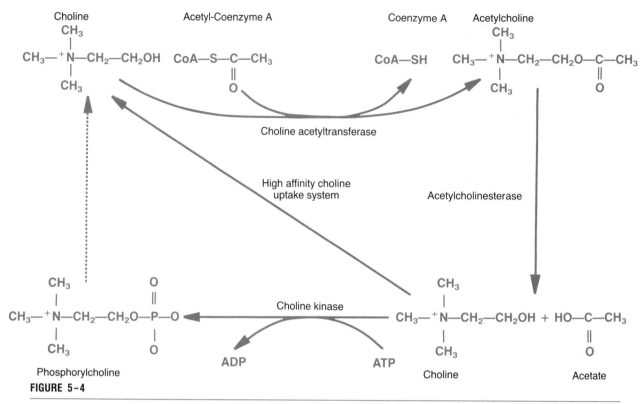

Choline acetyltransferase

High affinity choline uptake system

Acetylcholinesterase

Choline kinase

Phosphorylcholine

FIGURE 5–4

Principal steps in the biosynthesis and degradation of acetylcholine.

The availability of free choline regulates the rate of synthesis (Fig. 5–4).

Neurons do not synthesize choline. Because choline cannot cross the blood-brain barrier, the principal source of CNS choline is from the breakdown of the phospholipid, phosphatidylcholine. Cholinergic synapses are quite conservative and recycle over 50% of the choline. Following hydrolysis of ACh by acetylcholinesterase (see subsequent discussion), choline is taken up by the presynaptic terminal via a Na$^+$- and ATP-dependent *high affinity choline uptake system (HACU)*. Most cells and tissues, including neurons, have a low affinity choline uptake system, with K_ms ranging from 10 to 100 μM. However, cholinergic nerve terminals have an HACU with a K_m of 1 to 5 μM. Synaptic activity regulates the HACU. Greater stimulation increases the capacity of the HACU. After pharmacologically blocking the HACU, there is a corresponding decrease in both ACh synthesis and release.

ACh synthesis is in the cytoplasm of the axon terminal, and ACh is co-stored in synaptic vesicles with ATP. Two populations, or pools, of ACh-containing vesicles exist: (1) an active pool of vesicles that turn over rapidly and contain the newly synthesized ACh and (2) a reserve pool of vesicles that is used only when the demand for ACh exceeds the rate of synthesis.

When the action potential triggers the inward flow of calcium, there is a rapid (<200 μsec) exocytotic release of ACh. At rest, there is a slow, but constant release of ACh, in quantal units with each vesicle corresponding to one quantum and containing from 2000 to 10,000 molecules of ACh. First described for the neuromuscular synapse, this "quantal leak" phenomenon may be characteristic of central cholinergic synapses as well. At the neuromuscular synapse, each quantal release produces a miniature end-plate potential (MEPP), a depolarization of about 0.4 mV, or a miniature postsynaptic potential (MPSP) at other cholinergic synapses.

ACETYLCHOLINE RECEPTORS

The postsynaptic response depends on the properties of the postsynaptic receptor. For ACh, there are two families of receptors with quite different properties: the *nicotinic acetylcholine receptor (nAChR)* and the *muscarinic acetylcholine receptor (mAChR)*. The nAChRs are fast responding, ligand-gated ion channels with a short duration of activity (1 to 2 msec). The mAChRs couple to second messenger systems. They have long latencies (100 to 250 msec), and durations of activity measured in seconds.

NICOTINIC ACETYLCHOLINE RECEPTORS

Functionally, the nAChRs are more closely related to the $GABA_A$ receptor than to the mAChR. The nAChR has five subunits; two similar α-subunits; and single β-, γ- and δ-subunits (Fig. 5–5). All five subunits surround a central canal, the ion channel. Each α-subunit contains a binding site for ACh. When both binding sites are occupied, the ion channel opens, producing a rapid inward flow of cations (principally Na^+) with the generation of an EPSP. In the brain, at least four genes encode the α-subunit and two the β-subunit. The mRNAs for the α-subunits have a regional pattern of distribution in the CNS.

At least two subgroups of nAChRs (N_1-AChR and N_2-AChR) are known, with different patterns of distribution and pharmacological properties. N_1-AChRs, typified by those localized at the neuromuscular synapse, are activated by the agonist, phenyl trimethylammonium, reversibly blocked by D-tubocurarine, and irreversibly blocked by α-toxins from snake venoms (e.g., α-bungarotoxin). N_2-AChRs, typified by those localized at ganglionic synapses, are preferentially stimulated by the agonist, tetramethylammonium, and

blocked by the antagonists, trimethaphan and hexamethonium. They are resistant to the α-toxins.

MUSCARINIC ACETYLCHOLINE RECEPTORS

These 70 kDa receptor proteins are more closely related to the β-adrenergic receptors and other G-protein–coupled receptors than to nAChR. At least four genes encode the mAChRs and their mRNAs have regional patterns of distribution within the CNS.

Two classes of mAChRs exist, based on their binding properties. M_1-AChRs have a high affinity for pirenzepine, whereas M_2-AChRs have a low affinity for pirenzepine. The M_1-AChRs are typical of muscarinic receptors found in autonomic ganglia, and the M_2-AChRs are typical of those found on target organs of autonomic innervation (sweat glands, smooth muscle, and myocardium).

All mAChRs couple to a G-protein, and the nature of the G-protein determines the postsynaptic response. When coupled to one of the G_I-proteins, the inhibition of adenyl cyclase reduces the formation of cAMP. This response is more apparent when catecholamine stimulation of an adrenergic receptor has already activated the adenyl cyclase. When coupled to a G_P-protein, activation of phospholipase C leads to the hydrolysis of phosphatidylinositol; the mobiliza-

FIGURE 5–5

Structure of the nicotinic acetylcholine receptor. The receptor is a pentamere of five distinct subunits; α_1, α_2, β, γ, and δ. The γ-subunit may reside between the two α-subunits. The internal channel surrounded by the five subunits appears funnel-shaped, with the primary constriction at the membrane surface. Two α-toxin molecules bind to each receptor. Their binding surface primarily resides on the α-subunit, and these sites seem to be located near the outer perimeter of the molecule. The α-subunits also contain recognition sites for agonists, reversible antagonists, and coral lophotoxin. (Reproduced with permission from P. Taylor and J. H. Brown, Acetylcholine. In G., Siegel, B. Agranoff, R. W. Albers, and P. Molinoff (Editors), *Basic Neurochemistry*, 4th Edition, Raven Press, New York, 1989.)

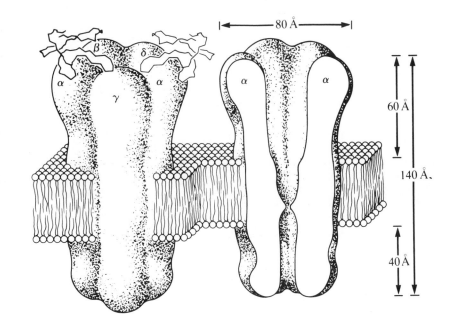

tion of Ca^{2+}; and the activation of Ca^{2+}-dependent protein kinases, including protein kinase C. When coupled to a G_K-protein, K^+ channels open and the membrane becomes hyperpolarized (e.g., mAChRs in the myocardium). The variety of second messenger systems coupled to muscarinic receptors makes generalizations difficult. Postsynaptic responses vary with the particular synapse or system.

CNS DISTRIBUTION OF AChRs

In the CNS, the spinal cord and the superior colliculus contain most of the nAChRs. The cholinergic synapses in higher centers are generally muscarinic. M_1-AChRs are dominant in the striatum, hippocampal formation, and cerebral cortex. M_2-AChRs are dominant in the cerebellum.

ACETYLCHOLINESTERASE AND ACh ACTION TERMINATION

The transmitter activity of ACh ends abruptly when the ester is hydrolyzed to choline and free acetate by the enzyme *acetylcholinesterase (AChE)*. AChE, one of a large family of esterases, is specific for ACh and is concentrated at neuronal and neuromuscular synapses. Many forms of AChE exist; however, most contain the same catalytic subunit, or multiples of the same subunit, with differences due principally to posttranslational modifications of the protein complex.

The AChE associated with presynaptic and postsynaptic membranes is often linked to a glycophospholipid, which binds the enzyme to the membrane surface. At the neuromuscular synapse, collagen-containing subunits bind the catalytic subunits to the basal lamina. These posttranslational modifications adapt the enzyme to specific locations and have little or no effect on the catalytic properties of the active site. During the cleavage of ACh, an acyl-AChE intermediate forms at the serine group of the active site. Configuration of the active site is such that water rapidly hydrolyzes the serine ester, which accounts for the very high catalytic efficiency of AChE.

Many reversible inhibitors, such as edrophonium, block substrate access to the active site. Others, classified as carbamoylating agents (e.g., neostigmine and physostigmine), form carbamoyl-serine intermediates at the active site. Because carbamoyl-serine is more stable than acetyl-serine and takes several minutes to hydrolyze, these agents inactivate the enzyme for brief periods. Alkyl phosphates, such as diisopropyl fluorophosphate (and many active components of nerve gas) form stable, covalent bonds with the serine and irreversibly inhibit AChE.

Responses to AChE inhibition vary with the synapses involved. Most ganglionic synapses of both the sympathetic and parasympathetic preganglionic fibers are facilitated as are the effects of postganglionic parasympathetic innervations and the cholinergic postganglionic sympathetic innervations. At neuromuscular synapses, there is a severe depolarization of motor end plates and a lack of coordinated muscle action potentials, which initially appear as muscle fasciculations, then as twitches, and eventually as flaccid paralysis.

Catecholamines

The *catecholamines (CAs)* are a family of neurotransmitters synthesized in nervous tissue from a common substrate, *tyrosine* (Fig. 5–6). *Norepinephrine (NE)* is the principal neurotransmitter for postganglionic sympathetic neurons and for several pathways in the CNS. These originate in the locus ceruleus of the brain stem and project to the cerebral cortex, the cerebellum, and the spinal cord. *Dopamine (DA),* the immediate precursor of NE, is also a neurotransmitter for several CNS pathways. The nigrostriatal pathway, motor system fibers from the substantia nigra to the caudate and putamen, accounts for approximately 80% of the brain's DA (see Chapter 16). Additional CNS dopaminergic pathways include the tuberoinfundibular pathway of the hypothalamus (Chapter 18) and the mesolimbic pathway projecting from the midbrain to forebrain and limbic structures (Chapter 22). *Epinephrine (EPI),* synthesized from NE, is the major hormone of the adrenal medulla and can stimulate most peripheral CA receptors. EPI is also the principal neurotransmitter for a small group of neurons in the brain stem projecting to the hypothalamus.

SYNTHESIS

Tyrosine hydroxylase (TH) is the initial and rate-limiting enzyme in the catecholamine pathway. This soluble enzyme is concentrated in the axon terminals of all CA-containing neurons. The product of the TH-catalyzed reaction is dihydroxyphenylalanine (L-*DOPA*). *DOPA decarbox-*

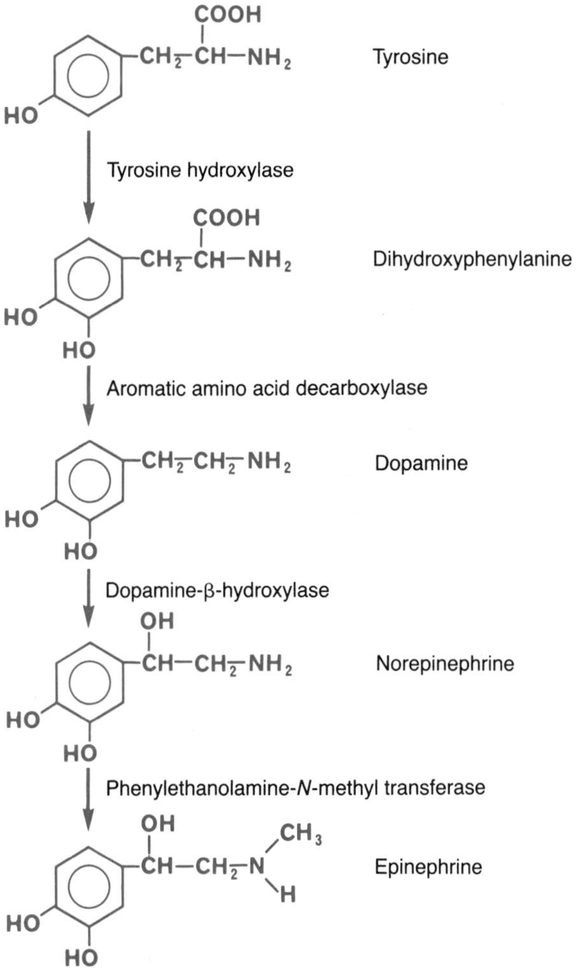

FIGURE 5-6

Principal steps in the biosynthesis of the catecholamines from tyrosine.

ylase rapidly decarboxylates L-DOPA to DA. Because dopa decarboxylase is not specific for L-DOPA and can decarboxylate 5-hydroxytryptophan and other aromatic amino acids, the preferred name for the enzyme is *aromatic amino acid decarboxylase (AADC)*. AADC is the last enzyme in the synthetic pathway for DA (see Fig. 5–6).

In NE- and EPI-containing neurons, the β-carbon on the side chain of DA is oxidized by the enzyme *dopamine-β-hydroxylase (DBH)* to yield NE. Unlike the soluble enzymes, TH and AADC, DBH is concentrated in the synaptic vesicles. DA is converted to NE as the CA is stored in the vesicle. The enzyme is also released with NE during synaptic transmission (see Fig. 5–6).

The final step in the CA synthetic pathway is the conversion of NE to the secondary amine, *epinephrine,* catalyzed by the methyl-transferring enzyme, *phenylethanolamine-N-methyltransferase (PNMT).* Only EPI-containing neurons and cells of the adrenal medulla contain PNMT (see Fig. 5–6).

STORAGE AND RELEASE

CAs are stored in synaptic vesicles as complexes with ATP and an acidic protein, chromogranin. Transport of the amine across the vesicle membrane is ATP- and Mg^{2+}-dependent and is coupled to a proton pump. The drug, reserpine, irreversibly blocks this storage process, thereby depleting the stores of CA available for release.

The CAs are released by exocytosis. This is a calcium-dependent process triggered by the action potential's activation of voltage-sensitive calcium channels. In addition to the CA, the other contents of the vesicle (ATP, chromogranin, and DBH) are released into the synaptic cleft.

REGULATION OF SYNTHESIS

The rate-limiting step in CA synthesis involves the enzyme TH. As levels of CA rise, the enzyme is increasingly inhibited by the reaction product. The kinetic properties of TH are coupled to nerve terminal depolarization. The affinity for the pteridine co-factor increases and end-product inhibition decreases with repeated nerve terminal depolarization. These changes are caused by a reversible phosphorylation of TH by protein kinase C, which is activated by the calcium influx associated with the depolarization. Prolonged stimulation of a CA neuron eventually increases the transcription of mRNA for TH and, hence, the rate of TH synthesis.

CATECHOLAMINE RECEPTORS

At least six groups of receptors are known for the CAs, two specific for DA and four for NE and EPI. A characteristic of CA synapses, as well as for serotonin and GABA, is the presence of *autoreceptors*. These are receptors located on the presynaptic terminal that are sensitive to the neurotransmitter released by that terminal. The autoreceptor modulates the release of additional transmitter. Except for the β-adrenergic autoreceptor, this modulation is one of negative feedback or inhibition.

Another feature of CA receptors is *denervation supersensitivity*. Following denervation, the CA receptors on the target (another neuron or a target organ) become hypersensitive to the ligand. All CA receptors couple to a second messenger system. Unlike the nAChRs, none of them are classified as ligand-gated ion channels.

DOPAMINE RECEPTORS

The two DA receptors are the D_1 receptors that activate adenyl cyclase and the D_2 receptors that inhibit adenyl cyclase. Although specific G-proteins have not been identified, these proteins probably mediate the activation and inactivation of adenyl cyclase.

Anatomically, the pattern of DA receptor distribution is complex. In some areas, both types of receptors have been identified on the same postsynaptic membrane. However, all of the autoreceptors are the inhibitory or the D_2 type.

NOREPINEPHRINE AND EPINEPHRINE RECEPTORS

The original concept of *α-adrenergic receptors* (*α-AR*) and *β-adrenergic receptors* (*β-AR*) distinguished between the opposite effects of excitation or contraction (α) and of inhibition or relaxation (β) in the sympathetic innervation of smooth muscle target organs. Today, the distinction is pharmacologically based. Isoproterenol is a selective β-AR agonist, propranolol is a β-AR antagonist, and phentolamine is an α-AR antagonist with little effect on β-AR receptors. NE and EPI act at both the α-AR and β-AR.

The β-AR is similar in structure to the mAChR. Two of the internal domains contain sites for a cAMP-dependent phosphorylation. When phosphorylated, the receptor becomes less sensitive to the ligand. The β-AR couples to a

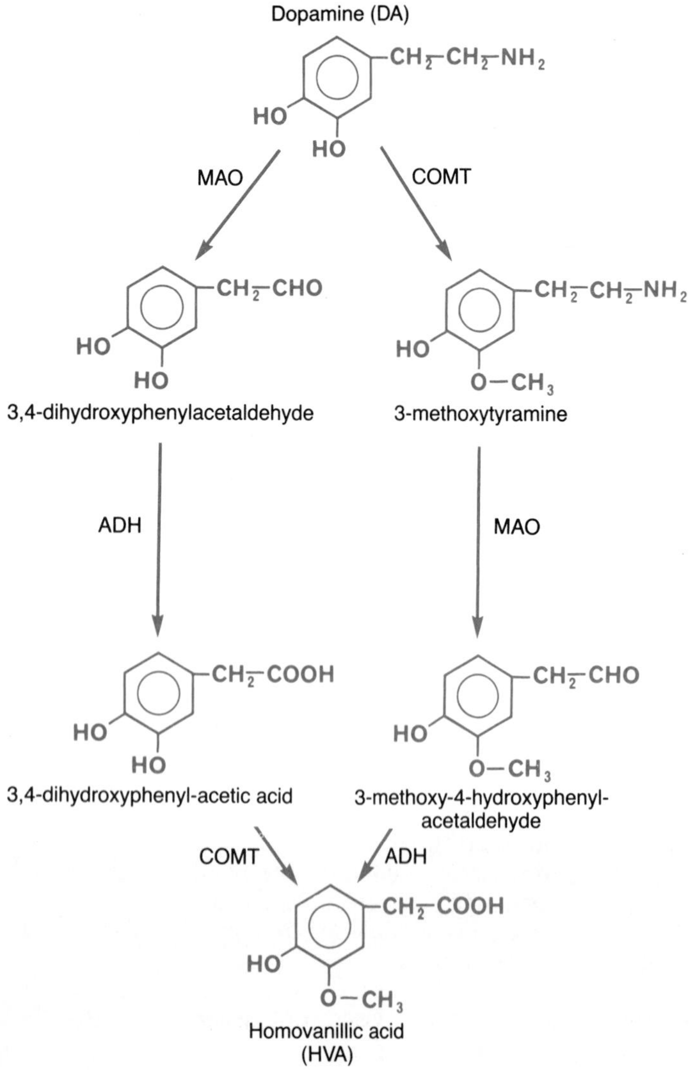

FIGURE 5-7

Principal steps in the catabolism of dopamine (DA). DA undergoes both an oxidative deamination (MAO) and an *O*-methylation (COMT). Regardless of which step is first, the final product is homovanillic acid (HVA) (see text). (ADH, aldehydedehydrogenase; COMT, catecholamine-O-methyl transferase; MAO, monoamine oxidase.)

G_S-protein and activates adenyl cyclase. Further stimulation activates the soluble *β-adrenergic receptor kinase (β-ARK)*. β-ARK also phosphorylates the β-AR, further desensitizing the receptor and reducing its ability to activate the G_S-protein. However, β-ARK only phosphorylates the receptor if the ligand is bound to the receptor. Both $β_1$-AR and $β_2$-AR activate adenyl cyclase, and both are in the CNS and the peripheral nervous system (PNS). The $β_1$-AR is equally sensitive to NE and EPI, whereas the $β_2$-AR has a higher affinity for NE. The *β-adrenergic autoreceptors* facilitate the release of additional transmitter, thus providing a positive feedback and an amplification of the original signal.

Binding properties of the $α_1$-AR and $α_2$-AR in the CNS and PNS are similar. The distinguishing features are pharmacological. NE and EPI bind to both receptors with comparable affinities. The effector coupling mechanisms are undefined, although $α_1$-ARs stimulate phosphoinositol turnover and the $α_2$-ARs may stimulate phospholipase A_2 and mobilize intracellular calcium stores. The *α-adrenergic autoreceptors* inhibit the release of additional transmitter, providing a negative feedback. Some tissues and areas of the brain have only one of the α-AR's, others have both. The pattern of distribution varies for different regions of the brain and for different peripheral tissues. For the distribution and function of some of these adrenergic receptors in peripheral tissue, see Table 18–1.

INACTIVATION THROUGH REUPTAKE AND CATABOLISM

Approximately 80% of the CAs are taken up by the presynaptic terminal and recycled via a Na^+- and ATP-dependent uptake system. Drugs that interfere with the Na^+ gradient (veratroidine, which opens sodium channels) or block Na^+/K^+-ATPase activity (ouabain) also inhibit CA uptake. Once in the presynaptic terminal, the CA is rapidly stored in the synaptic vesicles. Presynaptic CA terminals contain high levels of the mitochondrial enzyme *monoamine oxidase (MAO)* and, if the CA is not immediately sequestered in synaptic vesicles, it is rapidly oxidized.

The two principal enzymes involved in the catabolism of CAs are *monoamine oxidase (MAO)* and *catechol-O-methyl transferase (COMT)* (Figs. 5–7 and 5–8). This degradation consists of both a methylation of the hydroxyl group at the 3 position on the benzene ring (COMT) and an oxidative deamination of the side chain (MAO). Although glia contain most of the COMT, both neurons and glia contain MAO.

The principal metabolite of NE produced in

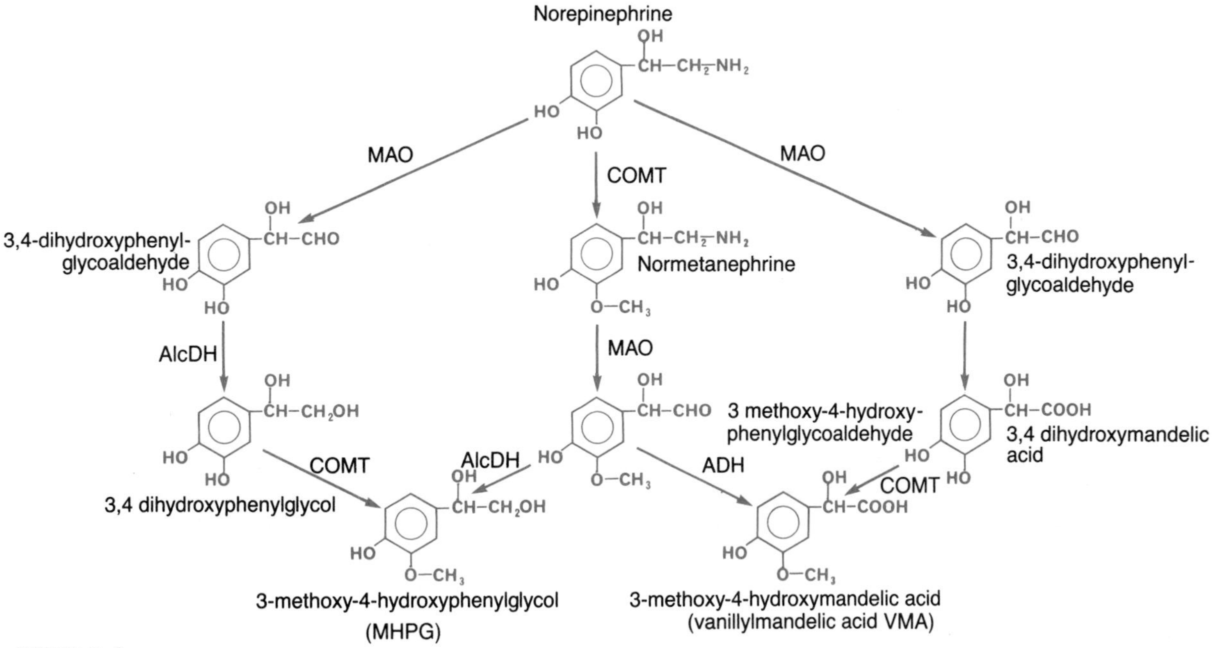

FIGURE 5–8

Principal steps in the catabolism of norepinephrine (NE). The two principal degradative products are 3-methoxy-4-hydroxyphenylglycol (MHPG) and 3-methoxy-4-hydroxymandelic acid (vanillylmandelic acid, VMA) (see text). (ADH, aldehydedehydrogenase; COMT, catecholamine-O-methyl transferase; MAO, monoamine oxidase; AlcDH, alcoholdehydrogenase.)

the brain is *3-methoxy-4-hydroxyphenylglycol (MHPG)*. *Vanillylmandelic acid (VMA)* is the principal metabolite from peripheral autonomic innervations (see Fig. 5–8). Brain DA catabolism leads to the formation of *homovanillic acid (HVA)* (see Fig. 5–7). All three metabolites are excreted by the kidneys. The levels of MHPG and HVA in the urine are indicators of CNS turnover of NE and DA, respectively (see Figs. 5–7 and 5–8). Characteristically, patients with reduced levels of brain DA, such as those with Parkinson's disease, have reduced levels of HVA in the urine.

Serotonin (5-Hydroxytryptamine)

Serotonin, or *5-hydroxytryptamine (5-HT)*, functions both as a neurotransmitter and as a modulator of neurotransmission. In the CNS, serotoninergic neurons are limited to a group of brain stem reticular formation nuclei, the *raphe nuclei*. Although few in number and restricted in localization, these neurons project to nearly all areas of the CNS. Neurons from midbrain raphe nuclei project to higher brain centers (cerebral cortex, hippocampus, thalamus, hypothalamus, basal ganglia, and cerebellum), whereas neurons from pontine and medullary raphe nuclei project to lower brain centers (medulla and spinal cord).

SYNTHESIS

L-Tryptophan is the natural substrate for the synthesis of 5-HT in the brain. *Tryptophan-5-hydroxylase* catalyzes the initial reaction with the formation of 5-hydroxytryptophan, which is rapidly decarboxylated by *aromatic amino acid decarboxylase (AADC)*, forming serotonin (5-HT) (Fig. 5–9).

Tryptophan hydroxylase is the rate-limiting step in 5-HT synthesis. Tryptophan hydroxylase activity is normally limited by the endogenous levels of tryptophan. Increased levels of neuronal activity activate a calcium/calmodulin–dependent protein kinase, leading to a reversible phosphorylation of tryptophan hydroxylase. This phosphorylation can produce a transient increase in the apparent V_{max} of the enzyme, providing endogenous levels of tryptophan are not limiting.

STORAGE, RELEASE, AND TERMINATION OF ACTIVITY

Serotonin is stored in synaptic vesicles and released in quantal units through a calcium-depen-

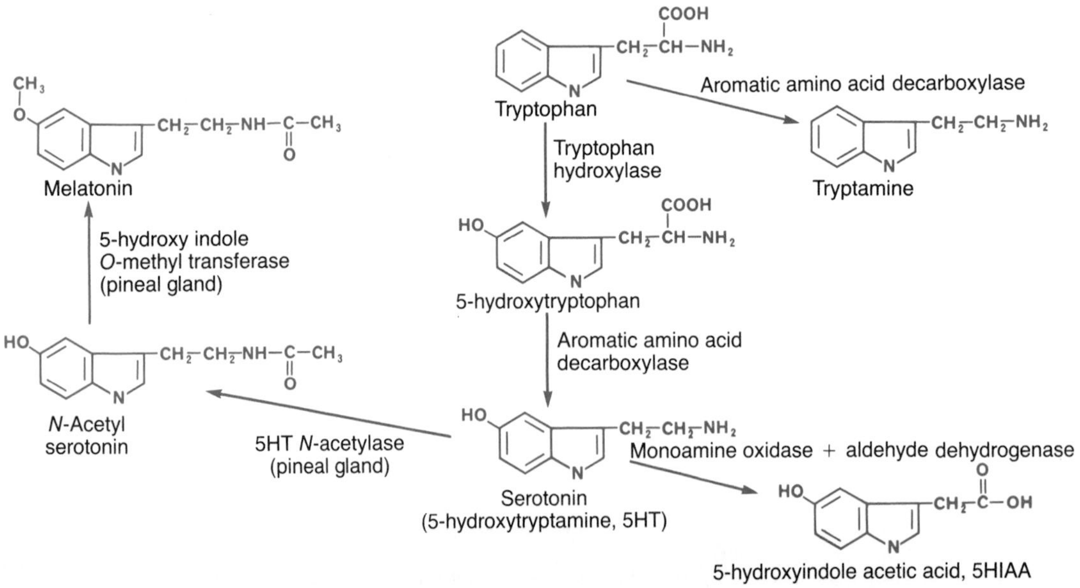

FIGURE 5-9

Principal pathway for the synthesis and degradation of serotonin (5-hydroxytryptamine, 5HT). The substrate for synthesis is tryptophan and the major metabolite is 5-hydroxyindol acetic acid (5HIAA). Serotonin is also converted to melatonin in the pineal gland (see text).

dent process of exocytosis. Serotonin may exist alone or in combination with other neurotransmitters (ACh, NE, DA, substance P, enkephalins, TRH, and prostaglandins) (see the discussion of Synaptic Transmission with Release of Multiple Neurochemical Transmitters later in this chapter).

The principal metabolite of serotonin is *5-hydroxyindole acetic acid* (*5-HIAA*). It is produced by the MAO catalyzed oxidative deamination of serotonin. This is followed by an oxidation of the aldehyde to the acid by aldehyde dehydrogenase (see Fig. 5–9). A minor product of serotonin catabolism is 5-hydroxytryptophol (not illustrated), the alcohol formed from a reduction of the aldehyde by alcohol dehydrogenase. 5-HIAA is the principal metabolite, and the level of 5-HIAA in cerebrospinal fluid is an index of serotonin turnover in the CNS.

As with the CAs, much of the serotonin is reused through a high-affinity, energy-dependent, uptake system. The serotonin uptake system is specific for serotonin and can be selectively blocked without affecting other biogenic amines.

RECEPTORS

At least seven receptors exist for serotonin: 5-HT_{1A}, 5-HT_{1B}, 5-HT_{1C}, 5-HT_{1D}, 5-HT_2, 5-HT_3, and 5-HT_4. Each has different pharmacological properties, distribution patterns, and biological responses.

Most serotonin responses are consistent with receptors coupled to a second messenger system —slow onset and long duration. The receptors 5-HT_{1B} and 5-HT_{1D} are autoreceptors, and they inhibit the further release of serotonin through the inhibition of adenyl cyclase. Both the 5-HT_{1C} and 5-HT_2 receptors activate phospholipase C, stimulating the phosphatidylinositol second messenger system. Stimulation of 5-HT_4 receptors activates adenyl cyclase postsynaptically, and stimulation of 5-HT_{1A} receptors inhibits adenyl cyclase. The activity of the 5-HT_{1A} receptor is more apparent when an adrenergic innervation has previously activated the adenyl cyclase. A subpopulation of 5-HT_{1A} receptors which activates adenyl cyclase may be present in the hippocampus.

The 5-HT_3 receptor differs from the other 5-HT receptors because it is a ligand-gated ion channel (like the nicotinic AChR) and not coupled to a G-protein. These receptors have a much faster response time. The 5-HT_3 receptors are found both in the PNS (sympathetic ganglia,

vagal afferents, and somatosensory neurons) and in areas of the CNS.

The actions of serotoninergic neurons are complex and functional generalizations are difficult to make. The physiological response to serotoninergic innervation reflects the nature of the postsynaptic receptor. Most serotoninergic synapses are inhibitory to the postsynaptic neuron, although some are excitatory. For example, serotoninergic fibers to the dorsal horn of the spinal cord inhibit the transmission of incoming somatosensory information, producing analgesia, whereas other descending serotoninergic fibers to the ventral horn facilitate motor activity.

Serotoninergic projections are associated with body temperature regulation, blood pressure, rapid eye movement (REM) sleep, circadian rhythm, and pain perception. Other studies have linked serotoninergic projections to human behavior, in particular to the inhibition of aggressive and impulsive behavior.

OTHER INDOLE AMINES

Melatonin, an *O*-methylated, *N*-acetylated derivative of serotonin (see Fig. 5–9), is the only other indole amine with a known biological function. Melatonin is synthesized in the pineal and has a role in human gonadal function, especially as it relates to puberal changes.

Histamine

The role of histamine both as a CNS neurotransmitter and a neuromodulator is now well established. The primary population of histaminergic neurons is in the ventral posterior portion of the hypothalamus. The distribution of terminals from this small population of neurons is vast, with terminals not only in the hypothalamus but also in nearly every other region of the brain and spinal cord.

Mast cells contain very high concentrations of histamine. Although the human CNS contains few mast cells under normal conditions, their role, if any, in neuronal modulation is unclear.

SYNTHESIS

Histamine does not cross the blood-brain barrier and is synthesized *in situ* from the decarboxylation of histidine by *histidine decarboxylase (HDC)*. Although AADC can decarboxylate histidine, HDC is specific for L-histidine and is localized only in histaminergic neurons. A combination of HDC and the normally low endogenous levels of histidine in the brain regulates the neuronal levels of histamine (Fig. 5–10).

STORAGE, RELEASE, AND TERMINATION OF ACTIVITY

The hypothalamic histaminergic neurons also contain other neurotransmitters: 5-HT, GABA, and adenosine. The peptides TRH, substance P, and galanin also have been co-localized with histamine. Histamine is stored in synaptic vesicles and released through a calcium-triggered exocytotic mechanism.

No uptake mechanism has been identified for histamine, and its neurochemical activity is terminated enzymatically. In the CNS, histamine is methylated in the postsynaptic area by the substrate-specific *histamine methyltransferase* and is subsequently oxidized by *MAO*. Both enzymes are glial. In the PNS, methylation is lacking and histamine is deaminated by *diamine oxidase* and further oxidized by *aldehyde dehydrogenase* to imidazole acetic acid (see Fig. 5–10).

HISTAMINE RECEPTORS

At least three histamine receptors are known: H_1, H_2, and H_3. The CNS contains both the H_1 and H_2 receptors. The highest concentration of the H_1 receptor is in the cerebral cortex and the lowest in the cerebellum. The H_2 receptor is the princi-

pal histamine receptor in the striatum. The H_3 receptor is an autoreceptor. When stimulated, it inhibits the release of additional histamine.

The H_2 receptor activates adenyl cyclase, whereas the H_1 receptor stimulates phospholipase C and phosphatidylinositol metabolism. H_1 receptor stimulation also may produce a calcium-dependent increase in cGMP and an indirect activation of adenyl cyclase. The multitude of responses observed with H_1 receptor stimulation may be the result of the activation of multiple second messenger systems triggered by the phosphatidylinositol metabolism cascade (see Modulators, Signal Transducers, and Second Messengers).

Neuronal responses to histamine are similar to other neurotransmitters coupled to second messenger systems. They have a long latency of response. In addition, they are of long duration, especially when compared with neurotransmitters coupled directly to ion channels. Histamine regulates a number of autonomic responses as well as behavioral and mental states.

Inhibitory Amino Acids: Gamma Aminobutyric Acid (GABA) and Glycine

GABA and *glycine* are the principal inhibitory neurotransmitters in the CNS. Postsynaptic receptors of both inhibitory amino acids are *lig-*

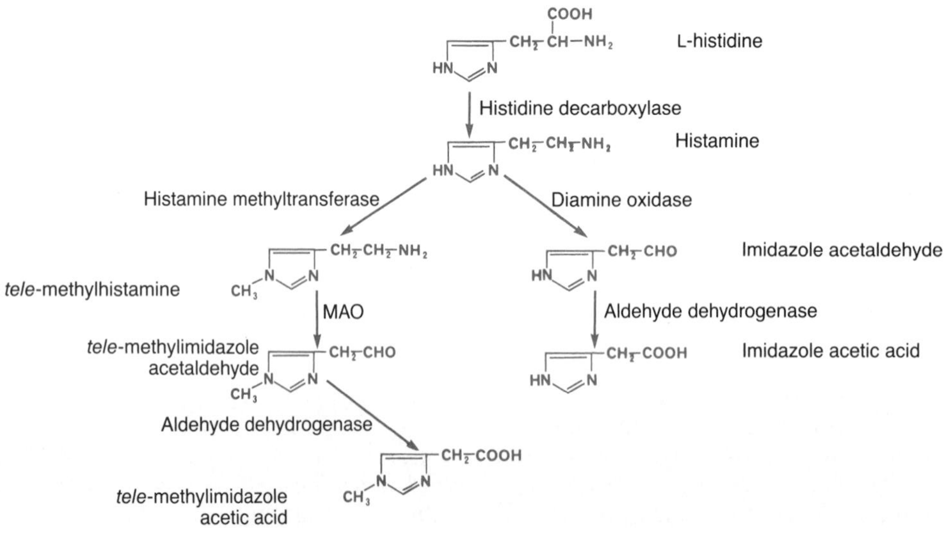

FIGURE 5–10

Principal pathway for the synthesis and degradation of histamine. Imidazole acetic acid is the primary metabolite in the peripheral nervous system and *tele*-methyimidazole acetic acid in the central nervous system (see text).

and-gated ion channels. Hence, when stimulated, the postsynaptic responses have short latencies and are of brief duration. Both neurotransmitters are found throughout the CNS. However, the neurotransmitter pool of glycine is more concentrated in the spinal cord and lower brain stem. In constrast, GABA is more concentrated at telencephalic and diencephalic levels.

GABA METABOLISM

The glutamate utilized for the *in vivo* synthesis of GABA comes principally from intermediates of glucose metabolism (Fig. 5–11). The tricarboxylic acid (TCA) cycle intermediate, α-ketoglutarate, is converted to glutamate. *Glutamic acid decarboxylase (GAD)* removes the carboxylic acid group adjacent to the α-amino group, forming *GABA*. The neurotransmitter is stored in vesicles and later released in quantal fashion, through the calcium-dependent exocytosis of synaptic vesicles.

Following release and interaction with the receptors, GABA is taken up either by adjacent glial cells or by the presynaptic nerve terminal. Both have *high-affinity GABA uptake systems*, but with differing properties. Antagonists can selectively inhibit either the glial or the neuronal uptake systems.

GABA transaminase (GABA-T) deaminates GABA with the formation of succinic semialdehyde. GABA-T is closely coupled to *succinic semialdehyde dehydrogenase (SSADH)* on the outer mitochondrial membrane. Hence, the succinic semialdehyde is rapidly oxidized to succinate. In the transamination reaction, GABA-T requires α-ketoglutarate, therefore, the deamination of GABA is coupled to the synthesis of the immediate precursor of GABA, glutamate. The metabolic path from α-ketoglutarate through GABA to succinate is called *the GABA shunt.*

Glia do not contain the neuron-specific GAD but do contain *glutamine synthetase.* They con-

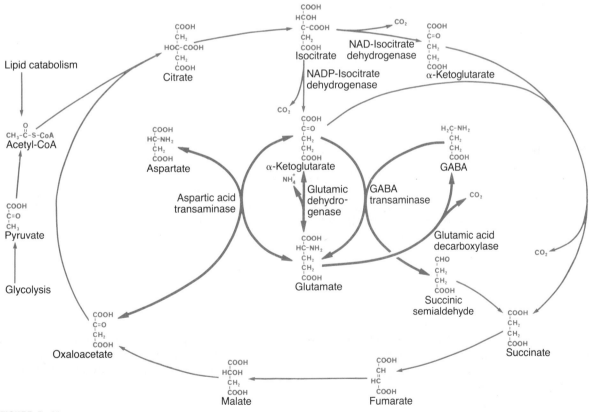

FIGURE 5-11

Relation of gamma amino butyric acid (GABA), aspartate, and glutamate metabolism to the tricarboxylic acid (TCA) cycle. Glutamate and aspartate are formed principally from transamination reactions with the TCA cycle intermediates α-ketoglutarate and oxaloacetic acid, respectively. The "GABA shunt" refers to the formation of glutamate from α-ketoglutarate and its decarboxylation to GABA, and to the subsequent degradation of GABA to succinic semialdehyde and its re-entry into the TCA cycle as succinate (see text).

vert the glutamate formed from the GABA-T reaction to *glutamine*. Glutamine is transported to the adjacent neuron terminal, deaminated by *glutaminase* to glutamate; and utilized for the synthesis of additional GABA, thus conserving the GABA precursor. Glutamine synthetase is found only in glia and GAD only in GABA-neurons. Glutaminase, GABA-T, and SSADH are found in both cell types.

GABA RECEPTORS

Two distinct populations of GABA receptors include $GABA_A$, a postsynaptic, ligand-gated chloride channel, and $GABA_B$, a presynaptic, second messenger–coupled receptor, functioning as a modulator of neurotransmitter release. These two families of receptor were originally differentiated on the basis of pharmacological properties. $GABA_A$ receptors respond to the agonist muscimol, are facilitated by the benzodiazepines, are blocked by the antagonist bicuculline, and are unresponsive to baclofen. In contrast, $GABA_B$ receptors, are specific for the agonist baclofen, weakly responsive to muscimol, and insensitive to bicuculline.

The $GABA_A$ receptors belong to the family of ion channel–coupled receptors and share many structural features in common with other ligand-gated ion channels, nAChR, glycine receptors, and glutamate receptors. $GABA_A$ receptors are tetramers composed of a mixture of α- and β-subunits. The subunits are arranged around the centrally located chloride channel. At least three different α-subunits exist. Different combinations of subunits produce receptors with slightly different pharmacological and physiological properties. Thus, differential gene expression can alter the properties of $GABA_A$ receptors and can provide a mechanism for synaptic plasticity.

The $GABA_B$ receptors are found at axoaxonal synapses in both the PNS and the CNS. These synapses are examples of presynaptic inhibition, similar to one illustrated in Figure 4–6. The inhibitory axoaxonal GABA synapse blocks or reduces the amount of NE, DA, 5-HT, or glutamate released at the primary synapse.

GLYCINE

Glycine, $CH_2(NH_3^+)COO^-$, is a simple two-carbon amino acid neurotransmitter. However, it exists in a number of metabolic pools in all cells of the nervous system, neurons and glia alike. Identifying the glycine neurotransmitter pool is difficult, because the enzymes involved in the synthesis and degradation of glycine are the same.

The glycine receptor is similar in many respects to the $GABA_A$ receptor—it is a ligand-gated chloride channel. However, the glycine receptor is specifically blocked by strychnine and the $GABA_A$ receptor is specifically blocked by bicuculline.

Excitatory Amino Acids: Glutamate and Aspartate

The dicarboxylic α-amino acids, *glutamate* and *aspartate*, are the principal excitatory neurotransmitters in the CNS. Both are released by way of a calcium-dependent process in response to electrical excitation and have receptors coupled to ion channels with short latencies of response. Neither amino acid can cross the blood-brain barrier; therefore, they are synthesized *in situ*. As with glycine, a number of problems developed in establishing their role as neurotransmitters, because they have major functions in protein and peptide syntheses, ammonia fixation, and as a precursor of GABA (glutamate). The most definitive data are from the identification of specific receptors and from ionophoretic studies.

BIOSYNTHESIS OF GLUTAMATE AND ASPARTATE

Glutamate is synthesized from the TCA cycle intermediate α-ketoglutarate by *glutamate dehydrogenase (GDH)* (see Fig. 5–11). Significant amounts of glutamate are formed from glutamine by the neuronal enzyme, glutaminase. Although some glutamate from the GABA-T reaction may enter the glutamate neurotransmitter pool, most is used for the synthesis of additional GABA. The principal source of *aspartate* is another TCA cycle intermediate, oxaloacetate, through a transamination reaction with glutamate (see Fig. 5–11). Asparagine and glutamine have been proposed as additional sources of aspartate.

Because both glutamate and aspartate exist in several metabolic pools, it has not been possible to identify the principal pathway of synthesis for the neurotransmitter pool. When the neuroanatomical pathways using these amino acids as neurotransmitters are destroyed, the synthetic pathways are not significantly altered, probably because the neurotransmitter pool is small compared with the other pools.

Glutamate is a potent excitatory neurotransmitter with as little as 10^{-14} moles sufficient to increase sodium conductance and decrease membrane resistance in the postsynaptic membrane. Aspartate is comparable in function, although less potent and not as widely distributed.

GLUTAMATE AND ASPARTATE RECEPTORS

Three principal families of receptors for the excitatory amino acids are grouped and defined by the action of specific agonists. *NMDA* receptors are selectively activated by N-methyl-D-aspartic acid and are sensitive to both aspartate and glutamate. *QA* receptors are selectively activated by quisqualic acid and KA receptors by kainic acid. Both receptors are more sensitive to glutamate than to aspartate. All three receptors are ligand-gated ion channels.

The NMDA receptors, however, have several unusual features. Activation of NMDA receptors is both voltage-dependent and ligand-dependent. Physiological concentrations of Mg^{2+}, at resting membrane potentials, block the postsynaptic receptor ion currents. Maximal activation of the NMDA receptor occurs when the membrane is depolarized to -20 to -30 mV. At these membrane potentials, Mg^{2+} loses its affinity for the receptor and no longer blocks the receptor-activated ion currents. In essence, at resting potentials, NMDA receptors are insensitive. When the membrane becomes depolarized to -30 mV, the receptors become sensitive to the ligand. At many of the synapses containing NMDA receptors, there is a co-localization of at least one other receptor, such as the QA or KA receptor. Thus, as glutamate is released, EPSPs generated from the stimulation of QA or KA receptors activate adjacent NMDA receptors.

Unlike other fast-acting excitatory synapses, those with NMDA receptors are biphasic. An initial short latency depolarization (from QA or KA receptors) is followed by an enhancement of the initial response as the voltage-gated mechanisms of the NMDA receptors are activated. NMDA-associated ion channels are permeable to Ca^{2+} as well as Na^+. The influx of calcium adds another dimension to the NMDA postsynaptic response. Calcium activates calcium/calmodulin-dependent protein kinases, triggering a number of secondary responses. These often lead to long term alterations in the synaptic physiology and are the basis for theories linking the NMDA synapse with memory, learning, and long-term potentiation.

Neuroactive Peptides

The study of neuroactive peptides has grown dramatically, stimulated by the technical advances in molecular biology, especially those in recombinant DNA. Neuroactive peptides are present in minute amounts, femtomoles or picomoles/gm of tissue. The classic neurotransmitters have concentrations measured in micromoles/gm of tissue. New techniques have provided the sensitivity necessary to study very small quantities. Synthesis of the neuroactive peptides requires the same steps as protein synthesis: DNA transcription, mRNA synthesis, assembly in the rough endoplasmic reticulum, and axonal transport for the finished product. Unlike the classic neurotransmitters, these steps are not unique. Therefore it is necessary to study the peptide, the specific mRNAs, and the peptide receptors rather than the synthetic enzymes.

BIOSYNTHESIS

Most neuroactive peptides are synthesized as large precursor molecules or *prohormones*. Second messenger systems, operating at the levels of both gene transcription and protein synthesis, regulate the synthesis of these large proteins. Once synthesized, specific *endopeptidases* cleave the precursor molecules forming the desired peptides from the parent molecule. *Aminopeptidases* and *carboxypeptidases* trim amino acids from the amino-terminal and carboxy-terminal ends of the peptides to yield the final neuroactive peptide.

In addition to "cutting" and "trimming," some peptides are modified, e.g., N-acetylation of β-endorphin and tyrosine sulfation of cholecystokinin. In theory, other peptides could be phosphorylated or O-methylated. The same prohormone, cleaved in a different pattern, can be the precursor for a different set of peptides in different areas of the CNS (Fig. 5–12).

Specific *synthetases*, however, form several of the smaller oligopeptides. Carnosine synthetase catalyzes the formation of *carnosine* (β-alanyl-L-histidine), and γ-glutamyl-L-cysteine synthetase forms *glutathione* (γ-L-glutamyl-L-cysteinylglycine).

CLASSIFICATION OF NEUROACTIVE PEPTIDES

The number of neuroactive peptides identified as neurotransmitters and as modulators of synaptic activity is increasing rapidly. As techniques

Prodynorphin

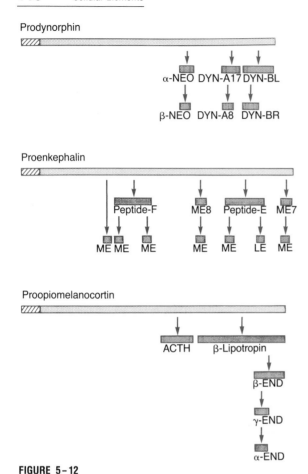

Proenkephalin

Proopiomelanocortin

FIGURE 5-12

Opioid peptide prohormones; prodynorphin, proenkephalin, and proopiomelanocortin and some of their products (see text and Table 5-2). (ACTH, adrenocorticotropic hormone; DYN-A8, dynorphin A$_{(1-8)}$; DYN-A17, dynorphin A$_{(1-17)}$; DYN-BL, dynorphin B (leumorphin); DYN-BR, dynorphin B (rimorphin); α-END, α-endorphin; β-END, β-endorphin; γ-END, γ-endorphin; LE, leu-enkephalin; ME, met-enkephalin; ME7, met-enkephalin-arg-phe; ME8, met-enkephalin-arg-gly-leu; α-NEO, α-neodynorphin; and β-NEO, β-neodynorphin.)

improve, the number identified will become higher. For convenience, the neuroactive peptides are grouped as *non-opioid peptides* (Table 5-1) and *opioid peptides* (Table 5-2).

Many of the non-opioid peptides were first identified in functional systems other than neurotransmission. The original name often relates to the discovery of the compound and usually bears little relation to its role as a neurotransmitter. Many pituitary tropic hormones, produced and released in the hypothalamus (TRH, CRH, GHRH, and SOM), are found in other areas of the CNS and have well defined roles as neurotransmitters or neuromodulators in addition to

TABLE 5-1

Examples of Non-opioid Neuroactive Peptides

NAME OF PEPTIDE	NUMBER OF AMINO ACIDS
Adrenocorticotropic hormone (ACTH)	24*
Angiotensin II (ATII)	8
Arginine vasopressin (AVP)	9
Arginine vasotocin (AVT)	9
Atrial natriuretic polypeptide (ANP)	28
Bradykinin	9
Calcitonin	32
L-Carnosine	2
Cholecystokinin (CCK)	8*
Calcitonin gene-related peptide (CGRP)	37
Corticotropin-releasing hormone (CRH)	41*
Galanin	29
Gonadotropin-releasing hormone (GRH) (luteinizing hormone–releasing hormone, LHRH)	10
Growth hormone–releasing hormone (GHRH)	44
Glucagon	29
Glutathione	3
α-Melanocyte stimulating hormone (α-MSH)	13
β-Melanocyte stimulating hormone (β-MSH)	18
Neuropeptide Y (NPY)	36
Neurotensin	13
Oxytocin	9
Somatostatin (SOM)	14*
Substance P (SubP)	11
Thyrotropin-releasing hormone (TRH)	3
Vasoactive intestinal peptide (VIP)	28*

* Other values have been reported.

that of tropic hormones. A discussion of the specific peptides and their location and function is beyond the scope of this text. However, they are discussed in relation to specific functional systems in subsequent sections of the text, i.e., the relation of SubP to somatosensory systems is considered in Chapter 10.

All opioid peptides share common pharmacological properties and are often called "the brain's own morphine." In the CNS, these peptides are associated with analgesia and euphoria and are found in abundance in the somatosensory pathways and the limbic system. Because of these commonalties, the opioid peptides are reviewed here as a group.

FORMATION OF OPIOID PEPTIDES

The human CNS contains at least 14 opioid peptides, all formed from three distinct prohormone proteins: *proenkephalin, proopiomelanocortin,* and *prodynorphin.* Three genes, regulated by a cAMP second messenger system, control the synthesis of these prohormones. Once synthe-

TABLE 5-2

Amino Acid Sequences of Opioid Peptides from Three Precursor Proteins*

	Proenkephalin
leu-Enkephalin	*Tyr-Gly-Gly-Phe-Leu*
met-Enkephalin	*Tyr-Gly-Gly-Phe-Met*
met-Enk-Arg-Phe	*Tyr-Gly-Gly-Phe-Met*-Arg-Phe
met-Enk-Arg-Gly-Leu	*Tyr-Gly-Gly-Phe-Met*-Arg-Gly-Leu
Peptide E	*Tyr-Gly-Gly-Phe-Met*-Arg-Arg-Val-Gly-Arg-Pro-Glu-Tyr-Trp-Met-Asn-Tyr-Gln-Lys-Arg-*Tyr-Gly-Gly-Phe-Leu*
	Proopiomelanocortin
β-Endorphin	*Tyr-Gly-Gly-Phe-Met*-Thr-Ser-Glu-Lys-Ser-Gln-Thr-Pro-Leu-Val-Thr-Leu-Phe-Lys-Asn-Ala-Ile-Lys-Asn-Ala-His-Lys-Lys-Gly-Gln
γ-Endorphin	*Tyr-Gly-Gly-Phe-Met*-Thr-Ser-Glu-Lys-Ser-Gln-Thr-Pro-Leu-Val-Thr-Leu
α-Endorphin	*Tyr-Gly-Gly-Phe-Met*-Thr-Ser-Glu-Lys-Ser-Gln-Thr-Pro-Leu-Val-Thr
	Prodynorphin
α-Neodynorphin	*Tyr-Gly-Gly-Phe-Leu*-Arg-Lys-Tyr-Pro-Lys
β-Neodynorphin	*Tyr-Gly-Gly-Phe-Leu*-Arg-Lys-Tyr-Pro
Dynorphin A $_{(1-17)}$	*Tyr-Gly-Gly-Phe-Leu*-Arg-Arg-Ile-Arg-Pro-Lys-Leu-Lys-Trp-Asp-Asn-Gln
Dynorphin A $_{(1-8)}$	*Tyr-Gly-Gly-Phe-Leu*-Arg-Arg-Ile
Dynorphin B (leumorphin)	*Tyr-Gly-Gly-Phe-Leu*-Arg-Arg-Gln-Phe-Lys-Val-Val-Thr-Arg-Ser-Gln-Gln-Asp-Pro-Asn-Ala-Tyr-Ser-Gly-Glu-Leu-Phe-Asp-Ala
Dynorphin B (rimorphin)	*Tyr-Gly-Gly-Phe-Leu*-Arg-Arg-Gln-Phe-Lys-Val-Val-Thr

*Italicized sequences represent the met-enkephalin and leu-enkephalin sequences embedded in the other opioid peptides (see text).

sized, the prohormones are subsequently cleaved and modified to form the neuroactive peptides (see Fig. 5-12). The second messenger, for the regulation of expression of the proenkephalin gene and probably the other genes as well, is cAMP.

Proopiomelanocortin (POMC) is composed of 263 amino acids and is the precursor of *β-lipotropin, ACTH*, and the several forms of *MSH*. The β-lipotropin is further cleaved to form *β-endorphin, α-endorphin,* or *γ-endorphin* (see Fig. 5-12 and Table 5-2). POMC is found principally in the pituitary gland, the arcuate nucleus of the hypothalamus, and the nucleus of the solitary tract. The neurons from the arcuate nucleus terminate in the preoptic area, the basal forebrain area, and the periaqueductal gray. The neurons from the nucleus of the solitary tract terminate in numerous pontine and medullary reticular nuclei, including the raphe nuclei and the locus ceruleus.

Proenkephalin is composed of 267 amino acids and is the precursor of the *enkephalins* and the enkephalin-related peptides (see Fig. 5-12 and Table 5-2). Proenkephalin has a broad distribution throughout the CNS as well as the adrenal gland. However, the processing of the prohormone is regionally specific. The highest levels of the enkephalins are found in the globus pallidus, with lesser amounts in the neocortex, diencephalon, pons, midbrain, mesencephalon, medulla,

and spinal cord. The cerebellum contains the least amount.

Prodynorphin is the precursor of the "dynorphin family" of peptides and consists of 256 amino acids. Prodynorphin is cleaved to form three leu-*enkephalin*-containing peptides, *neodynorphin, dynorphin A,* and *dynorphin B* (see Fig. 5-12 and Table 5-2). Depending on specific processing, neodynorphin is present as either an α- or a β-neodynorphin; dynorphin A as either an eight or a 17 amino acid-peptide; and dynorphin B as either a 29 amino acid-peptide (leumorphin) or a 13 amino acid-peptide (rimorphin). Prodynorphin is abundant in the posterior pituitary and hypothalamus, with very low concentrations in the cerebellum and neocortex. The amygdala, striatum, spinal cord, and limbic-forebrain areas contain moderate levels of the protein. The hippocampus, thalamus, and pons have relatively low levels.

The products from processing the same prohormone vary in different regions of the nervous system. The mechanisms that regulate the synthesis and post-translational processing are area specific. In the caudate nucleus, the principal products of proenkephalin are the pentapeptides, met-enkephalin and leu-enkephalin. However, in the adrenal medulla, the principal products of the same prohormone are higher molecular weight opioid peptides with met-enkephalin and leu-enkephalin constituting less than 5% of the total peptide pool. As varied as the products may be, the amino terminal sequence of all opioid peptides is either leu-*enkephalin* or met-*enkephalin* (see Table 5–2). This structural similarity probably accounts for the similarity in pharmacological properties.

RELEASE AND INACTIVATION

Most neuroactive peptides, opioid and non-opioid peptides alike, are stored and released in a conventional manner—a calcium-dependent exocytosis of the contents of the peptide-containing synaptic vesicle. No evidence exists that peptides are taken up by the presynaptic terminal. Instead, the principal route of inactivation is enzymatic. Often, a specific *exopeptidase* will terminate the activity by cleaving one or two amino acids from either the carboxy- or amino-terminal end of the peptide. Other specific *endopeptidases* cleave specific internal bonds, producing inactive peptides. For other peptides, *O*-methylation or *N*-acetylation reactions may inactivate the peptide. Inactivation can be as varied as the number of peptides.

RECEPTORS AND POSTSYNAPTIC RESPONSE

The opioid receptors are the best studied of the peptide receptors, principally because of the availability of agonists with relatively high binding affinity and of the specific antagonist, naloxone. Characteristic of all opioid receptors is the reversal of ligand binding by naloxone. Three principal classes of opioid receptors are as follows: (1) δ-*receptors* are selective for the enkephalins, (2) *k-receptors* bind the dynorphin family of peptides, and (3) μ-*receptors* appear specific for the endorphins. All appear to operate through an inhibition of the cAMP-second messenger system, coupled to a G_I-protein. The end result for μ- and δ-receptors is the activation of potassium channels, whereas k-receptors inactivate calcium channels. Both effects are inhibitory.

Several "mismatches" occur between opioid receptors and opioid peptides. The neocortex and caudate nucleus have the highest ligand binding but relatively low concentrations of peptide. The globus pallidus has the highest concentration of enkephalins but low ligand binding properties. It may be a question of the accessibility of the ligand to the receptor. Alternatively, postsynaptic receptors for peptides possibly have a low affinity for the ligand.

A similar situation exists for many of the non-opioid peptides. The release of a peptide in the restricted area of the synaptic cleft may be adequate. Most of the non-opioid peptide receptors also couple to a cAMP-second messenger system. However, they may be either excitatory or inhibitory.

Synaptic Transmission with Release of Multiple Neurochemical Transmitters

The coexistence of multiple neurotransmitters is well established for a large number of neurons and, with time, will probably become the rule rather than the exception. Several neurotransmitters coexisting in a single neuron add another dimension to our understanding of neuronal communication.

No set pattern for the coexistence of neurotransmitters exists. For some neurons, it is a combination of a classic (nonpeptide) neurotransmitter and a neuroactive peptide. For others, it is two or more classic neurotransmitters. For some, it is two or more neuroactive peptides with no classic neurotransmitter.

This diversity is not specific for a neurotransmitter or an anatomical location. For example, all NE neurons do not contain the same peptide as a co-transmitter, nor do all NE neurons in a single nucleus contain the same co-transmitter. Neurons of the locus ceruleus contain NE coupled with either NPY or galanin. However, neurons of the arcuate nucleus of the hypothalamus display a variety of combinations, representing at least ten neuroactive peptides and three classic neurotransmitters.

Usually, the same pattern of coexistence has been found in all species studied; however, some well-defined differences exist. The specific examples discussed in the following sections illustrate the potential of co-transmission rather than provide specific situations applicable to the human nervous system.

RELEASE OF COEXISTING NEUROTRANSMITTER MOLECULES

When a neuron contains more than one variety of neurotransmitter, the neurotransmitters can be released in several ways. In the simplest example, all transmitters are stored in the same vesicles and released together. In this case, the differential response resides in the type and distribution of receptors. An alternative scenario is the presence of several types of synaptic vesicles and a selective release of the different populations of vesicles. Both situations exist, but the last may be more common. In general, classic neurotransmitters are stored in small clear or small dense-core vesicles. Peptides are stored in large granular vesicles.

PLASTICITY OF COEXISTENCE

The existence of multiple neurotransmitters and the potential for the differential release of these transmitters create an added dimension to the variety of signals a single nerve ending can transmit. Second messenger systems can selectively activate the transcription of specific genes and, hence, the synthesis of specific proteins. Neurotransmitter combinations, therefore, have the potential to change or to become modulated, according to the physiological state of the neuron. Because many of the defined co-transmitter systems are the same from species to species, the specific combination of neurotransmitters is probably constant for most populations or subpopulations of neurons. However, the potential for plasticity is inherent in the system. Neurotransmitter combinations may be fixed, but the relative concentrations, ease of release, and responsiveness of receptors are all subject to modulation.

EXAMPLES OF COEXISTENCE AND RELEASE

The autonomic innervation of the cat salivary gland is a well-studied example of peripheral innervation. The parasympathetic nerve terminals contain ACh and VIP. The sympathetic nerve terminals contain NE and NPY. ACh alone induces secretion and increases the blood flow; VIP alone increases the blood flow but has no effect on secretion. In combination, ACh and VIP have an additive effect on the blood flow and VIP potentiates the ACh-induced secretion. Both NE and NPY produce vasoconstriction, but the effects are complementary: the NE response is rapid (several msec) and of brief duration (several sec), whereas the NPY effect develops slower and lasts for an extended period.

In the CNS, 5-HT projections from a medullary raphe nucleus to the ventral horn of the spinal cord contain, in addition to 5-HT, SubP and TRH. The nerve terminals have two types of vesicles: small clear vesicles containing 5-HT and large dense-core vesicles containing all three neurotransmitters (5-HT, SubP, and TRH). When applied ionophoretically, neither SubP nor TRH have any effect on the postsynaptic membrane.

During low frequency stimulation, only the small vesicles are released; 5-HT binds to the postsynaptic receptor and generates an EPSP. A slightly higher frequency of stimulation releases additional 5-HT (small vesicles) and is sufficient to stimulate the $5-HT_{1B}$ autoreceptor on the presynaptic membrane and to inhibit the release of additional 5-HT. However, at a very high frequency of stimulation, the large vesicles are activated, releasing SubP and TRH along with additional 5-HT. The TRH binds to the postsynaptic membrane at a site adjacent to or coupled with the 5-HT receptor. This facilitates the 5-HT receptor response, and the postsynaptic EPSP is greater than with 5-HT alone. At the same time, SubP binds to the 5-HT autoreceptor, blocking the 5-HT inhibition of further neurotransmitter release. Thus, the two peptides, having no defined effect by themselves, modulate the postsynaptic response of 5-HT by amplifying the postsynaptic receptor response and blocking the autoreceptor, which allows the release of additional 5-HT. The total postsynaptic response becomes much greater than that with the release of additional 5-HT alone — but *only* when the rate of firing is sufficient to activate the second population of synaptic vesicles, those containing the neuroactive peptides.

Nerve terminals of some primary sensory neurons in the spinal cord contain two neuroactive peptides, SubP and CGRP, and no classic transmitter. SubP alone produces a response that lasts for several minutes; CGRP alone does nothing. However, when co-released, the SubP response lasts for up to 30 minutes. In this system, CGRP may inhibit a SubP-specific endopeptidase, blocking the degradation of SubP and thereby prolonging its activity.

These few examples serve to illustrate the vast possibilities of interactions between multiple neurotransmitters and neuromodulators. We have only started to explore this exciting frontier of neurobiology. The number of interactions is almost unlimited. The potential for plasticity in the synapse, as modulated through the activation of selected gene transcription, makes the system even more adaptable to the changing physiology of the neuron.

SUGGESTED READING

Hökfelt, T., K. Fuxe, and B. Pernow (Editors) (1986). *Coexistence of Neuronal Messengers: A New Principle in Chemical Transmission. Progress in Brain Research,* Volume 68. Elsevier Publishing Company, Amsterdam.

This book presents a comprehensive discussion of the concept of multiple neurotransmitters. Although our knowledge has advanced since this symposium was held in 1985, it is still a valid introduction to the field. It places the concept in historical perspective and presents a frank discussion of the advantages and disadvantages of the techniques required.

McGeer, P. L., J. C. Eccles, and E. G McGeer (1987). *Molecular Neurobiology of the Mammalian Brain,* 2nd Edition. Plenum Press, New York, 774 pp.

A comprehensive review of the biochemistry of the mammalian brain. Approximately two thirds of the text is devoted to specific neurotransmitter systems and their synthesis, receptors, pharmacology, and mode of action. The remainder of the book is devoted to the application of the basic molecular mechanisms to specific integrative processes and functional systems.

Siegel, G., B. Agranoff, R. W. Albers, and P. Molinoff (Editors) (1989). *Basic Neurochemistry,* 4th Edition. Raven Press, New York, 984 pp.

As a comprehensive, multiauthored reference in the field of neurochemistry, this book has excellent sections devoted to neurotransmitter systems and the biochemical bases for many neurological disorders. The material is presented in a clear, concise, current, and well-referenced style.

Stryer, L. and H. R. Bourne (1986). G-Proteins: A family of signal transducers. Ann. Rev. Cell Biol., 2:391–419.

This review provides a good introduction to the G-proteins and their basic mechanism of action in the process of signal transduction. In this fast moving field, much has been added since this review was written, but the basic principles of action are still sound and still apply.

Part
III

MORPHOLOGY OF THE ADULT NERVOUS SYSTEM

Chapter

6

Spinal Cord

GENERAL FEATURES
SPINAL NERVES
WHITE MATTER
GRAY MATTER
REGIONAL DIFFERENCES

The spinal cord is a long, nearly cylindrical portion of the central nervous system (CNS). It is continuous rostrally with the brain stem and extends into the vertebral canal, where it ends at the level of the intervertebral disc between the first and second lumbar vertebrae. Although the spinal cord is only 6- to 12-mm wide, it has an average length of 42 cm in the adult female and 45 cm in the adult male. In total mass, the cord represents only 2% of the human CNS, yet it innervates the motor and sensory areas of the entire body, except for those areas that the cranial nerves innervate.

Terms for position are often a source of confusion, especially in reference to neuroanatomical structures. In general, *anterior* and *ventral* refer to the front of the body; *posterior* and *dorsal* to the back of the body; *cranial* and *superior* to the upper portion; and *caudal* and *inferior* to the lower portion. However, the terms *ventral, dorsal, cranial,* and *caudal* apply equally to animals with horizontal body positions.

In the human anatomical position (body erect, arms at the side, and palms forward), the neural axis bends at the level of the junction between the midbrain and diencephalon. Thus, in the spinal cord and brain stem through the level of midbrain, *anterior* is synonymous with *ventral;* *posterior* with *dorsal; cranial* with *superior;* and *caudal* with *inferior.* At the level of the diencephalon and telencephalon, however, *ventral* is a synonym for *inferior,* and *dorsal* is a synonym for *superior. Cranial* and *caudal* are rarely employed with reference to structures in the diencephalon and telencephalon. Because these synonyms are interchangeable in the neuroanatomical literature and textbooks, it is important to understand these distinctions.

General Features

Throughout its length, the spinal cord has an ordered and a segmental pattern of 31 pairs of *spinal nerves* (eight cervical, twelve thoracic, five lumbar, five sacral, and one coccygeal)—a segmental pattern not reflected in the internal organization of the spinal cord (Figs. 6–1 and 6–2). Each spinal nerve is composed of *dorsal roots*, sensory nerve fibers from neurons located in the *dorsal root ganglion*; and *ventral roots*, motor nerve fibers from neurons located mainly in the ventral portion of the spinal cord (Fig. 6–3). An exception may be the first cervical nerve, which has only ventral roots in about 50% of the cases.

117

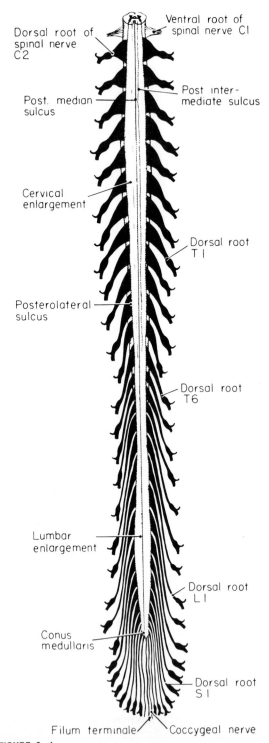

FIGURE 6-1

Posterior view of the spinal cord showing attached dorsal root filaments and spinal ganglia. Letters and numbers indicate corresponding spinal nerves. (Reproduced with permission from M. B. Carpenter, and J. Sutin, *Human Neuroanatomy*, 8th Edition, Williams & Wilkins, Baltimore, p. 233, 1983.)

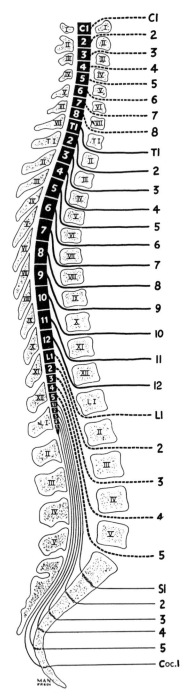

FIGURE 6-2

The alignment of spinal segments with the vertebrae. The bodies and spinous processes of the vertebrae are indicated by roman numerals. Spinal segments and spinal nerves are indicated by arabic numerals and letters. (Reproduced with permission from W. Haymaker, and B. Woodhall, *Peripheral Nerve Injuries; Principles of Diagnosis*, 2nd Edition, W. B. Saunders Co., Philadelphia, p. 32, 1953.)

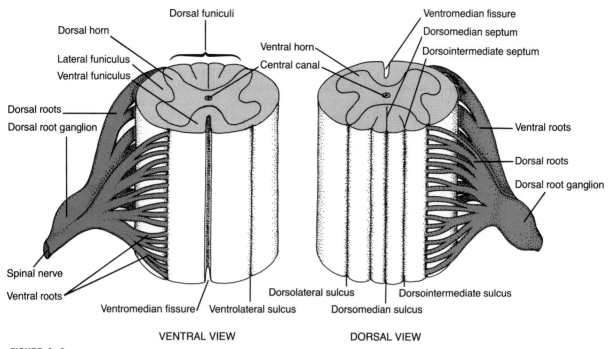

FIGURE 6-3

A typical spinal segment as seen from the ventral surface (left) and from the dorsal surface (right). Dorsal and ventral roots enter and exit, respectively, throughout the length of the spinal segment. These roots, in turn, collate to form the spinal nerve.

RELATION TO VERTEBRAL CANAL

The spinal cord is encased in the bony *vertebral canal,* and the spinal nerves exit through the *intervertebral foramina.* C-1 exits between the atlas and the occipital bone; C-2 through C-7 exit above the corresponding cervical vertebrae; and C-8 exits between the seventh cervical and first thoracic vertebrae. All thoracic, lumbar, and sacral nerves exit below the corresponding vertebrae (see Fig. 6-2).

In the adult, the caudal end of the spinal cord, the *conus medullaris,* is usually situated between the first and second lumbar vertebrae. Cervical nerves exit laterally; however, the more caudad the spinal nerve, the farther it travels within the vertebral canal before exiting at the appropriate intervertebral foramen.

In the embryo, all spinal nerves initially exit laterally. As development proceeds, the vertebral column grows at a faster rate than the spinal cord. A relative displacement of the spinal segments and the points of exit of the spinal nerves from the vertebral canal then develops (see Figs. 1-8 and 6-2).

Although the spinal cord ends at about the level of the first and second lumbar vertebrae, the dural sac continues to the level of the second sacral vertebra (see Chapter 9). The *conus medullaris* gives rise to the *filum terminale (filum terminale internum),* a filamentous thread of nonneuronal tissue extending to the base of the dural sac. The filum terminale passes through the dural sac and becomes the *coccygeal ligament (filum terminale externum),* anchoring both the spinal cord and the fluid-filled dural sac to the base of the vertebral canal. This lower portion of the dural sac (from L-2 to S-4) contains only nerve roots. Collectively, they are known as the *cauda equina.* Clinically, this area is of importance in the withdrawal of cerebrospinal fluid and the administration of spinal anesthetics (see Chapter 9).

MORPHOLOGY

The cylindrical spinal cord has two characteristic swellings, the *cervical* and *lumbosacral enlargements,* at the levels of origin of the spinal nerves that innervate the upper and lower extremities, respectively (see Fig. 6-1). These enlargements are caused by an increased number of neurons in the gray matter of the cord and reflect the larger peripheral field of innervation, the extremities.

The surface of the spinal cord is marked by several longitudinal grooves. On the anterior surface is the *ventromedian fissure*, 2 to 3 mm deep. On the posterior surface is the *dorsomedian sulcus*, continuous internally with the *dorsomedian septum*, a glial membrane. On the lateral surface is the *dorsolateral sulcus* (point of entry of the dorsal root fibers) and the *ventrolateral sulcus* (point of exit of the ventral root fibers). All these grooves extend the entire length of the cord. On the posterior surface, from the upper cervical to mid-thoracic levels, are the *dorsal intermediate sulci*. Each is continuous internally with a *dorsal intermediate septum*, also a glial membrane (Figs. 6–1 and 6–3).

The basic pattern of morphology laid down in the embryo is preserved in the adult, with the gray matter central and the white matter peripheral. The dorsal and ventral halves of the gray matter develop from the alar and basal plates, respectively, and are sensory (alar) and motor (basal) in general function (see Figs. 1–7 and 6–3).

The surrounding white matter is composed principally of longitudinally running nerve fibers, either ascending from the spinal cord to the brain or descending from the brain to various spinal cord levels. In addition, intersegmental spinospinal fibers ascend or descend for various distances. These form the *fasciculus proprius* (see Fig. 6–8). Thus, cervical segments have a greater number of fibers and a greater cross-sectional area of white matter than do lumbar levels. At any level of the cord, the white matter contains all the fibers descending from the brain to more caudal levels and all the fibers ascending to the brain from more caudal levels. The amount of gray matter, however, reflects the size of the peripheral field innervated by the spinal segment and is greatest in the cervical and lumbosacral enlargements.

In a transverse section of the spinal cord, the white matter is divided anatomically into six major areas or *funiculi*. The points of entry of the dorsal roots (the dorsolateral sulci), the dorsal horns, and the central gray matter are the boundaries of the paired *dorsal funiculi*. The *dorsal funiculi* are separated medially by the *dorsomedial septum*, extending centrally from the *dorsomedial sulcus*. The points of exit of the ventral roots (the ventrolateral sulci), the ventral horns, and the central gray matter are boundaries of the paired *ventral funiculi*. The *ventral funiculi* are separated medially by the ventromedial fissure. Laterally, between the dorsal and ventral roots of the each side and bounded internally by the gray matter of the dorsal and ventral horns, are the *lateral funiculi* (see Figs. 6–1 and 6–3).

The *dorsal funiculus* is further subdivided by the dorsal intermediate sulcus and the dorsal intermediate septum into the medially situated *fasciculus gracilis* and more lateral *fasciculus cuneatus*. This subdivision extends from C-1 to T-6. Below T-6, the dorsal funiculus contains only the fasciculus gracilis (see Figs. 6–1 and 6–3).

Spinal Nerves

Figure 6–4 illustrates a transverse section of the spinal cord at a mid-thoracic level, with its associated segmental nerve roots and spinal nerve. Peripherally, *dorsal* and *ventral roots* merge to form a mixed (sensory and motor) *spinal nerve*. The spinal nerve then splits to form the *posterior primary ramus* and the *anterior primary ramus*. The posterior primary ramus innervates the trunk musculature and the associated area of the back. The anterior primary ramus runs between the ribs, innervating the costal and abdominal musculature along with the anterior and lateral surfaces of the body. At the level of the cervical and lumbosacral enlargements, the anterior primary ramus participates in the formation of the *brachial plexus* and the *lumbosacral plexus*, respectively. These plexuses provide motor and sensory innervation to the upper and lower extremities.

The formation of somites during embryonic development establishes a segmental pattern of innervation for the adult. One segmental spinal nerve innervates each somite. The later division and migration of the somite and its derivatives determine, in large part, the pattern of peripheral innervation in the adult. Briefly, each somite forms a sclerotome, myotome, and dermatome. The sclerotome forms axial skeletal elements; the myotome, striated muscle; and the dermatome contributes to the subcutaneous connective tissue. In the adult, the pattern of innervation reflects this segmental pattern. Each cutaneous segment is called a *dermatome*. Although we think of one spinal nerve innervating each dermatome, in actuality an overlap exists with each nerve providing some innervation to each adjacent dermatome as well. Therefore, clinically, the loss of one spinal nerve is difficult to detect from the loss of cutaneous sensitivity.

Figures 6–5 (left) and 6–6 (left) depict the pattern of dermatomal cutaneous innervation in

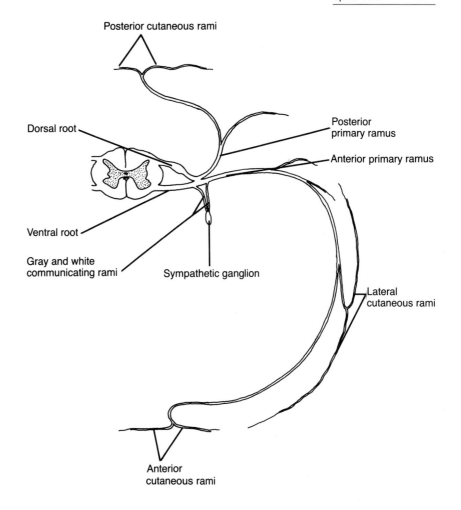

the adult. The anterior primary rami form major plexuses, notably the brachial and lumbosacral. This results in portions of several spinal nerves combining to form specific terminal peripheral nerves. The pattern of the cutaneous innervation of the peripheral nerves is represented in the right halves of Figures 6–5 and 6–6. The primary deviation from the segmental, dermatomal pattern is seen in the innervation of upper and lower extremities.

As discussed in Chapter 1, the "typical" spinal nerve contains fibers representing the four functional components: *general somatic efferent (GSE)*, motor to striated or skeletal muscle; *general somatic afferent (GSA)*, sensory to somatic tissue (muscle, skin, and joints); *general visceral efferent (GVE)*, autonomic or visceral motor; and *general visceral afferent (GVA)*, sensory to visceral structures. Figure 6–7 illustrates the relation of these four components to the segmental spinal nerve.

Somatic motor neurons (GSE) are situated in the *ventral horns* of the spinal cord. Their axons leave via the ventral root and distribute peripherally, with branches of the anterior and posterior primary rami of the spinal nerve to muscles of myotome origin (see Fig. 6–7).

Visceral motor neurons (GVE) reside in the *intermediolateral cell column* and their axons, *preganglionic sympathetic nerve fibers*, also join the spinal nerve via the ventral root. However, they soon leave the spinal nerve, forming the *white communicating ramus* of the *sympathetic* or *paravertebral ganglionic chain*. These *preganglionic* fibers either synapse with the neurons in the paravertebral sympathetic chain or pass through the chain, forming one of the *splanchnic nerves*. They end in one of the *prevertebral ganglia* (*superior mesenteric, inferior mesenteric,* or *celiac ganglion*).

Postganglionic fibers from the *paravertebral ganglia* form the *gray communicating ramus* and

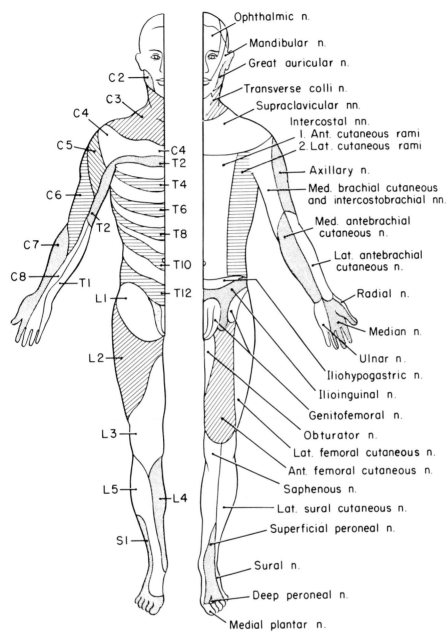

FIGURE 6-5

Anterior view of dermatomes (left) and cutaneous areas supplied by individual peripheral nerves (right). (Reproduced with permission from M. B. Carpenter, and J. Sutin, *Human Neuroanatomy*, 8th Edition, Williams & Wilkins, Baltimore, p. 190, 1983.)

re-join the spinal nerve to provide vasomotor, sudomotor, and pilomotor innervation to the trunk and extremities. *Postganglionic fibers* from the *prevertebral ganglia* innervate visceral target organs, such as the gastrointestinal tract and kidneys (see Fig. 6–7).

Sympathetic preganglionic fibers are present only in thoracic and lumbar spinal nerves. *Parasympathetic preganglionic nerve fibers* (also GVE) are found only in sacral and cranial nerves. The sacral preganglionic fibers do not enter the paravertebral sympathetic chain. They pass directly to the target organs and synapse with neurons located in *parasympathetic (or terminal) ganglia,* within or near the target organ. Chapter 18 reviews the visceral motor (GVE) or the *autonomic nervous system* in depth.

The cell bodies of both somatic afferent (GSA)

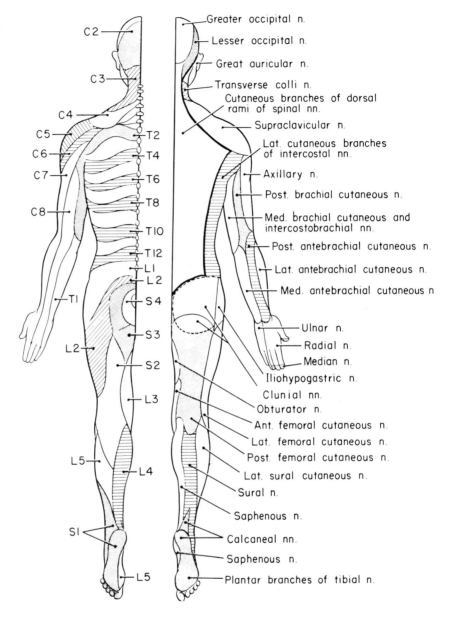

FIGURE 6-6

Posterior view of dermatomes (left) and cutaneous area supplied by individual peripheral nerves (right). (Reproduced with permission from M. B. Carpenter, and J. Sutin, *Human Neuroanatomy*, 8th Edition, Williams & Wilkins, Baltimore, p. 191, 1983.)

and visceral afferent (GVA) neurons reside in the *dorsal root ganglion*. The peripheral processes of the GSA neurons distribute with the spinal nerves and end in specialized sensory receptors. The central processes enter the spinal cord via the dorsal root. GVA fibers, with sensory receptors found in visceral structures, accompany the GVE preganglionic fibers through the sympathetic ganglia and subsequently to the target organs (see Fig. 6-7).

The principal function of the spinal cord is two-fold: (1) to receive sensory information from the body and transmit this information to the brain and (2) to provide motor innervation to somatic and visceral structures, much of which are under the control of higher brain centers. The spinal cord is also a reflexive center. Entering sensory fibers may synapse directly (or by way of an interneuron) on motor neurons thereby eliciting an immediate motor response or reflex. For more detail on somatic motor reflexes, see Chapter 14; for visceral motor reflexes, see Chapter 18.

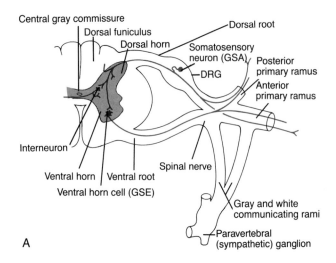

A

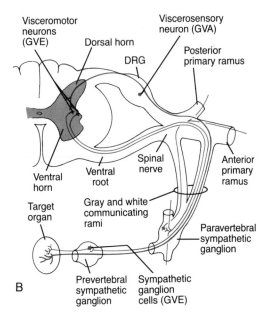

B

FIGURE 6-7

A typical thoracic spinal segment illustrating some of the major neuronal components. *A*, General somatic afferent and general somatic efferent components. *B*, General visceral afferent and general visceral efferent components.

White Matter

Within the dorsal, ventral, and lateral funiculi are literally millions of nerve fibers carrying sensory information from the spinal cord to the brain or carrying information associated with motor function from the brain to the spinal cord. In histological preparations, fibers from one pathway or tract are indistinguishable from those of another. Experimental studies with animals and postmortem comparisons of human spinal cord pathology with neurological history have been made to determine the relative positions of these specific pathways.

Ascending or descending groups of fibers, with a similar course and with a common function, are called *tracts* or *fasciculi*. In general, they are named according to origin and termination. For example, the spinotectal tract is made up of nerve fibers arising in the spinal cord and terminating in the tectum of the midbrain. Other examples are the descending corticospinal and rubrospinal tracts and the ascending spinoreticular and spinocerebellar tracts.

Figure 6–8 illustrates a number of the major ascending and descending tracts; however, considerable overlap and some individual variation occur. This is not a complete presentation of the

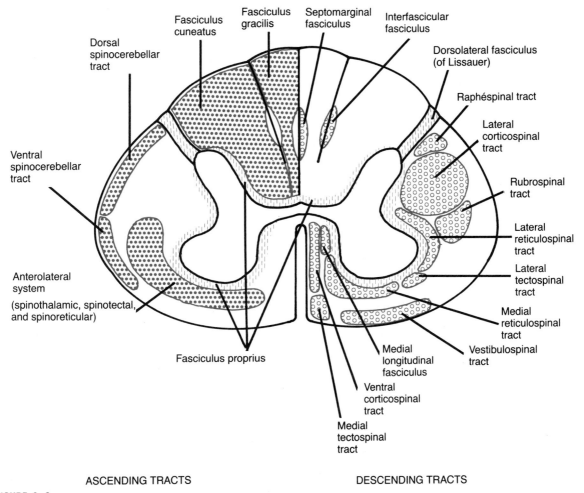

Dorsal
spinocerebellar
tract

Fasciculus
cuneatus

Fasciculus
gracilis

Septomarginal
fasciculus

Interfascicular
fasciculus

Dorsolateral fasciculus
(of Lissauer)

Raphéspinal tract

Lateral
corticospinal
tract

Rubrospinal
tract

Lateral
reticulospinal
tract

Lateral
tectospinal
tract

Medial
reticulospinal
tract

Vestibulospinal
tract

Medial
tectospinal
tract

Medial
longitudinal
fasciculus

Ventral
corticospinal
tract

Ventral
spinocerebellar
tract

Anterolateral
system
(spinothalamic, spinotectal,
and spinoreticular)

Fasciculus proprius

ASCENDING TRACTS   DESCENDING TRACTS

FIGURE 6-8

Some of the major fiber tracts of the spinal cord's white matter as represented at midcervical level. The ascending fiber tracts are on the left, the descending tracts on the right.

fasciculi and tracts, but it does contain the principal pathways. All are discussed in more detail in other chapters.

ASCENDING TRACTS

Ascending pathways generally transmit information about conditions in the environment surrounding the body—cutaneous sensory information—or about the body's movement and position in space—proprioceptive and position sense. These pathways relay the information to the thalamus and onto the cerebral cortex for conscious perception or to lower brain centers (cerebellum and tectum) for reflex activity.

The *dorsal funiculi* (*dorsal columns*), containing the *fasciculus gracilis* and *fasciculus cuneatus*, carry primary sensory information of proprioception, position and vibratory sense, and deep touch from the *ipsilateral* (same) side of the body. These are first order primary sensory neurons, and the fibers are uncrossed. The *fasciculus gracilis* carries information from spinal levels below T-6 and is present, therefore, at all spinal levels. The *fasciculus cuneatus* carries information from spinal levels above T-6 and is present only in cervical and upper thoracic levels. Collateral branches from these neurons form two small bundles of fibers that descend for a few segments before making synaptic connections within the spinal cord. These are the *septomarginal fasciculus* and the *fasciculus interfascicularis*. Although both are included in Figure 6-8, the septomarginal fasciculus is only in the lower half of the cord, at the levels of entry of the fibers that form the fasciculus gracilis. Similarly, the fasciculus interfascicularis is present only in the upper half of the spinal cord, at the levels of entry of fibers forming the fasciculus cuneatus.

In contrast, the *spinothalamic tract* carries pain, temperature, and light touch information to the thalamus but from the *contralateral* (opposite) side of the body. The *spinomesencephalic tract*, also a crossed pathway, ascends in association with the spinothalamic tract but carries nociceptive information to the midbrain region. Included in the *spinomesencephalic tract* are *spinotectal fibers* destined for the midbrain tectum and fibers carrying information to the periaqueductal gray and other midbrain structures. Collectively, the *spinothalamic, spinomesencephalic,* and *spinoreticular tracts* are known as the *anterolateral system (ALS)*.

The *dorsal spinocerebellar tract* contains uncrossed fibers from the *dorsal nucleus of Clarke* (see subsequent discussion) and carries proprioceptive information from the spinal cord to the cerebellum. The *ventral spinocerebellar tract*, which is much smaller than its dorsal counterpart, however, contains both crossed and uncrossed fibers en route to the cerebellum.

DESCENDING TRACTS

The largest and most prominent descending pathway is the *lateral corticospinal tract*, carrying information from the contralateral motor cortex of the telencephalon to the spinal cord. Because the lateral corticospinal tract has crossed or *decussated* in the lower medulla, these fibers innervate lower motor neurons on the same side of the spinal cord. A less prominent, uncrossed corticospinal pathway is the *ventral corticospinal tract*, a tract of minimal clinical importance because of its small size.

The *rubrospinal tract*, although quite prominent in some mammals, is relatively insignificant in humans. This motor pathway arises in the *red nucleus* and ends in relation to motor neurons throughout the spinal cord. Similarly, the *lateral* and *medial reticulospinal tracts* arise in nuclei of the medullary and pontine reticular formations, respectively, and end in relation to motor neurons in the spinal cord.

The *vestibulospinal tract*, originating exclusively in the lateral vestibular nucleus of the brain stem, modulates lower motor activity in response to vestibular sensory information. The

medial longitudinal fasciculus and the *medial* and *lateral tectospinal tracts* also alter motor function and carry information from brain stem nuclei.

The *raphespinal tract* arises principally from the nucleus raphe magnus of the medulla and ends in the external laminae of the dorsal horn. This pathway inhibits the transmission of entering sensory signals at the level of the spinal cord.

INTERSEGMENTAL FIBERS

Although most of the pathways mentioned thus far carry information between the brain and the spinal cord, extensive fiber connections occur between spinal segments. Most of these short-range fibers ascend or descend adjacent to the gray matter and collectively are called the *fasciculus proprius*. Primary sensory fibers, carrying pain, temperature, and touch information, bifurcate upon entering the spinal cord. Their branches ascend and descend for several spinal segments in the *dorsolateral fasciculus of Lissauer*, before synapsing in the dorsal horn (see Fig. 6–8). Intrasegmental fibers, establishing connections with neurons in the opposite half of the spinal cord, cross the midline in the *anterior white commissure*.

Gray Matter

The neuronal organization in the gray matter is one of longitudinally arranged columns and laminae. Two sets of nomenclature are in use. The first is the traditional columnar and nuclear organization. The second, the laminae of Rexed, is a cytoarchitectonic map of the spinal cord, a map that correlates well with synaptic connections and neurophysiological data. Figures 6–9, 6–10, and 6–11 illustrate both sets of nomenclature, as they apply to three representative levels of the spinal cord: lower cervical, mid-thoracic, and lumbar.

NUCLEI AND COLUMNS

The dorsal horn is one site of termination for primary sensory fibers and functions to (1) integrate and modulate sensory information; (2) relay sensory information to higher centers, e.g., thalamus, cerebellum, and brain stem; and (3) establish reflex arcs. Three dorsal horn nuclei or columns are present at all levels of the spinal cord. They include the *posteromarginal nucleus*, the

FIGURE 6-9

Section through the fifth or sixth cervical segment of the adult spinal cord. Major nuclear groups are identified on the left. Rexed's spinal laminae are illustrated on the right.

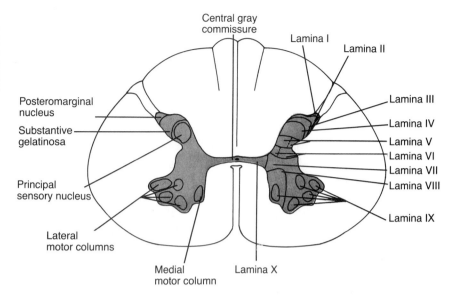

substantia gelatinosa, and the *principal sensory nucleus (nucleus proprius)*. Limited to spinal segments C-8 through L-3 is the *dorsal nucleus of Clarke (nucleus dorsalis* or *Clarke's column)*.

The ventral horn contains lower motor neurons for the innervation of striated muscle. The *medial motor column*, extending the entire length of the spinal cord, innervates the axial musculature. The *lateral motor columns*, present in the cervical enlargement (C-5 to T-1) and the lumbo-sacral enlargement (L-1 to S-3), innervate muscles of their respective extremities. In reality, this is not a single column, but a series of small columns or nuclei arranged according to the muscle groups innervated.

The *intermediolateral cell column* contains preganglionic sympathetic (GVE) neurons and is limited to thoracic and lumbar levels (T-1 to L-3). The *intermediomedial cell column* is associated with visceral motor reflexes and has a

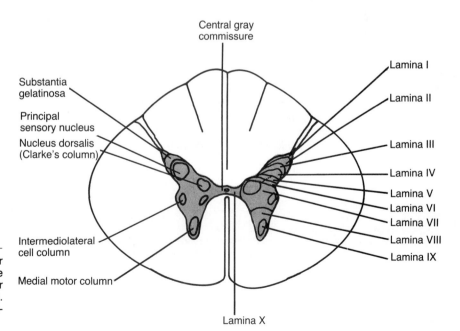

FIGURE 6-10

Section through the second or third thoracic segment of the adult spinal cord. Major nuclear groups are identified on the left. Rexed's spinal laminae are illustrated on the right.

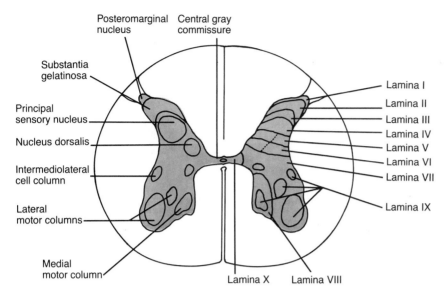

FIGURE 6-11

Section through the second lumbar segment of the adult spinal cord. Major nuclear groups are identified on the left. Rexed's spinal laminae are illustrated on the right.

similar distribution (Table 6–1). The gray matter, crossing the midline and surrounding the central canal, is the *central gray matter* or the *gray commissure*.

LAMINAE OF REXED

Rexed's laminae I, II, III, and IV encompass most of the dorsal horn. Lamina I corresponds to the posteromarginal nucleus and lamina II to the substantia gelatinosa. Laminae III and IV include most of the principal sensory nuclei.

Laminae V and VI occupy the base of the dorsal horn and are subdivided into medial and lateral compartments. These subdivisions are based principally on neuronal connections and electrophysiological data. Both laminae are important for the integration of somatic motor information and as reflex centers and major sources of spinocerebellar fibers.

Laminae VII and VIII are more complex. They include the dorsal nucleus of Clarke and the intermediolateral and intermediomedial cell columns. They extend throughout the zona intermedia and ventral portions of the gray matter. These laminae are important in motor reflex activity. Lamina IX includes the lateral and medial motor columns and lamina X the central gray of the spinal cord.

TABLE 6-1

Major Spinal Cord Nuclei or Columns

NUCLEUS OR COLUMN	SPINAL LEVEL	FUNCTION
Posteromarginal nucleus	All levels	All three receive primary sensory information. The first two appear to modulate this
Substantia gelatinosa	All levels	information, whereas the principal sensory nucleus is associated more with transmis-
Principal sensory nucleus (nucleus proprius)	All levels	sion to higher centers and with reflex connections.
Dorsal nucleus of Clarke (nucleus dorsalis)	C8–L3	Nucleus of origin of the dorsal spinocerebellar tract.
Intermediomedial nucleus	T1–L3	A center for autonomic reflexes.
Intermediolateral nucleus	T1–L3	Nucleus of origin of sympathetic preganglionic fibers.
Medial motor columns	All levels	Lower motor neurons innervating axial musculature.
Lateral motor columns	C5–T1 and	Lower motor neurons innervating muscles of the upper extremity.
	L1–S3	Lower motor neurons innervating muscles of the lower extremity.

FIGURE 6-12

Weigert-stained, transverse section of the human spinal cord at the C-1 level. Lateral corticospinal fibers are now located medially toward the pyramidal decussation. At this level, fibers of the spinal trigeminal tract interdigitate with those of the dorsolateral fasciculus. Bar = 3.0 mm. (Reproduced with permission from D. E. Haines, *Neuroanatomy: An Atlas of Structures, Sections, and Systems*, 3rd Edition. Urban & Schwarzenberg, Baltimore-Munich, 1991.)

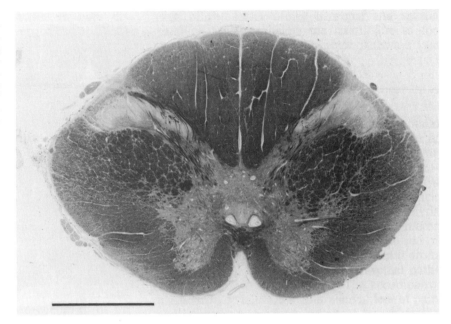

Regional Differences

Gross regional differences exist in the size of the spinal cord. Most notable are the swellings produced by the cervical and lumbosacral enlargements (see Fig. 6-1). However, the organization of the gray matter and the presence or absence of specific nuclear groups are most valuable for identifying the specific level of the cord from which a section has been taken. In addition, the relative abundance of white matter and the presence or absence of a fasciculus cuneatus are helpful.

In upper cervical levels, the white matter is relatively abundant and the fasciculus cuneatus is well developed. The dorsal horns are quite small.

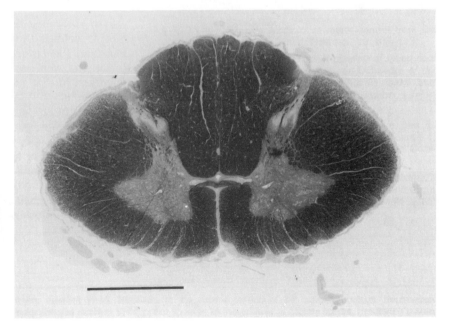

FIGURE 6-13

Weigert-stained, transverse section of human spinal cord showing its characteristic appearance at lower cervical levels (C-7). The ventral horn is large. Proportionately and absolutely, a large amount of white matter is noted. The general shape of the cord is oval. Bar = 3.0 mm. (Reproduced with permission from D. E. Haines, *Neuroanatomy: An Atlas of Structures, Sections, and Systems*, 3rd Edition. Urban & Schwarzenberg, Baltimore-Munich, 1991.)

No dorsal nuclei of Clarke, no lateral motor columns, and no intermediolateral cell columns are found. However, the accessory nucleus, associated with cranial nerve XI, is found in the upper cervical cord. The spinal tract and nucleus of the trigeminal nerve interdigitate with the dorsal lateral fasciculus of Lissauer and the substantia gelatinosa. The large corticospinal tracts have decussated and are more medial than in the lower levels of the spinal cord (Fig. 6–12).

At the level of the cervical enlargement (C-7), there is still a relatively large amount of white matter with prominent fasciculi cuneatus and gracilis. The general shape of the cord is oval. Lateral motor columns are very conspicuous as are the dorsal horns. No dorsal nuclei of Clarke or intermediolateral cell columns are seen (Fig. 6–13).

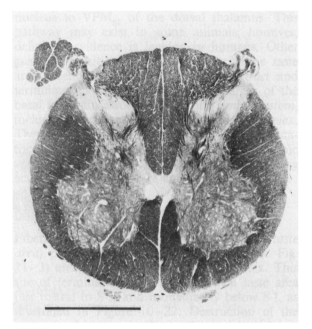

FIGURE 6–15

Weigert-stained, transverse section of human spinal cord showing its characteristic appearance at lumbar level L-4. Dorsal and ventral horns are large in relation to a modest amount of white matter. Fibers of the medial division of the dorsal root directly enter the gracile fasciculus. Bar = 3.0 mm. (Reproduced with permission from D. E. Haines, *Neuroanatomy: An Atlas of Structures, Sections, and Systems*, 3rd Edition. Urban & Schwarzenberg, Baltimore-Munich, 1991.)

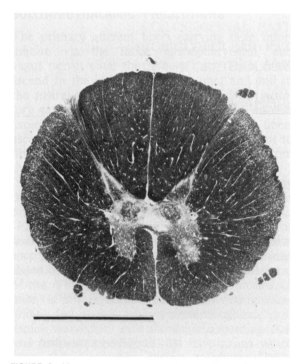

FIGURE 6–14

Weigert-stained, transverse section of human spinal cord showing its characteristic appearance at thoracic level T-4. The white matter appears large in relation to the rather small amount of gray matter. Dorsal and ventral horns are small, especially when compared with lower cervical and lumbar levels. The shape of the cord is round. Bar = 3.0 mm. (Reproduced with permission from D. E. Haines, *Neuroanatomy: An Atlas of Structures, Sections, and Systems*, 3rd Edition. Urban & Schwarzenberg, Baltimore-Munich, 1991.)

In mid-thoracic levels (T-4), the profile of the cord is round, the white matter is reduced in area, and the fasciculus cuneatus is smaller. The dorsal and ventral horns are small, but a very prominent dorsal nucleus of Clarke and an intermediolateral cell column are noted. Lateral motor columns are absent, and small medial motor columns occupy the ventral horns (Fig. 6–14).

In the lumbosacral enlargement (L-4), the cord is round to slightly oval, the fasciculus cuneatus is absent, and the relative amount of white matter is reduced, especially in comparison with the gray matter. Both dorsal and ventral horns are large, and very prominent lateral motor columns are visible. The dorsal nucleus of Clarke and the intermediolateral cell columns are absent (Fig. 6–15).

In lower sacral levels, the cord becomes very small and the white matter sparse, limited to a thin circumferential mantle. The gray matter now

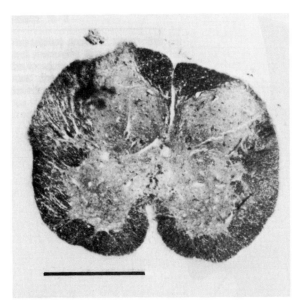

FIGURE 6-16

Weigert-stained, transverse section of human spinal cord showing the characteristics of a low sacral level. Gray matter occupies most of the cross section. The H-shaped appearance is not obvious at the sacral-coccygeal levels. The white matter is a comparatively thin mantle. Bar = 1.0 mm. (Reproduced with permission from D. E. Haines, *Neuroanatomy: An Atlas of Structures, Sections, and Systems*, 3rd Edition. Urban & Schwarzenberg, Baltimore-Munich, 1991.)

occupies most of the cross-sectional area, although the H-shaped pattern, characteristic of higher levels, is not as apparent. Lateral motor columns are small but present, and the dorsal horns are well developed (Fig. 6-16).

SUGGESTED READING

Clark, R. G. (1984). Anatomy of the mammalian cord. In *Handbook of the Spinal Cord*, Volume 2. R. A. Davidoff (Editor). Marcel Dekker, Inc., New York, pp. 1-46.

A well-referenced overview of the morphology of the mammalian spinal cord.

Hardy, A. G. and A. B. Rossier (1975). *Spinal Cord Injuries.* Georg Thieme Publishers, Stuttgart.

A brief synopsis of the clinical aspects of spinal cord injury is presented. Although considerable text is devoted to the treatment of the disorders, ample text is given to the anatomical basis of the symptoms.

Mountcastle, V. B. (1974). Effects of spinal transection. In *Medical Physiology*, Volume 1, 13th Edition. V. B. Mountcastle (Editor). C. V. Mosby Co., St. Louis, MO, pp. 662-667.

A concise discussion of the traumatic effect of spinal cord transection with special emphasis on spinal shock and the functional capacity of the isolated spinal cord.

Rexed, B. (1964). Some aspects of the cytoarchitectonics and synaptology of the spinal cord. In *Progress in Brain Research*, Volume 11. *Organization of the Spinal Cord.* J. C. Eccles and J. P. Schade (Editors). Elsevier Publishing Company, Amsterdam, pp. 58-92.

A review by Rexed of his laminar organization for spinal cord gray matter and the relation of this nomenclature to the more traditional nuclear organization.

Scheibel, A. B. (1984). The organization of the spinal cord. In *Handbook of the Spinal Cord*, Volume 2. R. A. Davidoff (Editor). Marcel Dekker, Inc., New York, pp. 47-78.

An excellent review of the current state of knowledge of neuronal organization and connectivity in the mammalian spinal cord.

Chapter
7

Brain Stem and Cerebellum

EXTERNAL FEATURES
MEDULLA, PONS, AND MIDBRAIN
DIENCEPHALON
CEREBELLUM

External Features

GENERAL BOUNDARIES

In the adult human brain, the *brain stem* makes up only 4.4% of the brain's weight, the *cerebellum* 10.5%, and the *telencephalon* 85.1%. Extending from the spinal cord to the lamina terminalis, the *brain stem* has four main subdivisions: *medulla, pons, midbrain,* and *diencephalon.*

The *medulla,* or more properly, *medulla oblongata,* is the smallest and the most caudal portion of the brain stem. A derivative of the embryonic myelencephalon, the medulla is continuous inferiorly with the spinal cord and superiorly with the *pons* (Fig. 7–1). The *pons,* clearly visible as a large elevation on the ventral or anterior surface of the brain stem, is situated between the medulla and the *midbrain*. The *midbrain,* shortest of the brain stem subdivisions, extends rostrally from the pons to the *diencephalon.* The *diencephalon,* consisting of the *dorsal thalamus, hypothalamus, epithalamus,* and *ventral thalamus* (or *subthalamus*), is best seen in the midsagittal plane, because it is buried beneath large telencephalic structures, the *cerebral cortex* and the *basal ganglia.* From the basal surface, only a portion of the *hypothalamus* (the *mammillary bodies* and the *tuber cinereum*) is visible (Figs. 7–1 and 7–2).

The *cerebellum* is dorsal to the pons and is connected to the brain stem by three pairs of peduncles: the *inferior cerebellar peduncles* (*restiform* and *juxtarestiform bodies*) connect the cerebellum with the medulla, the *middle cerebellar peduncles* (*brachia pontis*) with the pons, and the *superior cerebellar peduncles* (*brachia conjunctivum*) with the midbrain (Figs. 7–1, 7–3, 7–4, and 7–5).

MEDULLA

The medulla forms a transitional zone, connecting the less differentiated regions of the nervous system, the spinal cord, with the more highly differentiated regions of the brain. The sulci and fissures on the surface of the cervical spinal cord and many of the underlying nuclear columns and fiber pathways extend for varying distances into the medulla.

On the ventral surface (see Fig. 7–2), the ventrolateral sulci extend the length of the medulla to the base of the pons and are the point of exit for motor rootlets of the *hypoglossal nerve* (cranial nerve XII). The ventral funiculi of the spinal cord extend into the lower medulla and, rostral to the *pyramidal decussation,* are replaced by enlarged elevations known as the *medullary pyramids.* The ventromedian fissure becomes

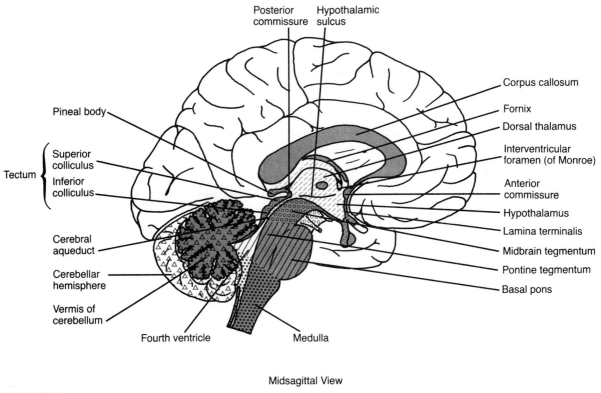

Posterior commissure   Hypothalamic sulcus

Corpus callosum

Fornix

Dorsal thalamus

Interventricular foramen (of Monroe)

Anterior commissure

Hypothalamus

Lamina terminalis

Midbrain tegmentum

Pontine tegmentum

Basal pons

Pineal body

Superior colliculus

Inferior colliculus

Tectum

Cerebral aqueduct

Cerebellar hemisphere

Vermis of cerebellum

Fourth ventricle   Medulla

Midsagittal View

FIGURE 7-1

Midsagittal view of the brain illustrating the major subdivisions of the brain stem. Gray shaded areas represent cut surfaces.

partially obliterated by the decussating fibers but reappears rostral to the decussation. Lateral to the pyramids and extending for approximately 2 cm below the pons are two ovoid mounds, the *olives* (or *olivary eminences*), a reflection of the underlying *inferior olivary nuclei* (see Figs. 7–9 and 7–10). In the sulcus, dorsal (posterior) to the olive, are rootlets of the *glossopharyngeal nerve* (cranial nerve IX) and the *vagus nerve* (cranial nerve X). Caudal to the rootlets of the vagus nerve, but along a line continuous with these rootlets and extending into the upper cervical spinal cord along the lateral surface of the lateral funiculus, are rootlets of the *spinal accessory nerve* (cranial nerve XI) (see Figs. 7–2 and 7–3).

The *olives* are seen more clearly in a lateral view of the brain stem (see Fig. 7–3) along with an elevation, just dorsal to the olive, the *tuberculum cinereum*. This is related to the underlying descending *spinal tract* and *nucleus of the trigeminal nerve* (cranial nerve V). The spinal tract of V and the accompanying spinal nucleus of V extend the entire length of the medulla and interdigitate caudally with the dorsolateral fasciculus of

Lissauer and the substantia gelatinosa of the upper cervical spinal cord.

The dorsal columns of the cervical spinal cord, the *fasciculus gracilis* and *fasciculus cuneatus*, extend rostrally into the medulla (see Fig. 7–4). At the *obex*, the inferior margin of the *fourth ventricle*, the dorsomedian sulcus splits to form the inferior boundaries of the fourth ventricle. With the opening of the fourth ventricle, the fasciculus gracilis and fasciculus cuneatus are spread laterally. Additionally, nuclei (*gracile* and *cuneate*) associated with each fasciculus produce small bulges on the dorsolateral surface of the medulla known as the *gracile tubercle* (or *clava*) and the *cuneate tubercle* (see Figs. 7–4, 7–8, and 7–9).

The *restiform bodies* form on the dorsolateral surfaces of the medulla—principally from a collation of fibers from the dorsal spinocerebellar tract, olivocerebellar and reticulocerebellar fibers, along with cuneocerebellar fibers from the external cuneate nucleus—and swing dorsad toward the central portions of the cerebellum (see Figs. 7–10 and 7–11). At the base of the cerebellum,

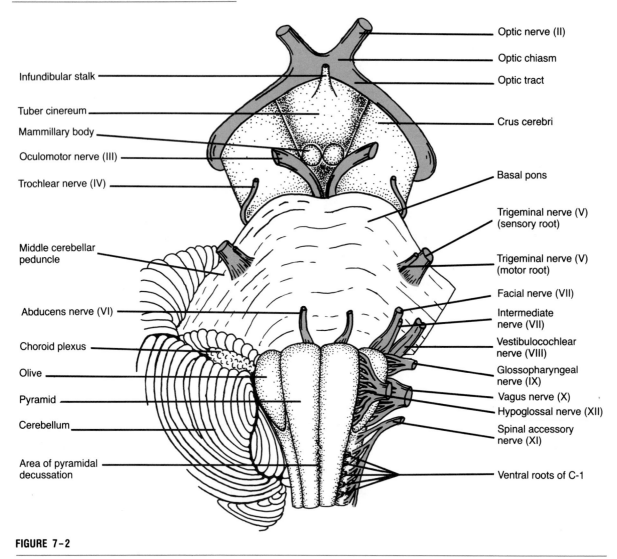

FIGURE 7-2

Ventral (anterior) view of the brain stem.

the restiform body is joined by a bundle of vestibulocerebellar and cerebellovestibular fibers, the *juxtarestiform body*, to form the *inferior cerebellar peduncle*. Often, however, the term inferior cerebellar peduncle is used as a synonym for restiform body.

Three cranial nerves exit (motor) or enter (sensory) the brain stem at the *medullopontine junction*: the *abducens nerve* (cranial nerve VI) exits between the pyramids and the pons; the *facial nerve* (cranial nerve VII) exits between the olive and the pons; and the *vestibulocochlear (statoacoustic) nerve* (cranial nerve VIII) enters the brain stem at the medullopontine angle, with the cochlear portion on the dorsolateral surface of

the restiform body and the vestibular portion entering the medulla beneath the restiform body (see Figs. 7–2 and 7–3).

PONS

Derived from the basal portion of the embryonic metencephalon, the *pons* is situated between the medulla and the midbrain. Its most striking feature is a large ovoid mass on the ventral surface of the brain stem, the *basal pons* (see Fig. 7–1). The size of the basal pons varies among mammals and is proportional to the degree of neocortical development. The *pontine nuclei* of the basal pons relay information from the neocortex to the

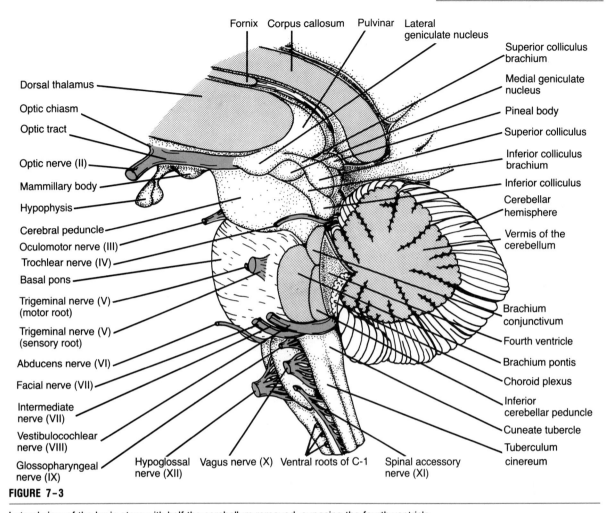

FIGURE 7-3

Lateral view of the brain stem with half the cerebellum removed, exposing the fourth ventricle.

cerebellum. Corticopontine fibers terminate in the pontine nuclei, and pontocerebellar fibers arise from these nuclei and enter the cerebellum as the *middle cerebellar peduncle* (see Figs. 7–2, 7–3, and 7–4). That portion of the brain stem between the basal pons and the floor of the fourth ventricle is known as the *pontine tegmentum* (see Fig. 7–1). The pontine tegmentum is continuous with the midbrain tegmentum above and the central core or *reticular formation* of the medulla below. The superior and inferior margins of the basal pons are utilized to approximate the indistinct boundaries of the pontine tegmentum (see Fig. 7–1).

Although nuclei associated with several cranial nerves are located in the pontine tegmentum, the *trigeminal nerve* (cranial nerve V) is the only nerve to exit and enter the pons and it does so through the central portion of the middle cere-

bellar peduncle. The trigeminal nerve has two components: a large sensory root, the *portio major*, and a smaller motor root, the *portio minor*. Both are visible as distinct roots on the lateral surface of the middle cerebellar peduncle (see Figs. 7–2 and 7–3).

CEREBELLUM

The cerebellum develops from the alar portion of the embryonic metencephalon, in the rostral margin of the roof of the fourth ventricle (the *rhombic lip*), and grows in a posterior and inferior direction, ultimately covering most of the fourth ventricle (see Fig. 1–15). The *cerebellar cortex*, thrown into a series of tiny folds or *folia*, can be divided laterally into *hemispheres* and a central portion known as the *vermis* (see Fig. 7–5).

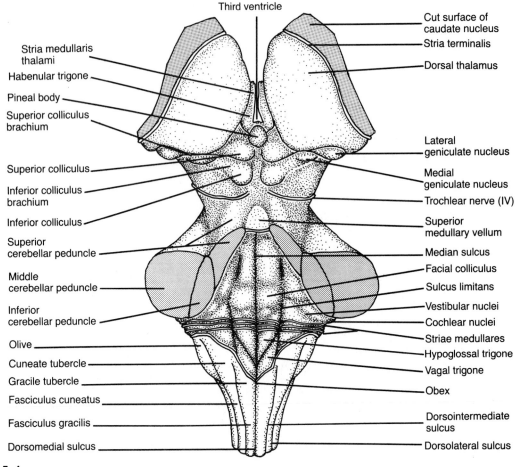

Third ventricle

Stria medullaris thalami

Habenular trigone

Pineal body

Superior colliculus brachium

Superior colliculus

Inferior colliculus brachium

Inferior colliculus

Superior cerebellar peduncle

Middle cerebellar peduncle

Inferior cerebellar peduncle

Olive

Cuneate tubercle

Gracile tubercle

Fasciculus cuneatus

Fasciculus gracilis

Dorsomedial sulcus

Cut surface of caudate nucleus

Stria terminalis

Dorsal thalamus

Lateral geniculate nucleus

Medial geniculate nucleus

Trochlear nerve (IV)

Superior medullary vellum

Median sulcus

Facial colliculus

Sulcus limitans

Vestibular nuclei

Cochlear nuclei

Striae medullares

Hypoglossal trigone

Vagal trigone

Obex

Dorsointermediate sulcus

Dorsolateral sulcus

FIGURE 7-4

Dorsal (posterior) view of the brain stem with the cerebellum removed, exposing the floor of the fourth ventricle.

Five deep fissures further subdivide the hemispheres into lobes and lobules: the *primary fissure, posterior superior fissure, horizontal fissure, prepyramidal fissure,* and *posterolateral fissure.* The *flocculonodular lobe,* or *archicerebellum,* is phylogenetically the oldest portion and is found on the ventral surface, separated from the rest of the cerebellum by the posterolateral fissure. The *anterior lobe,* or *paleocerebellum,* is on the anteroinferior portion of the cerebellum and is bounded by the primary fissure. The remainder of the cerebellum, extending from the rostrally located primary fissure to the posterolateral fissure, constitutes the *posterior lobe,* or *neocerebellum* (Fig. 7–5).

FOURTH VENTRICLE

With the development of the fourth ventricle, those portions of the embryonic neural tube de-

rived from the alar plate are spread laterally (see Fig. 1–14). In the adult, the floor of the fourth ventricle has several notable bumps (the *facial colliculus,* the *vagal trigone,* and the *hypoglossal trigone*) and grooves (the *median sulcus* and the more laterally situated *sulcus limitans*) (see Fig. 7–4). The facial colliculus marks the point where the *facial nerve* (cranial nerve VII) courses over the *abducens nucleus* (nucleus of cranial nerve VI), prior to exiting from the brain stem (see Fig. 1–25). The vagal and hypoglossal trigones reflect the underlying nuclei of the *vagus nerve* (cranial nerve X) and the *hypoglossal nerve* (cranial nerve XII). The sulcus limitans continues to mark the separation of the underlying nuclei into motor (medial) and sensory (lateral) components as it did in the embryonic neural tube.

The *superior medullary velum* is a thin sheet of tissue underlying the cerebellum and extending between the superior cerebellar peduncles. The

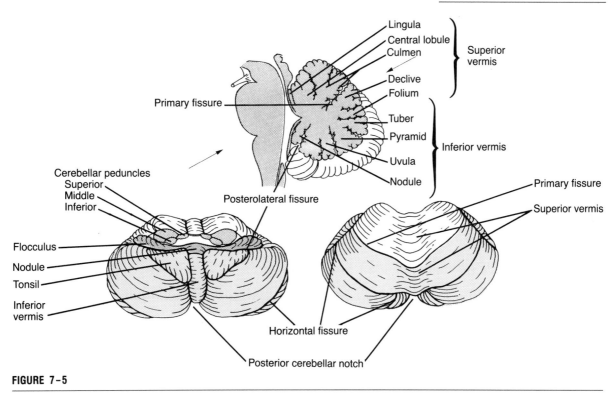

FIGURE 7-5

Midsagittal, dorsal, and ventral views of the cerebellum.

inferior medullary velum (or *tela choroidea of the fourth ventricle*) is the very thin, delicate choroid plexus covering the inferior portion of the fourth ventricle. Together, with the cerebellum, the superior medullary velum and inferior medullary velum form the roof of the fourth ventricle (see Figs. 7–4, 7–5, 7–10, and 7–13).

MIDBRAIN

The shortest segment of the brain stem, the *midbrain*, extends from the pons to the diencephalon and third ventricle. The dorsal (posterior) portion or roof of the midbrain, the *tectum*, consists of four small elevations, the pairs of *inferior colliculi* and *superior colliculi*. The *cerebral aqueduct of Sylvius* lies ventral to the tectum and connects the third ventricle of the diencephalon to the fourth ventricle of the pons and medulla. Ventral to the cerebral aqueduct, continuous with the pontine tegmentum and extending rostral to the third ventricle, is the *midbrain tegmentum* (see Figs. 7–1, 7–3, and 7–4).

Two massive elevations, the *crus cerebri* (or *pes pedunculi*), embrace a midline depression, the *interpeduncular fossa*, and form the most ventral portion of the midbrain (see Fig. 7–2). The *crus*

cerebri contains millions of fibers of neocortical origin (the corticospinal, corticobulbar, and corticopontine fibers). These fibers terminate in lower centers of the brain stem and spinal cord. The crus cerebri (pes pedunculi) together with the large, underlying nucleus, the *substantia nigra*, form the *basis pedunculi*. The basis pedunculi and the midbrain tegmentum form the *cerebral peduncles* (see Fig. 7–17). Often, these neuroanatomical terms are applied loosely. For example, *cerebral peduncle* often is used as a synonym for *crus cerebri*.

Two cranial nerves exit the midbrain: the *trochlear nerve* (cranial nerve IV) from the dorsal surface, just caudal to the inferior colliculus, and the *oculomotor nerve* (cranial nerve III) through the interpeduncular fossa (see Figs. 7–2, 7–3, and 7–4).

DIENCEPHALON

The *diencephalon*, a paired structure separated medially by the third ventricle, is continuous inferiorly with the midbrain and extends anteriorly to the lamina terminalis (see Fig. 7–1). It contains four subdivisions: the *epithalamus*, the *thalamus* (*dorsal thalamus*), the *hypothalamus*, and the *ventral thalamus* (*subthalamus*). From the ventral surface, only portions of the *hypothalamus* are visible (see Fig. 7–2). When the cerebral hemispheres are removed, the thalamus and epithalamus are more clearly visible beneath the corpus callosum (see Figs. 7–3 and 7–4).

The relatively small, dorsally situated epithalamus consists of the *pineal gland*, the *habenula*, and the *stria medullaris thalami* (see Figs. 7–1 and 7–4). Anterior to the epithalamus and on either side of the third ventricle is the relatively large, ovoid *thalamus*, bounded medially by the third ventricle, laterally by the internal capsule of the telencephalon, dorsally by the transverse cerebral fissure (immediately beneath the corpus callosum), and ventrally by the hypothalamus, as indicated by the presence of the *hypothalamic sulcus* in the wall of the third ventricle. On its medial surface, the thalamus extends from the *interventricular foramen* (*of Monroe*) to the *posterior commissure* (see Figs. 7–1, 7–3, and 7–4). The *hypothalamus* forms the ventral and lateral walls of the third ventricle, ventral to the hypothalamic sulcus and extending from the lamina

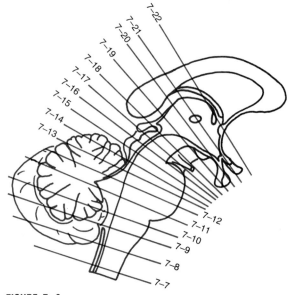

FIGURE 7–6

Midsagittal outline of the brain stem with lines representing the planes of the transverse, Weigert-stained sections in Figures 7–7 through 7–22.

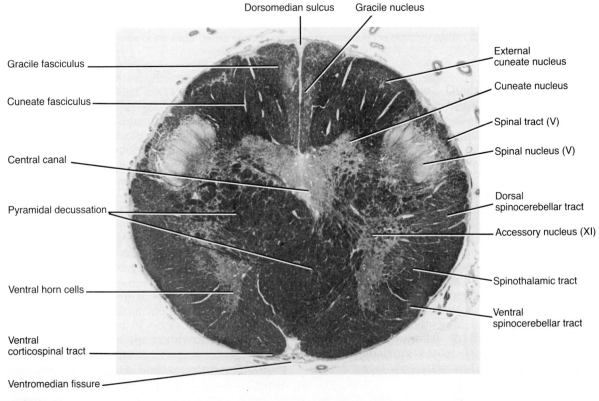

FIGURE 7–7

Transverse section through the lower medulla at the level of the pyramidal decussation. Human brain stem; Weigert stain.

terminalis to the posterior boundaries of the *mammillary bodies* (see Figs. 7–1 and 7–2).

The *ventral thalamus*, situated ventral to the thalamus, lateral to the hypothalamus, medial to the internal capsule, and dorsal to the crus cerebri, is not visible from the exterior.

One cranial nerve, the *optic nerve* (cranial nerve II), is associated with the diencephalon and, although it is not a true nerve but a pathway within the central nervous system (CNS), it is traditionally considered a cranial nerve. The optic nerve was formed during embryonic development when axons of retinal ganglion cells grew into the primitive optic stalk (see Chapter 1 and Figs. 7–1 and 7–2).

Medulla, Pons, and Midbrain

ASCENDING SENSORY PATHWAYS

Primary sensory fibers, ascending from the spinal cord and traveling in the *fasciculus gracilis* and *fasciculus cuneatus*, extend into the medulla and synapse on neurons of the *gracile* and *cuneate nuclei*. These nuclei, located deep to their respective fasciculi, relay tactile, vibratory, and deep pressure sense from the body to the cerebral cortex by way of the thalamus. The secondary sensory fibers from these nuclei sweep across the central portion of the medulla, as the *internal arcuate fibers*, and ascend to the thalamus, as the *medial lemniscus*. In the medulla, the medial lemnisci are visible as a pair of heavily myelinated fiber tracts, oriented vertically, and situated adjacent to the midline, between the very prominent *inferior olivary nuclei*. Fibers in the fasciculi gracilis and cuneatus carry sensory information from the ipsilateral side of the body. However, the internal arcuate fibers cross the midline. The remainder of the pathway, from the medial lemniscus through the thalamus to the cerebral cortex, carries information from the contralateral side of the body (Figs. 7–6 through 7–10, 7–24, and 7–25).

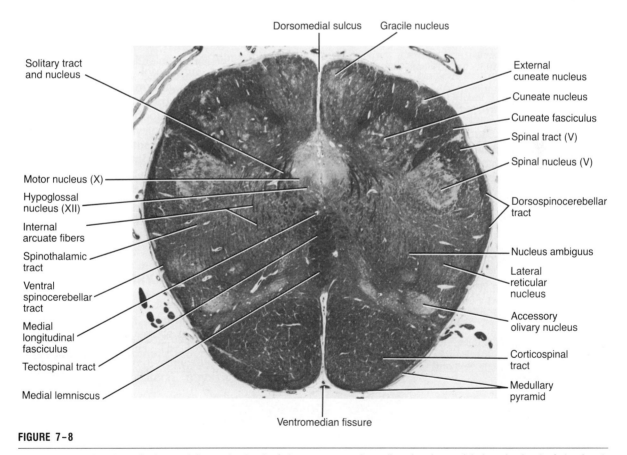

FIGURE 7–8

Transverse section through the medulla at the level of the cuneate and gracile tubercles and below the level of the fourth ventricle. Human brain stem; Weigert stain.

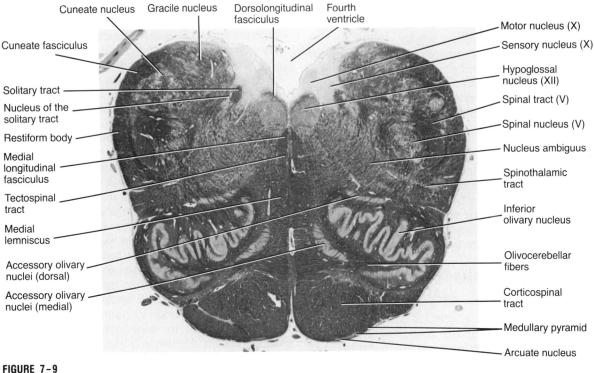

FIGURE 7–9

Transverse section through the medulla at the level of the olive and the lower portion of the fourth ventricle. Human brain stem; Weigert stain.

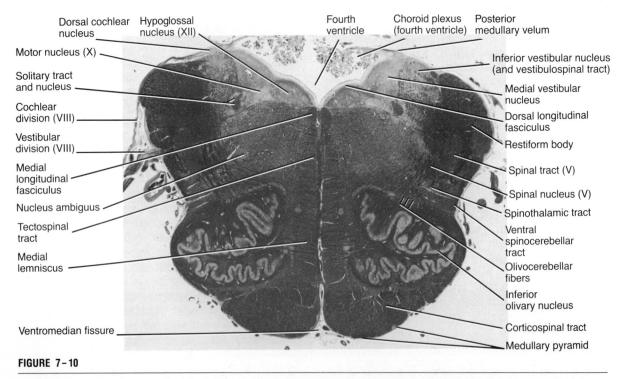

FIGURE 7–10

Transverse section through the upper end of the medulla, just below the medullopontine junction. Human brain stem; Weigert stain.

The *anterolateral system*, the spinothalamic and spinotectal tracts, continues without interruption through the medulla, pons, and midbrain to the thalamus. Initially, these tracts are located in the ventrolateral portion of the medulla, a position comparable to that in the spinal cord. With the appearance of the inferior olivary nuclei, the anterolateral system is displaced to a position dorsolateral to the inferior olivary nuclei and ventral to the restiform bodies (see Figs. 7–7 through 7–10 and 7–24).

At the level of the pons, the medial lemniscus is found in the ventral portion of the pontine tegmentum, just dorsal to the basal pons. With the absence of the inferior olivary nuclei, the medial lemniscus shifts from a vertical to a horizontal orientation and gradually moves to a more lateral and dorsolateral position, as it ascends through the midbrain. At the base of the diencephalon, the medial lemniscus occupies a position immediately below the ventral posterolateral nucleus of the thalamus, its nucleus of termination (Figs. 7–11 through 7–18, 7–26, and 7–27).

As the *anterolateral system* (principally the spinothalamic and spinotectal pathways) ascends

in the pontine tegmentum, it remains in a lateral location. The spinotectal tract terminates in the *superior colliculus* of the midbrain. However, the spinothalamic tract continues to the thalamus and terminates in the ventral posterolateral nucleus. At the level of the midbrain, the spinothalamic and medial lemniscal pathways gradually merge prior to terminating in the same thalamic nucleus (see Figs. 7–11 through 7–18).

DESCENDING PATHWAYS

Corticospinal, corticobulbar (cortex to brain stem nuclei), and *corticopontine* fibers originate in the cerebral cortex, descend through the *internal capsule* of the telencephalon, lateral to the thalamus, and emerge on the ventral surface of the midbrain, as the *crus cerebri*. As the fibers continue to descend, they enter the basal pons where the pontine nuclei and associated pontocerebellar fibers separate the descending cortical fibers into a number of smaller fascicles. The corticopontine fibers terminate in the basal pons, but the corticospinal fibers continue to descend, without interruption, through the basal pons. They emerge

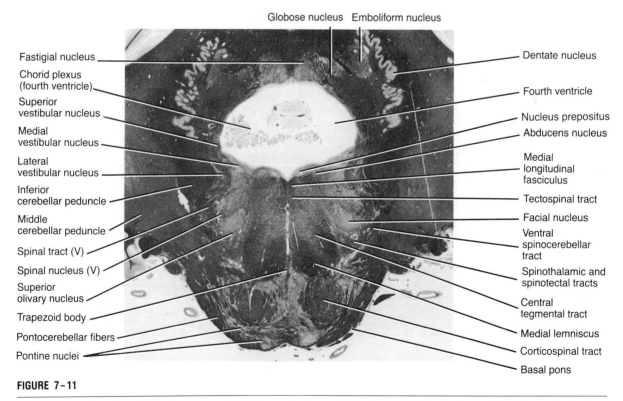

Globose nucleus Emboliform nucleus

Fastigial nucleus
Chorid plexus (fourth ventricle)
Superior vestibular nucleus
Medial vestibular nucleus
Lateral vestibular nucleus
Inferior cerebellar peduncle
Middle cerebellar peduncle
Spinal tract (V)
Spinal nucleus (V)
Superior olivary nucleus
Trapezoid body
Pontocerebellar fibers
Pontine nuclei

Dentate nucleus
Fourth ventricle
Nucleus prepositus
Abducens nucleus
Medial longitudinal fasciculus
Tectospinal tract
Facial nucleus
Ventral spinocerebellar tract
Spinothalamic and spinotectal tracts
Central tegmental tract
Medial lemniscus
Corticospinal tract
Basal pons

FIGURE 7–11

Transverse section through the lower pons. Note the cerebellar nuclei in the roof of the fourth ventricle. Human brain stem; Weigert stain.

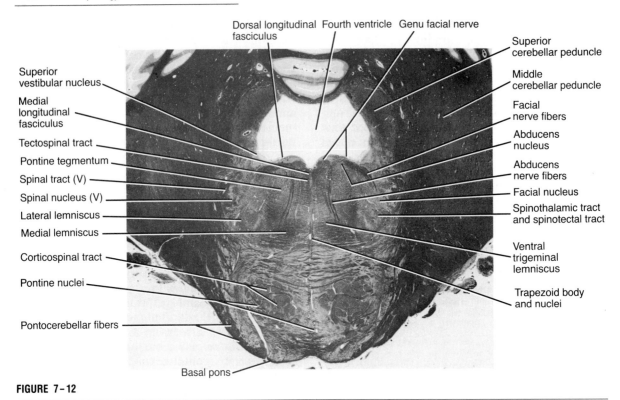

Dorsal longitudinal fasciculus — Fourth ventricle — Genu facial nerve

Superior cerebellar peduncle

Middle cerebellar peduncle

Facial nerve fibers

Abducens nucleus

Abducens nerve fibers

Facial nucleus

Spinothalamic tract and spinotectal tract

Ventral trigeminal lemniscus

Trapezoid body and nuclei

Superior vestibular nucleus

Medial longitudinal fasciculus

Tectospinal tract

Pontine tegmentum

Spinal tract (V)

Spinal nucleus (V)

Lateral lemniscus

Medial lemniscus

Corticospinal tract

Pontine nuclei

Pontocerebellar fibers

Basal pons

FIGURE 7–12

Transverse section through the pons, at the level of the facial colliculus and facial nucleus. Human brain stem; Weigert stain.

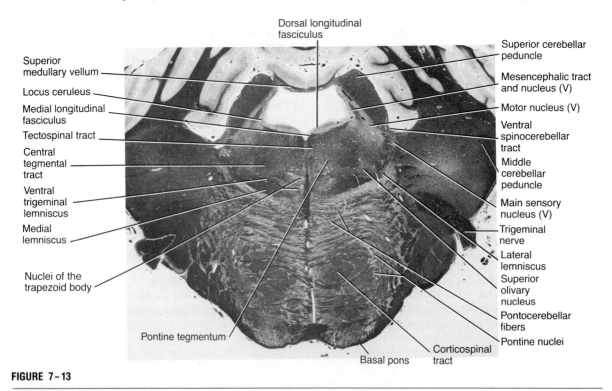

Dorsal longitudinal fasciculus

Superior cerebellar peduncle

Mesencephalic tract and nucleus (V)

Motor nucleus (V)

Ventral spinocerebellar tract

Middle cerebellar peduncle

Main sensory nucleus (V)

Trigeminal nerve

Lateral lemniscus

Superior olivary nucleus

Pontocerebellar fibers

Pontine nuclei

Superior medullary vellum

Locus ceruleus

Medial longitudinal fasciculus

Tectospinal tract

Central tegmental tract

Ventral trigeminal lemniscus

Medial lemniscus

Nuclei of the trapezoid body

Pontine tegmentum

Basal pons

Corticospinal tract

FIGURE 7–13

Transverse section through the upper pons at the level of the entrance of the trigeminal nerve. Human brain stem; Weigert stain.

on the ventral surface of the medulla as the medullary pyramids, or *pyramidal tract*. Some of these fibers are axons of giant pyramid-shaped, cortical neurons, hence, the names pyramidal tract and medullary pyramids. As the descending corticospinal fibers reach the lower medulla, they decussate (the *pyramidal decussation*) and assume a position in the lateral funiculus of the spinal cord (Figs. 7–7 through 7–19).

Above the decussation, fibers from the left cerebral hemisphere, destined to innervate lower motor neurons on the right side of the body, descend on the left side of the brain stem. Below the decussation, the *lateral corticospinal tract* is ipsilateral to the lower motor neurons. About 15% of the corticospinal fibers do not decussate and continue in the ventral funiculus of the spinal cord as the uncrossed, *ventral corticospinal tract* (see Fig. 7–8). Corticobulbar fibers descend through the brain stem in the "company" of the corticospinal tract but "peel off" to innervate motor nuclei of cranial nerves throughout the brain stem.

Two descending motor pathways arise in the midbrain. The *rubrospinal tract* arises from the *red nucleus*. The fibers immediately cross to the opposite side as the *ventral tegmental decussation* and descend through the midbrain, pons, and medulla in the vicinity of the ascending spino-thalamic tract. Once in the spinal cord, the rubrospinal tract assumes a position adjacent to the lateral corticospinal tract. The *tectospinal tract* originates in the *superior colliculus* of the midbrain. Its fibers cross ventral to the periaqueductal gray as the *dorsal tegmental decussation* and descend through the brain stem immediately ventral to the *medial longitudinal fasciculus*. Once in the lower medulla and upper cervical cord, the fibers split to form the *medial* and *lateral tectospinal tracts* of the spinal cord (see Figs. 7–8 through 7–19).

CEREBELLAR RELAY NUCLEI AND ASSOCIATED PATHWAYS

The *pontine nuclei*, collectively, are the largest of the cerebellar relay nuclei. Located in the *basal pons*, these nuclei receive corticopontine fibers

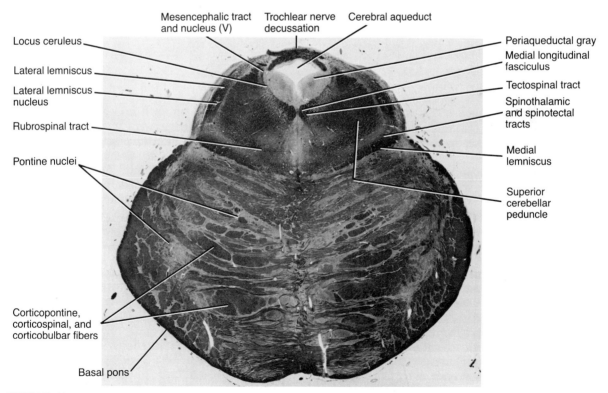

FIGURE 7-14

Section through the upper pons at the level of the decussation and the exit of the trochlear nerve. Human brain stem; Weigert stain.

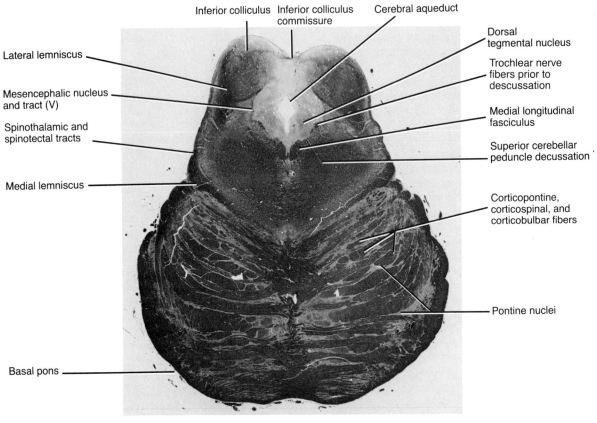

Inferior colliculus — Inferior colliculus commissure — Cerebral aqueduct

Lateral lemniscus

Mesencephalic nucleus and tract (V)

Spinothalamic and spinotectal tracts

Medial lemniscus

Basal pons

Dorsal tegmental nucleus

Trochlear nerve fibers prior to descussation

Medial longitudinal fasciculus

Superior cerebellar peduncle decussation

Corticopontine, corticospinal, and corticobulbar fibers

Pontine nuclei

FIGURE 7-15

Section through the upper pons (ventrally) and the midbrain (dorsally) at the level of the inferior colliculus and the decussation of the brachium conjunctivum. Human brain stem; Weigert stain.

and axons from the pontine neurons, cross the midline, and enter the opposite cerebellar hemisphere via the middle cerebellar peduncle. The small *arcuate nuclei*, situated on the ventral surface of the medullary pyramids, are functionally related to the pontine nuclei and are part of the same corticocerebellar system; however, their fibers cross and enter the cerebellum via the restiform body (see Figs. 7–9 and 7–11 through 7–16).

The prominent *inferior olivary nuclei* of the medulla have a cerebellar relay function. These nuclei receive *rubro-olivary* and *cortico-olivary* fibers as well as a contribution from the *central tegmental tract*. *Olivocerebellar fibers* cross the medulla and enter the restiform body of the opposite side (see Figs. 7–9, 7–10, 7–25, 7–26, and 7–27).

The ascending *dorsal spinocerebellar tract* gradually assumes a dorsolateral position on the surface of the medulla and is joined by the olivocerebellar fibers to make up the bulk of the

restiform body. The *external (accessory) cuneate nucleus* also contributes *cuneocerebellar fibers* to the restiform body. The *ventral spinocerebellar tract*, however, does not enter the restiform body or the inferior cerebellar peduncle but continues to ascend through the medulla and pons, before entering the cerebellum via the superior cerebellar peduncle (see Figs. 7–8, 7–9, 7–10, 7–13, and 7–26).

CRANIAL NERVE NUCLEI AND ASSOCIATED PATHWAYS

Spinal nerves contain four functional components: general somatic efferent (*GSE*), general visceral efferent (*GVE*), general somatic afferent (*GSA*), and general visceral afferent (*GVA*). The *cranial nerves* contain these four plus three others: *special visceral efferent (SVE)*, *special somatic afferent (SSA)*, and *special visceral afferent (SVA)*. However, no one cranial nerve contains more than five components and some contain only one.

The motor neurons innervating striated muscle derived from the embryonic branchial or visceral arches are *SVE*. Fibers carrying sensory information from the organs of special sense derived from embryonic ectoderm (the eye and ear) are *SSA*, whereas those carrying sensory information from special sensory receptors of visceral or endodermal origin (the olfactory mucosa and the taste buds) are *SVA*.

The nuclei of the cranial nerves form columns, similar to the motor and sensory columns of the spinal cord (see Chapter 6); however, they lack the continuity found in the spinal cord. In addition, with the formation of the fourth ventricle and the subsequent migration of the SVE neurons, the position of some of the columns has shifted (see Figs. 1–9, 1–14, and 1–25 and Chapter 19). These nuclei and the cranial nerves with which they are associated are summarized in

Table 1–2. Although a functional component may be present in a number of cranial nerves, it often shares a common nucleus within the brain stem. For example, the GSA components of cranial nerves V, VII, IX, and X enter the spinal tract of V and synapse in the spinal nucleus of V.

GENERAL SOMATIC EFFERENT NUCLEI

The *hypoglossal nuclei* are found on either side of the midline, just ventral to the central canal in the lower medulla and on either side of the midline in the floor of the fourth ventricle. The *abducens nuclei* occupy a similar position in the floor of the fourth ventricle, but at the level of the pontine tegmentum. The *trochlear nuclei* are found near the midline of the midbrain tegmentum and just caudal to the level of the *oculomotor nuclei* (see Figs. 7–8 through 7–12, 7–16, 7–17, 7–24, and 7–25).

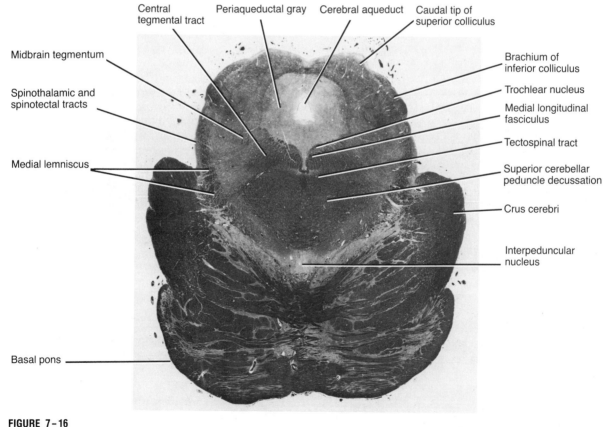

FIGURE 7–16

Section through the midbrain between the superior and inferior colliculi. The plane of section includes the rostral tip of the basal pons. Human brain stem; Weigert stain.

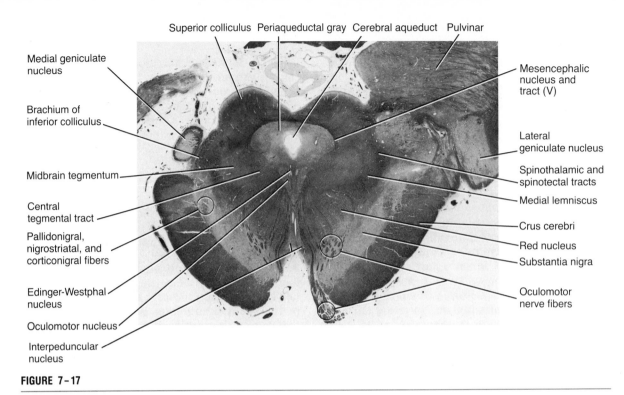

Superior colliculus Periaqueductal gray Cerebral aqueduct Pulvinar

Medial geniculate nucleus

Brachium of inferior colliculus

Midbrain tegmentum

Central tegmental tract

Pallidonigral, nigrostriatal, and corticonigral fibers

Edinger-Westphal nucleus

Oculomotor nucleus

Interpeduncular nucleus

Mesencephalic nucleus and tract (V)

Lateral geniculate nucleus

Spinothalamic and spinotectal tracts

Medial lemniscus

Crus cerebri

Red nucleus

Substantia nigra

Oculomotor nerve fibers

FIGURE 7-17

Section through the midbrain at the level of the superior colliculus and the exit of the oculomotor nerve. The more posterior portions of the diencephalon are also visible. Human brain stem; Weigert stain.

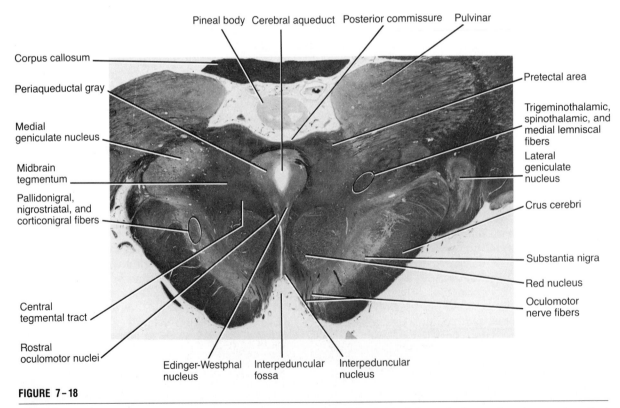

Pineal body Cerebral aqueduct Posterior commissure Pulvinar

Corpus callosum

Periaqueductal gray

Medial geniculate nucleus

Midbrain tegmentum

Pallidonigral, nigrostriatal, and corticonigral fibers

Central tegmental tract

Rostral oculomotor nuclei

Edinger-Westphal nucleus

Interpeduncular fossa

Interpeduncular nucleus

Pretectal area

Trigeminothalamic, spinothalamic, and medial lemniscal fibers

Lateral geniculate nucleus

Crus cerebri

Substantia nigra

Red nucleus

Oculomotor nerve fibers

FIGURE 7-18

Section through the rostral midbrain and the posterior diencephalon at the level of the pretectum, red nucleus, and cerebral peduncles. Human brain stem; Weigert stain.

Third ventricle Habenulointerpeduncular tract Habenular nucleus Centromedian nucleus Pulvinar

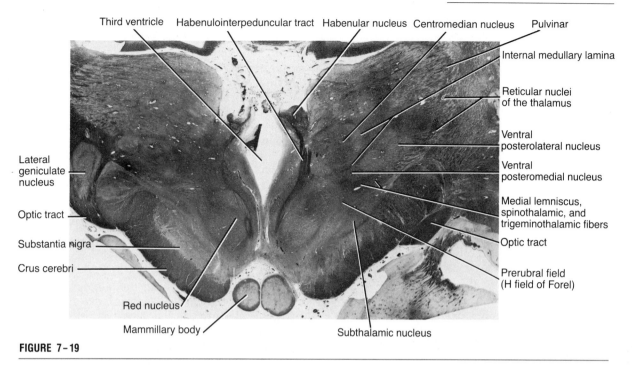

Internal medullary lamina

Reticular nuclei of the thalamus

Ventral posterolateral nucleus

Ventral posteromedial nucleus

Medial lemniscus, spinothalamic, and trigeminothalamic fibers

Optic tract

Prerubral field (H field of Forel)

Lateral geniculate nucleus

Optic tract

Substantia nigra

Crus cerebri

Red nucleus

Mammillary body

Subthalamic nucleus

FIGURE 7-19

Section through the diencephalon at the level of the habenula, ventral thalamus, and posterior portions of the dorsal thalamus. Human brain stem; Weigert stain.

SPECIAL VISCERAL EFFERENT NUCLEI

All of the SVE nuclei have migrated during development and occupy a ventrolateral position in the adult brain stem (see Fig. 1–25). The small *accessory nucleus* extends from the upper cervical segments of the spinal cord into the lower levels of the medulla. The *nucleus ambiguus* is a slender column of neurons extending from the accessory nucleus into the more rostral levels of the medulla. The large prominent *facial nucleus* is situated in the caudal portion of the pontine tegmentum, and the *motor nucleus of V* (*trigeminal*) is in the rostral pontine tegmentum (see Figs. 7–7 through 7–13, 7–26, and 7–27).

GENERAL VISCERAL EFFERENT NUCLEI

The large *motor nucleus of X* (*vagus*), located in the floor of the fourth ventricle beneath the vagal trigone, provides parasympathetic preganglionic innervation to all of the thoracic and most of the abdominal viscera (see Figs. 7–8, 7–9, 7–10, 7–24, and 7–25). The *inferior* and *superior salivatory nuclei* provide parasympathetic preganglionic fibers to the glossopharyngeal and facial nerves, respectively. These two nuclei are proba-

bly superior extensions of the motor nucleus of X, but they are not easily identified in Weigert-stained preparations. The *Edinger-Westphal nucleus* of the midbrain (parasympathetic innervation to the eye) is located in the superomedial portion of the oculomotor complex (see Figs. 7–17 and 7–18).

GENERAL VISCERAL AFFERENT AND SPECIAL VISCERAL AFFERENT NUCLEI

Two medullary nuclei receive visceral afferent information: (1) the *solitary nucleus* (*nucleus of the solitary tract*), a tubular-shaped nucleus surrounding the primary sensory fibers that form the *solitary tract*, and (2) the *sensory nucleus of X*, located immediately lateral to the motor nucleus of X. Taste fibers (*SVA*) terminate in the superior portion of the solitary nucleus, whereas *GVA* fibers terminate in the remainder of the solitary nucleus and in the dorsal sensory nucleus of X (see Figs. 7–8, 7–9, 7–10, 7–25, and 7–26). This is another example of a single brain stem nucleus receiving sensory input from several cranial nerves—the facial, glossopharyngeal, and vagus.

GENERAL SOMATIC AFFERENT NUCLEI

The *spinal nucleus of V*, extending from the point of entry of the trigeminal nerve in the midpons caudally to the cervical spinal cord where it interdigitates with the substantia gelatinosa, is the major *GSA* nucleus of the brain stem. The nucleus is located in the dorsolateral portion of the pons and medulla and is accompanied by the *spinal tract of V*, the primary *GSA* fibers destined to terminate within the nucleus (see Figs. 7–7 through 7–13, 7–25, 7–26, and 7–27). One additional *GSA* nucleus is associated with the trigeminal nerve: the *main sensory nucleus of V*, located near the point of entry of the trigeminal nerve in the pons (see Figs. 7–13 and 7–27). Secondary fibers from both the spinal nucleus of V and the main sensory nucleus of V cross the midline and ascend to the ventral posteromedial nucleus of the thalamus via the *ventral trigeminal lemniscus*, in a position adjacent to the medial lemniscus.

The *mesencephalic nucleus of V* is not a true *GSA* nucleus because the neurons are primary sensory neurons, similar to those of dorsal root ganglia. The mesencephalic nucleus of V is accompanied by the *mesencephalic tract of V* (the central *and* peripheral processes of these unipolar sensory neurons). This nucleus extends from the point of entry of the trigeminal nerve, rostral through the midbrain, along the lateral margin of the periaqueductal gray (see Figs. 7–13 through 7–16).

SPECIAL SOMATIC AFFERENT NUCLEI

The *vestibulocochlear nerve* (cranial nerve VIII) carries special sensory information from the cochlea and the vestibular apparatus. The nerve, upon reaching the medulla at the medullopontine angle, splits into cochlear and vestibular divisions. The cochlear division, attached to the dorsolateral surface of the restiform body (see Fig. 7–3), contains the *dorsal* and *ventral cochlear nuclei*—the inferior margins of which are visible in Figure 7–10.

A number of nuclei and fiber tracts of the ascending auditory pathway are visible in Weigert-stained brain stem sections. Fibers from the cochlear nuclei ascend in the ventrolateral portion of the pontine tegmentum, with many synapsing in the *nuclei of the trapezoid body* and the *superior olivary nuclei*. Ascending fibers of the auditory pathway become collated to form the *lateral lemniscus* and some make further synaptic connections in the *nuclei of the lateral lemniscus*. On reaching the upper pons, the lateral lemniscus moves dorsad to enter the *inferior colliculus* of the midbrain. Auditory fibers from the inferior colliculus form the *brachium of the inferior colliculus* and enter the diencephalon to terminate in the *medial geniculate nucleus* (see Figs. 7–11 through 7–17).

At the point of separation from the cochlear division, the vestibular division enters the brain stem deep to the restiform body and terminates in the *superior, medial, lateral* and *inferior vestibular nuclei*. Fibers from the vestibular nuclei ascend in the brain stem and descend into the spinal cord. Descending fibers from the *medial vestibular nucleus* form the centrally located *medial longitudinal fasciculus* (*medial vestibulospinal tract*) and those from the *lateral vestibular nucleus* form the *lateral vestibulospinal tract*. The last descends through the substance of the inferior vestibular nucleus to eventually assume a position in the ventral funiculus of the spinal cord. Other vestibular fibers have extensive connections with the cerebellum, especially with the flocculonodular lobe and the fastigial nuclei (see Figs. 7–10, 7–11, and 7–12).

BRAIN STEM RETICULAR FORMATION

The brain stem reticular formation is a complex organization of over 100 separate nuclei forming the central core of the midbrain tegmentum, pontine tegmentum, and medulla. The most clearly visible are the *lateral reticular nuclei* of the medulla (see Figs. 7–8 and 7–9). Although their functions are many, the nuclei of the reticular formation can be grouped into three major categories: those associated with (1) regulation of the level of consciousness and cortical alertness, the *reticular activating system* (*RAS*); (2) the control of somatic motor movements via efferents to the cranial nerve nuclei and the motor columns of the spinal cord, the *motor reticular formation*; and (3) the regulation of visceral motor or autonomic functions, such as the groups of nuclei forming the *cardiovascular* and *respiratory centers*. Principal descending pathways include the *medial* and *lateral reticulospinal tracts* and the *raphespinal tract*. More detailed analyses of the reticular formation and its nuclei and pathways are included in Chapters 12, 14, 15, and 21.

Diencephalon

EPITHALAMUS

The *pineal gland*, the *habenular nuclei*, and the *stria medullaris thalami* are the major structures of the epithalamus. Also included in the epithalamus, although non-neuronal, is the roof, or *tela choroidea*, of the third ventricle. This very thin, ependymal layer and its associated choroid plexus is attached to the medial margin of the stria medullaris and extends forward from the suprapineal recess and the habenular nuclei to the interventricular foramen (see Figs. 7–18, 7–19, 7–20, 7–24, and 7–25).

The *habenular nuclei* are a principal relay station for information from the limbic forebrain areas to the midbrain. Limbic system information, from septal and hypothalamic–preoptic areas, travels to the habenular nuclei via the stria medullaris thalami. This information is subsequently conveyed to the *interpeduncular nucleus* of the midbrain via the *habenulointerpeduncular tract* (*fasciculus retroflexus of Meynert*) (Figs. 7–19, 7–25, and 7–26; see Chapter 22).

The *pineal gland* contains no direct CNS connections in humans; however, its rich vascular supply carries sympathetic fibers from the superior cervical ganglia. This innervation is responsible for the circadian activity of the gland, in particular, the cyclic production of hormones, such as melatonin. The gland is not photosensitive in humans but receives light cycle information relayed indirectly from the suprachiasmatic nucleus of the hypothalamus by way of the superior cervical sympathetic ganglia (see Chapter 18).

VENTRAL THALAMUS

Principally motor in function, the *ventral thalamus* is not sharply delineated from the midbrain with which it functionally shares two prominent midbrain nuclei, the *red nucleus* and the *substantia nigra*. In more anterior levels of the ventral thalamus, the substantia nigra is replaced with a light-staining, ovoid nucleus, the *subthalamic nucleus*. Immediately dorsomedial to the subthalamic nucleus is the flattened *zona incerta* and the heavily myelinated *prerubral field* (*H field of*

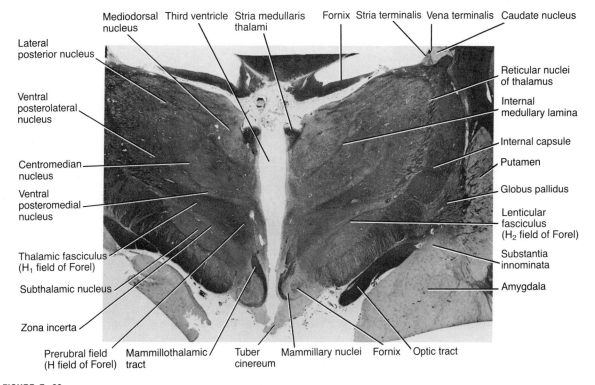

FIGURE 7–20

Section through the diencephalon including the mammillary and tuberal regions of the hypothalamus, the dorsal thalamus, and portions of the ventral thalamus. Human brain stem; Weigert stain.

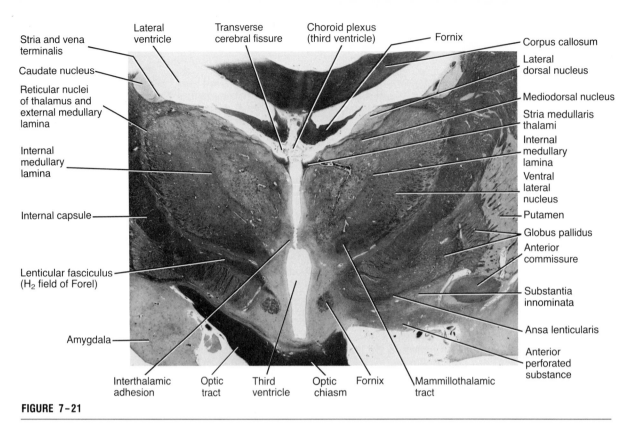

FIGURE 7-21

Section through the diencephalon including the anterior portions of the hypothalamus and the central portion of the dorsal thalamus. Human brain stem; Weigert stain.

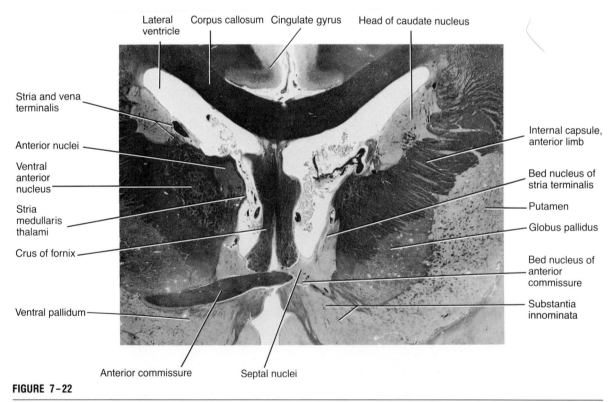

FIGURE 7-22

Section through the rostral diencephalon including the anterior commissure and the genu of the fornix. Human brain stem; Weigert stain.

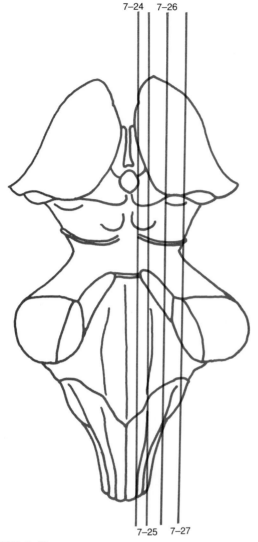

7–24 7–26

7–25 7–27

FIGURE 7–23

Outline of the dorsal surface of the brain stem with lines representing the planes of the parasagittal, Weigert-stained sections in Figures 7–24 through 7–27.

Forel) with its associated nuclei. These structures are lateral to the hypothalamus, medial and dorsal to the internal capsule and crus cerebri, and ventral to the thalamus (see Figs. 7–19, 7–20, and 7–24 through 7–27). The extensive interconnections of these structures with the basal ganglia, cerebellum, and thalamus and their role in motor function are discussed in Chapter 16.

THALAMUS

The *thalamus* (*dorsal thalamus*) functions principally as a cortical relay station and, with few exceptions, information cannot reach the cerebral cortex unless it is relayed by a thalamic nucleus. The nature of these connections is discussed in Chapter 20 and in other chapters dealing with motor, sensory, and limbic systems.

A sheet of myelinated fibers, the *internal medullary lamina*, roughly divides each half of the thalamus into medial and lateral regions. Within the internal medullary lamina are a number of *intralaminar nuclei*, the most prominent of which is the *centromedian nucleus*. Anteriorly, the lamina splits. Situated within the cleavage are a group of nuclei, collectively known as the *anterior nuclei* (Figs. 7–19 through 7–22 and 7–24 through 7–27).

The most prominent nucleus of the medial region is the *mediodorsal nucleus*, situated medial to the internal medullary lamina and separated from the surface of the third ventricle by the *midline nuclei*, which include the *interthalamic adhesion* (see Figs. 7–20, 7–21, 7–26, and 7–27).

The lateral region is subdivided into two divisions: a lateral division and a ventral division. The lateral division, which actually is located dorsally rather than laterally, contains two nuclei, the *lateral dorsal nucleus* and the *lateral posterior nucleus*. The ventral division is divided into three nuclear groups: the *ventral anterior nucleus*, the *ventral lateral nucleus*, and the *ventral posterior nucleus*. The *ventral posterior nucleus* is commonly subdivided into lateral and medial components, the *ventral posterolateral* and *ventral posteromedial nuclei* (Figs. 7–19 through 7–22, 7–25, 7–26, and 7–27).

In the posterior portion of the dorsal thalamus are three prominent nuclei: the *pulvinar* and the *medial* and *lateral geniculate nuclei*. In some classifications, the medial and lateral geniculate nuclei are grouped together as the *metathalamus* (see Figs. 7–17, 7–18, and 7–19). The lateral surface of the thalamus is covered by the *external medullary lamina*, containing a collection of small nuclei, the *reticular nuclei of the thalamus*, which are functionally unrelated to the brain stem reticular formation (see Chapter 20; Figs. 7–19, 7–20, and 7–21).

HYPOTHALAMUS

The numerous hypothalamic nuclei are not easily differentiated in Weigert-stained material. However, the heavily myelinated *fornix*, as it passes from the *anterior commissure* through the hypothalamus to the *mammillary nuclei*, roughly di-

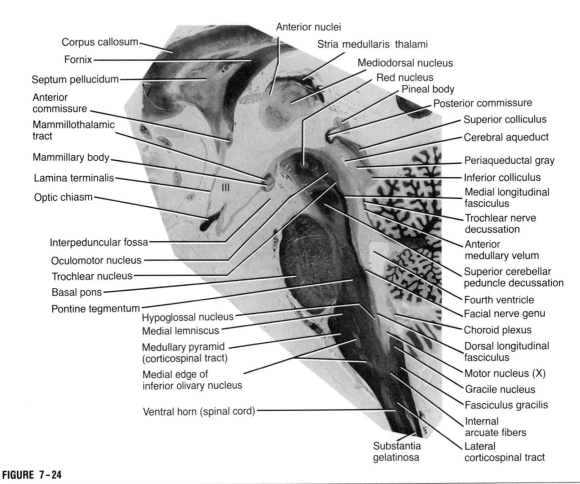

Anterior nuclei
Corpus callosum
Fornix
Septum pellucidum
Anterior commissure
Mammillothalamic tract
Mammillary body
Lamina terminalis
Optic chiasm
Interpeduncular fossa
Oculomotor nucleus
Trochlear nucleus
Basal pons
Pontine tegmentum
III
Hypoglossal nucleus
Medial lemniscus
Medullary pyramid (corticospinal tract)
Medial edge of inferior olivary nucleus
Ventral horn (spinal cord)

Stria medullaris thalami
Mediodorsal nucleus
Red nucleus
Pineal body
Posterior commissure
Superior colliculus
Cerebral aqueduct
Periaqueductal gray
Inferior colliculus
Medial longitudinal fasciculus
Trochlear nerve decussation
Anterior medullary velum
Superior cerebellar peduncle decussation
Fourth ventricle
Facial nerve genu
Choroid plexus
Dorsal longitudinal fasciculus
Motor nucleus (X)
Gracile nucleus
Fasciculus gracilis
Internal arcuate fibers
Lateral corticospinal tract
Substantia gelatinosa

FIGURE 7–24

Parasagittal section, just lateral to the midline and through the medial margins of the inferior olivary nucleus, the red nucleus, and the mammillary body. Human brain stem; Weigert stain.

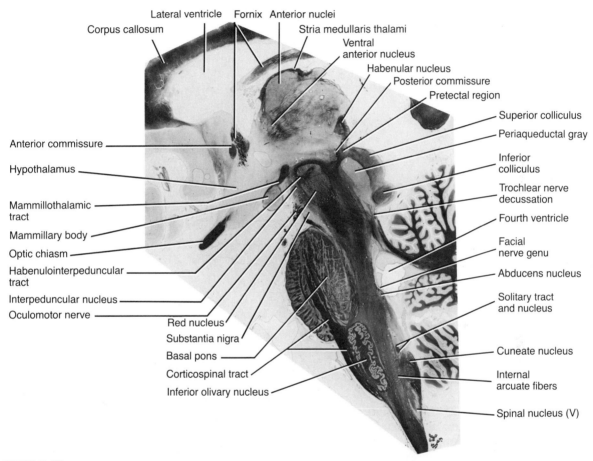

Corpus callosum
Lateral ventricle Fornix Anterior nuclei
Stria medullaris thalami
Ventral
anterior nucleus
Habenular nucleus
Posterior commissure
Pretectal region
Superior colliculus
Periaqueductal gray
Anterior commissure
Hypothalamus
Inferior
colliculus
Mammillothalamic
tract
Trochlear nerve
decussation
Mammillary body
Fourth ventricle
Optic chiasm
Facial
nerve genu
Habenulointerpeduncular
tract
Abducens nucleus
Interpeduncular nucleus
Solitary tract
and nucleus
Oculomotor nerve
Red nucleus
Substantia nigra
Basal pons
Cuneate nucleus
Corticospinal tract
Internal
arcuate fibers
Inferior olivary nucleus
Spinal nucleus (V)

FIGURE 7-25

Parasagittal section through the abducens nucleus, medullary pyramids, and the medial nuclei of the dorsal thalamus. Human brain stem; Weigert stain.

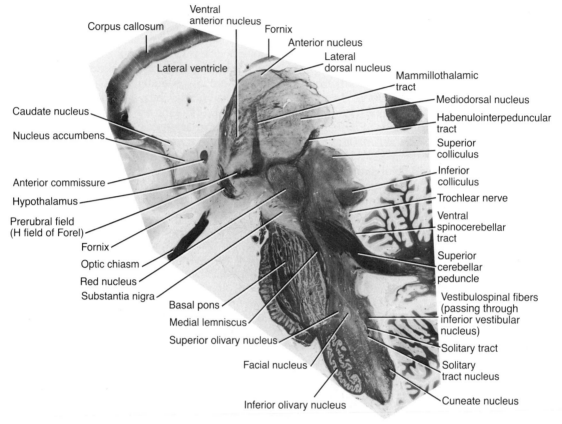

FIGURE 7-26

Parasagittal section through the facial nucleus and the lateral hypothalamus. Human brain stem; Weigert stain.

vides the hypothalamus into a *medial zone* and a *lateral zone*. The anterior third of the hypothalamus, from the optic chiasm anterior, is known as the *chiasmatic region*; the middle third, containing the *tuber cinereum* and the *hypophyseal stalk*, is the *tuberal region*; and the posterior third, including the *mammillary bodies*, is the *mammillary region*. Although this nomenclature may seem arbitrary, these traditional divisions of the hypothalamus have a practical application (see Chapter 18 and Figs. 7–19, 7–20, 7–21, and 7–23 through 7–27).

Cerebellum

Motor and sensory information is processed or integrated in the cerebellar cortex. The integrated information is relayed to four pairs of cerebellar nuclei located in the roof of the fourth ventricle, the *fastigial*, *globose*, *emboliform*, and *dentate*

nuclei (see Fig. 7–11). The internal structure and organization of the cerebellum are discussed in depth in Chapter 17. Efferent fibers leave the cerebellum via the superior cerebellar peduncles and, after crossing to the opposite side as the *decussation of the brachium conjunctivum*, they terminate in the *red nucleus*, in the nuclei of the *ventral thalamus*, and in the *ventral anterior* and *ventral lateral nuclei* of the thalamus.

In addition to efferent fibers from the cerebellar nuclei, the *superior cerebellar peduncle* contains afferent fibers from the ascending ventral spinocerebellar tract; the *middle cerebellar peduncle* contains afferent fibers from the cerebral cortex by way of the corticopontocerebellar pathway; and the *inferior cerebellar peduncle* contains principally afferents to the cerebellum from vestibular, somatosensory, and olivary sources (vestibulocerebellar, dorsal spinocerebellar, cuneocerebellar, and olivocerebellar fibers) (see Figs. 7–3, 7–4, and 7–5).

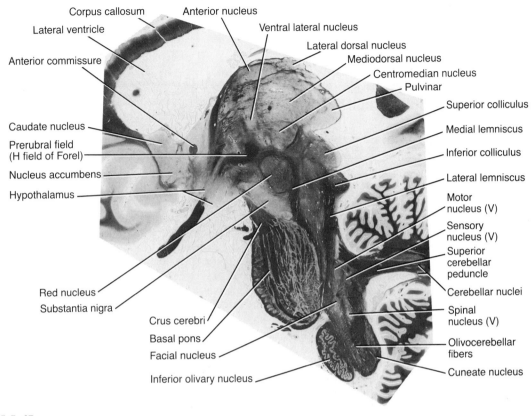

Corpus callosum
Anterior nucleus
Lateral ventricle
Ventral lateral nucleus
Lateral dorsal nucleus
Anterior commissure
Mediodorsal nucleus
Centromedian nucleus
Pulvinar
Superior colliculus
Caudate nucleus
Medial lemniscus
Prerubral field (H field of Forel)
Inferior colliculus
Nucleus accumbens
Lateral lemniscus
Hypothalamus
Motor nucleus (V)
Sensory nucleus (V)
Superior cerebellar peduncle
Red nucleus
Cerebellar nuclei
Substantia nigra
Spinal nucleus (V)
Crus cerebri
Basal pons
Olivocerebellar fibers
Facial nucleus
Cuneate nucleus
Inferior olivary nucleus

FIGURE 7-27

Parasagittal section through the motor and main sensory nuclei of the trigeminal nerve and the centromedian nucleus of the thalamus. Human brain stem; Weigert stain.

SUGGESTED READING

Haines, D. E. (1991). *Neuroanatomy. An Atlas of Structures, Sections and Systems*, 3rd Edition. Urban & Schwarzenberg, Baltimore-Munich, 252 pp.

A thorough, yet concise atlas and guide to the organization and structure of the human central nervous system. Slices, Weigert-stained sections, and diagrams provide an excellent reference to the organization of the brain stem as well as other portions of the nervous system.

Netter, F. H. (1983). *The Ciba Collection of Medical Illustrations*. Volume 1, *Nervous System*. Part I, *Anatomy and Physiology*. CIBA Pharmaceutical Company, West Caldwell, New Jersey.

An excellent compendium of illustrations of the brain and brain stem. Especially suitable for understanding the three-dimensional relationships between specific tracts and nuclei within the human central nervous system.

Chapter

8

Telencephalon

CEREBRAL CORTEX
BASAL GANGLIA
BASAL FOREBRAIN

The *telencephalon*, or the paired *cerebral hemispheres*, is the largest subdivision of the human brain. Each *cerebral hemisphere* consists of an outer mantle of gray matter, the *pallium* or *cerebral cortex*; an extensive underlying *white matter*; and a large aggregation of deep nuclei, the *basal ganglia* and *basal forebrain*. The hemispheres develop from the telencephalic vesicles, growing laterally from the embryonic prosencephalon or forebrain (see Chapter 1). At the ventral attachment of the vesicle to the brain stem, large aggregations of telencephalic neuroblasts give rise to the basal ganglia. As the basal nuclei increase in size, the remainder of the telencephalic vesicle continues to balloon outward and backward, forming the *cerebral cortex* with the lumen of the balloon becoming the *lateral ventricle* (see Fig. 1–19).

In the adult, the hemispheres are separated from each other by a deep midline cleft, the *longitudinal cerebral fissure*, and from the underlying brain stem and cerebellum by the *transverse cerebral fissure*. Both fissures contain meninges and thick folds of dura, the *falx cerebri* (longitudinal cerebral fissure) and *tentorium cerebelli* (posterior portion of the transverse cerebral fissure) (see Chapter 9).

Cerebral Cortex

As the cerebral hemisphere grows backward, downward, and then forward, the cortex immediately superficial to the basal ganglia, the *insula* (or *island of Reil*), becomes buried beneath the overgrowing hemispheres. The prominent *lateral sulcus* (*fissure of Rolando*) is thus formed (see Figs. 1–19, 1–20, and 8–1 through 8–3). The large folds of overgrowing cortex, known as *opercula*, are named for the cortical lobe of which they are a part (*frontal operculum*, *parietal operculum*, and *temporal operculum*). As the hemispheres continue to grow, the cortex is thrown into a series of folds—increasing the surface area with a minimal change in volume—the ridges are *gyri* and the grooves *sulci*.

The overall pattern of gyri and sulci is quite variable. However, certain primary sulci appear early in development, are consistent from brain to brain, and are used as boundaries for the division of the cortex into lobes. The cortex can be subdivided into as many as 200 histologically distinct areas and, although the secondary sulci and gyri vary considerably from brain to brain, these histologic areas are remarkably constant.

FIGURE 8-1

Lateral view of the brain.

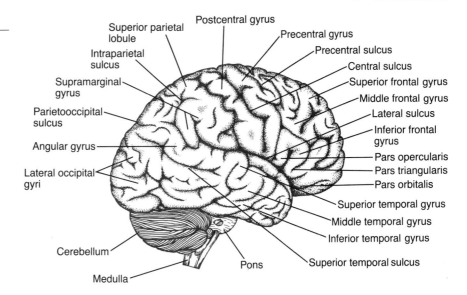

Postcentral gyrus
Superior parietal lobule
Intraparietal sulcus
Supramarginal gyrus
Parietooccipital sulcus
Angular gyrus
Lateral occipital gyri
Precentral gyrus
Precentral sulcus
Central sulcus
Superior frontal gyrus
Middle frontal gyrus
Lateral sulcus
Inferior frontal gyrus
Pars opercularis
Pars triangularis
Pars orbitalis
Superior temporal gyrus
Middle temporal gyrus
Inferior temporal gyrus
Superior temporal sulcus
Cerebellum
Pons
Medulla

PRIMARY SULCI AND GYRI

On the lateral surface of the hemisphere, in addition to the lateral sulcus, a prominent and consistent landmark is the *central sulcus*, separating the *precentral gyrus* (primary somatomotor cortex) from the *postcentral gyrus* (primary somatosensory cortex). At their ventrolateral margins, the postcentral and precentral gyri are in continuity, forming a blind end to the central sulcus (see Fig. 8–1).

On the medial surface of the hemisphere, the prominent *calcarine sulcus* separates the inferior

lingual gyrus from the superior *cuneus*. The anterior portion of the calcarine sulcus is sometimes continuous with the less prominent *collateral sulcus*. Branching from the calcarine sulcus and running in a posterosuperior direction is the deep *parietooccipital sulcus*. The *cingulate gyrus* extends over the entire length of the corpus callosum, anteriorly from beneath the genu to the posterior margin of the splenium, where it becomes the *isthmus of the cingulate gyrus*, or simply the *isthmus*. The cingulate gyrus is separated from the remainder of the cortex by the *cingulate sulcus* (Figs. 8–4 and 8–6).

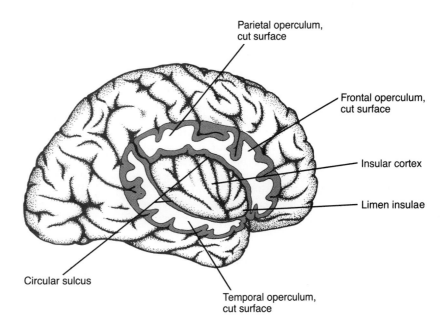

Parietal operculum, cut surface
Frontal operculum, cut surface
Insular cortex
Limen insulae
Circular sulcus
Temporal operculum, cut surface

FIGURE 8-2

Lateral view of the right cerebral hemisphere. Frontal, parietal, and temporal opercula have been removed to expose the insular cortex.

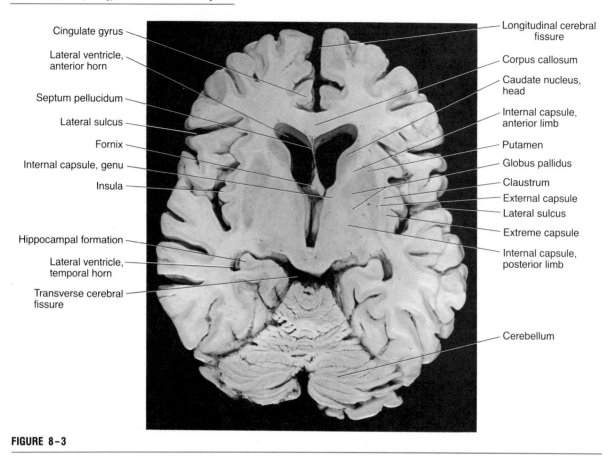

Cingulate gyrus

Lateral ventricle, anterior horn

Septum pellucidum

Lateral sulcus

Fornix

Internal capsule, genu

Insula

Hippocampal formation

Lateral ventricle, temporal horn

Transverse cerebral fissure

Longitudinal cerebral fissure

Corpus callosum

Caudate nucleus, head

Internal capsule, anterior limb

Putamen

Globus pallidus

Claustrum

External capsule

Lateral sulcus

Extreme capsule

Internal capsule, posterior limb

Cerebellum

FIGURE 8–3

A horizontal section through the cerebral hemispheres at the level of the internal capsule and basal ganglia. Unstained.

PRINCIPAL LOBES OF CEREBRAL HEMISPHERES

The adult cerebral cortex is subdivided into six regions: the *frontal, parietal, occipital, temporal,* and *limbic lobes* and the *insula* (Figs. 8–2, 8–5, and 8–6).

On the lateral surface of the hemisphere, the *frontal lobe* is separated from the remainder of the cortex posteriorly by the *central sulcus* and inferiorly by the *lateral sulcus.* The *parietal lobe* is immediately behind the *central sulcus,* and the *temporal lobe* is inferior to the *lateral sulcus.* The posterior boundary of the *parietal* and *temporal lobes* and the anterior border of the *occipital lobe* is formed by a line drawn from the superior margin of the *parietooccipital sulcus* to the *preoccipital notch* (an indentation in the ventrolateral margin of the hemisphere produced by the underlying temporal bone). The preoccipital notch

is not always present, in which case the position of the line is approximated. A second line, drawn at a right angle to the first and extending to the lateral sulcus, forms the boundary between the posterior portions of the temporal and parietal lobes (see Fig. 8–5).

On the medial surface of the hemisphere, the *central sulcus* continues to separate the *frontal* and *parietal* lobes; the *parietooccipital sulcus* separates the *parietal* and *occipital lobes;* and a line from the *preoccipital notch* to the anterior portion of the *calcarine sulcus* separates the *occipital* and *temporal lobes,* on the medial and inferior surfaces of the hemispheres (see Fig. 8–6). The *limbic lobe* forms an inner ring of cortical tissue on the medial surface of the hemispheres, separated from portions of the frontal and parietal lobes by the *cingulate sulcus* and from portions of the temporal lobe by the *collateral sulcus* (see Fig. 8–6).

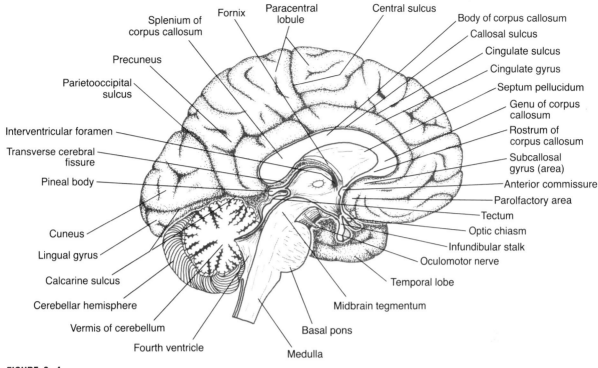

FIGURE 8-4

Midsagittal view of the brain.

FRONTAL LOBE

Extending forward from the central sulcus, the frontal lobe makes up about a third of the total cortical tissue. On the lateral surface and anterior to the *precentral gyrus*, the frontal lobe is tradi- tionally divided into *superior, middle,* and *inferior frontal gyri*. "Areas" is a more descriptive term, because the sulci separating them are not present consistently. The *inferior frontal gyrus* is further subdivided into the *pars opercularis, pars triangularis,* and *pars orbitalis* (see Fig. 8–1).

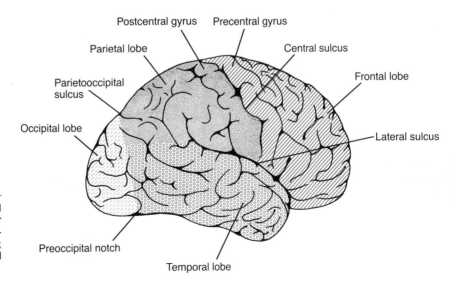

FIGURE 8-5

Lateral view of the right cerebral hemisphere illustrating the major cortical lobes. Frontal lobe, diagonal lines; parietal lobe, stipple; occipital lobe, dashed lines; and temporal lobe, circles.

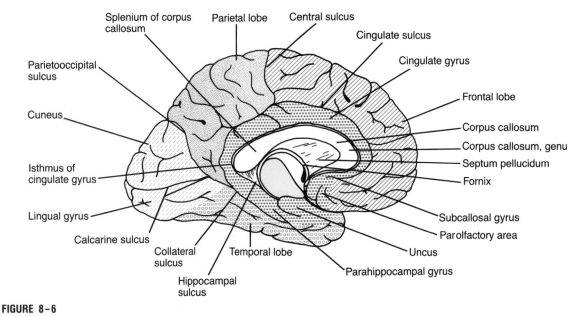

FIGURE 8-6

Midsagittal view of the left cerebral hemisphere illustrating the major cortical lobes. Frontal lobe, diagonal lines; parietal lobe, stipple; occipital lobe, dashed lines; temporal lobe, open circles; and limbic lobe, filled circles.

The precentral gyrus forms the *primary motor area*. The area immediately anterior to the precentral gyrus is the *premotor area*, and the most anterior portion of the frontal lobe is the *prefrontal area* (see Chapters 15 and 21). A region of the inferior frontal gyrus on the dominant hemisphere, usually the left hemisphere in right-handed individuals, is known as *Broca's area* and is associated with the expressive or motor mechanisms of speech.

The ventral surface of the frontal lobe rests on the bony roof of the orbit. Those frontal lobe gyri lateral to the *olfactory bulb* and *olfactory tract* are known as the *orbital gyri*. Deep to the olfactory bulb and tract is the *olfactory sulcus*, which forms the lateral margin of the more medially located *gyrus rectus*. Posteriorly, the olfactory tract divides into *medial* and *lateral olfactory striae*, forming a small triangular area known as the *olfactory trigone*. Both the medial and lateral olfactory striae are covered with a thin layer of primitive cortical tissue, the *medial* and *lateral olfactory gyri*. Immediately posterior to the olfactory trigone is the *anterior perforated substance* (Fig. 8-7).

PARIETAL LOBE

The lateral aspect of the parietal lobe, posterior to the *postcentral gyrus*, is subdivided into *supe-

rior* and *inferior parietal lobules* by an often indistinct *intraparietal sulcus*. The inferior lobule is further subdivided into two gyri: the *supramarginal gyrus,* capping the superior margin of the lateral sulcus, and the *angular gyrus*, lying above the posterior portion of the *superior temporal sulcus*. The supramarginal and angular gyri, together, compose *Wernicke's area*, an area associated with receptive or comprehensive speech. The *postcentral gyrus*, which extends onto the medial surface of the hemisphere, is the *primary somesthetic area*, receiving primary somatosensory information from the opposite half of the body (see Figs. 8-1 and 8-5).

On the medial surface, the area of the parietal lobe anterior to the *parietooccipital sulcus* is known as the *precuneus*. The more rostral portion, surrounding the central sulcus, is known as the *paracentral lobule*. Anterior portions of the *paracentral lobule* are actually a medial continuation of the precentral gyrus, and posterior portions are the medial aspect of the postcentral gyrus (see Figs. 8-4 and 8-6).

OCCIPITAL LOBE

The *calcarine sulcus* runs horizontally across the medial aspect of the occipital lobe, dividing it into the superior *cuneus* and the inferior *lingual gyrus*. Cortical tissue of the cuneus and that of

FIGURE 8-7

View of the ventral surface of the cerebral hemispheres with the cerebellum and most of the brain stem removed.

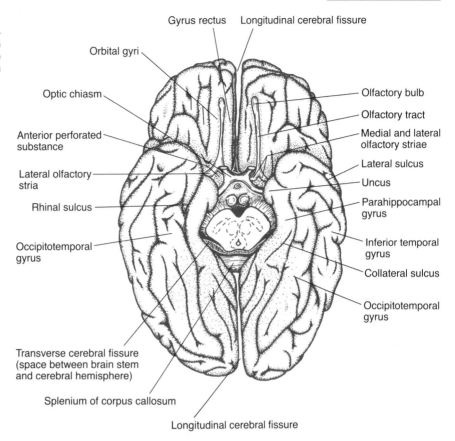

the lingual gyrus immediately adjacent to and extending into the depths of the calcarine sulcus constitute the *primary visual cortex* and are collectively referred to as the *striate* or *calcarine cortex* (see Figs. 8–4 and 8–6). The lateral surface of the occipital lobe is subdivided into several small, ill-defined *lateral occipital gyri* (see Figs. 8–1 and 8–5).

TEMPORAL LOBE

On the lateral surface of the brain, the temporal lobe lies ventral to the *lateral sulcus* and contains three principal gyri running parallel to the lateral sulcus: the *superior, middle,* and *inferior temporal gyri* separated by the *superior* and *middle temporal sulci,* when present. On the superior surface of the temporal lobe, in the depths of the *lateral sulcus,* are a series of oblique-running gyri, the *transverse temporal gyri (of Heschl).* These form the primary *auditory cortex* (see Figs. 8–1 and 8–5).

On the ventral surface of the temporal lobe, the broad *occipitotemporal gyrus* lies adjacent to

the *inferior temporal gyrus.* The *rhinal* and *collateral sulci* separate the occipitotemporal gyrus from the more medially located *parahippocampal gyrus* (a component of the limbic lobe) (see Figs. 8–6 and 8–7).

LIMBIC LOBE

The *limbic lobe* forms an inner ring of cortical tissue on the medial surface of the hemisphere, completely surrounding the corpus callosum and diencephalon. Beneath the rostrum of the corpus callosum is the *subcallosal gyrus* and proceeding anteriorly from the lamina terminalis are the *preterminal* and *parolfactory gyri.* Collectively, the preterminal, parolfactory, and subcallosal gyri are known as the *parolfactory area* or *subcallosal area* (see Figs. 8–4 and 8–6).

The parolfactory area is continuous with the *cingulate gyrus,* which extends over the corpus callosum, separated from it by the *callosal sulcus* and from the adjacent frontal and parietal areas by the *cingulate sulcus.* Posteriorly, the *cingulate gyrus* curves behind and beneath the splenium of the corpus callosum, forming the *isthmus* of the *cingulate gyrus*. The *isthmus* continues anteriorly as the *parahippocampal gyrus*. The anterior, fist-shaped end of the parahippocampal gyrus forms the *uncus* (see Figs. 8–6 and 8–7). The uncus, the anterior third of the parahippocampal gyrus, and the lateral olfactory gyrus, superficial to the lateral olfactory stria, constitute the *piriform area*, much of which is olfactory in function.

The *hippocampal formation* (*hippocampus* and *dentate gyrus*) parallels the parahippocampal gyrus and is separated from it by the *hippocampal sulcus*. The hippocampal formation is deep within the temporal lobe and is best seen in sectioned preparations (see Figs. 8–3 and 8–11).

INSULA

The *insula*, buried in the depths of the lateral sulcus and immediately superficial to the basal ganglia, is visible only when the overlying *frontal*, *parietal*, and *temporal opercula* are spread apart or cut away (see Figs. 8–2 and 8–3). The roughly triangular surface of the insula is surrounded by the *circular sulcus*. The ventroanterior margin of the insula, the *limen insulae*, is continuous in a ventromedial direction with the *anterior perforated substance*.

CORTICAL WHITE MATTER

The cortical white matter can conveniently be considered in three categories: *projection fibers*, *commissural fibers*, and *association fibers*. In general, *projection fibers* pass between the cortex and lower levels of the nervous system; *commissural fibers* interconnect comparable areas of one hemisphere with the other; and *association fibers* connect different areas within the same hemisphere.

Most of the *cortical projection fibers* are contained within the *internal capsule*, and they consist of *thalamocortical*, *corticothalamic*, *corticostriate*, *corticobulbar*, *corticopontine*, and *corticospinal* fibers. The *internal capsule* is divided into an *anterior limb* (between the head of the caudate nucleus and the lentiform nucleus); a *posterior limb* (between the thalamus and the lentiform nucleus); and a *genu* (between the lentiform nucleus and the junction between the head of the caudate nucleus and the dorsal thalamus medially) (see Fig. 8–3). Continuing posteriorly, the *retrolenticular* portion of the internal capsule is posterior to the lentiform nucleus and the

sublenticular portion of the capsule lies beneath the lentiform nucleus.

The *fornix* is a cortical projection bundle, consisting principally of fibers projecting from the hippocampal formation to the hypothalamus and basal forebrain area as well as carrying fibers from the septal complex to the hippocampus.

The largest of the *commissural* fiber systems is the *corpus callosum*, reciprocally connecting comparable neocortical areas of one hemisphere with the other. The *corpus callosum* is divided into a bulbous posterior portion, the *splenium*; a large middle section, the *body*; an anterior curved portion, the *genu*; and a portion extending from the genu to the lamina terminalis, the *rostrum* (see Fig. 8–4).

The *anterior commissure* runs from amygdala to amygdala, crossing the midline in the lamina terminalis and interconnecting olfactory bulbs, amygdaloid nuclei, anterior perforated substances, parahippocampal gyri, and other cortical areas of the anterior temporal area (see Fig. 8–4).

The *hippocampal commissure*, a part of the fornix situated below the splenium of the corpus callosum, consists mostly of fornix fibers from the hippocampus, which enter the contralateral fornix for distribution with the fornix fibers of the opposite side.

The white matter of the hemispheres contains a vast number of *cortical association fibers*, connecting cortical areas within the same hemisphere. These range from short fibers connecting adjacent gyri (*arcuate fibers*) to bundles of association fibers extending from one pole of the hemisphere to the other (see Fig. 8–8).

The *uncinate fasciculus* connects the uncus and anterior temporal areas with frontal lobe areas and lies immediately ventral to the *inferior frontooccipital fasciculus*, which runs along the inferior part of the extreme capsule and interconnects lateral and ventrolateral areas of the frontal lobe with the occipital cortex, as well as making other connections along the way. The *inferior longitudinal fasciculus* is in the ventrolateral portion of the temporal lobe, interconnecting areas of occipital and temporal lobes (see Fig. 8–8).

The *superior longitudinal fasciculus* extends along the dorsolateral border of the putamen, lateral to the internal capsule, and interconnects areas of the frontal, parietal, and occipital lobes. This fasciculus then arches ventroanteriorly to make connections in the temporal lobe. Also in the lateral portion of the hemisphere is the *lateral occipital fasciculus*, a thin sheet of fibers running vertically through the anterior portion of the

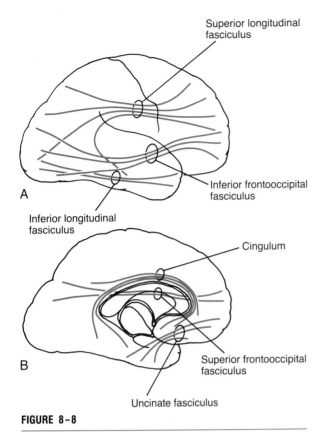

Superior longitudinal fasciculus

A

Inferior longitudinal fasciculus

Inferior frontooccipital fasciculus

Cingulum

B

Superior frontooccipital fasciculus

Uncinate fasciculus

FIGURE 8-8

Diagram of the brain illustrating the major cortical association bundles. *A*, Lateral view. *B*, Midsagittal view.

occipital lobe and the posterior portions of the parietal and temporal lobes. These fibers, interconnecting areas of the temporal and parietal lobes, are sometimes called *Wernicke's fasciculus.*

The *superior frontooccipital fasciculus* is found medial to the internal capsule, between the caudate nucleus and the interdigitating fibers of the internal capsule and corpus callosum. This fasciculus interconnects areas of occipital and temporal cortex with frontal and insular cortex (see Fig. 8–8).

The *cingulum* is a large cortical association bundle located deep to the cingulate gyrus. It runs from the septal and basal forebrain areas to the parahippocampal gyrus as well as interconnecting adjacent areas of frontal, parietal, and occipital cortices along the way (see Fig. 8–8).

FUNCTIONAL LOBES AND AREAS

Most of the cerebral cortex in humans is classified as *neopallium* (*neocortex*) or *isocortex*. Phylogenetically, it is the newest area and contains six distinct histological layers.

The oldest cortical area is the *archipallium* (*archicortex*), a three-layered cortex associated with the limbic system and involved in such diverse functions as emotion, influence of emotion on the function of visceral motor systems, and memory. This cortical area includes the *hip-*

TABLE 8-1

Limbic Lobe and the Rhinencephalon

RHINENCEPHALON	**Subcortical Structures** Olfactory bulb and tract Anterior olfactory nucleus Medial and lateral olfactory striae Medial and lateral olfactory gyri* Anterior perforated substance Septal nuclei Nucleus of the diagonal band of Broca Bed nucleus, stria terminalis Bed nucleus, anterior commissure
	Cortical Regions Parolfactory area Hippocampal formation Parahippocampal gyrus* Uncus* Subcallosal gyrus Cingulate gyrus Isthmus of the cingulate gyrus

LIMBIC LOBE†

* The term *piriform area* is often used to refer collectively to the lateral olfactory gyrus, the anterior portion of the parahippocampal gyrus, and the uncus.

† The *limbic system* is a term used to refer to the limbic lobe plus a number of subcortical forebrain structures and portions of the brain stem that are functionally related (see Chapter 22).

pocampal formation (*hippocampus* and *dentate gyrus*).

The next oldest cortical area, the *paleopallium* (*paleocortex*), is olfactory in nature and may have from one to five cortical layers; this includes the *piriform area* (the *lateral olfactory gyrus*, the *uncus*, and the *anterior* portion of the *parahippocampal gyrus*). Together, the *paleopallium* and *archipallium* are classified as *allocortex*. The allocortical areas are reviewed in Chapters 13 and 22; the isocortex, in Chapter 21.

Both the *limbic lobe* and the *rhinencephalon* include cortical areas defined by a functional system. Although the *rhinencephalon* includes only those telencephalic structures, cortical and subcortical, immediately associated with olfaction, the *limbic lobe* is strictly cortical (Table 8–1).

Basal Ganglia

Five major nuclear groups compose the basal ganglia: the *caudate nucleus*, the *putamen*, the *globus pallidus*, the *amygdala* (or *amygdaloid complex*, because it is composed of a number of small, discrete nuclei), and the *claustrum* (Table 8–2). Singly, and in various combinations, these nuclei are referred to by other names. Together, the putamen and globus pallidus are known as the *lentiform nucleus* (*lenticular nucleus*). The caudate and putamen constitute the *neostriatum*. The globus pallidus is known as the *paleostriatum*, and the amygdala as the *archistriatum* (Figs. 8–3 and 8–9).

TABLE 8–2

Basal Ganglia

Lentiform nucleus	1. Caudate nucleus	Neostriatum	Striatum*
	2. Putamen		
	3. Globus pallidus — Paleostriatum		
	4. Amygdala —— Archistriatum		
	5. Claustrum		

* The term *striatum* is used in a narrow sense to refer only to the neostriatum and in a broader sense to refer to neo-, paleo-, and archistriatum.

The term *striatum* (or *corpus striatum*) usually is a synonym for neostriatum (caudate and putamen). Sometimes, however, it refers collectively to the neostriatum, paleostriatum, and archistriatum (caudate, putamen, globus pallidus, and amygdala). The term *basal ganglia* is sometimes employed in a more global fashion to include functionally related nuclear groups in the ventral thalamus and midbrain, such as the *subthalamic nucleus*, the *zona incerta*, and the *substantia nigra*.

CAUDATE NUCLEUS AND PUTAMEN

The *caudate* and *putamen* are the newest components of the basal ganglia. In the human brain, and in other primates and mammals with a well-developed cerebral cortex, the two nuclei are separated by the *anterior limb* of the *internal capsule*, a massive aggregation of fibers connecting the cortex with lower levels of the brain stem and spinal cord. The putamen processes sensorimotor information, whereas the caudate processes

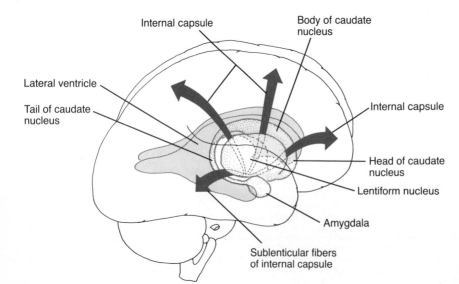

Internal capsule

Body of caudate nucleus

Lateral ventricle

Tail of caudate nucleus

Internal capsule

Head of caudate nucleus

Lentiform nucleus

Amygdala

Sublenticular fibers of internal capsule

FIGURE 8–9

Diagram of the brain illustrating the relative position of the basal ganglia and the lateral ventricles within the cerebral hemispheres.

information destined for association areas of the prefrontal cortex (see Chapter 16). In mammals lacking a well-defined internal capsule, these fibers pass through the neostriatum as small fascicles. The two nuclei (caudate and putamen) are not identifiable as separate structures. When these brains are sectioned, the fascicles give the neostriatum a striped or striated appearance—hence, the term "striatum" (Figs. 8–3, 8–10, and 8–11).

GLOBUS PALLIDUS

The *globus pallidus* lies deep (medial) to the putamen but lateral to the internal capsule. In Weigert-stained sections, the globus pallidus is darker than the adjacent putamen. It is separated from the putamen by a layer of dark-staining, myelinated fibers, the *external lamina*. The globus pallidus is further subdivided into *internal* and *external divisions* (GPi and GPe) by an

internal lamina of myelinated fibers (see Figs. 7–21 and 8–11). In unstained slices, these laminae appear white (see Fig. 8–3).

The putamen and globus pallidus are closely associated with the integration of motor activity. The caudate and putamen receive extensive cortical, thalamic, and brain stem connections, whereas the principal afferent connections to the globus pallidus are from the caudate and putamen. The globus pallidus is the major efferent nucleus of the group with extensive projections to the thalamus, ventral thalamus, hypothalamus, and midbrain (see Chapter 16).

AMYGDALA

The *amygdala*, a large well-defined nuclear complex situated in the tip of the temporal lobe deep to the uncus, is in anatomical continuity with the ventrolateral portion of the putamen (see Figs. 1–19, 8–9, and 8–11). The principal connec-

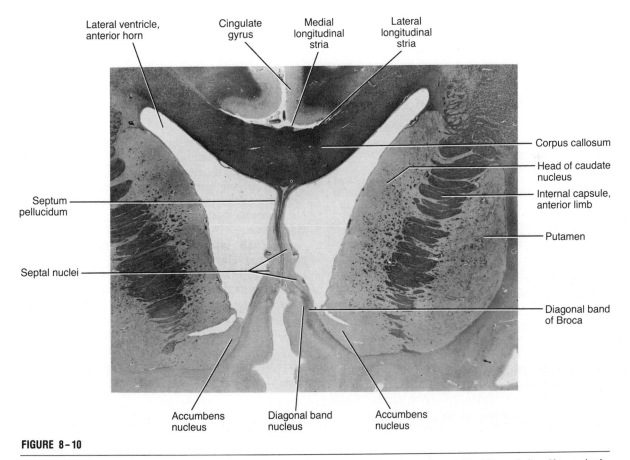

FIGURE 8–10

Transverse section through the anterior limb of the internal capsule and the septal region of the telencephalon. Human brain; Weigert stain.

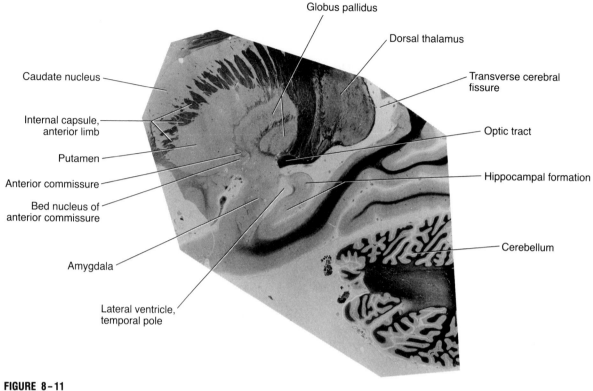

FIGURE 8–11

Parasagittal section through the basal ganglia, thalamus, and temporal horn of the lateral ventricle illustrating the continuity between the striatum and the amygdaloid complex. Human brain; Weigert stain.

tions of the amygdala are associated with the limbic and olfactory systems.

CLAUSTRUM

The *claustrum* is a flattened, sheet-like aggregation of neurons lying deep to the insular cortex and lateral to the putamen. It is bounded laterally by the *extreme capsule*, a sheet of white matter beneath the insular cortex, which follows the contours of the gyri. The medial boundary is the *external capsule*, a smooth sheet of white matter separating the claustrum from the putamen (see Fig. 8–3). Afferent and efferent connections of the claustrum are poorly understood; however, well-defined reciprocal connections between this nucleus and sensory areas of the cerebral cortex have been described. In many ways, these connections are more similar to those of the thalamus than to other nuclei of the basal ganglia.

Basal Forebrain

The basal forebrain is an oft neglected area with ill-defined landmarks. Its functions appear di-

verse, and the connections are for the most part poorly understood. Many of the basal forebrain structures are located deep to the *anterior perforated substance*, anterior and lateral to the hypothalamus, and ventral to the striatum. Table 8–3 lists those structures composing the basal forebrain area.

Although the basal forebrain constitutes less than 1% of the human brain, its collective size, relative to total body mass, is larger than that for any other primate. Many of the nuclei and fiber pathways associated with this area are part of the limbic and olfactory systems. These are covered in depth in Chapters 22 and 13, respectively.

ANTERIOR PERFORATED SUBSTANCE

The *anterior perforated substance* is visible on the ventral surface of the brain, bounded anteriorly by the medial and lateral olfactory striae, lateral to the optic tract, and continuous with the ventroanterior margin of the insular cortex, the *limen insulae* (see Figs. 7–21 and 8–7). The anterior perforated substance is readily identifiable from the numerous small perforations in its

TABLE 8–3

Basal Forebrain Structures

Anterior perforated substance
Nucleus accumbens
Substantia innominata (basal nucleus of Meynert)
Septal complex
  Septal nuclei
    Dorsal septal nucleus
    Lateral septal nucleus
    Medial septal nucleus
  Nucleus of the diagonal band of Broca
  Bed nucleus of the anterior commissure
  Bed nucleus of the stria terminalis

surface produced by small penetrating branches of the anterior and middle cerebral arteries. The histological organization of the anterior perforated substance actually is that of a trilaminar cortex and is often referred to as the cortex of the anterior perforated substance.

SEPTAL COMPLEX

The most visible part of the septum in a midsagittal view of the forebrain is the *septum pellucidum*. This is a thin sheet of non-neuronal elements stretching from the fornix to the corpus callosum and forming most of the medial wall of the anterior horn of the lateral ventricle (see Figs. 8–3, 8–4, and 8–10). The inferior portion, the "true septum" or *septum verum*, contains a number of prominent nuclei, comparable to septal nuclei found in lower forms. Of the many *septal nuclei* within the true septum (above the subcallosal gyrus, anterior and superior to the fornix), the *dorsal, lateral,* and *medial septal nuclei* are the most prominent (see Figs. 7–22 and 8–10 and Table 8–3).

The *diagonal band of Broca* originates in the parolfactory area and the medial portion of the septum and extends along the posterior margin of the anterior perforated substance, immediately lateral to the optic tract. Closely associated with the diagonal band is the *nucleus of the diagonal band of Broca* (see Fig. 8–10).

The *stria terminalis* runs along the inner curvature of the caudate nucleus, as it extends from the septal complex of the basal forebrain area to the *amygdala* of the temporal lobe. In the basal forebrain area, the stria terminalis has a prominent nucleus associated with it, the *bed nucleus of the stria terminalis*. In the vicinity of the lamina terminalis, adjacent to the septal nuclei and immediately anterior to the *anterior commissure*, is the *bed nucleus of the anterior commissure* (see Fig. 7–22 and Table 8–3).

NUCLEUS ACCUMBENS

The *nucleus accumbens* (sometimes referred to as the *nucleus accumbens septi*) extends from the base of the septal complex laterally to the junction of the caudate and putamen, where it becomes continuous with the striatal nuclei (see Fig. 8–10). Anatomically, the nucleus accumbens receives afferents from the amygdala, projects to the globus pallidus, and appears to functionally link the limbic system with the basal ganglia.

SUBSTANTIA INNOMINATA

The *substantia innominata* (or *basal nucleus of Meynert*) is situated ventral to the lentiform nuclei and extends anteriorly toward the amygdala and nucleus accumbens. The rostral portion of the substantia innominata lies deep to the anterior perforated substance (see Fig. 7–21). Anatomically, the connections of the substantia innominata are similar to those of the globus pallidus. The substantia innominata appears to be more closely related in function to the basal ganglia than to the limbic or olfactory systems.

SUGGESTED READING

Haines, D. E. (1991). *Neuroanatomy. An Atlas of Structures, Sections and Systems*, 3rd Edition. Urban & Schwarzenberg, Baltimore-Munich, 252 pp.

A thorough, yet concise atlas and guide to the organization and structure of the human central nervous system. Slices, Weigert-stained sections, and diagrams provide an excellent reference source to the organization of the telencephalon.

Netter, F. H. (1983). *The Ciba Collection of Medical Illustrations*. Volume 1, *Nervous System*. Part I, *Anatomy and Physiology*. Ciba Pharmaceutical Company, West Caldwell, New Jersey.

An excellent compendium of illustrations of the human brain. Especially suitable for understanding the three-dimensional relationships between specific structures and nuclei within the human central nervous system.

Chapter

9

Meninges, Ventricular System, and Vasculature

MENINGES
VENTRICULAR SYSTEM
SPINAL CORD VASCULATURE
CEREBRAL ARTERIAL SUPPLY
CEREBRAL VENOUS RETURN
IN SITU VISUALIZATION

During development, the embryonic neural canal is modified to form a system of ependymal-lined, interconnected chambers, the *ventricles* of the brain (see Chapter 1; Figs. 1–16 and 1–19). Later, capillaries from the meninx primitivum invade the thinned, ependymal walls of the ventricles, forming the delicate *choroid plexus.* This plexus begins to produce *cerebrospinal fluid* (*CSF*), filling the ventricular system and the space immediately surrounding the brain and spinal cord, the *subarachnoid space.*

With the production of *CSF*, the brain and spinal cord become suspended in a fluid-filled chamber. The bony *cranial vault* and the *vertebral canal*, along with three layers of protective membranes, the *meninges*, physically protect the delicate nervous tissue and insure the integrity of its fluid environment.

Meninges

DURA MATER

In the cranium, the dense connective tissue of the *dura mater* can be divided into two layers: an outer or *periosteal layer* and an inner or *meningeal layer.* The periosteal layer is rich in nerve fibers and blood vessels and serves as the periosteum of the cranial vault. The meningeal layer is avascular and covered with a layer of flattened, squamous-like mesothelial cells. Except for those sites where the two dural layers separate to form an endothelial-lined *dural venous sinus*, the two layers are fused (Fig. 9–1).

At several locations, the meningeal layer of dura mater is reflected on itself, forming prominent dural folds, the largest of which is the *falx cerebri.* Extending posteriorly from the crista galli in the floor of the anterior cranial fossa, the line of attachment of the *falx cerebri* arches posteriorly along the midline of the inner surface of the calvaria to the internal occipital protuberance. This separates the two cerebral hemispheres and effectively divides the cranial cavity into two lateral compartments. Extending along the line of attachment of the falx cerebri, just beneath the periosteal layer of the dura, is the *superior sagittal sinus*, the largest of the dural venous sinuses. The *inferior sagittal sinus* runs along the inferior, free margin of the falx cerebri and is surrounded

FIGURE 9-1

FIGURE 9-1

A transverse section through the calvaria, the superior sagittal sinus, and the falx cerebri. Note the relationships among the cerebral cortex and the meninges, the dura mater, the arachnoid (red), and the pia mater. Arachnoid granulations pierce the dura mater, providing points of exit for cerebrospinal fluid (CSF) from the subarachnoid space. Arachnoid trabeculae span the CSF-filled, subarachnoid space. The pia mater closely adheres to the surface of the brain, held tight by a glial membrane.

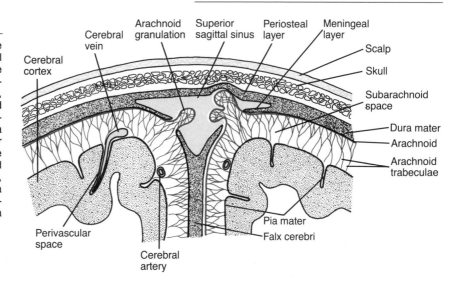

by the meningeal layer of the dura (Figs. 9-1, 9-2, and 9-3).

Posteriorly, the vertically oriented *falx cerebri* is continuous with the nearly horizontal *tentorium cerebelli* at their junction along the *straight sinus*. The tentorium arises anterolaterally from the petrous ridge of the temporal bone and extends posteromedially to join the falx cerebri in the midline. This forms a partial roof over the posterior cranial fossa, with the cerebellum and most of the brain stem located beneath this roof (see Figs. 9-2 and 9-3). The small *superior*

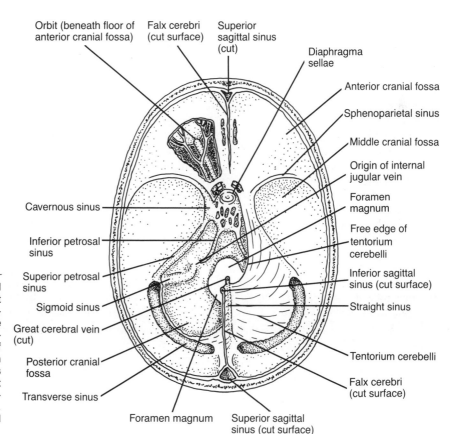

FIGURE 9-2

A view into the base of the skull with the brain removed. The cut ends of the falx cerebri are indicated, and the left half of the tentorium cerebelli has been removed. The superior surface of the transverse sinus has been removed on both sides as has the roof of the orbit on the left side. Anterior, middle, and posterior cranial fossae are indicated. Most blood vessels and cranial nerves have been omitted.

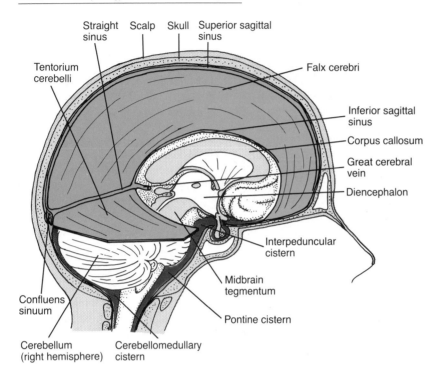

Straight sinus · Scalp · Skull · Superior sagittal sinus

Tentorium cerebelli

Falx cerebri

Inferior sagittal sinus

Corpus callosum

Great cerebral vein

Diencephalon

Interpeduncular cistern

Midbrain tegmentum

Pontine cistern

Confluens sinuum

Cerebellum (right hemisphere) · Cerebellomedullary cistern

FIGURE 9-3

Midsagittal view of the skull illustrating the relationships among the dural folds (falx cerebri and tentorium cerebelli, in red), the brain, and the cranial vault. The right cerebral hemisphere, along with the diencephalon and midbrain, have been removed to expose the falx cerebri. However, the medulla, pons, and cerebellum remain intact beneath the tentorium cerebelli.

petrosal sinus is located along the line of attachment of the *tentorium cerebelli* to the petrous portion of the temporal bone (see Fig. 9-2). The free anteromedial edges of the tentorium cerebelli embrace the midbrain at the level of the tectum and crus cerebri, forming the *tentorial notch.*

The *straight sinus* runs horizontally in the midline at the junction between the falx cerebri and the tentorium cerebelli; the *transverse sinus* runs along the posterolateral margin of the tentorium; and the *superior petrosal sinus* runs along the anterolateral attachment of the tentorium (see Fig. 9-2). Dural venous sinuses are discussed in Cerebral Venous Return.

Two other dural folds of note are the *diaphragma sellae,* forming a roof over the pituitary fossa (see Fig. 9-2), and the *falx cerebelli,* a small vertically oriented fold beneath the tentorium cerebelli. The free edge of the falx cerebelli extends forward into the small, interhemispheric depression on the cerebellum.

The dural blood supply (see Cerebral Arterial Supply) is principally of extracranial origin. The sensory innervation of the supratentorial dura (all dura above the level of the tentorium) is provided by the trigeminal nerve. The infratentorial dura is innervated by branches of the upper cervical and vagus nerves.

The cranial dura, through its periosteal layer, is closely adherent to the inside of the skull—there is no epidural space. At the level of the foramen magnum, however, the meningeal layer separates from the periosteal layer and forms a tube-shaped sac of *spinal dura,* extending into the vertebral canal and surrounding the spinal cord. The *spinal dural sac* extends from the foramen magnum to the second sacral vertebra, where it abruptly tapers to surround the *filum terminale* of the spinal cord (*filum terminale internum*) and forms the *coccygeal ligament* (*filum terminale externum*). This anchors the dural sac to the base of the vertebral canal (see Fig. 1-8).

Both external and internal surfaces of the spinal dura mater are covered with flattened, squamous-like mesothelial cells. Within the vertebral canal, the dural sac is surrounded by an *epidural space* filled with fatty areolar tissue. In addition to its clinical importance for the administration of epidural anesthetics, the *epidural space* contains the major venous drainage of the spinal cord, the *epidural venous anastomosis,* and lymphatic vessels.

As the spinal nerves pierce the spinal dura mater at their points of exit from the vertebral canal, the dura is reflected over the exiting nerve and blends imperceptibly with the thick connective tissue sheath composing the epineurium of the peripheral nerve.

ARACHNOID

Closely adherent to the inner surface of the dura mater is the *arachnoid membrane*. This avascular layer follows the contour of the inner surface of the dura mater and gives rise to numerous *arachnoid trabeculae*, which span the *subarachnoid space* between the dura mater and the pia mater on the surface of the brain. The CSF-filled *subarachnoid space* is in continuity with the CSF of the fourth ventricle of the brain through three foramina in the roof of the ventricle, the *medial foramen of Magendie* and the *lateral foramina of Luschka* (Fig. 9–4).

In addition to forming the arachnoid trabecu-lae, many of the irregular, interdigitating cells of the arachnoid retain the potential of rounding up, detaching from the arachnoid membrane, and becoming macrophages.

At numerous points along the superior sagittal sinus, tufts of the arachnoid membrane protrude through the dura mater and into the venous sinus as *arachnoid granulations* (see Figs. 9–1 and 9–4). These are sites of exit for the CSF and are most numerous in the superior sagittal sinus. They are found in other dural venous sinuses as well. The number of arachnoid granulations increases with age as does their tendency to become calcified. Whether the two processes are related is not known.

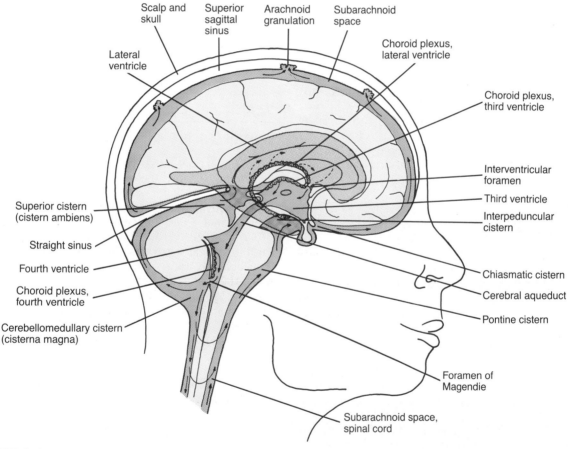

FIGURE 9–4

Production and flow pattern of the cerebrospinal fluid (CSF) within the ventricles of the brain and the surrounding subarachnoid space. The CSF is produced by the choroid plexus of the lateral, third, and fourth ventricles. Fluid flow is from the lateral ventricle, through the interventricular foramen, through the third ventricle, and into the fourth ventricle via the cerebral aqueduct. The CSF leaves the fourth ventricle, via the medial foramen of Magendie and the lateral foramina of Luschka (not illustrated), enters the subarachnoid space, and ultimately empties into the venous blood of the superior sagittal sinus through arachnoid granulations.

SUBARACHNOID SPACE

The cranial dura and the adherent arachnoid follow the contour of the cranial vault, whereas the pia mater follows that of the brain. As a result, the subarachnoid space is not uniform. Areas where the subarachnoid space is especially large are known as *subarachnoid cisterns*. The largest cistern, the *cerebellomedullary cistern* (*cisterna magna*), is located immediately dorsal to the medulla and extends vertically from the foramen magnum to the inferior surface of the cerebellum (Figs. 9–3 and 9–4).

Other cranial cisterns of significance are the *pontine*, *interpeduncular*, *chiasmatic*, and *superior cisterns*. The last cistern is of clinical importance because of its contents: the posterior, superior, and lateral surfaces of the midbrain; the great cerebral vein; the pineal; and the posterior and superior cerebellar arteries (see Figs. 9–3 and 9–4).

The *lumbar cistern* is located in the lower portion of the spinal dural sac, extending from the first lumbar to the second sacral vertebra. The cistern contains the filum terminale, the nerve roots of the cauda equina, and CSF (see Fig. 1–8). In the adult, samples of CSF usually are withdrawn from the *lumbar cistern*—the lumbar spinal tap—because there is a relative abundance of CSF, no central nervous system (CNS) tissue, and minimal potential for damage to the nerve roots.

PIA MATER

The *pia mater* is a thin, connective tissue layer closely following the contours of the brain and separated from the *subpial astrocytic membrane* by only a basement membrane. The arachnoid trabeculae are anchored to the fine collagenous network on the free surface of the pia mater, where cells from the two layers blend together.

As blood vessels spread over the surface of the brain, small penetrating branches enter the substance of the brain. They pierce the pia and carry a perivascular cuff of pia and arachnoid into the brain, forming a small but identifiable *perivascular* (*Virchow-Robin*) *space*, between the vessel and the pia, which remains in continuity with the subarachnoid space (see Fig. 9–1). It was believed that the perivascular space extended into the depths of the brain along the vascular tree and provided a channel for movement of CSF. However, electron microscopic studies have failed to confirm this hypothesis. Instead, after the vessel penetrates for a short distance, the pia mater

and the connective tissue sheath of the vessel blend together and the space is obliterated.

At spinal levels, small flattened "tabs" of pial tissue, the *denticulate ligaments*, extend from the lateral surface of the spinal cord to the dura mater and arachnoid. The denticulate ligaments, alternating with the exit of spinal nerves from the dural sac, contribute to the fixation of the spinal cord within the subarachnoid space.

Pia mater also is reflected over the rootlets of emerging nerve fibers of the brain stem and spinal cord, investing them with a thin coat of mesodermal cells, as they traverse the subarachnoid space.

From the base of the spinal cord, the *pia mater* forms a long slender tube running caudally to attach to the inner surface of the dural sac. This tube, extending from the *conus medullaris* of the cord, is the *filum terminale* (*filum terminale internum*), and it anchors the spinal cord to the dural sac. The dural sac, in turn, is anchored to the bony coccyx by the *coccygeal ligament* (*filum terminale externum*).

Ventricular System

VENTRICLES OF THE BRAIN

The ependymal-lined cavities of the cerebral hemispheres form the paired *lateral ventricles*. Each of these large, C-shaped cavities is connected with the unpaired *third ventricle* through a short canal, the *interventricular foramen* (*of Monroe*). The vertically orientated, slit-shaped third ventricle separates the two halves of the diencephalon and is continuous posteroinferiorly with the *cerebral aqueduct* (*of Sylvius*). The narrow, tubular cerebral aqueduct passes through the midbrain, opening into the *fourth ventricle* at the level of the pons and medulla. The rhomboid-shaped fourth ventricle, with its paired lateral recesses, is in continuity with the subarachnoid space through the *medial foramen of Magendie* and the paired *lateral foramina of Luschka* (Figs. 9–4 and 9–5).

Lateral Ventricles

The *lateral ventricle* extends forward into the frontal lobe as the *anterior horn*. This portion is devoid of choroid plexus and bounded medially by the septum pellucidum. The *body* of the lateral ventricle stretches from the interventricular foramen posteriorly to the splenium of the corpus callosum. The choroid fissure and its associated

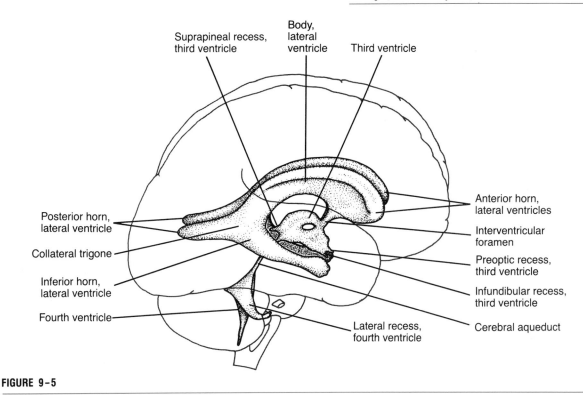

FIGURE 9-5

The ventricles of the brain illustrating their relative position.

choroid plexus are located along the anteromedial concavity of the body. The *inferior horn* (or *temporal horn*) is a continuation of the body, as it swings inferolaterally and then anteriorly toward the tip of the temporal lobe, where it ends adjacent to the amygdaloid complex. The choroid fissure and its associated choroid plexus are located on the superomedial concavity of the inferior horn. The *posterior horn* is a finger-like projection, extending posteriorly into the occipital lobe. It does not contain any choroid plexus. The triangular area of the lateral ventricle where the body, inferior horn, and posterior horn meet is sometimes referred to as the *collateral trigone* (see Figs. 9–4 and 9–5).

Third Ventricle

Except for the infundibulum and interthalamic adhesion, the hypothalamus and thalamus are completely separated from their counterparts on the opposite side by the *third ventricle*. The anterior margin of the third ventricle is the lamina terminalis; the posterior margin, the midbrain tegmentum. The choroid plexus of the lateral ventricles extends through the interventricular foramina and into the roof of the third ventricle.

The lateral margin of the roof of the third ventricle is attached to the thalamus along a slight elevation produced by the stria medullaris thalami, extending from the habenular complex forward to the interventricular foramen (see Figs. 9–4 and 9–5).

The contour of the third ventricle, as seen in midsagittal plane, is characterized by several notable recesses: the *preoptic recess* lies above the optic chiasm; the *infundibular recess* extends into the base of the infundibular stalk; and the *suprapineal recess* extends posteriorly, above the habenular commissure and the pineal gland. The smaller *pineal recess* (not illustrated) extends posteriorly above the posterior commissure and into the base of the pineal gland (see Fig. 9–5).

Cerebral Aqueduct

The narrowest segment of the ventricular system is the *cerebral aqueduct*. Situated ventral to the tectum and dorsal to the tegmentum, it is also the most vulnerable to obstruction. Pressure on the tectum from a tumor of the pineal gland can block the normal flow of CSF and produce a form of noncommunicating hydrocephalus (see Fig. 9–4).

Fourth Ventricle

The cerebral aqueduct spreads open at the level of the rostral pons to form the rhomboid-shaped *fourth ventricle*. After reaching maximum width at the level of the inferior margin of the middle cerebellar peduncle, the fourth ventricle begins to narrow, tapering to a slender canal in the lower medulla. On each side, a lateral recess extends from the widest portion of the ventricle, around the cerebellar peduncles, adjacent to the flocculus of the cerebellum. The choroid plexus of the posterior medullary vellum extends along the roof of the lateral recess and often herniates into the subarachnoid space through the lateral foramina of Luschka (see Fig. 9–5). The single *medial foramen of Magendie*, in the posterior medullary vellum, and the two *lateral foramina of Luschka* are the only openings between the ventricular system and the subarachnoid space. These are essential for the normal flow of the CSF.

CHOROID PLEXUS

The choroid plexus of the lateral and the third and fourth ventricles produces over 70% of the CSF. The remainder is produced from unidentified sites within the ventricular system. The ventricular surface of the choroid plexus is lined with a cuboidal epithelium, continuous with and of similar origin to the ependyma of the ventricles (see Fig. 2–23).

With the surface epithelium thrown into a series of folds and trabeculae, the choroid plexus has the appearance of a delicate sponge. Loose connective tissue and fenestrated capillaries fill the folds, but the cuboidal epithelium lining the ventricular surface is responsible for the regulation and production of the CSF. Microvilli project from these cells, and the basal surface, with its basal infoldings, is in close contact with a prominent basement membrane. These cuboidal cells are held together with intercellular tight junctions, forming an anatomical barrier between the blood plasma and the CSF of the ventricles (see Figs. 2–24 and 9–6).

CEREBROSPINAL FLUID COMPOSITION AND PRODUCTION

The CSF is clear and colorless with a total volume of approximately 150 ml, of which only about 23 ml is in the ventricles. The remaining 127 ml fill the subarachnoid space surrounding the brain and spinal cord. In the supine position, CSF pressure in the adult varies from 50 to 150 mm of H_2O. Because the specific gravity of the brain is 1.040 and that of the CSF is 1.007, an adult brain of 1400 gm has an apparent weight of less than 50 gm when suspended in CSF.

Under normal conditions, CSF is virtually cell free, with a leukocyte count of 0 to 5 cells per μl. Relative to serum levels, the CSF is low in protein, glucose, K^+, and Ca^{++}, but high in Na^+, Mg^{++}, and Cl^-. These differences are greater than would be expected if the CSF were merely a dialysate of the plasma (Table 9–1).

Active, ATP-dependent pump mechanisms are present in the choroidal epithelium for the secretion of Na^+ and the removal of K^+ from the CSF. Other, energy-dependent mechanisms regulate the levels of the divalent cations, Ca^{++} and Mg^{++}. The slightly lower osmolality of the CSF (289 mOsm/L compared with 290 to 300 in serum) facilitates the transport of small molecules, metabolic products, and drugs from the surrounding brain tissue into the CSF.

In humans, the rate of production of CSF is quite rapid with average values ranging from 500 to 750 ml per day, or a four- to five-volume turnover per day. Feedback mechanisms do not exist for the regulation of the rate of CSF production, and the choroid plexus continues to produce CSF even though the ventricles and subarachnoid spaces are filled and the pressure is high. Thus, obstructions to the normal flow, either within the ventricular system or at the level of the arachnoid granulations, produce high CSF pressure and brain damage.

CEREBROSPINAL FLUID FLOW

The lateral ventricles contain the largest amount of choroid plexus and produce the greatest volume of CSF. Fluid produced in the lateral ventricles flows through the interventricular foramen into the third ventricle and mixes with the CSF produced there. CSF from the third ventricle flows through the cerebral aqueduct and into the fourth ventricle, mixing further with the fluid produced therein. All CSF exits the ventricular system through the foramina of the fourth ventricle and enters the subarachnoid space. On entering the subarachnoid space, CSF moves over the surface of the spinal cord and brain to ultimately leave the subarachnoid space and to enter the dural venous sinuses, through the arachnoid granulations (see Fig. 9–4).

The movement of CSF through the arachnoid

Cuboidal epithelium
of choroid plexus

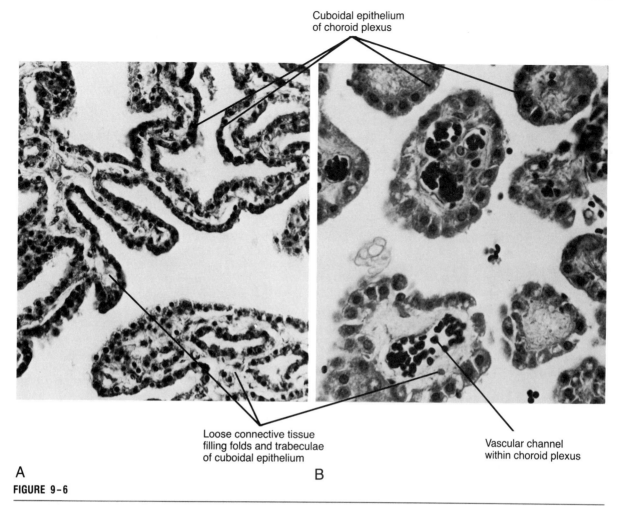

Loose connective tissue
filling folds and trabeculae
of cuboidal epithelium

Vascular channel
within choroid plexus

A   B

FIGURE 9-6

Choroid plexus. *A,* Anastomosing villus-like structures, covered with a cuboidal epithelium and containing a rich vascular plexus, are characteristics of the choroid plexus.

B, The choroid plexus at higher magnification. Human tissue; hematoxylin and eosin stain.

TABLE 9-1

Comparison of Cerebrospinal Fluid and Serum*

	CEREBROSPINAL FLUID	SERUM
Protein, total (mg/L)	150–450	60,000–78,000
Albumin (mg/L)	100–300	35,000–50,000
Immunoglobulins (mg/L)	5–69	7,000–23,250
Glucose (mmol/L)	2.2–3.9	3.9–5.8
Chloride (mmol/L)	118–132	98–106
Calcium (mmol/L)	1.05–1.35	2.1–2.55
Magnesium (mmol/L)	0.78–1.26	0.65–1.05
Potassium (mmol/L)	2.8–3.2	4.0–5.1
Sodium (mmol/L)	147–151	136–146

* Serum is the fluid portion of coagulated blood after removal of the fibrin clot and blood cells, whereas plasma is the fluid (noncellular) portion of circulating, noncoagulated blood.

granulations into the blood stream is a passive, pressure-dependent, one-way process. The CSF flows through a system of microscopic tubules within the epithelial cells of the arachnoid, across the basement membrane, and between the endothelial cells lining the sinus. When venous pressure exceeds that of the CSF, the tubules collapse and the flow stops.

Blockage of the movement of CSF into the dural venous sinuses, at the arachnoid granulations, leads to *communicating hydrocephalus.* If CSF cannot leave the ventricular system (i.e., blockage of the foramina of the fourth ventricle or obstruction of the cerebral aqueduct), the condition is termed *noncommunicating hydrocephalus.*

BLOOD-BRAIN, BLOOD-CSF, AND CSF-BRAIN EXCHANGES

Three separate fluid compartments exist within the CNS: the blood; the CSF; and the fluid in the extracellular spaces, or for purposes of discussion, the "brain." In CNS tissue, there is a constant exchange of ions, small molecules, and macromolecules between these compartments. These exchanges, in many cases, are highly selective and often carrier-mediated transfers.

This selective transfer from one compartment to the other is functionally a "*barrier.*" In the case of the *blood-CSF barrier* and the *blood-brain barrier,* anatomical structures can be identified that form a physical barrier. However, no anatomical barrier separates the CSF and brain compartments. Any functional barrier to the transfer of molecules is one of diffusion gradients only.

The *blood-CSF barrier* is anatomically defined by the tight junctions between the epithelial cells of the choroid plexus. The capillaries of the choroid plexus are fenestrated, permitting macromolecules to diffuse through the connective tissue stroma of the plexus. However, transfer through the epithelium is quite selective (see Fig. 2–24). Although some circulating peptides and plasma proteins are found in the CSF, these are transported by specific carrier mechanisms.

The anatomical basis of the *blood-brain barrier* resides in the endothelial cells of the capillary beds within the brain. The capillaries are surrounded by a smooth basement membrane and the dense *perivascular glia limitans* (see Fig. 2–17). Unlike the endothelial cells of the choroid plexus, these endothelial cells are not fenestrated, have few pinocytotic vesicles, and are held together by tight junctions. Specific areas known as *circumventricular organs* are exceptions (see subsequent discussion).

The tight junctions and the plasma membrane of the endothelial cells combine to form a continuous physical barrier to intercellular diffusion of substances. Macromolecules injected into the brain diffuse through the perivascular glia limitans and the basement membrane but do not enter the capillary. Similarly, macromolecules from the blood stream do not readily pass through the endothelial cell barrier. The passage of ions and molecules through the endothelium, from the blood stream to the extracellular spaces, is a highly selective process. It is limited to carrier-mediated mechanisms or to the diffusion of highly lipophilic compounds, because compounds soluble in the plasma membrane of en-

dothelial cells pass into the brain. The kinetics for the passage of different substances between the blood and brain is variable and depends on a number of factors, including the capacity of specific carrier mechanisms.

In the case of the *CSF-brain barrier,* no physical barrier exists and compounds appear free to diffuse from one compartment to the other. The ciliated ependymal cells do not have tight junctions. Movement of the cilia is believed to facilitate the mixing of CSF and extracellular fluids. Large macromolecules injected into either the substance of the brain or the CSF diffuse, unimpeded, from one compartment to the other (see Figs. 2–22 and 2–23).

Included in areas of exception to the blood-brain barrier are specific sites known collectively as the *circumventricular organs.* These highly vascular areas with fenestrated capillaries and abundant perivascular spaces include the following: the pineal gland, the neurohypophysis, the area postrema, the subfornical organ, the organum vasculosum of the lamina terminalis, and the median eminence of the hypothalamus. Except for the area postrema, situated at the junction of the fourth ventricle and the spinal canal, all are midline structures associated with the diencephalon. When macromolecules are injected into the blood stream, they diffuse into the neural tissue surrounding these areas.

The *pineal gland* is associated with the secretion of biogenic amines and melatonin and contains significant amounts of neuroactive peptides, such as thyrotropin-releasing hormone (TRH), luteinizing hormone–releasing hormone (LHRH), and somatostatin. Functionally, the pineal is associated with the mechanisms that regulate circadian rhythm. The *neurohypophysis* is involved in the release of neurohormones, such as oxytocin, vasopressin, and neurophysin, into the systemic circulation. The *area postrema* is believed to be a chemoreceptive area, triggering vomiting reflexes in response to circulating emetic substances. The *subfornical organ* is anatomically associated with the choroid plexus adjacent to the interventricular foramen and functions in the regulation of body fluids. The *organum vasculosum* of the lamina terminalis is, among other things, a chemosensory area, responding to circulating peptides and macromolecules. The *median eminence* is associated with the neuroendocrine functions and the regulation of the anterior pituitary through the release of peptide neurohormones into the hypothalamohypophyseal portal circulation. All of these structures con-

Meninges, Ventricular System, and Vasculature **177**

cerned with neurohumoral, chemoreceptive, or autonomic reflex activities are discussed in greater detail in Chapter 18.

Spinal Cord Vasculature

ARTERIAL SUPPLY

The blood supply to the spinal cord is from two primary sources: (1) the paired *vertebral arteries* and (2) the small, segmental *radicular arteries*, branches of various segmental arteries.

Each *vertebral artery* arises as a branch of the subclavian artery, ascends in the neck to the sixth cervical vertebra, enters the foramen of the transverse process of the sixth cervical vertebra, and continues to ascend through the foramina of the transverse processes of the upper cervical vertebrae. Immediately above the first cervical vertebra, the vertebral artery passes posterior to the atlanto-occipital articulation and swings anteriorly to pass through the dura, entering the posterior cranial fossa through the *foramen magnum*, lateral to the medulla. At this level, the vertebral artery moves to the anterior surface of the medulla, where it subsequently fuses with the verte-

bral artery of the opposite side near the base of the pons, to form the *basilar artery* (see Fig. 9–8).

Before fusion, the vertebral arteries give rise to the *posterior* and *anterior spinal arteries*, although the posterior spinal artery may be a branch of the posterior inferior cerebellar artery. The *posterior spinal arteries* descend along the posterolateral surface of the medulla and onto the posterior surface of the spinal cord, just medial to the point of entry of the dorsal roots. The *anterior spinal arteries* fuse to form a single *anterior spinal artery*, which descends along the surface of the anterior median fissure. Both the anterior spinal artery and the posterior spinal arteries extend the entire length of the spinal cord (Fig. 9–7).

Throughout their length, the anterior and posterior spinal arteries receive anastomotic branches from segmental spinal arteries known as *radicular arteries*. Typically, *radicular arteries* enter the spinal canal through an intervertebral foramen in the company of a spinal nerve; branch to form *anterior* and *posterior radicular arteries* which, in turn, anastomose with the anterior and posterior spinal arteries, respectively (see Fig. 9–7). Thus, the anterior and posterior spinal arteries become

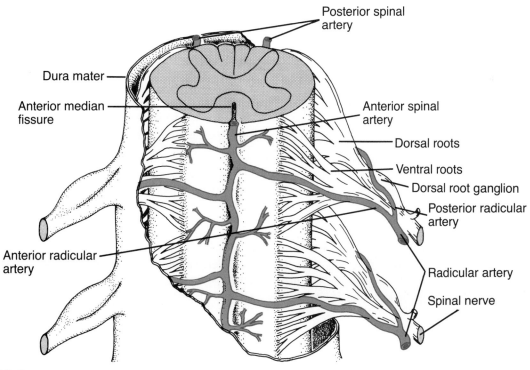

FIGURE 9–7

Arterial supply of the spinal cord.

anastomotic channels of the segmental radicular arteries. The vertebral arteries are the major arterial supply for cervical levels of the spinal cord; however, in thoracic, lumbar, and sacral levels the spinal arteries receive a significant contribution of arterial blood from the radicular arteries.

Although all spinal nerves are accompanied by radicular arteries, most of these arteries are too small to contribute significantly to the blood supply of the spinal cord. Normally, there are six to eight radicular arteries with major anastomotic contributions to the spinal arteries. These are quite variable, although the contributions generally are greater in the upper and lower levels of the spinal cord and least in the mid-thoracic region.

Radicular arteries may contribute small branches to the dorsal and ventral roots and to spinal cord tissue, but their primary role is that of a feeder to the system of spinal arteries. The *anterior spinal artery* has numerous small branches, with many entering the anterior median fissure. These supply most of the gray matter of the spinal cord, along with the white matter of the anterior funiculus. The *posterior spinal arteries* provide small, circumferential branches that pass over the lateral surface of the cord and penetrate the substance of the cord. Although some overlap occurs in the pattern of blood supply, the anterior spinal artery supplies the anterior funiculus and all of the gray matter except some portions of the dorsal horn. The posterior spinal arteries supply the lateral and posterior funiculi and parts of the dorsal horn (see Fig. 9–12).

VENOUS RETURN

The venous drainage of the spinal cord is similar, in principle, to the arterial supply but has a greater variability and a greater number of anastomoses. *Anteromedian* and *anterolateral veins* drain into *anterior radicular veins*. *Posteromedian* and *posterolateral veins* drain into *posterior radicular veins*. The radicular veins, in turn, penetrate the dura mater and drain into the *epidural venous anastomosis*. This is located in the fatty tissue between the dural sac and the periosteum of the vertebral canal. This venous plexus drains into segmental veins of the thorax and abdomen.

Cerebral Arterial Supply

The brain receives its entire arterial blood supply from two pairs of arteries: the *internal carotid arteries* and the *vertebral arteries*. The vertebral arteries, after entering the cranial vault, merge to form the single *basilar artery*. This subsequently divides, forming two terminal branches, the *posterior cerebral arteries*. Each internal carotid forms two terminal branches, the *anterior cerebral artery* and the *middle cerebral artery*. The internal carotid, after entering the cranial vault, immediately gives rise to an *ophthalmic artery,* which enters the orbit along with the optic nerve. The internal carotid subsequently gives rise to a *posterior communicating artery* and the *anterior choroidal artery* before forming its terminal branches (see Figs. 9–8 through 9–11).

The two anterior cerebral arteries are in communication via a short *anterior communicating artery*. Each internal carotid artery communicates with the posterior cerebral artery of the same side via a *posterior communicating artery*. These anastomotic arterial vessels complete a ring around the base of the brain, surrounding the interpeduncular fossa, the base of the hypothalamus, and the optic chiasm, known as the *cerebral arterial circle*, or the *circle of Willis* (see Fig. 9–9).

In theory, this arterial ring can equalize the pressure between the major arteries and can insure adequate blood flow, if any one of the four primary vessels becomes obstructed. With normal levels of blood pressure in all four primary vessels, little blood exchange occurs between the two halves of the brain. Usually, the communicating arteries are quite small. The anastomoses are insufficient to provide adequate blood supply following an acute, unilateral occlusion of one of the four principal vessels. If the occlusion is gradual and over an extended period, the communicating arteries may enlarge, providing an adequate anastomotic blood supply.

The paired *vertebral arteries* supply the cervical spinal cord, medulla, pons, and cerebellum, and portions of the diencephalon along with the medial surface of the occipital lobes and the inferomedial surface of the temporal lobes. The paired *internal carotid arteries* supply the remainder of the diencephalon and telencephalon. Normally, those portions of the brain superior to the tentorial notch are supplied by the *cerebral arterial circle*, those below the notch by the *vertebral-basilar system*.

VERTEBRAL-BASILAR SYSTEM

In addition to the *anterior* and *posterior spinal arteries*, the *vertebral arteries* give rise to the *posterior meningeal arteries* (not illustrated) and

FIGURE 9-8

Major cerebral arteries as seen on the base of the brain. Left half of the cerebellum and the tip of the left temporal lobe have been removed.

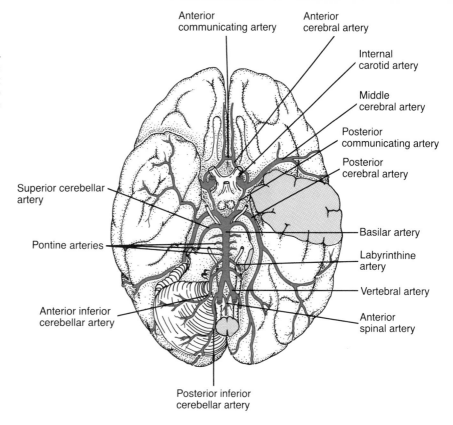

Anterior communicating artery

Anterior cerebral artery

Internal carotid artery

Middle cerebral artery

Posterior communicating artery

Posterior cerebral artery

Superior cerebellar artery

Basilar artery

Pontine arteries

Labyrinthine artery

Vertebral artery

Anterior inferior cerebellar artery

Anterior spinal artery

Posterior inferior cerebellar artery

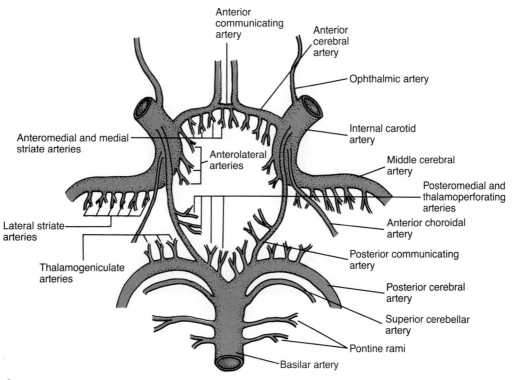

Anterior communicating artery

Anterior cerebral artery

Ophthalmic artery

Anteromedial and medial striate arteries

Internal carotid artery

Anterolateral arteries

Middle cerebral artery

Posteromedial and thalamoperforating arteries

Lateral striate arteries

Anterior choroidal artery

Thalamogeniculate arteries

Posterior communicating artery

Posterior cerebral artery

Superior cerebellar artery

Pontine rami

Basilar artery

FIGURE 9-9

The cerebral arterial circle of Willis and its principal branches.

179

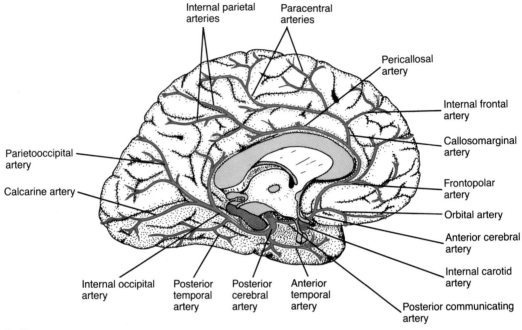

FIGURE 9-10

The cerebral arteries as seen from a midsagittal view of the hemisphere.

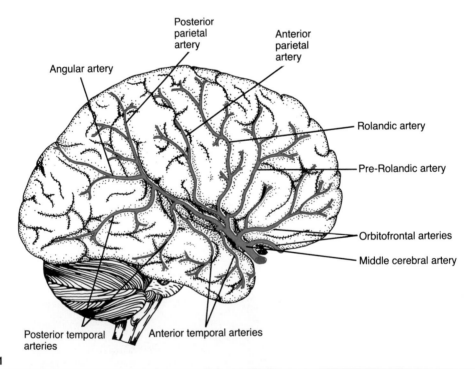

FIGURE 9-11

The course of the middle cerebral artery as seen from the lateral surface of the hemisphere with the temporal lobe depressed to expose part of the insular cortex.

the *posterior inferior cerebellar arteries* (see Fig. 9–8).

The *basilar artery* gives rise to the *anterior inferior cerebellar arteries*, the *labyrinthine arteries* (*internal auditory arteries*), numerous *circumferential* and *paramedian pontine arteries* (or *rami*), and the *superior cerebellar arteries* before terminating in the paired *posterior cerebral arteries* (see Figs. 9–8 and 9–9).

Anterior Spinal Artery

In the medulla, the *anterior spinal arteries* supply the ventromedial region, including the pyramids; pyramidal decussation; medial lemniscus; medial longitudinal fasciculus; hypoglossal nucleus, except the most rostral portion; dorsal motor nucleus of the vagus; medial accessory olivary nuclei; and lower portions of the solitary tract and nucleus. In the upper medulla, comparable areas are supplied by paramedian branches of the vertebral and basilar arteries (Fig. 9–12).

Posterior Spinal Artery

Although limited to the lower portion of the medulla, the *posterior spinal arteries* supply the dorsal column tracts and nuclei (gracile and cuneate fasciculi and their associated nuclei), along with the dorsal portion of the restiform body (see Fig. 9–12).

Bulbar Branches of the Vertebral Artery

The *vertebral arteries* give rise to numerous *bulbar branches*, which supply a wedge-shaped portion of the lateral medulla. Below the level of the pyramidal decussation, this wedge occupies the broad region between the anterior funiculus and the fasciculus cuneatus. At higher levels, the wedge becomes narrower, extending from the medullary pyramids to the dorsal surface of the inferior olive. Included in the supply area of these bulbar branches are the roots of the glossopharyngeal and vagus nerves, most of the inferior olivary nucleus, inferior portions of the nucleus ambiguus; and much of the lateral medullary reticular formation. At higher levels, the bulbar branches of the vertebral arteries overlap with the paramedian branches of the basilar artery (see Fig. 9–12).

Posterior Inferior Cerebellar Artery

The medullary branches of the *posterior inferior cerebellar artery* supply the dorsolateral region of the medulla from the level of the inferior olive to the medullopontine angle, immediately dorsolateral to the area supplied by the bulbar branches of the vertebral arteries. This region includes such structures as the spinothalamic pathways; rubrospinal tract; spinal nucleus and tract of the trigeminal; descending autonomic pathways; most of the inferior cerebellar peduncle; and the cochlear nuclei; as well as rostral portions of the nucleus ambiguus and the dorsal motor nucleus of the vagus, including their rootlets (see Fig. 9–12).

After giving off the medullary branches, the *posterior inferior cerebellar artery* swings onto the inferior surface of the cerebellum to supply the inferior portion of the vermis, the tonsil, and the inferolateral surface of the hemisphere. Branches also supply part of the choroid plexus of the fourth ventricle.

Paramedian and Circumferential Branches of the Basilar Artery

Paramedian branches of the *basilar artery* supply medial portions of the basal pons and overlap in the upper medulla with the bulbar branches of the vertebral artery. The area supplied includes such structures as the pontine nuclei and the corticospinal, corticobulbar, and corticopontine fibers. Some of the more deeply penetrating branches reach areas of the pontine tegmentum and include part of the medial lemniscus (Figs. 9–12 and 9–13).

The *short circumferential branches* of the *basilar artery* supply a wedge of the basal pons, lateral to that supplied by the paramedian branches, including variable amounts of the corticospinal tract and medial lemniscus, some pontine nuclei, pontocerebellar fibers and portions of the spinal tract, and nucleus of the trigeminal nerve as well as portions of the facial nucleus and associated fibers (see Fig. 9–13).

The *long circumferential branches* of the *basilar artery* swing around the basal pons to supply most of the pontine tegmentum. These vessels anastomose freely with bulbar branches of the anterior inferior cerebellar and superior cerebellar arteries.

Anterior Inferior Cerebellar Artery

Bulbar branches of the *anterior inferior cerebellar artery* supply most of the pontine tegmentum in the lower pons (see Fig. 9–13). The cerebellar portion swings around the lateral margin of the

Abbreviations used in Figures 9–12 through 9–15. AbdNr, abducens nerve; *AbdNu,* abducens nucleus; *AC,* anterior commissure; *ALS,* anterolateral system (spinal thalamic pathways); *AMV,* anterior medullary velum; *AmyNu,* amygdaloid nucleus (complex); *AntNu,* anterior nucleus of thalamus; *APS,* anterior perforated substance.

BP, basilar pons; *CaNu,B,* caudate nucleus, body; *CaNu,H,* caudate nucleus, head; *CaNu,T,* caudate nucleus, tail; *CC,* crus cerebri; *Cl,* claustrum; *CM,* centromedian nucleus of thalamus; *CorCl,B,* corpus callosum, body; *CorCl,Spl,* corpus callosum, splenium; *CS,* chief sensory trigeminal nucleus; *CSp,* corticospinal fibers; *CTT,* central tegmental tract.

DMNu, dorsal motor nucleus of vagus (Fig. 9–12) or dorsomedial nucleus of thalamus (Fig. 9–15); *DCNu,* dorsal cochlear nucleus; *DSCT,* dorsal spinocerebellar tract; *EWNu,* Edinger-Westphal nucleus; *FacNr,* facial nerve; *FacNu,* facial nucleus; *FCu,* cuneate fasciculus; *FGr,* gracile fasciculus; *For,B,* fornix, body; *For,Col,* fornix, column; *For,Cr,* fornix, crus.

GP, globus pallidus; *Hip,* hippocampal formation; *HyNr,* hypoglossal nerve; *HyNu,* hypoglossal nucleus; *HyTh,* hypothalamus; *IAF,* internal arcuate fibers; *IC,* inferior colliculus; *IntCap,AL,* internal capsule, anterior limb; *IntCap,PL,* internal capsule, posterior limb; *IntCap,RL,* internal capsule, retrolenticular limb.

LCSp, lateral corticospinal tract; *LGB,* lateral geniculate body (nucleus); *LL,* lateral lemniscus; *MB,* mammillary body; *MCP,* middle cerebellar peduncle; *MesNu,* mesencephalic trigeminal nucleus; *MGB,* medial geniculate body (nucleus); *ML,* medial lemniscus; *MLF,* medial longitudinal fasciculus; *Mo,* motor trigeminal nucleus.

NuAm, nucleus ambiguus; *NuCu,* cuneate nucleus; *NuGr,* gracile nucleus; *NuPp,* nucleus prepositus; *OcNr,* oculomotor nerve; *OcNu,* oculomotor nucleus; *OpTr,* optic tract; *Pi,* pineal; *PonNu,* pontine nuclei; *Pul,* pulvinar; *Put,* putamen; *Py,* pyramid; *PyDec,* pyramidal decussation.

RB, restiform body; *RetF,* reticular formation; *RNu* and *RN,* red nucleus; *RuSp,* rubrospinal tract; *SC,* superior colliculus; *SCP,* superior cerebellar peduncle; *SCP,Dec,* superior cerebellar peduncle decussation; *Sep,* septum pellucidum; *SN,* substantia nigra; *SolNu,* solitary nucleus; *SpTNu,* spinal trigeminal nucleus; *SpTT&Nu,* spinal trigeminal tract and nucleus; *SThNu,* subthalamic nucleus; *StTer,* stria terminalis.

TecSp, tectospinal tract; *TrapB,* trapezoid body; *TriNr,* trigeminal nerve; *TriTh,* trigeminothalamic tracts; *TroNr,* trochlear nerve; *TroNu,* trochlear nucleus; *VA,* ventral anterior nucleus of thalamus; *Ven,* ventricle; *VesNu,* vestibular nucleus; *VL,* ventral lateral nucleus of thalamus; *VSCT,* ventral spinocerebellar tract.

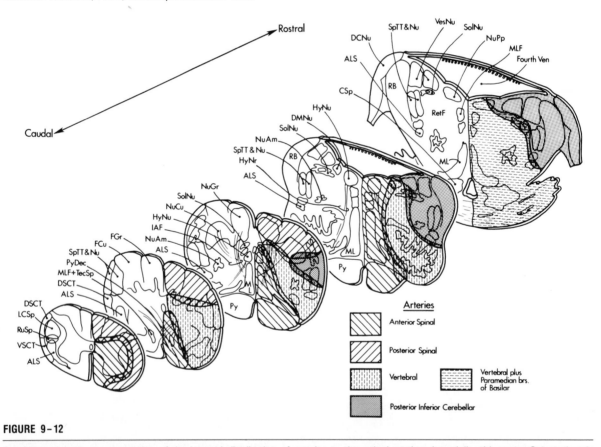

FIGURE 9–12

Semidiagrammatic representation of the internal distribution of arteries to the spinal cord and medulla oblongata. Selected main structures are labeled on the left side of each section, and the general pattern of arterial distribution overlies these structures on the right. (Reproduced with permission from D. E. Haines, *Neuroanatomy: An Atlas of Structures, Sections, and Systems,* 3rd Edition. Urban & Schwarzenberg, Baltimore-Munich, 1991.)

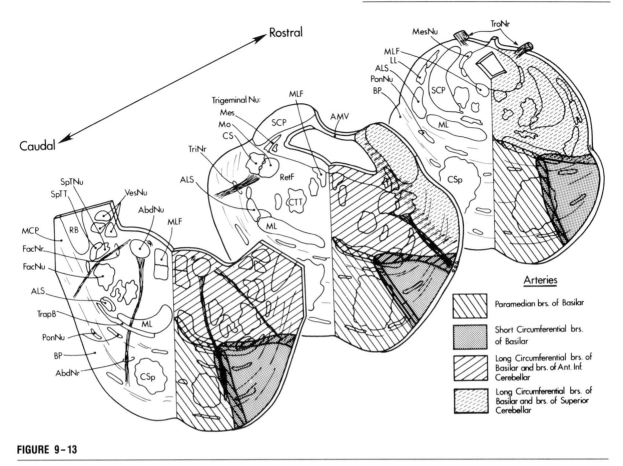

FIGURE 9-13

Semidiagrammatic representation of the internal distribution of arteries to the pons. Selected main structures are labeled on the left side of each section, and the general pattern of arterial distribution overlies these structures on the right. (Reproduced with permission from D. E. Haines, *Neuroanatomy: An Atlas of Structures, Sections, and Systems*, 3rd Edition. Urban & Schwarzenberg, Baltimore-Munich, 1991.)

pons toward the cerebellopontine angle, near the facial and vestibulocochlear nerves; turns laterally above the flocculus; and spreads over the inferior surface of the cerebellar hemisphere. Superficial branches supply the flocculus, the inferior surface of the hemisphere, and portions of the vermis; deep penetrating branches supply the dentate nucleus of the cerebellum.

Labyrinthine Artery

The *labyrinthine (internal auditory) artery* may arise either as a branch of the basilar artery or as a branch of the anterior inferior cerebellar artery. This vessel travels in close association with the *facial* and *vestibulocochlear nerves* (cranial nerves VII and VIII), passes through the internal audi-

tory meatus of the temporal bone, and supplies structures of the inner and middle ear.

Superior Cerebellar Artery

The area supplied by the *superior cerebellar artery* includes much of the pontine tegmentum, above the level supplied by the anterior inferior cerebellar artery, and extends into the midbrain to include portions of the tegmentum, the tectum, and the crus cerebri (Figs. 9-13 and 9-14). The *superior cerebellar artery* courses around the brain stem at the pontomesencephalic junction, caudal to the oculomotor and trochlear nerves and rostral to the trigeminal nerve, toward the free margin of the tentorium cerebelli where it passes beneath it and onto the superior surface of

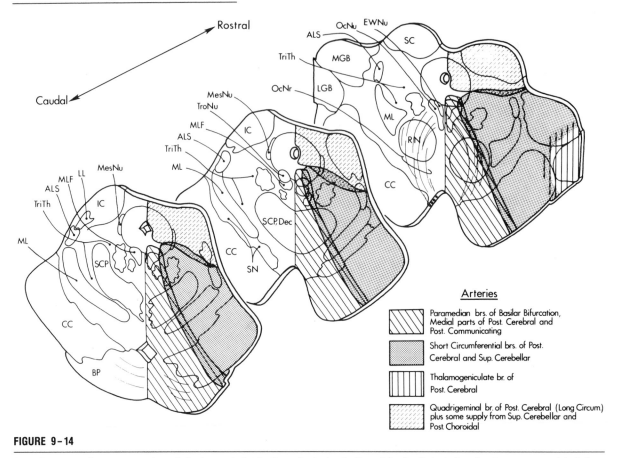

FIGURE 9-14

Semidiagrammatic representation of the internal distribution of arteries in the midbrain. Selected main structures are labeled on the left side of each section, and the general pattern of arterial distribution overlies these structures on the right. (Reproduced with permission from D. E. Haines, *Neuroanatomy: An Atlas of Structures, Sections, and Systems*, 3rd Edition. Urban & Schwarzenberg, Baltimore-Munich, 1991.)

the cerebellar hemisphere. Hemispheric branches supply the tentorial (superior) surface of the cerebellar hemisphere and portions of the lateral surface; penetrating branches supply the cerebellar nuclei and the middle and superior cerebellar peduncles.

Collectively, the bulbar branches of the *anterior inferior* and *superior cerebellar arteries* and the *long circumferential branches* of the *basilar artery* provide the major arterial supply to the following: the oculomotor, trochlear, trigeminal, abducens, and facial nuclei; portions of the vestibular and cochlear nuclei as well as the medial longitudinal fasciculus; medial lemniscus; spinothalamic pathways; ventral spinocerebellar tract; and reticular formation and portions of the middle and superior cerebellar peduncles. As a result, obstruction of one or more of the terminal branches of these arteries can lead to symptoms associated with one or more of these structures. Complete

obstruction of the basilar artery is nearly always fatal.

CEREBRAL ARTERIAL CIRCLE

The branches from the arterial circle are divided into two groups: the *central* or *penetrating arteries* and the larger *cortical arteries*. The *central arteries* arise from the arterial circle or proximal portions of the cerebral arteries and penetrate the basal portion of the forebrain, providing the arterial blood supply to the diencephalon, the internal capsule, the basal forebrain nuclei, and the basal ganglia. Although extensive anastomoses occur between the central arteries, they are often called "end-arteries," because the anastomoses are not sufficient for adequate circulation following an acute occlusion. The larger *cortical arteries* ramify over the surface of the hemispheres, giving off smaller branches that penetrate the pia mater and supply the more superficial areas of the cortex. Anastomoses occur between these terminal branches; however, most are functionally inadequate.

Central Arteries

The *anteromedial arteries*, branches of the anterior cerebral and anterior communicating arteries, supply most of the anterior hypothalamus and the basal forebrain area, including the septal nuclei. Also arising from the anterior cerebral artery are the *medial striate arteries*. These have a similar origin to that of the anteromedial arteries; however, they penetrate much deeper, vascularizing the head of the caudate nucleus and part of the anterior limb of the internal capsule (Figs. 9–9 and 9–15).

The *anterolateral arteries*, branches of the anterior cerebral and middle cerebral arteries, supply portions of the anterior perforated substance, the substantia innominata, and basal portions of the globus pallidus. The *lateral striate arteries*, of the middle cerebral artery, supply most of the lentiform nucleus and internal capsule (see Figs. 9–9 and 9–15).

The *posteromedial arteries*, branches of the posterior cerebral and posterior communicating arteries, supply the posterior half of the hypothalamus, much of the ventral thalamus, and the area surrounding the interpeduncular fossa. *Thalamoperforating arteries* are a deeper-penetrating

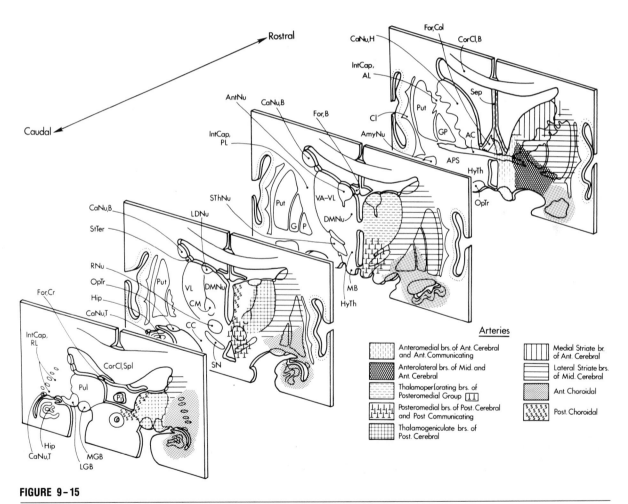

FIGURE 9–15

Semidiagrammatic representation of the internal distribution of arteries to the diencephalon, basal ganglia, and internal capsule. Selected main structures are labeled on the left side of each section, and the general pattern of arterial distribution overlies these structures on the right. (Reproduced with permission from D. E. Haines, *Neuroanatomy: An Atlas of Structures, Sections, and Systems*, 3rd Edition. Urban & Schwarzenberg, Baltimore-Munich, 1991.)

group of posteromedial arteries, which supply the anterior and medial portions of the thalamus and some of the hypothalamus. Arising from the posterior cerebral artery are the *thalamogeniculate arteries*. These vessels supply the posterior and lateral portions of the thalamus, including the pulvinar and the medial and lateral geniculate nuclei (see Figs. 9–9, 9–14, and 9–15).

The *anterior choroidal artery*, a branch from the internal carotid artery and occasionally from the middle cerebral artery, passes posteriorly over the optic tract and swings laterally toward the anteromedial portion of the temporal lobe, where it enters the choroid fissure. This artery supplies the choroid plexus of the lateral ventricle and numerous structures in the vicinity of the choroid fissure, such as the hippocampal formation, the ventral portions of the globus pallidus, the amygdala, the tail of the caudate nucleus, and the retrolenticular and sublenticular portions of the internal capsule. The *posterior choroidal arteries* are branches of the posterior cerebral artery. The *medial branches* supply the choroid plexus of the third ventricle, the superior and medial surfaces of the thalamus, the area of the pineal, and portions of the dorsal midbrain. *Lateral branches* enter the choroid fissure and anastomose with branches of the anterior choroidal artery (see Figs. 9–14 and 9–15).

Cortical Arteries

The *anterior cerebral artery*, after giving off its central branches, spreads over the medial surface of the frontal and parietal lobes with terminal branches extending onto the convexity of the hemisphere. The *orbital artery* is the first cortical branch, leaving the anterior cerebral artery immediately beneath the corpus callosum and supplying the orbital area and inferomedial surface of the frontal lobe. The *frontopolar artery* arises next and supplies the medial surface of the prefrontal area. The anterior cerebral bifurcates, forming the *callosomarginal* and *pericallosal arteries*. The callosomarginal artery runs dorsal to the cingulate gyrus, terminating in the *internal frontal* and *paracentral arteries*. The pericallosal artery terminates as the *internal parietal arteries* in the precuneus area on the medial surface of the parietal lobe (see Fig. 9–10).

The *middle cerebral artery* enters the lateral fissure and sends numerous branches to the insular cortex, before "fanning out" over the lateral surface of the hemisphere. The branch arteries, named for the cortical area supplied, have termi-

nal anastomoses with branches of the anterior and posterior cerebral arteries supplying the medial and inferior surfaces of the hemisphere. These anastomoses tend to reduce the extent of the damaged area following an acute occlusion of one of the major branches; however, they are not sufficient to provide adequate circulation to the entire deprived area.

Principal branches of the middle cerebral artery dorsal to the lateral sulcus are one or more *orbitofrontal arteries* to the anteroinferior portion of the frontal lobe; the *pre-rolandic artery* anterior to the precentral gyrus; the *rolandic artery* immediately over the central sulcus (fissure of Rolando); the *anterior parietal artery* (or *post-rolandic artery*) posterior to the postcentral gyrus; and the *posterior parietal artery*, extending over the area of the supramarginal gyrus. Branches of the middle cerebral artery ventral to the lateral sulcus include one or more *anterior temporal arteries*; one or more *posterior temporal arteries*; and the terminal branch of the middle cerebral artery, the *angular artery*, extending over the area of the angular gyrus (see Fig. 9–11).

The *posterior cerebral artery* passes around the lateral margin of the crus cerebri, dorsal to the tentorium cerebelli, to supply the inferior and medial surfaces of the temporal and parietal lobes. The principal branches of the posterior cerebral artery include the *anterior* and *posterior temporal arteries*, spreading over the anteroinferior and posteroinferior surfaces of the temporal lobe; the *internal occipital artery*, with two terminal branches; the *calcarine artery;* and the *parieto-occipital artery*, passing over the calcarine and parieto-occipital sulci, respectively (see Fig. 9–10).

MENINGEAL ARTERIES

Most of the arterial supply to the meninges is provided by vessels other than those that supply the substance of the brain. The major meningeal vessel is the *middle meningeal artery*, a branch of the maxillary artery. After entering the calvaria through the foramen spinosum, this artery supplies most of the supratentorial dura mater. Dura mater in the anterior and posterior cranial fossae is supplied by a number of small meningeal arteries, collectively known as the *anterior meningeal* and *posterior meningeal arteries*. Normally, there are two small anterior meningeal arteries, both branches of the posterior ethmoidal artery. The posterior meningeal arteries consist of one or more branches of the occipital artery; several from the ascending pharyngeal artery;

and, usually, a small meningeal branch from the vertebral artery.

Cerebral Venous Return

The venous return from the brain, unlike that from other parts of the body, does not follow the arterial supply. Very small venous channels arise from the capillary plexuses within the substance of the brain and enter the subarachnoid space as small veins (see Fig. 9–1) or enter an anastomotic plexus of venous channels deep to the pia mater, ultimately to emerge as small cerebral veins. Venous blood flows through these *cerebral veins* into a unique system of *dural venous sinuses,* finally exiting the cranium by way of the *internal jugular veins.*

The *deep cerebral veins* drain the central or medullary core of the brain (the basal ganglia, internal capsule, and diencephalon). *Superficial cerebral veins* receive venous blood from the cortex, brain stem, and cerebellum. Throughout the cerebral venous system, there are extensive anastomoses, not only between adjacent veins but also between the superficial systems and deep drainage systems within the substance of the brain. With extensive anastomoses, a gradual occlusion of a venous channel rarely produces more than a transitory effect.

DURAL VENOUS SINUSES

The dura mater of the cranium forms an elaborate series of venous channels, the *dural venous sinuses* (Figs. 9–1, 9–2, and 9–16). These sinuses, endothelial-lined channels between the periosteal and meningeal layers of the dura mater, have no valves and lack the elasticity of peripheral veins, because of the dense, connective-tissue nature of the dura mater.

The *superior sagittal sinus* runs along the superior margin of the falx cerebri, extending from its attachment to the frontal crest, near the foramen cecum, to the internal occipital protuberance. As the superior sagittal sinus flows from the front to the back, it increases in size, being largest at its termination, the *confluence of the sinuses,* or *confluens sinuum* (see Fig. 9–16). Throughout its course, the wall of the superior sagittal sinus is

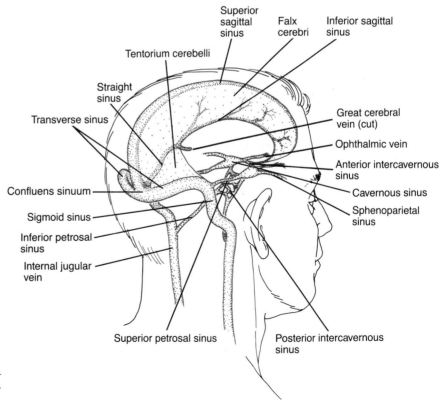

FIGURE 9-16

The venous sinuses of the cranium.

penetrated by a series of *arachnoid villi*, and by numerous superficial cerebral veins (see Fig. 9–1). The arachnoid villi are protrusions of the arachnoid into the venous channel for the drainage of CSF.

The *inferior sagittal sinus* runs caudally, along the free inferior border of the falx cerebri. At the junction of the free border of the tentorium cerebelli with the falx, the inferior sagittal sinus and the *great cerebral vein* join the *straight sinus*. Located along the dural seam formed by the posteroinferior margin of the falx cerebri and the midline of the tentorium cerebelli, the *straight sinus* flows posteriorly to terminate in the *confluens sinuum*, along with the superior sagittal sinus (see Figs. 9–2 and 9–16).

From the point of confluence of the superior sagittal and straight sinuses, the venous flow continues laterally and forward in a horizontal plane along the inner surface of the occipital bone, as the left and right *transverse sinuses*. The pattern of venous flow usually is not symmetrical. Normally, most of the blood from the superior sagittal sinus enters the right transverse sinus and that from the straight sinus enters the left transverse sinus. Also entering the confluens from below is the *occipital sinus*, a small sinus located in the free margin of the falx cerebelli. At the occipital-petrosal junction, the transverse sinus becomes the S-shaped *sigmoid sinus*, curving downward and medially toward the jugular foramen. Near the foramen, the sigmoid sinus leaves the cranial vault as the *internal jugular vein* (see Figs. 9–2 and 9–16).

The *cavernous sinuses* are a pair of large, irregular venous spaces in the anterior portion of the middle cranial fossa, extending from the petrous portion of the temporal bone to the superior orbital fissure. The cavernous sinus surrounds the internal carotid artery as well as the oculomotor, trochlear, and abducens nerves and the ophthalmic division of the trigeminal nerve, as these nerves pass through the dura mater to enter the orbit. Irregular networks of small venous channels interconnect the two cavernous sinuses, anterior and posterior to the sella turcica, the *anterior intercavernous sinus* and the *posterior intercavernous sinus*. Blood enters the cavernous sinus from the *ophthalmic vein* and the *sphenoparietal sinus* and exits via the *superior* and *inferior petrosal sinuses*. The superior petrosal sinus drains into the transverse sinus and the inferior petrosal sinus into the jugular vein (see Figs. 9–2 and 9–16).

DEEP CEREBRAL VEINS

A number of small *deep cerebral veins* form in the floor of the lateral ventricle and are named for the areas drained. The *thalamostriate vein* (*vena terminalis*), adjacent to the stria terminalis, between the thalamus and caudate nucleus, drains the striatum, internal capsule, and portions of the corpus callosum. The *choroidal vein* runs along the choroid fissure and drains the choroid plexus of the lateral ventricle. The *septal vein* drains the septal area and the basal forebrain area. These veins converge near the interventricular foramen to form a pair of large *internal cerebral veins*.

The *internal cerebral veins* run posteriorly and superiorly within the transverse cerebral fissure from the interventricular foramen. Initially, these veins pass over the lateral margin of the choroid plexus of the third ventricle and, subsequently, lateral and superior to the pineal gland.

Posterior to the pineal gland and beneath the splenium of the corpus callosum, the paired cerebral veins fuse to form the *great cerebral vein* (*of Galen*), a short vein of large diameter, which enters the straight sinus (see Fig. 9–16). A number of smaller veins contribute to the internal cerebral veins, as they pass over the third ventricle. These drain the epithalamus and posterior portions of the thalamus.

The large *basal vein* (*of Rosenthal*) drains the anterior and medial surfaces of the temporal lobe, along with the insular cortex, the ventral striatum, and the anterior perforated substance. The basal vein then courses caudally around the cerebral peduncles to empty directly into the *great cerebral vein*. Venous drainage, from the inferior and medial portions of the occipital lobe, is carried by the *occipital vein* to the great cerebral vein. Although both the *basal* and the *occipital veins* drain superficial cortical areas, they are usually grouped with the deep cerebral veins, because they terminate in the great cerebral vein.

SUPERFICIAL CEREBRAL VEINS

Usually, ten to 15 *superior cerebral veins* drain the medial and lateral surfaces of the cerebral hemispheres and enter the superior and inferior sagittal sinuses. A number of *inferior cerebral veins* drain the basal surface of the hemispheres and the inferior portion of the lateral surface. A large *superficial middle cerebral vein* can often be identified. This vein runs along the lateral sulcus and drains into the sphenoparietal or cavernous sinus.

EMISSARY VEINS

In addition to venous drainage from the brain, the *dural venous sinuses* also receive blood from the surface of the face and scalp via a series of *emissary veins*. The principal emissary veins include *frontal* and *nasal emissary veins* passing through the skull to the superior sagittal sinus; *parietal* and *occipital emissary veins*, to the confluens sinuum; and *mastoid emissary veins*, to the transverse sinus. These vessels are small and quite variable; however, they are potential routes for the spread of infection to the meninges from superficial areas of the face and scalp.

In Situ Visualization

Modern techniques now permit the visualization *in situ* of the gross morphology, the ventricular system, the vasculature, and even many of the principal nuclear and fiber structures within the gray and white matter of the living brain.

With *magnetic resonance imaging* (*MRI*) leading the way, the neurologist and neurosurgeon are now able to see images of the living brain once seen only by the pathologist at postmortem examination. *MRI* produces "slices" through the brain and head (or portions of the body) in nearly any plane. By altering various parameters, areas of tissue with very small differences in fluid content can be recognized. For example, gray and white matter are readily differentiated with *MRI*. This visualization is possible without contrast media injection or potentially damaging irradiation. Tumors, areas of infarction, and signs of disease processes can be observed and, more importantly, can be identified at earlier stages. Although often limited to major medical centers, *MRI* is the diagnostic tool of the future (Figs. 9–17 and 9–18*B*).

Computed tomography (*CT*) utilizes irradiation for similar, multiplanar scans of the brain. Now in widespread use, *CT* scanning will probably be replaced in the future by *MRI*, because the latter has greater versatility, higher resolution, increased differentiation, and absence of harmful radiation (Fig. 9–18*A*).

For many years, the ventricular system of the brain had been visualized by *pneumoencephalography*, a radiation procedure in which air was

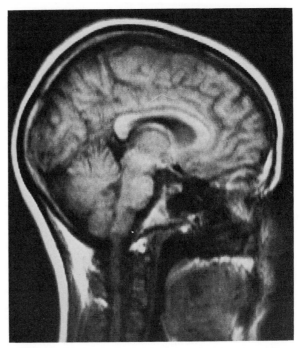

FIGURE 9–17

Magnetic resonance imaging scan in the midsagittal plane of a normal human brain. (Courtesy of Dr. Leon Partain, Department of Radiology and Radiological Sciences, Vanderbilt University Medical Center, Nashville.)

injected into the ventricular system, displacing the CSF and thereby increasing the density differential between the ventricular cavities and the surrounding brain tissue. This procedure has virtually been replaced by the safer, less traumatic, noninvasive *CT* and *MRI* techniques (Fig. 9–19).

For the study of most cerebrovascular diseases, however, *angiography* (radiographic visualization of the vasculature following contrast media injection) is still the method of choice. The technique is best suited for demonstrating intracranial vascular stenosis or occlusion, delineating patterns of collateral circulation, identifying abnormalities in the blood flow, and visualizing small aneurysms. Subtraction techniques have dramatically improved resolution and detail in angiography (Fig. 9–20).

Positron emission tomography (*PET*) utilizes the same principles of detection and data processing as *CT* scanning, but in place of x-rays, the sensors detect the emission of positrons. Short-lived, positron-emitting isotopes are incorporated into drugs or other compounds to be studied, and injected into the patient. The *PET*

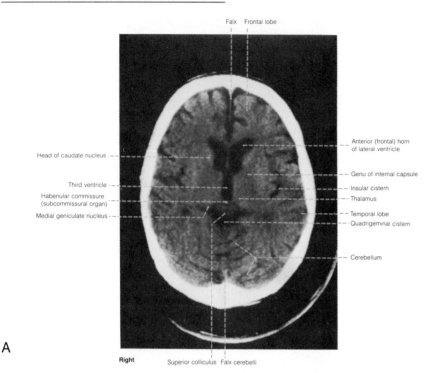

Falx   Frontal lobe

Head of caudate nucleus --

Third ventricle --

Habenular commissure
(subcommissural organ) --

Medial geniculate nucleus --

Anterior (frontal) horn
of lateral ventricle

Genu of internal capsule

Insular cistern

Thalamus

Temporal lobe

Quadrigeminal cistern

Cerebellum

A

Right   Superior colliculus   Falx cerebelli

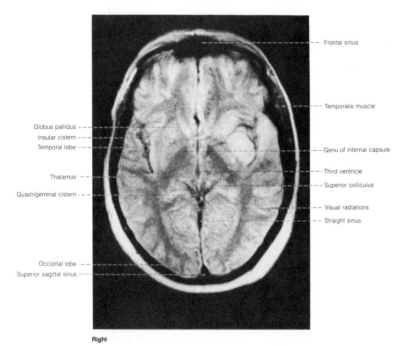

Frontal sinus

Temporalis muscle

Globus pallidus --

Insular cistern --

Temporal lobe --

Thalamus --

Quadrigeminal cistern --

Genu of internal capsule

Third ventricle

Superior colliculus

Visual radiations

Straight sinus

Occipital lobe --

Superior sagittal sinus --

B

Right

FIGURE 9-18

A, Computed tomography (CT) scan and *B*, magnetic resonance imaging (MRI) scan, from the same general region of a normal human brain. The plane of section for the MRI scan is nearly parallel to an imaginary line from the lateral margin of the orbit to the external auditory meatus. The CT scan deviates approximately 15 degrees from this plane. (Reproduced with permission from H. N. Schnitzlein and F. R. Murtagh, *Imaging Anatomy of the Head and Spine*. Urban & Schwarzenberg, Baltimore, 1985.)

scan localizes the isotope. Although *PET* is still in the experimental stages, applications have included the differentiation between types of tumors based on the relative uptake of specific amino acids and the localization of binding sites of specific drugs. Positron-emitting isotopes have half-lives measured in minutes and an on-site cyclotron is needed to generate the isotopes—a few of the major drawbacks for the widespread utilization of these techniques.

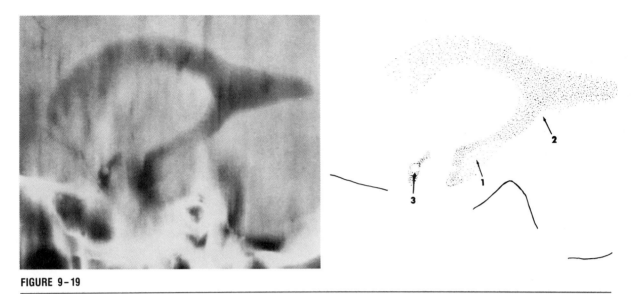

FIGURE 9-19

Pneumoencephalogram. *1*, Pes hippocampi. *2*, Collateral trigone. *3*, Middle cerebral artery. (Reproduced with permission from G. Di Chiro, *An Atlas of Detailed Normal Pneumoencephalographic Anatomy*, 2nd Edition. Charles C Thomas, Springfield, IL, 1971.)

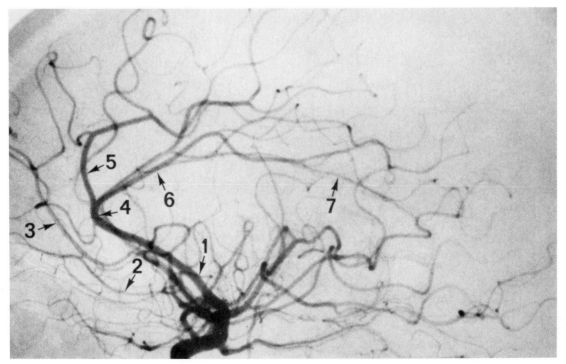

FIGURE 9-20

Left internal carotid angiogram, arterial phase, lateral view. *1*, Anterior cerebral artery in the cistern of the lamina terminalis. *2*, Orbitofrontal artery. *3*, Frontopolar artery. *4*, Anterior cerebral artery in front of the genu of the corpus callosum. *5*, Callosomarginal artery. *6*, Pericallosal artery in the cingulate sulcus. *7*, Pericallosal artery in the cingulate sulcus just above the corpus callosum. (Reproduced with permission from A. G. Osborn, *An Introduction to Cerebral Angiography*. Harper & Row, Hagerstown, 1980.)

SUGGESTED READING

Haines, D. E. (1991). *Neuroanatomy. An Atlas of Structures, Sections and Systems*, 3rd Edition. Urban & Schwarzenberg, Baltimore-Munich, 252 pp.

A thorough, yet concise, atlas and guide to the organization and structure of the human CNS. The relations between the ventricular system and the gross morphology of the brain are illustrated. Detailed illustrations of the blood supply to the deep structures of the brain stem and cerebrum are provided along with angiograms demonstrating the major cerebral vessels.

Osborn, A. G. (1980). *Introduction to Cerebral Angiography.* Harper & Row, Publishers, Hagerstown, Maryland, 436 pp.

As a concise introduction to the field of angiography, this text is rich in illustrative material, including some excellent angiograms of the cerebral vasculature, both normal and pathological.

Partain, C. L., R. R. Price, J. A. Patton, M. V. Kulkarmi, and A. E. James, Jr. (1988). *Magnetic Resonance Imaging*, 2nd Edition. Volume I, *Clinical Principles.* Volume II, *Physical Principles and Instrumentation.* W. B. Saunders Co., Philadelphia, 1808 pp.

In the rapidly developing field of noninvasive imaging, MRI has become the standard. Any text or reference in this fast-moving field is soon out of date; however, this two-volume series is on the "cutting edge" of the field. In addition to state-of-the-art clinical applications, this series includes excellent discussions of the history of MRI, its physical principles, comparisons with other imaging techniques, and future directions and potentials.

Schnitzlein, H. N. and F. R. Murtagh (1985). *Imaging Anatomy of the Head and Spine.* Urban & Schwarzenberg, Baltimore-Munich.

A photographic atlas, principally of the head and neck region, including MRI and CT scans along with both gross and microscopic sections in the standard planes. This atlas is an excellent reference and guide for the interpretation of CT and MRI scans as well as providing a direct side-by-side comparison of the two procedures.

Stephens, R. B. and D. L. Stilwell (1969). *Arteries and Veins of the Human Brain.* Charles C Thomas, Springfield, Illinois.

An outstanding atlas of the arterial and venous supply of the human brain. A complete and coherent set of photographs and a concise explanatory text are presented. The vasculature of the brain was injected with various media. Photographs were made of whole, dissected, and sliced brain preparations. This atlas illustrates the pattern and distribution of the superficial arteries and veins as well as the pattern and distribution of deep, penetrating branches.

Part
IV

SENSORY SYSTEMS

Chapter
10

General Somatic and General Visceral Afferent Pathways

GENERAL FEATURES OF AFFERENT PATHWAYS

PRIMARY AFFERENT NERVES AND PERIPHERAL RECEPTORS

SPINAL CORD PROCESSING OF GENERAL SOMATIC AFFERENT INFORMATION

DORSAL COLUMNS AND RELATED AFFERENT PATHWAYS

ANTEROLATERAL SYSTEM AND COMPONENT PATHWAYS

GENERAL SOMATIC AFFERENT COMPONENTS OF THE CRANIAL NERVES

THALAMIC RELAY OF SOMATOSENSORY INFORMATION

SOMATOSENSORY CORTEX

GENERAL VISCERAL AFFERENT PATHWAYS

MODULATION OF NOCICEPTIVE SIGNALS

CLINICAL CORRELATIONS

General Features of Afferent Pathways

Sensory, or *afferent pathways*, are the brain's principal source of information about the outside world, the internal functioning of the body, and the position and movement of the body in space. The *general sensory systems* are subdivided into *general somatic afferent* (GSA), the sensory innervation of somatic structures (developed from embryonic ectoderm and somatic mesoderm), and *general visceral afferent* (GVA), the sensory innervation of the viscera (developed from embryonic endoderm and splanchnic mesoderm).

The five *special sensory systems* (*visual, auditory, vestibular, taste, and olfaction*) are discussed in Chapters 11, 12, and 13.

GENERAL SOMATIC AFFERENT (GSA) PATHWAYS

GSA pathways share many features (Fig. 10–1). *First*, all have a *peripheral receptor*, a specialization for the conversion (transduction) of a sensory stimulus (pressure, heat, stretch, and so forth) into an action potential. Receptors vary in complexity from the simple "naked" nerve ending to the more complex, self-adjusting, servomechanism of the muscle spindle. Most receptors

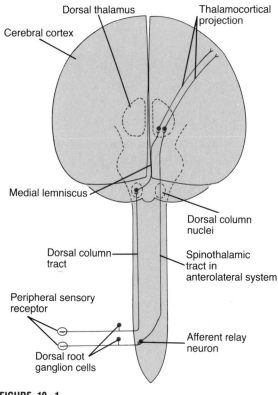

FIGURE 10-1

The general features of two principal general somatic afferent (GSA) pathways: the spinothalamic system for pain and temperature and the dorsal column system for tactile discrimination and proprioception (see text).

have a low threshold for a specific modality and high thresholds for all others. Some, however, are multimodal and respond to more than one modality. *Second*, a *primary afferent neuron (first-order sensory neuron or 1° sensory neuron)* transmits the action potential generated at the receptor into the central nervous system (CNS). The cell bodies of these neurons reside in *dorsal root ganglia* (or cranial nerve sensory ganglia). *Third*, on entering the CNS, the primary sensory neurons synapse with *second-order neurons (2° neurons)*, relaying the signal to higher centers and establishing *reflex* connections with the motor systems. In some instances, an interneuron may be situated between the primary afferent fiber and the second-order or relay neuron. *Fourth*, as a general rule, the axons of second-order sensory neurons cross the midline of the spinal cord or brain stem and ascend to the contralateral *thalamus*. Here, thalamic neurons relay the signal to the *somatosensory* portion of the *cerebral cortex* (see Fig. 10-1). Hence, signals generated from

stimulation of primary afferent neurons on the left side of the body ultimately reach the right cerebral hemisphere, because of the crossing or *decussation* of the second-order neuron.

Several GSA pathways carry different sensory information. These pathways cross to the contralateral side of the CNS at different levels of the neural axis. For example, the second-order neurons, relaying pain and temperature signals, cross immediately in the ventral white commissure at the entry level of the primary afferent fibers and ascend to the contralateral thalamus. Axons of primary afferent neurons carrying tactile information, however, ascend in the ipsilateral dorsal column before synapsing with relay neurons in the dorsal column nuclei. Axons from these second-order neurons cross the midline in the lower medulla and ascend to the contralateral thalamus. Pathway differences such as these are useful in the clinical evaluation of damage to the CNS.

LOCALIZATION OF PRIMARY AFFERENT STIMULI

As noted in Chapter 6, individual spinal nerves innervate specific areas or dermatomes of the body surface (see Figs. 6-5 and 6-6). Spinal nerves have a highly organized pattern of innervation—a pattern retained after the central processes of the individual sensory neurons enter the CNS. The entire central pathway retains this pattern of *topographic organization*. Hence, each body point innervated is represented on a "map" at each level of relay in the sensory pathway, e.g., the relay nuclei in the dorsal horn of the spinal cord, the dorsal column (gracile and cuneate) nuclei, and the dorsal thalamus. These *somatotopic maps* are present in the ascending tracts as well. Thus, a point-to-point representation occurs from the receptor to the cortex. An earlier representation of the cortical localization is the now classic "homunculus," of Penfield and Rasmussen. This is a representation of the body as projected on the somatosensory cortex (Fig. 10-2). Although at least four separate representations of the body occur in the primary somatosensory area of the cortex (see the following discussion), the homunculus serves to illustrate the general features of somatotopic organization. Note the distorted representation of the body and body parts. The amount of cortical representation for a specific body part is directly related to the density of innervation, a feature preserved from the periphery to the cortex.

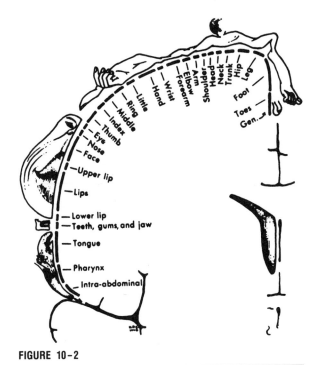

FIGURE 10-2

Sensory "homunculus." A schematic representation of the sensory organization of the postcentral gyrus in the human. (Reproduced with permission from W. Penfield, and T. Rasmussen, *The Cerebral Cortex of Man*. Macmillan, New York, 1950.)

SPECIFICITY OF AFFERENT SIGNALS

The detection of different sensory modalities is a function of the differential sensitivity of individual sensory receptors, e.g., heat versus touch to the glabrous surface of the index finger. Specific receptors respond to different sensory stimuli with different levels of sensitivity. Although all sensory information enters the CNS as an action potential, the connections within the CNS segregate the signals for the different modalities. Thus, within the somatotopic organization of the pathways is a suborganization based on sensory modality.

Primary Afferent Nerves and Peripheral Receptors

NERVE FIBER CLASSIFICATION

Peripheral nerve fibers vary in size, ranging from very large diameter, heavily myelinated fibers to very small diameter, nonmyelinated fibers (see Figs. 2–25 and 2–26). Action potential conduction is much faster for large, myelinated fibers

(see Chapter 3); however, more information can be transmitted, per unit of cross-sectional area, with slower, smaller-diameter fibers. Nerve fibers are classified according to size and conduction velocity. Two sets of terminology are used to classify nerve fibers. Both classifications are illustrated in Figure 10–3, along with some of the sensory and motor functions associated with each fiber type.

In the general classification, all myelinated fibers are type A and nonmyelinated fibers are type C. Type-A fibers are subdivided into types $A\alpha$, $A\beta$, $A\gamma$, and $A\delta$; often, they are simply referred to as α, β, γ, and δ fibers. Sensory

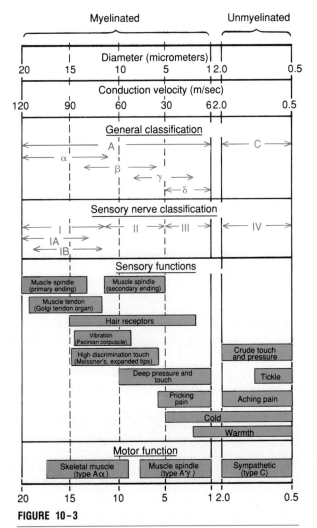

FIGURE 10-3

Physiological classifications and functions of nerve fibers. (Reproduced with permission from A. C. Guyton, *Textbook of Medical Physiology*, 7th Edition. W. B. Saunders Co., Philadelphia, 1986.)

physiologists employ an additional classification with myelinated fibers divided into groups I, II, and III and with nonmyelinated fibers placed into group IV. Group I fibers consist of I-A (afferents from the annulospiral endings of muscle spindles) and I-B (afferents from the Golgi tendon organs). Both I-A and I-B correspond to type-Aα fibers in the general classification. Fibers from "flower-spray" endings of muscle spindles and many cutaneous tactile receptors are group II (type-Aβ of the general classification). Group III fibers carry crude touch, temperature, and some pain sensation. These correspond to type-Aδ fibers. The nonmyelinated fibers of group IV (type-C) also carry temperature, crude touch, and pain sensation (see Fig. 10–3).

SENSORY TRANSDUCTION

The conversion of a sensory stimulus into an action potential is *sensory transduction*. Receptors are sensitive to specific stimuli, whether it be specific frequencies of sound vibrations (hearing) or electromagnetic radiation (vision); specific chemical compounds (taste, olfaction, and some pain); or physical changes to the body (pressure, touch, stretch, movement, or vibration (mechanoreceptors)). Nerve fibers relay the sensory signal to the CNS as an action potential—a simple frequency-modulated signal. The specificity of the signal for a particular sensory modality resides (1) in the sensitivity of the receptor for a specific stimulus and (2) in the segregation of the signals during processing in the CNS.

Consider the generation of an action potential from pressure stimulation of a pacinian corpuscle as an example of sensory transduction. This receptor often is a prototype for mechanosensory transduction because the receptor is large, readily dissectable, and thus amenable to experimental manipulation. The nerve terminal within the corpuscle (see Fig. 10–5) is similar to the postsynaptic membrane of a neuron. This terminal maintains a resting potential and has all the properties of an excitable membrane. Physical deformation of the terminal depolarizes the neuronal membrane, generating a *receptor potential*. The receptor potential spreads passively over the nerve terminal, in a manner similar to an excitatory postsynaptic potential (*EPSP*) on the dendrite of a neuron. Once the *trigger zone* reaches threshold, it generates an action potential through the same mechanism as the initial segment of an axon (sequential activation of voltage-sensitive Na^+ and K^+ channels). The only difference between the generation of an action potential in a primary sensory neuron and a multipolar motor neuron is the location of the trigger zone (see Fig. 2–2D).

The higher the receptor potential is above threshold, the greater the *rate* of action potential generation. Theoretically, the rate of transition of voltage-sensitive Na^+ channels from the inactivated state to the resting state limits the firing rate (see Fig. 3–4). Most mechanoreceptors have a very large range of sensitivity, and some are able to detect pressure differences over a 10,000- to 100,000-fold range. This sensitivity is possible because small changes in stimulus strength at low levels of stimulation produce greater alterations in the amplitude of the receptor potential than similar changes in stimulus strength at a more intense level of stimulation. For a given receptor, very small differences in stimulus strength are detectable only when the *total stimulus is small*; these very small differences are undetectable when the *total stimulus is large*.

RECEPTOR CLASSIFICATION

Three broad categories of sensory receptors are based on the origin of the stimulus: *exteroceptors*, *proprioceptors*, and *interoceptors*. *Exteroceptors* provide information about the external environment and include GSA receptors associated with the external body surface and sensitive to modalities, such as heat, touch, pressure, and vibration. In a broad sense, exteroceptors also include the receptors associated with the special senses of vision, hearing, and smell. *Proprioceptors* provide information about the position and movement of the body in space and include GSA receptors in muscles, tendons, and joint capsules in addition to the vestibular apparatus of the inner ear. *Interoceptors* provide sensory information from the internal organs of the body, general visceral afferent (GVA) receptors. They are discussed later in this chapter.

This classification reveals little of the sensory modality of the GSA receptors. Therefore, we also employ a classification based on the type of stimulation to which a receptor responds: *mechanoreceptors*, *thermoreceptors*, and *nociceptors*. *Mechanoreceptors* respond to some form of mechanical deformation of the tissue or the receptor, e.g., stretch, vibration, pressure, and touch. These receptors range in complexity from the simple naked nerve ending to the complex muscle spindle. The sensations detected range from discriminatory touch to body position and orientation in space. The mechanoreceptors include both exteroceptors and proprioceptors. The second group, *thermoreceptors*, responds to warmth or cold. The third group, *nociceptors*, or *pain receptors*, responds to noxious or painful stimuli.

Mechanoreceptors

The simplest mechanoreceptor, anatomically, is the *naked nerve ending* (Fig. 10–4). As the name implies, these are bare nerve terminals, devoid of myelin or Schwann cell ensheathment. Found in the epidermis of the skin and the cornea of the eye and in other areas, such as the pinna of the ear, these terminal nerve branches can respond to pressure and touch stimuli. Naked nerve endings with tactile properties also are found in the deeper layers of the skin. Other populations of naked nerve terminals are sensitive to different sensory modalities, with some functioning as specific nociceptors and others as thermoreceptors (see subsequent discussion). Those terminal branches of type-Aδ or type-C nerve fibers with a sensitivity to mechanical stimulation generate receptor potentials in response to a physical distortion of the nerve ending.

The second type of mechanoreceptor is the *expanded-tip tactile receptor*, an example of which is *Merkel's disc* (see Fig. 10–4). These receptors, specialized for high resolution, discriminatory touch, are on the terminal branches of large, myelinated, type-Aβ nerves. The nerve ending of each terminal branch forms a flattened, disc-like structure capped by a modified epithelial cell known as *Merkel's cell*. Merkel's discs are concentrated in nonhairy or *glabrous* skin, although significant numbers are found in hairy skin. The greatest concentrations are in those areas more sensitive to touch. Physiologically, these receptors are slow adapting. Stimulation triggers a volley of high frequency action potentials that continue at a high "unadapted" rate during stimulation.

Meissner's corpuscles are a third type of mechanoreceptor (see Fig. 10–4). These encapsulated receptors are in dermal papillae and account for nearly half the tactile receptors on the glabrous surface of the digits and hand. Meissner's corpuscles are also abundant on the foot, the front of the forearm, the lips, and the mucosa of the tongue. The cylindrical-shaped receptors, roughly 80-μm long and 25- to 30-μm in diameter, contain an outer capsule of connective tissue. The capsule is continuous at the base with the perineurium of one or more large, myelinated, type-Aβ nerve fibers innervating each capsule. The core of the capsule contains a stack of disc-like epithelioid cells, partially separating the profusely branching nerve fibers as they spiral toward the top of the capsule. These sensitive tactile receptors are rapidly adapting. With the continuous application of a single stimulus, the receptors respond with an immediate burst of activity followed by a rapid attenuation of the signal. The receptive field of these receptors is small and well suited for the detection of shape and intensity information during *active* touch. The ability to adapt rapidly makes them especially sensitive to the movement of objects or the

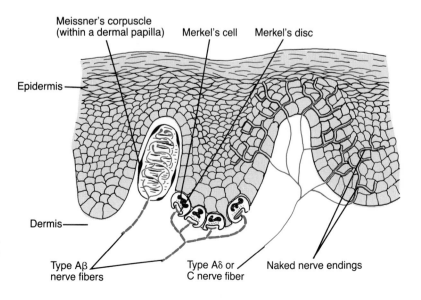

FIGURE 10–4

Three types of cutaneous general somatic afferent (GSA) receptors: Meissner's corpuscle, Merkel's disc, and naked nerve endings. The basal lamina of the epithelium is not illustrated. Usually, more than one nerve fiber innervates each Meissner's corpuscle.

Meissner's corpuscle (within a dermal papilla)   Merkel's cell   Merkel's disc

Epidermis

Dermis

Type Aβ nerve fibers   Type Aδ or C nerve fiber   Naked nerve endings edges of objects over the skin surface and the detection of low frequency vibrations.

The very sensitive *peritrichial nerve endings* are the terminal branches of type-Aβ fibers wrapped around the base and shaft of the hair follicle (Fig. 10–5). Physical distortion of the nerve endings from movement of the hair is sufficient to generate receptor potentials. The properties of these receptors are similar to those of Meissner's corpuscles in glabrous skin: both are very sensitive, have small receptive fields, adapt rapidly, and are innervated by myelinated type-Aβ nerve processes.

The encapsulated *Ruffini's end organs* are found both in the dermis of the skin and in the deeper connective tissue layers, including joint capsules (see Fig. 10–5). These large receptors, 0.5 to 1.0 mm long and up to 0.2 mm in diameter, contain a capsule of 4 to 5 layers of lamellar cells and a core of longitudinally arranged collagen fibers. Highly branched, nonmyelinated fiber terminals interdigitate with the collagen fibers. The single type-Aβ fiber innervating each receptor loses its myelin sheath upon entering the capsule. The surrounding connective tissue anchors each end of the capsule, accounting for the high sensitivity of the receptor to the

stretching of the skin or joint capsule. These end organs, with a large, poorly defined receptive field, are concentrated in nail beds and in the folds of the skin near joints of the extremities. Those Ruffini end organs found in joint capsules provide information on joint rotation. All Ruffini end organs show very little adaptation with prolonged stimulation, i.e., they are classified as slow adapting.

Pacinian corpuscles are large ovoid, onion-shaped receptors found beneath the skin and in deep fascial tissues (Fig. 10–5). These rapidly adapting receptors have a poorly defined receptive field and are sensitive to both pressure and vibration, in the 200 to 400 Hz range. A single type-Aβ fiber innervates each corpuscle, shedding its myelin sheath upon entry and remaining unbranched, as it runs the length of the central core of the capsule. The corpuscle contains an inner core of about 60 layers of lamellar cells, each layer separated by fluid; an outer portion of about 30 layers of less dense lamellar cells; and an external shell of connective tissue.

Included in the group of *mechanoreceptors* are the *Golgi tendon organs* and the *muscle spindles.* These two proprioceptors, located in deep tissues (tendons and muscles), provide sensory information essential for spinal cord reflexes and the control of motor function via the cerebellum. In addition, some of the sensory information generated by these receptors reaches the cerebral cortex via the dorsal column-medial lemniscal system and contributes to a conscious awareness of posture and the movement of the limbs and body in space. A detailed description of the structure and mechanism of action of these receptors is in Chapter 14.

Golgi tendon organs, located in the tendons of muscles, are innervated by large, heavily myelinated type-Aα fibers. These receptors respond both to stretch and to tension on the tendon.

Muscle spindles are dynamic receptors found in somatic muscle tissue. These complex receptor organs have several types of sensory endings and a motor component. Through the continual readjustment of their length, these receptors provide uninterrupted information about the rate of change in muscle length during muscle relaxation and contraction.

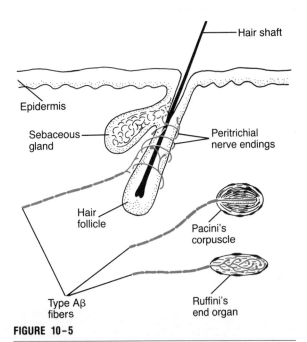

FIGURE 10–5

Three types of cutaneous and subcutaneous general somatic afferent (GSA) receptors: peritrichial nerve endings, Pacini's corpuscle, and Ruffini's end organ. Both Pacini's corpuscle and Ruffini's end organ are found in deeper tissues as well (see text).

Thermoreceptors

The three basic types of thermoreceptors, are *cold receptors*, *warmth receptors*, and temperature-sensitive *nociceptors* that respond to extremes of heat or cold. A specific receptor organ has not been identified for nerve fibers responding to warm stimuli, and the *warmth receptors* are presumed to be naked nerve endings of small nonmyelinated, C-fibers sensitive to *increases* in temperature. *Cold receptors*—naked nerve endings of small, myelinated, type-Aδ nerve fibers—branch and penetrate the basal layers of the epidermis. Thermoreceptors respond to temperature changes of about 2°C, with a burst of activity that diminishes to about a fifth of the initial response within 10 seconds. The sensory transduction mechanism is unknown, and these receptors do not appear to respond to direct physical stimulation. One working hypothesis proposes that changes in temperature alter the rate or rates of specific biochemical reactions that, in turn, result in the generation of the receptor potential. Most enzymatic rates change as much as two–fold, with a temperature change of 10°C.

Nociceptors

Nociceptors, as a group, are naked nerve endings of type-Aδ (acute pain) or type-C (chronic pain) fibers. Nociceptors fall into three categories: *mechanosensitive nociceptors* respond to excessive mechanical stress or mechanical damage to the tissues; *thermosensitive nociceptors* respond to extremes of heat and cold; and *chemosensitive nociceptors* respond to specific chemical compounds, such as histamine, bradykinin, serotonin, prostaglandins, proteolytic enzymes, K^+, and acids. Most pain receptors respond to a specific stimulus, although some are sensitive to more than one noxious stimulus. Most nociceptors are either

nonadapting or very slow-adapting. Mechanonociceptors and thermonociceptors respond *only* to noxious levels of stimuli and are not sensitive to "normal" levels of mechanical or thermal stimulation.

Many somatic afferent receptors are naked nerve endings with little apparent anatomical specialization, yet they respond selectively to specific sensory modalities, e.g., tactile stimulation, temperature, and noxious stimuli. The only GSA receptors in the cornea of the eye, for example, are naked nerve endings, yet they are able to differentiate between several forms of mechanical, thermal, and nociceptive stimulation. With the lack of apparent morphological differences, the selective responsiveness probably represents a molecular differentiation.

Spinal Cord Processing of General Somatic Afferent Information

The spinal cord is the first level of GSA processing in the CNS. The central processes of neurons in the dorsal root ganglia, carrying signals from the peripheral receptors, enter the spinal cord by way of the *dorsal roots*. At this point, sensory information is partially segregated by modality and area of innervation.

Each dorsal root contains fibers from an anatomical region or a *dermatome* of the body (see Figs. 6–5 and 6–6). Fibers from the more distal portion of the dermatome occupy the more rostral portion of the dorsal root, and those from the

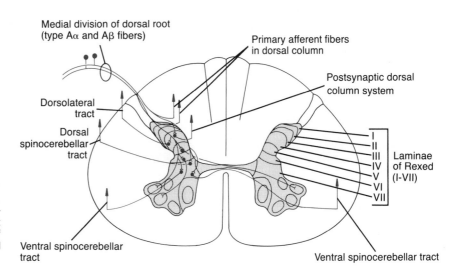

FIGURE 10-6

Medial division of the dorsal root. Some of the principal connections made by primary afferent fibers from the medial division of the dorsal root are illustrated (see text).

proximal portions of the dermatome are caudal. Fibers transmitting signals from nociceptors and thermoreceptors (type-Aδ and type-C fibers) form the *lateral division of the dorsal root*, whereas the large type-Aα and type-Aβ fibers, transmitting signals from mechanoreceptors, form the *medial division of the dorsal root* (Figs. 10–6 and 10–7).

The dorsal root fibers form two major ascending afferent systems. First, fibers entering through the medial division of the dorsal root form the ipsilateral *dorsal column system*. Second, those in the lateral division contribute to the contralateral *anterolateral system*. Each of these systems consists of several distinct tracts or pathways (see subsequent discussion).

After entering the spinal cord, primary afferent fibers bifurcate into ascending and descending branches. Those from the lateral division ascend and descend in the *dorsolateral fasciculus of Lissauer*, and those from the medial division do so in the *ventrolateral margin of the dorsal column*, immediately adjacent to the dorsal horn. The ascending and descending arms of the primary afferents branch profusely with the formation of terminals that synapse (1) with interneurons or motor neurons for reflex connections at the spinal level, (2) with neurons projecting to higher levels of the CNS for the modulation of motor function, and (3) with neurons projecting to brain stem centers for the modulation of the sensory signals (see Figs. 10–6 and 10–7). Chapter 14 provides an in-depth discussion of those pathways associated with motor reflexes (spinal reflexes and spinoreticular and spinotectal systems). Chapter 17 discusses those associated with

cerebellar function (dorsal and ventral spinocerebellar tracts).

Dorsal Columns And Related Afferent Pathways

DORSAL COLUMN-MEDIAL LEMNISCAL PATHWAY

Large, myelinated fibers (type-Aα and type-Aβ) from the medial division of the dorsal root enter the *ipsilateral dorsal column* (*dorsal funiculus*) and ascend to the inferior portion of the medulla in either the *fasciculus gracilis* or *fasciculus cuneatus* (see Figs. 10–6 and 10–13). These fibers carry information from the slow-adapting receptors (Merkel's discs, Ruffini's corpuscles, and Golgi tendon organs), the rapidly adapting receptors (Meissner's corpuscles, peritrichial endings, and pacinian corpuscles), and muscle spindles.

Medial division fibers entering the spinal cord below the mid-thoracic level form the fasciculus gracilis; those from cervical and upper thoracic levels form the fasciculus cuneatus. These primary afferent fibers enter the dorsal funiculus and begin their ascent immediately adjacent to the dorsal horn. Fibers from more rostral levels enter and ascend in the same fashion, displacing the fibers from caudal levels to a more medial position. Thus, a primary afferent fiber from L-2, for example, enters the spinal cord via the medial division of the dorsal root and ascends to the brain stem. As fibers from sequentially higher spinal levels enter and ascend, the fibers from L-2

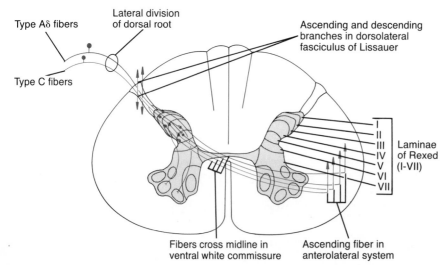

Type Aδ fibers

Type C fibers

Lateral division of dorsal root

Ascending and descending branches in dorsolateral fasciculus of Lissauer

I
II
III
IV
V
VI
VII

Laminae of Rexed (I-VII)

Fibers cross midline in ventral white commissure

Ascending fiber in anterolateral system

FIGURE 10–7

Lateral division of the dorsal root. Some of the principal connections made by primary afferent fibers from the lateral division of the dorsal root are illustrated (see text).

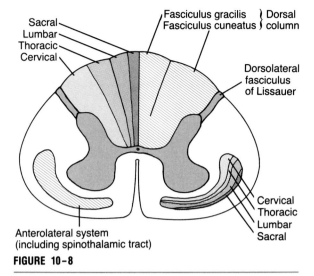

FIGURE 10-8

A section through the upper cervical spinal cord illustrates the somatotopic organization of the dorsal columns (gracile and cuneate fasciculi) and the anterolateral system.

move to a more medial position in the ever increasing dorsal column. This results in the laminated pattern of somatotopic representation seen in Figure 10-8. Below the level of T-6, the dorsal funiculus contains only the fasciculus gracilis; above T-6, it contains both the fasciculus gracilis and fasciculus cuneatus.

Fibers from the gracile and cuneate fasciculi end in the lower medulla, synapsing in the *gracile* and *cuneate nuclei*, respectively. Axons of relay neurons in the gracile and cuneate nuclei arch

ventromedially through the medullary reticular formation as the *internal arcuate fibers*, cross the midline, and form the contralateral *medial lemniscus* (Fig. 10-9). The gracile nucleus is lower in the medulla than is the cuneate nucleus. (Note the relative positions of the cuneate and gracile tubercles in Figure 7-4.) In an ascending series of sections through the medulla, the gracile nucleus appears first; then both nuclei; and, finally, only the cuneate nucleus.

Fibers of the medial lemniscus ascend through the brain stem ending in the *ventral posterolateral nucleus (VPL)* of the thalamus (see following discussion). In the medulla, the paired medial lemnisci are central in the brain stem with a vertical orientation (see Figs. 10-9 and 10-10). At the level of the pons, the medial lemnisci assume a horizontal orientation and gradually shift to a more lateral position but remain dorsal to the pontine nuclei (Fig. 10-11). The medial lemnisci continue to shift in a lateral and dorsolateral direction, as they ascend through the brain stem. At the level of the midbrain and superior colliculus, they lie dorsolateral to the red nucleus and dorsomedial to the substantia nigra (Fig. 10-12).

Throughout their ascent in the brain stem, fibers of the medial lemnisci retain a well-organized somatotopy as illustrated in Figures 10-9 through 10-12. In the medulla, fibers representing the back of the head and arms are in the dorsal portion of the vertically oriented, medial lemniscus. Those from the leg are ventral. When the medial lemniscus assumes a horizontal orien-

FIGURE 10-9

The somatotopic organization of the medial lemniscus and the anterolateral system at the level of the lower medulla are illustrated, caudad to the obex and below the level of the fourth ventricle. Level comparable to the Weigert-stained section in Figure 7-8. The internal arcuate fibers, projecting from the gracile and cuneate nuclei to the contralateral medial lemniscus, are illustrated in red.

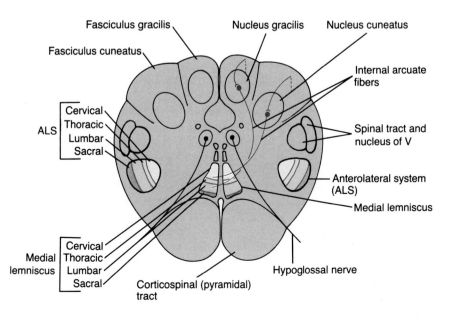

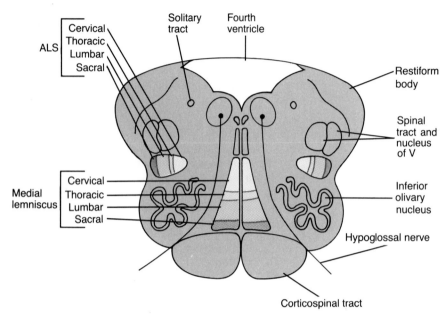

FIGURE 10-10

The somatotopic organization of the medial lemniscus and the anterolateral system at the level of the inferior olivary nucleus in the medulla are illustrated. Level comparable to the Weigert-stained section in Figure 7-10. Note the shift in position of the anterolateral system with the appearance of the inferior olivary nucleus.

tation, head and arm fibers are medial and leg fibers are lateral. When the medial lemniscus reaches the upper portion of the midbrain, the somatotopic orientation of the fibers matches that of the ventral posterolateral nucleus of the thalamus (see subsequent discussion).

In summary, primary Aα- and Aβ-fibers, organized somatotopically, ascend in the ipsilateral dorsal column, carrying somatosensory information to the ipsilateral gracile and cuneate nuclei. Relay neurons from these nuclei cross the mid-

line at the level of the lower medulla and ascend to the contralateral thalamus via the contralateral medial lemniscus (Fig. 10-13).

ALTERNATIVE DORSAL COLUMN PATHWAYS

The preceding pathway transmits sensory information, without a synapse, from peripheral receptors to the dorsal column nuclei. However, the dorsal column nuclei also receive second-

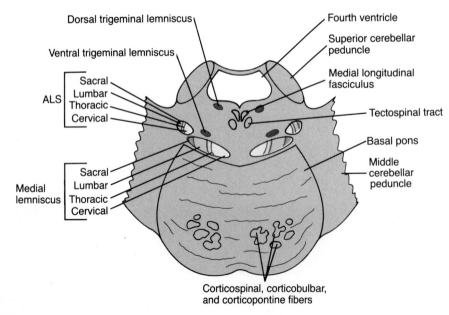

FIGURE 10-11

The somatotopic organization of the medial lemniscus and the anterolateral system at the level of the pons are illustrated. Level comparable to the Weigert-stained section in Figure 7-13. Note the 90-degree rotation of the medial lemniscus. Representation from the lumbar and sacral levels are now lateral to the cervical level.

FIGURE 10-12

The somatotopic organization of the medial lemniscus and the anterolateral system at the level of the superior colliculus of the midbrain are illustrated. Level comparable to the Weigert-stained section in Figure 7–17. Note the lateral displacement of the medial lemniscus and the interdigitation of the lemniscal fibers with those of the spinothalamic pathways. When the ascending fibers reach the level of the ventral posterior thalamic nuclei, the two pathways will be in somatotopic register.

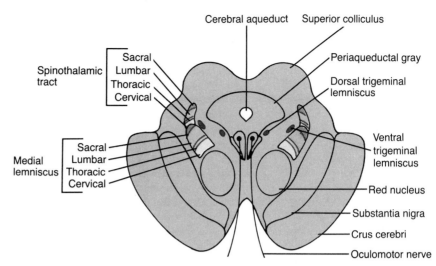

FIGURE 10-12

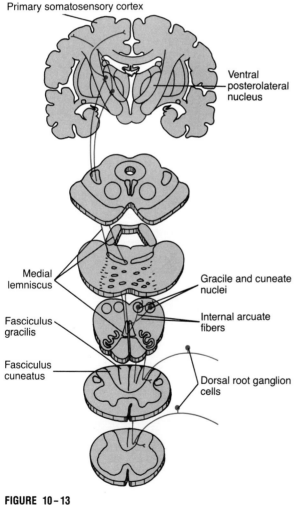

FIGURE 10-13

A simplified schematic illustrates the course of the ascending dorsal column/medial lemniscal pathway, from the spinal cord to the primary somatosensory cortex.

order sensory information. This alternative dorsal column-medial lemniscal pathway is known as the *postsynaptic dorsal column system*. Collaterals of primary afferent neurons synapse with neurons located mainly in *lamina IV* of the dorsal horn. These second-order relay neurons enter the ipsilateral dorsal funiculus and ascend to the medulla in the *dorsal columns*, ending in either the gracile or cuneate nucleus. From here, information is relayed to the contralateral, ventral posterolateral nucleus of the thalamus via the medial lemniscus (Fig. 10–14). A few of these relay fibers from lamina IV also ascend in the *dorsolateral tract* (see Fig. 10–6); however, the dorsolateral tract contains principally spinocervicothalamic fibers (see subsequent discussion). In either case, the fibers of the postsynaptic dorsal column system ascend to the medulla and end in the dorsal column nuclei (see Fig. 10–14).

Afferents from muscle spindles also use an alternative pathway from the dorsal columns to the thalamus. Muscle spindle afferents from the lower extremity ascend several segments in the *fasciculus gracilis*, synapse in *lamina VII*, and ascend to the medulla in the *dorsolateral tract*. These ascending fibers then synapse in a small nuclear group, situated immediately rostral to the nucleus gracilis, *nucleus Z*. Projections from nucleus Z join the contralateral *medial lemniscus* and ascend to the thalamus, ending almost exclusively in the *ventral posterosuperior nucleus (VPS)* (see subsequent discussion). In a comparable pathway from the upper extremity, primary afferents from muscle spindles ascend in the ipsilateral *fasciculus cuneatus* and synapse in the *external cuneate nucleus*. Projection fibers from the external cuneate nucleus join the contralateral

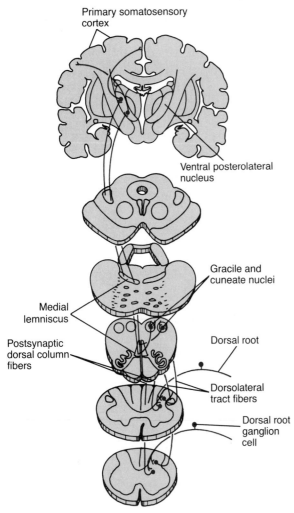

FIGURE 10-14

A simplified schematic illustrates the course of the postsynaptic dorsal column system, from the spinal cord to the primary somatosensory cortex. This pathway is often referred to as the second-order dorsal column pathway.

medial lemniscus and end in the *VPS* of the thalamus.

SPINOCERVICOTHALAMIC TRACT

A third pathway carrying somatosensory information to the brain is the *spinocervicothalamic tract*. This system, although quite prominent in some animals (e.g., the cat), appears to be rudimentary in the human nervous system. The spinocervicothalamic pathway carries signals from rapidly adapting receptors (Meissner's corpuscles and peritrichial nerve endings), although the dor-

sal column system relays most of this information. Primary sensory fibers enter the medial division of the dorsal root and synapse with relay neurons of *lamina IV* and the adjacent laminae. The axons of these relay neurons ascend in the ipsilateral *dorsolateral tract* of the spinal cord but end in the *lateral cervical nucleus*, a slender column of multipolar neurons in the lateral funiculus, immediately ventrolateral to the dorsal horn at spinal levels C-1 and C-2. Axons from relay neurons in the lateral cervical nucleus join the ascending fibers of the contralateral medial lemniscus and continue to the ventrobasal complex of the thalamus (Fig. 10-15).

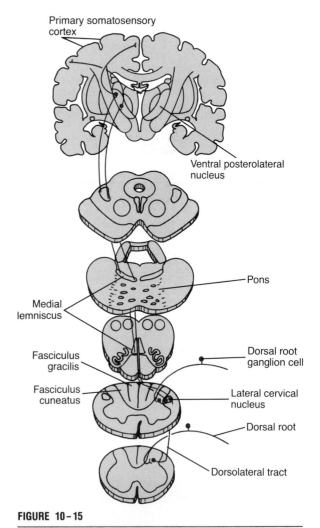

FIGURE 10-15

A simplified schematic illustrates the course of the spinocervicothalamic tract, from the spinal cord to the primary somatosensory cortex.

All three pathways have several features in common.

1. Sensory information carried by type-Aα and type-Aβ fibers enters the CNS via the medial division of the dorsal root.

2. Information ascends to the medulla on the ipsilateral side of the spinal cord.

3. All three pathways cross to the contralateral medial lemniscus in the medulla and ascend to the ventrobasal complex of the thalamus.

4. All three pathways are somatotopically organized.

SPINOCEREBELLAR PATHWAYS

Only a small component of the proprioceptive information carried by the medial division of the dorsal root is relayed to the thalamus via the dorsal column-medial lemniscal system. The remainder is carried to the cerebellum in one of four pathways. These are presented briefly here and in depth in Chapter 17.

The *dorsal (posterior) spinocerebellar tract* carries information to the cerebellum from the trunk and lower extremities. Primary afferent fibers enter the medial division of the dorsal root, ascend a few segments in the fasciculus gracilis, and terminate in the *nucleus dorsalis (Clarke's column)*. This nucleus is located in lamina VII of the spinal cord from C-8 to L-3 (see Figs. 6–10 and 10–6). Axons from this nucleus ascend in the ipsilateral *dorsal spinocerebellar tract* (see Fig. 6–8), joining the *restiform body* in the lower medulla and entering the cerebellum as part of the *inferior cerebellar peduncle.*

The *cuneocerebellar tract* (the upper extremity, head and neck equivalent of the dorsal spinocerebellar tract) forms from proprioceptive fibers of the fasciculus cuneatus that synapse in the *external (accessory) cuneate nucleus* (see Fig. 7–8). Fibers from neurons of the external cuneate nucleus enter the *restiform body* and then the cerebellum as part of the *inferior cerebellar peduncle.* The cuneocerebellar tract also is uncrossed with fibers entering the ipsilateral inferior cerebellar peduncle.

The *ventral (anterior) spinocerebellar tract* carries information from the lower extremities and trunk, but unlike the dorsal spinocerebellar tract, the fibers are both crossed and uncrossed (see Figs. 6–8 and 10–6). This pathway arises from neurons of lamina VI and VII of the spinal cord and ascends through the medulla and pons to enter the cerebellum as part of the *superior cerebellar peduncle (brachium conjunctivum).*

The *rostral spinocerebellar tract* is considered by many as the arm and head equivalent of the ventral spinocerebellar tract. Fibers forming this poorly delineated pathway arise from neurons in lamina VII of spinal segments C-4 through C-8. These projection fibers are mostly uncrossed and enter the cerebellum as components of both the *restiform body* and the *superior cerebellar peduncle.*

Anterolateral System and Component Pathways

The *anterolateral system (ALS)* is a composite of three major ascending pathways (the *spinothalamic tract*, the *spinoreticular tract*, and the *spinotectal tract*) located in the ventrolateral margin of the anterior quadrant of the spinal cord (see Fig. 10–8). Although somatotopically arranged, the organization of this tract is much cruder than that of the dorsal columns. As the ALS ascends through the brain stem, spinoreticular fibers end in the reticular formation of the medulla, pons, and midbrain. Spinotectal fibers end in the superior colliculus, and at this point the ALS becomes simply the spinothalamic tract. Throughout the brain stem, many fibers of the spinothalamic tract give off collateral branches to the brain stem reticular formation and the tectum.

The *spinotectal tract* is a crossed pathway relaying sensory information to the tectum, principally the *superior colliculus.* These fibers end in a somatotopic fashion in the deep layers of the tectum and are associated principally with reflex motor function of the head and upper body. The *spinoreticular tract*, also a crossed pathway, ascends to the brain stem reticular formation. This pathway is discussed in detail in Chapter 14. The role of the spinoreticular tract in the modulation of primary afferent signals is discussed later in this chapter.

The *spinothalamic tract* is a crossed pathway of second- and third-order sensory relay fibers, transmitting pain, temperature, and crude touch information to the thalamus. These relay neurons cross the midline in the ventral white commissure and ascend to the brain stem in the contralateral ALS (see Fig. 10–7).

MULTIPLE PAIN PATHWAYS

Nociceptive signals reach the brain by two distinct pathways: one carrying *fast, acute pain* and the other *slow, chronic pain.* Small, myelinated type-

Aδ fibers carry acute pain information. Although these fibers have slow conduction velocities compared with those of the dorsal columns, they are more than ten times faster than type-C fibers carrying slow, chronic pain signals (see Fig. 10–3). Both fiber types are components of the lateral division of the dorsal root. After entering the CNS at the *dorsolateral fasciculus of Lissauer,* the fibers branch, ascending and descending for one to three segments before entering the dorsal gray (see Fig. 10–7). Once in the dorsal horn, the pathways diverge.

ACUTE PAIN PATHWAY

Acute pain fibers (type-Aδ) synapse with relay neurons in both *lamina I* and *lamina V.* Axons from these second-order relay neurons cross to the opposite side of the spinal cord in the *ventral white commissure* and ascend through the spinal cord and brain stem to the thalamus in the contralateral *ALS* (see Figs. 10–7 and 10–16). This pathway is often referred to as the *neospino-thalamic pathway.* In addition to synapses with relay neurons, there are many synapses with interneurons at the spinal level (see Fig. 10–7). Some are involved in motor reflexes, such as the withdrawal reflex.

At the level of the lower medulla, the *ALS* remains in a ventrolateral position, dorsolateral to the medullary pyramids and ventral to the spinal tract and nucleus of the trigeminal nerve (see Fig. 10–9). At midmedullary levels (see Fig. 10–10), the ALS remains ventral to the spinal tract and nucleus of the trigeminal nerve but dorsolateral to the inferior olivary nucleus. In the pons, the ALS remains in the same relative position and is now immediately dorsolateral to the reoriented medial lemniscus (see Fig. 10–11). When the ALS reaches the midbrain at the level of the superior colliculus (see Fig. 10–12), it contains only the spinothalamic tract and remains dorsolateral to the medial lemniscus, although the fibers of the two pathways begin to interdigitate. The medial lemniscus and spinothalamic tract merge before they reach the level of the ventrobasal complex of the thalamus. The combined pathways end there in a precise, three-dimensional, somatotopic map with the different sensory modalities segregated as subunits within the map.

Only 10 to 20% of the pain fibers in the ALS reach the thalamus directly, the remainder ending throughout the brain stem reticular formation. Signals carried by these fibers, however, project to the thalamus by diffuse, multisynaptic pathways. The pain relay fibers of the ALS that do reach the thalamus are primarily associated with acute pain. These end in both the *intralaminar nuclei* and in the *ventrobasal complex* of the thalamus.

CHRONIC PAIN PATHWAY

The type-C fibers, carrying chronic pain information, synapse in the *substantia gelatinosa* (*laminae II* and *III*). In contrast to the acute pain pathway, where most of the primary sensory neurons synapse with thalamic relay neurons, the primary sensory neurons of the chronic pain pathway terminate on interneurons, which in turn, transmit the sensory information to thalamic relay neurons in *lamina V* (see Fig. 10–7). The chronic pain pathway is often referred to as the *paleospinothalamic pathway.* Most of the axons from lamina V relay neurons cross the midline and ascend toward the brain stem and thalamus in the contralateral *ALS.* A few ascend in the ipsilateral *ALS* (not illustrated).

The somatotopic pattern for chronic pain is less well defined than that for acute pain. In addition, fewer of the ALS fibers relaying chronic pain information reach the thalamus. Most leave the ALS and end in areas of the brain stem reticular formation. Much of the chronic pain information reaches the thalamus through diffuse multisynaptic pathways that terminate in the *intralaminar nuclei* of the thalamus (see Fig. 10–19 and Fig. 20–3). The relative paucity of chronic pain fibers terminating in the ventrobasal complex accounts for the lack of a precise localization of this sensory modality.

PAIN PATHWAYS AND THE BRAIN STEM RETICULAR FORMATION

The many collateral and terminal connections from both pain pathways with the brain stem reticular formation are of major importance. Connections with the reticular formation and brain stem areas, such as the periaqueductal gray and nucleus raphe magnus, are important in the modulation of painful stimuli (see subsequent discussion). These brain stem centers form part of the ascending *extrathalamic cortical modulatory systems* discussed in Chapter 21. These systems are involved in the regulation of behavioral responses, such as arousal, excitability, defense, and aversion.

Temperature

Small, unmyelinated, type-C fibers carry the signals from warm-sensitive receptors, whereas the small, myelinated, type-Aδ fibers carry the signals from cold sensitive receptors. Both fibers enter the *dorsolateral fasciculus of Lissauer* and branch, ascending and descending one to three spinal segments before synapsing in *laminae I, II,* and *III* of the dorsal horn. Thermal information is transmitted by one or more interneurons to the relay neurons of *lamina V*. Axons from lamina V neurons cross the spinal cord in the ventral white commissure to the contralateral *ALS* in parallel with the pain fibers (Figs. 10–7 and 10–16). Thermal fibers ascend through the brain stem in the ALS. Although a number end in the brain stem reticular formation, a significant number end in the ventrobasal complex of the thalamus. This information is relayed to the somatosensory cortex. This small but identifiable cortical representation is sufficient for the localization of thermal stimuli but not with the precision of the mechanoreceptor pathways of the dorsal columns.

Crude Touch

Most of the crude touch sensory information is from naked nerve endings, principally C-fibers. These signals enter the spinal cord via the lateral division of the dorsal root and follow a course through the spinal cord and brain stem to the thalamus that is identical to the temperature pathway. As with pain and temperature, somatotopic organization is present within the ALS, but precision in tactile discrimination is lacking.

Some of the crude touch sensation is from peritrichial nerve endings. These fibers are typical dorsal column afferents (see previous discussion); however, they give off collateral branches that synapse with thalamic relay neurons of lamina V. These, in turn, cross to the opposite side in the ventral white commissure and enter the contralateral ALS. Peritrichial information carried by the dorsal column system maintains a high degree of spatial resolution, a feature apparently lost in the peritrichial information transmitted in the ALS. This loss probably is due to a relative paucity of representation of this pathway in the cortex.

General Somatic Afferent Components of the Cranial Nerves

Of the cranial nerves, the *trigeminal (cranial nerve V)* provides the major GSA innervation to the face. Spinal nerves C-2 through C-5 innervate the neck and occipital portion of the head. The trigeminal nerve innervates the entire face from the lower margin of the mandible to the top of the scalp and laterally to the anterior portion of the pinna of the ear, including the anterior wall of the external auditory meatus (Fig. 10–17). In addition, the trigeminal innervates most of the dura mater, except for the infratentorial portion

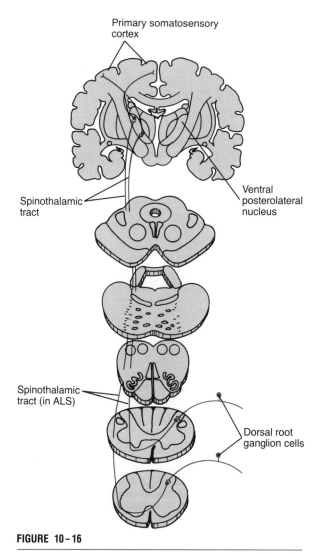

FIGURE 10–16

A simplified schematic illustrates the course of the spinothalamic tract, from the spinal cord to the primary somatosensory cortex. The spinothalamic, the spinotectal and the spinoreticular tracts make up the anterolateral system (ALS).

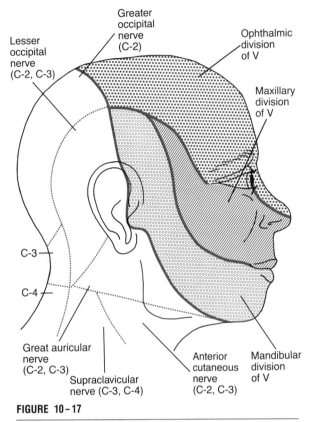

Lesser occipital nerve (C-2, C-3)

Greater occipital nerve (C-2)

Ophthalmic division of V

Maxillary division of V

C-3

C-4

Great auricular nerve (C-2, C-3)

Supraclavicular nerve (C-3, C-4)

Anterior cutaneous nerve (C-2, C-3)

Mandibular division of V

FIGURE 10-17

The cutaneous innervation of the the head and neck. Areas innervated by the three divisions of the trigeminal nerve are shaded in red, and the areas innervated by branches of cervical nerves C-2 through C-5 are outlined in red.

that is supplied by the *vagus nerve* (*cranial nerve X*). The *facial* (*cranial nerve VII*), *glossopharyngeal* (*cranial nerve IX*), and *vagus nerves* also innervate very small areas of the external auditory meatus and the pinna.

TRIGEMINAL GANGLION

The primary sensory neurons, corresponding to the dorsal root ganglion cells of the spinal cord, of the trigeminal nerve reside in the cranial vault in the *trigeminal ganglion* (*semilunar*, or *gasserian ganglion*). The trigeminal nerve has three divisions, each arising as a major trunk from the trigeminal ganglion. The *ophthalmic division* innervates the upper portion of the face, the *maxillary division* innervates the middle portion, and the *mandibular division* innervates the lower portion (see Fig. 10-17). For details of the peripheral distribution of these fibers see Chapter 19.

TRIGEMINAL NUCLEI

The trigeminal system has three sensory nuclei: the *spinal nucleus of V*; the *main sensory nucleus of V* (*chief*, or *principal nucleus of V*); and the *mesencephalic nucleus of V*, in addition to the *motor nucleus of V* (Fig. 10-18). The motor nucleus of V innervates the muscles of mastication (see Chapter 19).

The *spinal nucleus of V* is a long column of neurons in the dorsolateral brain stem extending caudad from the point of entry of the trigeminal nerve in the midpontine region to the upper cervical spinal cord (see Figs. 10-9 and 10-10). In the upper cervical spinal cord, the spinal nucleus of V merges with and becomes indistinguishable from the substantia gelatinosa (laminae I through IV) of the dorsal horn. The spinal tract of V merges with the dorsolateral fasciculus of the spinal cord (see Figs. 7-7 through 7-12).

Based on cytoarchitectural studies, the spinal nucleus of V contains three subdivisions: the *pars oralis* makes up the rostral third of the nucleus; the *pars interpolaris*, the middle third; and the *pars caudalis*, the caudal third (see Fig. 10-18). The caudal portion of the spinal nucleus of V is associated with pain and thermal sensations, whereas the more rostral portions are associated with tactile sense. A dorsal-ventral somatotopic organization to the spinal nucleus exists with fibers from the ophthalmic division ending throughout the ventral portion of the nucleus, the mandibular division in the dorsal portion, and the maxillary division in the middle.

The *main sensory nucleus of V* is rostral to the spinal nucleus of V in the midpontine region (see Figs. 7-13 and 10-18). Anatomically and functionally, the main sensory nucleus is the homologue of the dorsal column nuclei. The main sensory nucleus of V also is somatotopically organized, similar to that of the spinal nucleus of V.

The *mesencephalic nucleus of V* is unusual for a CNS nucleus. It consists of pseudounipolar, primary sensory neurons but, unlike the dorsal root ganglion cells, it is within the CNS. Because these are pseudounipolar sensory neurons, there are no synapses in this nucleus. These neurons, together with their central and peripheral processes, form the *mesencephalic tract and nucleus of V*, a thin column of neurons adjacent to a small bundle of myelinated nerve fibers extending rostrally from the point of entry of the trigeminal nerve to the level of the oculomotor nuclei and superior colliculi in the midbrain. This nucleus and associated fiber tract lie along the lateral

FIGURE 10-18

The trigeminal nuclei. The distribution and course of the primary afferent fibers and some of the principal thalamic projection systems are shown. The contributions of the spinal nucleus of V to the dorsal trigeminal lemnisci and the ipsilateral ventral trigeminal lemniscus are not illustrated (see text).

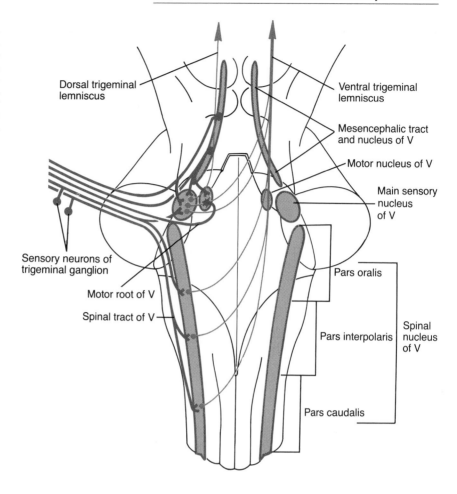

margin of the periaqueductal gray (see Figs. 7–13 through 7–17). The peripheral processes of the primary sensory neurons exit the CNS with the motor root of the trigeminal nerve and accompany the motor branches to the muscles of mastication, where they end in proprioceptive receptors. The central processes project to the *main sensory nucleus of V* and to the *motor nucleus of V*, for reflex connections with the motor neurons (see Fig. 10–18).

PRIMARY AFFERENT FIBERS

Approximately half the afferent fibers of the trigeminal nerve descend in the *spinal tract of V*. In general, these are small fibers, comparable to type-Aδ and type-C fibers in the spinal cord. Most are concerned with the sensations of pain and temperature. The remaining fibers, mostly large, myelinated type-Aβ fibers bifurcate with an

ascending branch ending in the *main sensory nucleus of V* and a descending branch ending in the more rostral levels of the *spinal nucleus of V*, principally the *pars oralis*. These fibers are comparable to the medial division of the dorsal root and transmit various mechanoreceptive-mediated sensations, principally discriminative touch.

AFFERENT PROJECTIONS

Relay fibers from the *spinal nucleus of V*, carrying principally pain, temperature, and touch information, cross the midline, form the *ventral trigeminal lemniscus,* and ascend to the contralateral *ventral posteromedial nucleus* of the thalamus (see Figs. 10–11, 10–12, and 10–18). Other fibers leave the *spinal nucleus of V*, enter the adjacent *brain stem reticular formation*, and ascend to the thalamus by way of a diffuse, multisynaptic pathway. These multisynaptic projections end bilaterally in both the *ventral poster-*

omedial nuclei and the *intralaminar nuclei* of the thalamus (Fig. 10–19).

Many of the relay fibers from the *main sensory nucleus of V* decussate in the pontine tegmentum, join the *ventral trigeminal lemniscus*, and ascend to the contralateral *ventral posteromedial nucleus* of the thalamus. The uncrossed projections from the main sensory nucleus form a smaller, less well-defined pathway, the *dorsal trigeminal lemniscus* (see Figs. 10–11, 10–12, and 10–18). Thus, fibers from the main sensory nucleus terminate in both the ipsilateral and contralateral ventral posteromedial nuclei of the thalamus: the uncrossed fibers ascending in the dorsal trigeminal lemniscus and the crossed fibers ascending in the ventral trigeminal lemniscus in the company of relay fibers from the spinal nucleus of V.

In summary, the *ventral trigeminal lemniscus* contains primarily crossed nerve fibers from both the spinal nucleus of V and the main sensory nucleus of V. This pathway carries pain, temperature, and crude touch information from the spinal nucleus as well as mechanoreceptor information for discriminatory tactile and pressure sense from the main sensory nucleus. Both the nuclei of origin (main sensory and spinal nuclei of V) and the target nucleus in the contralateral thalamus are organized somatotopically. The *dorsal trigeminal lemniscus*, however, carries principally uncrossed mechanoreceptor information from the main sensory nucleus of V to the ipsilateral ventral posteromedial nucleus of the thalamus.

GENERAL SOMATIC AFFERENT COMPONENTS OF OTHER CRANIAL NERVES

The *facial, glossopharyngeal,* and *vagus nerves* have a GSA component, albeit small. For all three, GSA fibers innervate a very small area on the pinna of the ear and in the external auditory meatus. Primary sensory neurons reside in the *geniculate ganglion* (facial nerve), *superior ganglion* (glossopharyngeal nerve), and *jugular ganglion* (vagus nerve). The central processes of these neurons enter the CNS with their respective nerves and join the descending *spinal tract of V* to end in the *spinal nucleus of V* (see Figs. 19–8, 19–9, and 19–10). When these fibers join the spinal tract of V, they course in the dorsal most portion, immediately adjacent to the fibers of the mandibular division of V. These fibers carry sensory information for pain, temperature, and touch.

Four cranial nerves generally regarded as "pure" motor nerves contain a few primary sensory neurons: the *oculomotor, trochlear, abducens,* and *hypoglossal nerves* (*cranial nerves III, IV, VI,* and *XII*). These small aggregations of sensory neurons, embedded within the nerve trunks near the brain stem, are not sufficient to be recognized as a ganglion and are often disregarded. These neurons carry a portion of the proprioceptive information from the muscles innervated by the respective nerves. The principal route for GSA information from these muscles,

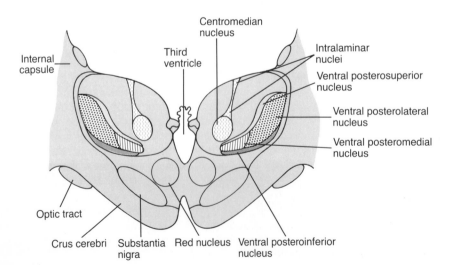

Internal capsule
Third ventricle
Centromedian nucleus
Intralaminar nuclei
Ventral posterosuperior nucleus
Ventral posterolateral nucleus
Ventral posteromedial nucleus
Optic tract
Crus cerebri
Substantia nigra
Red nucleus
Ventral posteroinferior nucleus

FIGURE 10–19

The components of the ventrobasal complex and the intralaminar nuclei including the centromedian nucleus of the dorsal thalamus are illustrated. Level comparable to the Weigert-stained section in Figure 7–19.

however, is via the ophthalmic division of V (extraocular muscles) and the upper cervical nerves (tongue musculature).

Thalamic Relay of Somatosensory Information

VENTROBASAL COMPLEX

The *ventrobasal complex*, a group of nuclei in the posterior portion of the ventral tier of the thalamic nuclei, is the principal thalamic relay center for ascending somatosensory pathways (see Chapter 20 for the overall organization of the thalamus). The largest and most prominent nucleus is the *ventral posterior nucleus (VP)*, which is subdivided into lateral and medial components; the *ventral posterolateral nucleus (VPL)*; and the *ventral posteromedial nucleus (VPM)*. The *ventral posterosuperior nucleus (VPS)* forms a thin shell or cap over the dorsal surface of the *VP*, and the *ventral posteroinferior nucleus (VPI)* is a narrow nuclear zone immediately ventral or inferior to VP (see Fig. 10–19). Together these four nuclei, VPL, VPM, VPS, and VPI, compose the ventrobasal complex.

VP relays signals from both *rapidly adapting* and *slowly adapting mechanoreceptors* to the *anterior parietal cortex*, specifically *Brodmann's area 3b* and *area 1* of the *primary somatosensory cortex, S-I* (Fig. 10–20; for Brodmann's areas, see Fig. 21–3). Within the *VP*, the *VPL* receives a dense input from the *medial lemniscus*, and *VPM* from the *main sensory nucleus of V*. Fiber terminations from the *spinothalamic tract* in *VPL* and from the *spinal nucleus of V* in *VPM* are less dense and more uneven than those from the medial lemniscus.

The *VP* contains a highly organized, somatotopic representation of the body parts. The detailed, three-dimensional map from the squirrel monkey is a good example (Fig. 10–21). The human VP is not mapped in this detail, but with a few differences, such as the lack of a tail region, the general pattern is probably the same. Within the somatotopic organization is a suborganization of terminals according to sensory modality. Thus, within each body-part "block" of VP is a mosaic of terminals, segregated according to the sensory information transmitted.

Specific *nociceptive* fibers, originating in *laminae I* and *V* of the spinal cord and traveling in the contralateral *spinothalamic tract*, as well as nociceptive fibers from the *spinal nucleus of V*

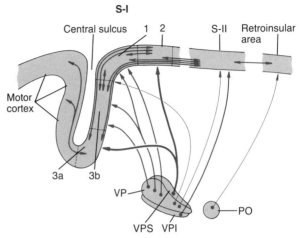

FIGURE 10–20

Thalamocortical projections to the somatosensory areas. Note the relation of areas 3a, 3b, 1, and 2 to the central sulcus. Major thalamic projections to S-I, S-II, and the retroinsular area as well as some of the major intracortical connections are indicated. Nociceptive projections from ventral posterior (VP) nucleus and posterior complex (PO) are thin red lines; muscle spindle projections from ventral posterosuperior (VPS) nucleus are thick red lines; and tactile projections from VP and ventral posteroinferior (VPI) nuclei are intermediate in thickness. (Modified with permission from J. H. Kaas, The somatosensory system. In G. Paxinos (Editor), *The Human Nervous System.* Academic Press, New York, 1990.)

project to the *VP*. Small thalamic neurons relay the nociceptive signal to the somatosensory cortex, both to area *S-I*, along the margin between areas 3b and 1, and to the *secondary somatosensory area (S-II)* (see Fig. 10–20).

The *VPS* receives sensory input exclusively from *proprioceptors* (muscle spindles, joint receptors, and other deep tissue receptors) and projects to both *area 3a* and *area 2* of S-I, with some of the thalamic relay neurons projecting to both areas via collaterals (see Fig. 10–20). VPS also is highly organized somatotopically with a pattern of body representation paralleling that of the adjacent VP: the head representation is medial; the leg, lateral; and the arm, between the head and leg. Both active and passive movement of limbs and joints and compression of muscle and joint tissues activate relay neurons of VPS; they do not respond to tactile stimuli.

The functional organization of *VPI* is not as well understood as that of VP and VPS. The *VPI* receives numerous terminals from the *spinothalamic tract* and from the relay neurons in the *spinal nucleus of V*. The major cortical projections from VPI are to *S-II*, with a minor component to *S-I* (not illustrated) (see Fig. 10–20).

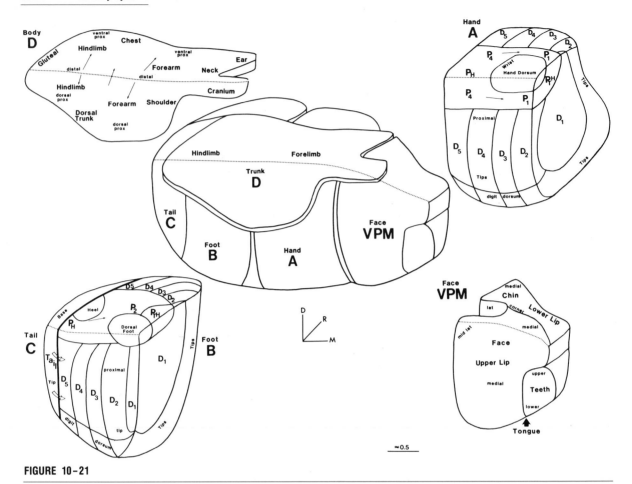

FIGURE 10-21

The somatotopic organization of the ventral posterior (VP) nucleus of squirrel monkeys. Except for the lack of a lateral region devoted to the tail, a similar organization exists in the human VP. Traditionally, VP has two divisions, ventral posteromedial (VPM) for the face and ventral posterolateral (VPL) for the body.

VPL is further divided here into subnuclei for the hand (A), foot (B), tail (C), and trunk and proximal limbs (D). The figure shows where body parts are represented in the subnuclei and how the subnuclei fit together. (Reproduced with permission from J. Kaas, R. J. Nelson, M. Sur, R. W. Dykes, and M. M. Merzenich, J. Comp. Neurol., 226: 111–140, 1984.)

POSTERIOR COMPLEX

The *posterior complex* (*PO*) lies just behind the ventrobasal complex, immediately rostral to the medial geniculate nucleus. Principal projections to PO are nociceptive, from laminae I and IV through VII of the contralateral spinal cord. Thalamic relay neurons of the PO project to a third somatosensory area, the *retroinsular area* (Figs. 10–20 and 10–22). Some somatotopic organization exists both in the PO and in the retroinsular cortical area; however, it is not as well defined as VP and S-I.

INTRALAMINAR NUCLEI

The pain pathways terminate in a number of *intralaminar nuclei*, including the *centrolateral*,

centromedian, and *parafascicular nuclei*. The precise somatotopic localization seen in the VP nuclei is not present, and the receptive fields of relay neurons projecting to these nuclei are usually large and bilateral. These nuclei receive some terminals from the *spinothalamic tract*, but the diffuse multisynaptic relays within the *brain stem reticular formation* convey much of this ascending nociceptive information. Functionally and anatomically, the intralaminar nuclei are a diencephalic extension of the brain stem reticular formation. Intralaminar neurons project both to the striatum and to widespread areas of the cortex, including the somatosensory areas. These connections suggest a role in sensorimotor integration. In addition, many of the widespread cortical projections of intralaminar relay neurons are part of a general cortical arousal mechanism.

THALAMIC NUCLEI INDIRECTLY RELATED TO THE SOMATOSENSORY SYSTEM

Three nuclei, *anterior pulvinar*, *medial pulvinar*, and *lateral posterior nucleus* (*LP*), have major projections to the parietal cortex. All have extensive reciprocal connections with the somatosensory areas and with adjacent parietal and temporal areas, but they do not receive direct, ascending somatosensory information. Because of the widespread parietal and temporal connections, including the somatosensory areas, their function is considered modulatory or integrative.

Somatosensory Cortex

Three areas of the cerebral cortex receive significant projections from the somatosensory relay nuclei: the *primary somatosensory cortex* (*S-I*) (the postcentral gyrus of the parietal lobe), the *secondary somatosensory cortex* (*S-II*) (a small area in the parietal operculum, just caudad to the central sulcus), and the *retroinsular area* (an even

smaller area in the depths of the lateral fissure at the posterosuperior margin of the insula) (see Fig. 10–22).

Other cortical areas with significant somatosensory representation include several areas of the insular cortex, additional regions of the parietal operculum, most of the posterior parietal cortex, and an area of the cingulate gyrus near the medial margin of the postcentral gyrus. These areas are concerned primarily with higher-order cortical processing of somatosensory information. The cortical cytoarchitectonics, the structural organization of the neurons in the cortex, is discussed in Chapter 21.

PRIMARY SOMATOSENSORY CORTEX, S-I

The primary somatosensory area, *S-I*, the *postcentral gyrus*, consists of four separate parallel representations of the body parts, each with a distinguishing cytoarchitecture, *Brodmann's areas 3a, 3b, 1,* and *2* (see Fig. 21–3). Area 3a lies deep within the central sulcus, area 3b occupies most of the middle half of the posterior wall of the central sulcus, area 1 the crest of the postcen-

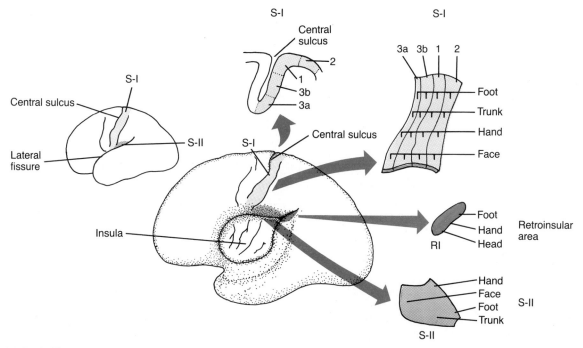

FIGURE 10–22

Somatosensory cortical areas. S-I, S-II, and the retroinsular cortex are three areas known to receive somatosensory projections from the thalamus. The small figure (left) illustrates the areas visible from the lateral surface of the brain. In the center, spreading the lateral fissure exposes the underlying insular cortex, S-II and the retroinsular area.

At the top, a cross section through the central sulcus and S-I illustrates the relative position of the S-I components, cortical areas 3a, 3b, 1, and 2. If the somatosensory areas were removed and laid out as flat sheets, they would appear as illustrated on the right. This view is used for somatotopic maps, such as in Figure 10–23.

tral gyrus, and area 2 lies immediately caudad to area 1 (see Fig. 10–22). Each of the somatotopic maps is organized in a pattern similar to that in the classic homunculus of Penfield and Rasmussen (see Fig. 10–2). The foot and leg areas are located medially, followed by the trunk, upper extremity, hands, and face, as one moves laterally and inferiorly over the surface of the postcentral gyrus, in the anterior parietal cortex.

The most precise maps of the somatosensory cortex have been constructed for monkeys (Fig. 10–23); however, with a few obvious anatomical differences, human studies support the same general pattern of organization.

Area 3b, often called "S-I proper," is essential for tactile discrimination and the appreciation of shape. These functions are lost if the area is damaged. Nearly 70% of the neurons in VP project to this area, with information from cutaneous mechanoreceptors of both the fast- and slow-adapting types. Area 3b has reciprocal connections with areas 1 and 2 and with S-II.

Area 1, immediately adjacent to 3b and con-

taining a body map that parallels and mirrors the one in 3b, also receives cutaneous mechanoreceptor information relayed by neurons in VP, many of which are from collaterals of neurons projecting to 3a. Area 1 has reciprocal projections to areas 2 and 3b and to area S-II.

Area 2 has a complex representation from both cutaneous and deep receptors, receiving muscle spindle afferent information from VPS, some cutaneous information from VP, and projections from cortical areas 3b and 1. This combination of position and tactile sense is probably important for stereognosis and other discriminations during active touch.

The fourth body representation is in *Area 3a*, located deep in the central sulcus. Signals from muscle spindles and deep receptors relayed in VPS provide the major input with roughly half the neurons projecting to both 3a and 2. Besides reciprocal projections to area 2 and S-II, area 3a has strong connections with motor and premotor areas of the adjacent frontal cortex. These associations along with descending fibers terminating in

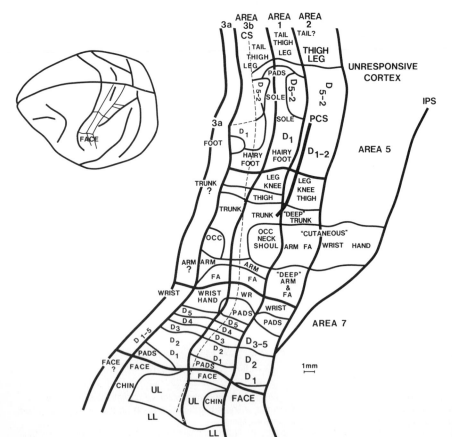

FIGURE 10–23

A summary diagram of the somatotopic organization of the primary somatosensory cortex (S-I) in macaque monkeys. A dorsolateral view of the brain (upper left) shows the location of the depicted cortex (right). A dashed line marks the crown of the central sulcus (CS). For reference also note the postcentral sulcus (PCS) and the intraparietal sulcus (IPS). (D1–D5, digits of hand (lateral) or foot (medial); UL, upper lip; LL, lower lip; FA, forearm; SHOUL, shoulder; OCC, occiput; WR, wrist.) (Reproduced with permission from T. P. Pons, P. E. Garraghty, C. G. Cusick, and J. H. Kaas, J. Comp. Neurol., 241: 445–466, 1987.)

the basal ganglia, pons, and dorsal column nuclei suggest roles for area 3a in the modification of motor behavior and the modulation of ascending afferent signals.

Although less precise, somatotopically, than the mechanoreceptor maps, there are nociceptive projections from VP to the junction of 3b and 1. The somatotopic organization is not as precise as that for the mechanoreceptors. The nociceptive signals may use the existing tactile map to add the dimension of localization to the painful stimulus.

SECONDARY SOMATOSENSORY CORTEX, S-II

Somatosensory area *S-II*, often termed the somatosensory cortex of the lateral sulcus, is not as well defined as S-I. Lesions to the area seldom produce the sensory deficits observed in S-I. However, S-II is part of the corticolimbic projection system and is important for memory and recall of somatosensory information. S-II receives projections from all four areas of S-I and direct somatosensory information from the spinothalamic tract by way of VPI and some tactile projections from VP. Thalamic projections to S-II are somatotopically organized, albeit crudely in comparison with S-I (see Fig. 10–22).

RETROINSULAR AREA

The *retroinsular area*, deep in the upper portion of the lateral fissure at the posterosuperior margin of the insular cortex, receives direct somatosensory projections from the thalamus, principally nociceptive projections from PO along with some light touch information, probably of spinothalamic tract origin. These terminals also are localized somatotopically as illustrated in Fig. 10–22.

General Visceral Afferent Pathways

The *general visceral afferent (GVA) system* innervates those structures developed from embryonic endoderm and splanchnic mesoderm. These include the mucosal-lined cavities of the head and neck and the contents of the thoracic, abdominal, and pelvic cavities.

The pharyngeal and nasal cavities and the tongue are richly innervated. Sensory information is relayed with a high degree of resolution to the somatosensory cortex for the conscious apprecia-

tion of the sensation (principally pain, temperature, and touch). Conversely, the visceral organs of the body cavities are sparsely innervated, and the perception of a sensory stimulus is quite different.

The peripheral receptors are limited to naked nerve endings and pacinian corpuscles. Although many sensory modalities can be detected in the nasal, oral, and pharyngeal cavities, selectivity for the modality resides in the relative sensitivity of the receptor.

CRANIAL NERVE COMPONENTS

The *facial nerve* innervates the nasal and sinus cavities and the soft palate; the *glossopharyngeal nerve* innervates the pharyngeal mucosa and the posterior third of the tongue (the anterior two thirds is somatic and therefore innervated by the GSA component of the trigeminal nerve); and the *vagus nerve* innervates the laryngeal mucosa and the viscera of the thorax and most of the abdomen.

The *primary sensory neurons* of the *facial nerve* are in the *geniculate ganglion*, those for the *glossopharyngeal nerve* are in the *petrosal (inferior) ganglion*, and those of the *vagus nerve* are in the *nodose (inferior) ganglion* (see Figs. 19–8, 19–9, and 19–10). The central processes of the GVA neurons for all three enter the brain stem with their respective nerves, join the *solitary tract (fasciculus)*, and synapse in the *solitary nucleus (nucleus of the solitary tract)* or in both the solitary nucleus and the *dorsal sensory nucleus of the vagus* (the glossopharyngeal and vagus nerves) (Figs. 7–8, 7–9, 7–10, and 7–25). The secondary connections of the solitary nucleus and the dorsal sensory nucleus of the vagus are complex, with most associated with autonomic reflexes. Discrete fiber projections from either the solitary nucleus or the sensory nucleus of the vagus to the thalamus have not been identified. However, it is likely that such connections exist because information related to taste is relayed through the solitary nucleus and is appreciated and interpreted at the cortical level. Those visceral afferent fibers associated with a high degree of discrimination, i.e., from the nasal cavities, tongue, and pharyngeal cavity, appear to synapse in the spinal nucleus of V.

SPINAL COMPONENTS

At the spinal level, GVA neurons innervating the thoracic, abdominal, and pelvic viscera travel with the sympathetic nerves and enter the spinal cord in the lateral division of the dorsal root (see Fig. 6–7B). Most are small, type-C fibers, although some pacinian corpuscles are located in the mesentery. These are innervated by the larger, type-Aβ fibers. As with the brain stem GVA components, many of the spinal visceral afferents are concerned with reflex mechanisms.

REFERRED PAIN

The most common visceral sensory modality is pain. Unlike somatic afferents, visceral afferents do not have a well-defined ascending sensory pathway. Instead, the stimulus frequently is perceived as originating from a somatic area, a phenomenon known as *referred pain*. Primary GVA fibers transmit the noxious signal from the viscera to the spinal cord, where one of two events happens: Either (a) the *GVA* fibers synapse with the same relay neurons as incoming GSA fibers and the GSA pathway carries the signal to the thalamus or (b) the constant bombardment of GSA relay neurons by stimulated GVA fibers lowers the threshold of the relay neurons and basal levels of GSA input now transmit the noxious signal to higher centers. In each case, the ascending GSA system carries the signal and the brain perceives the stimulus as coming from the peripheral field of the GSA neuron.

An alternative explanation of referred pain involves a viscero-viscero-somatic sequence, in which visceral pain literally produces somatic pain through the activation of peripheral vasoconstrictors. At the spinal level, the GVA signals activate peripheral vasoconstrictor neurons—GVE sympathetic preganglionic neurons—leading to a localized ischemia in the spinal dermatome. The ischemia, in turn, activates GSA nociceptors and the somatic pain signal is then perceived as originating in the somatic dermatome.

During development, growing tips of the GVA fibers enter the early primordia of the target organs. Hence, the spinal segments of origin of GVA fibers reflect the early embryonic location of the organ primordium and not the final position of the organ in the adult. For example, the fetal diaphragm develops in the mid cervical region and, in later development, migrates caudally carrying the sensory and motor innervation with it. Thus, referred pain from the diaphragm is usually felt in the C-4 dermatome, even though the adult diaphragm is situated along the lower margin of the rib cage. Listed in Table 10–1 are

TABLE 10–1

Referred Pain Dermatomes for Some of the Major Organs

ORGANS	DERMATOMES*
Diaphragm	C-3 to C-4
Heart	T-1 to T-8
Gallbladder	T-6 to T-8
Stomach	T-6 to T-9
Small intestine	T-9 to T-10
Appendix	T-10
Large intestine	T-11 to L-2
Rectum	S-2 to S-4
Testes and ovaries	T-10 to T-12
Prostate	T-10 to T-12
Uterus	T-10 to T-12
Adrenal gland	T-8 to L-1
Kidneys	T-10 to L-1
Urinary bladder	T-11 to L-2
Renal pelvis and ureter	L-1 to L-2

* For a dermatomal map, see Figures 6–5 and 6–6.

the dermatomes associated with referred pain from some of the major visceral organs (also refer to Figs. 6–5 and 6–6).

"FALSE VISCERAL PAIN" OR PARIETAL PAIN

During embryonic development, the mesoderm of the lateral plate splits into the *splanchnopleure* and the *somatopleure*. The former forming the walls and serosa of the visceral organs, the latter forming the body musculature and the peritoneal lining of the body cavities. GVA fibers innervate the splanchnopleure and its derivatives, whereas GSA fibers innervate derivatives of the somatopleure. When a visceral organ becomes diseased or inflamed to the point of impinging on the wall of the body cavity, a noxious stimulus may arise from the lining of the cavity, the parietal layer. The sensory fibers stimulated are GSA, small, myelinated type-Aδ fibers. This pain, known as *parietal pain*, is perceived as originating from the spinal segments stimulated and is not referred. Hence, with appendicitis, the initial pain will be "true" visceral pain—originating from the appendix—and referred to dermatome T-10 in the umbilical area. As inflammation increases, nociceptors in the adjacent parietal layer lining the abdominal cavity are stimulated and the pain shifts to the lower right quadrant of the abdominal wall. This is *parietal pain* and is actually a GSA sensory signal, acute pain carried by GSA type-Aδ fibers. Parietal pain is very sharp, with a prickling quality as compared with the deep chronic pain associated with the initial pain referred to the umbilical area.

Modulation of Nociceptive Signals

The CNS has the capacity to suppress or attenuate incoming sensory signals, not only nociceptive signals but other sensory modalities as well. If the CNS did not have the capacity to filter selectively incoming information, the constant barrage of afferent signals from the external environment would be overwhelming. The modulation of sensory information originally was considered a cortical function with the incoming afferent signals transmitted, unimpeded, from the periphery to the cerebral cortex.

However, several subcortical systems have been identified that selectively *impede* or even *amplify* afferent signals. This is not to say there is no cortical suppression of afferent signals. Our ability to *consciously* suppress afferent information, i.e., concentrating on a particular signal and ignoring others, is a cortical-*initiated* function. Whether the suppression actually takes place in the cortex or at a subcortical level is unknown.

Most of our understanding of the subcortical modulation of afferent signals relates to the suppression of noxious or painful stimuli. Under certain situations the CNS can "ignore" painful stimuli. The athlete experiencing the excitement of the contest and the combat soldier fighting during battle often are unaware of severe and normally painful injuries during the contest or battle. In both instances, painful stimuli were not perceived. The information was either inhibited or "short circuited" at some point before reaching a conscious center.

MODULATION OF NOXIOUS STIMULI BY TACTILE STIMULATION

The repetitive stimulation of type Aβ fibers attenuates the relay, at the spinal level, of the noxious signals carried by the primary afferent type-Aδ and type-C fibers. A theory developed to explain these observations is the *gate theory*. This theory proposes the existence of "gate cells" in laminae II and III. Collaterals from type-Aβ tactile fibers excite these cells, and collaterals from type-Aδ and type-C pain fibers inhibit them. The gate cells, in turn, project to lamina V and form excitatory axoaxonal synapses on the axon terminals of the primary afferent fibers (type-Aβ, -Aδ, and -C) as they synapse with the spinothalamic relay neurons (Fig. 10–24). Because the amount of transmitter released by an action potential is proportional to the change in membrane potential, the depolarization of the primary afferent axon terminal from the excitatory axoaxonal syn-

FIGURE 10–24

The major components in the gate theory for the modulation of pain through type Aβ fiber stimulation. The gate cell, itself inhibited by pain fibers and excited by type Aβ fibers, inhibits the transmission of primary sensory information through primary afferent depolarization (see text).

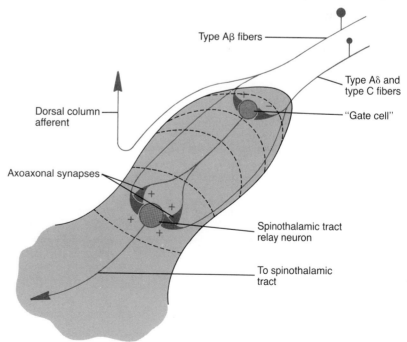

Type Aβ fibers

Type Aδ and type C fibers

"Gate cell"

Dorsal column afferent

Axoaxonal synapses

Spinothalamic tract relay neuron

To spinothalamic tract

apse reduces the primary afferent signal to the thalamic relay neuron—an inhibitory mechanism known as *primary afferent depolarization* (see Chapter 4).

Although little direct evidence supports the theory and the identity of the gate cell is equivocal, they help explain, for example, the relief one experiences from a painful stimulus to the hand when the area is rubbed or the arm is shaken. They also explain the relief from chronic pain experienced by patients following dorsal column stimulation.

DESCENDING SEROTONINERGIC-OPIOID PEPTIDE ANALGESIC PATHWAY

High concentrations of opioid peptides are in the *periaqueductal gray* (*PAG*) of the midbrain (endorphins) and in the *substantia gelatinosa* of the spinal cord (enkephalins and dynorphins). Endorphin-containing neurons from the PAG project to

the rostral medullary reticular formation, principally the *nucleus raphe magnus* (*NRM*) and the *nucleus gigantocellularis* (*NGC*). Serotoninergic neurons from these nuclei form a descending pathway to the dorsal horn of the spinal cord. The pathway descends immediately dorsolateral to the inferior olivary nucleus in the medulla and enters the dorsolateral portion of the lateral funiculus of the spinal cord near the ascending spinocervicothalamic tract. These fibers reach all levels of the spinal cord and synapse on small, enkephalin-containing and dynorphin-containing neurons in the substantia gelatinosa. These interneurons form axoaxonal synapses on the primary afferent terminals of type-Aδ and type-C pain fibers resulting in the attenuation of the nociceptive signal at the level of entry (Fig. 10–25).

Stimulation of the PAG, the NRM, the NGC, or the substantia gelatinosa blocks the afferent signals from painful but not tactile stimuli. The morphine antagonist, naloxone, reverses the ef-

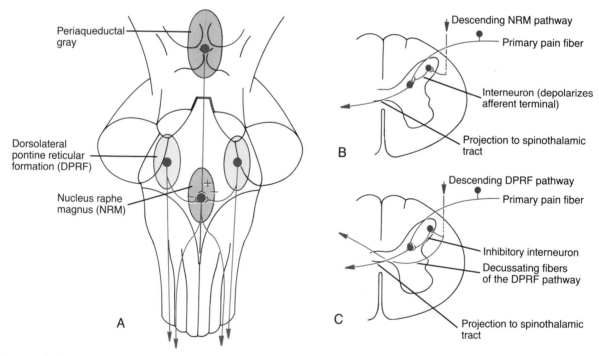

FIGURE 10–25

Simplified schematic of two descending analgesic pathways. *A*, Enkephalin-containing fibers project from the periaqueductal gray to the nucleus raphe magnus (NRM). Serotoninergic fibers from the NRM descend bilaterally to the spinal cord. Adrenergic fibers from the dorsolateral pontine reticular formation (DPRF) descend ipsilaterally to the spinal cord after giving off inhibitory collaterals to NRM.

B, Serotoninergic fibers from NRM synapse with the enkephalin- and dynorphin-containing interneurons of the substantia gelatinosa. These interneurons attenuate the pain signal through primary afferent depolarization.

C, Adrenergic fibers from the DPRF synapse with inhibitory interneurons of the substantia gelatinosa on both sides of the spinal cord. The interneurons inhibit projection neurons of the spinothalamic tract in lamina V (see text for details of both systems).

fect. Direct stimulation of primary pain afferents releases the neurotransmitter, substance P; however, the simultaneous stimulation of the descending serotoninergic pathway blocks this release. Naloxone prevents this blockade. These findings are consistent with opioid peptide–containing interneurons of the substantia gelatinosa inhibiting the release of substance P by the primary afferent neurons. This inhibition by the interneurons is through primary afferent depolarization (PAD).

Only two thirds of the descending projections from the NRM are serotoninergic, and peptides (substance P and TRH) colocalize in most of the terminals. These findings are similar to those of the projections from the raphe to the ventral horn discussed in Chapter 5. The remaining third of the projections are peptidergic fibers containing somatostatin, enkephalins, and other peptides, either singly or in combination.

DESCENDING ADRENERGIC ANALGESIC PATHWAY

In addition to the serotoninergic-opioid peptide analgesic system, an adrenergic analgesic pathway projects from the reticular formation to the spinal cord. *Adrenergic neurons* in the *dorsolateral pontine reticular formation* descend in the dorsolateral portion of the lateral funiculus of the spinal cord and end in the *substantia gelatinosa*. The norepinephrine receptors in the dorsal horn are primarily of the α_2-type. Stimulation of this descending adrenergic pathway inhibits the nociceptive relay neurons in lamina V and the analgesia produced is insensitive to naloxone, indicating an absence of opioid peptides in this pathway. The neurochemical transmitter of the interneurons relaying the signal from laminae II and III to lamina V is unknown, although gamma-aminobutyric acid (GABA) is a leading candidate. Collaterals from the descending adrenergic system also inhibit the serotoninergic projection neurons in the NRM (see Fig. 10–25).

REGULATION OF DESCENDING ANALGESIC PATHWAYS

Both analgesic pathways originate in the brain stem reticular formation. This central core of nuclei receives collaterals from descending motor systems. Sensory pathways have direct spinoreticular projections, and collaterals from the ascending spinothalamic tract end in the reticular formation. This includes the PAG and intrala-

minar nuclei of the thalamus. In addition, the cerebral cortex, limbic system, and hypothalamus have rich projections to the reticular formation.

The basic circuitry is available for reflex, conscious, behavioral, and autonomic influences on the modulation of nociceptive signals. All these systems probably influence the basal level of activity of these nociceptive pathways, with the degree of modulation the sum of their relative contributions.

GENERAL ASPECTS OF DESCENDING ANALGESIC PATHWAYS

At this time, a consensus has been made on several points.

1. Medial areas of the rostral medullary reticular formation (NRM and NGC) form a descending serotoninergic-opioid peptide modulatory pathway. Although opioid peptide neurons from the PAG project to these reticular formation nuclei, they are not the final path to the spinal cord.

2. The dorsolateral pontine reticular formation forms a descending adrenergic modulatory pathway, a nonopioid peptide pathway.

3. The modulatory pathways project to all levels of the spinal cord and descend in the dorsolateral portion of the lateral funiculus.

4. No single neurotransmitter is totally responsible for the serotoninergic-opioid peptide pathway.

Clinical Correlations

A knowledge of the different somatosensory pathways and their divergent courses through the spinal cord and brain stem is needed for the localization and assessment of damage to the CNS. Many of the correlations discussed subsequently involve other functional systems. However, this discussion is limited to the somatosensory components included in this chapter.

DORSAL ROOT AND PERIPHERAL NERVE INJURY

Damage to either a dorsal root or a peripheral nerve interrupts all modalities of somatosensory information. The sensory deficits from damage to either a dorsal root or a spinal nerve always follow a segmental pattern. In comparison, peripheral nerve damage may involve portions of several spinal segments. Compare the dermatome and cutaneous nerve distributions in Figures 6–5 and 6–6. The peripheral fields of both spinal and peripheral nerves overlap with those of the adjacent segments or nerves. Because of this, it is difficult to detect deficits from the loss of a single dorsal root or spinal nerve. The deficits from the loss of a cutaneous nerve are more restricted than those illustrated. Irritative lesions to a dorsal root or peripheral nerve often produce a burning and tingling sensation in the area of innervation and are clinically identifiable.

SPINAL CORD INJURY

Different sensory modalities follow separate pathways throughout the spinal cord. Pain and temperature senses ascend in the contralateral ventrolateral quadrant whereas tactile and proprioceptive senses ascend in the ipsilateral dorsal columns.

A classic example of spinal cord injury, although rare in its pure form, is the *Brown-Séquard syndrome*, a *hemisection of the spinal cord*. Because all ascending and descending fibers are severed in the damaged half of the cord, all sensory pathways ascending on the damaged side are affected. One sees a loss of pain and temperature sensation on the contralateral side of the body below the level of the lesion and a loss of tactile and proprioceptive sensation on the ipsilateral side of the body below the level the lesion. In addition, an ipsilateral loss of motor function occurs below the level of the lesion, principally because of the destruction of the corticospinal tract. Because this is an "upper motor neuron" lesion, spastic paralysis of the muscles is involved (see Chapter 15).

In terms of sensory deficit, hemisection of the left half of the cord at T-6, for example, produces a loss of pain and temperature sense on the right side of the body below T-6 and a loss of tactile and proprioceptive sense on the left side of the body below T-6. More restrictive lesions of the cord will reduce the deficits accordingly, e.g., damage to the left ventral quadrant produces only a contralateral loss of pain and temperature sense, with tactile and proprioceptive sense intact.

In some diseases, *syringomyelia* for example, a cavitation of the central gray of the spinal cord occurs. This disease is characterized by a bilateral loss of pain and temperature sense for all spinal segments involved, because the lesion destroys the ventral white commissure containing the crossing spinothalamic fibers from both sides but

spares most of the fibers already ascending in the white matter. If the cavitation extends from C-4 through C-8, a total loss of pain and temperature sense takes place in both arms, except for the inner surface of the arm innervated by upper thoracic segments. All proprioceptive and tactile sense would be intact. As the disease progresses, the cavitation increases in the rostrocaudal axis and involves more spinal segments. In the later stages, it extends laterally and involves the somatic motor columns and the symptoms increase accordingly.

Occlusion of the *anterior spinal artery* may spare both major ascending sensory pathways in the spinal cord but involves both medial lemnisci in the lower medulla (see Fig. 9–12). Occlusion of one *posterior spinal artery* damages the dorsal column pathways and usually involves the ALS as well. At the spinal level, this effect produces an ipsilateral loss of tactile and proprioceptive sense and a contralateral loss of pain and temperature sense. In the lower medulla, only the dorsal columns and dorsal column nuclei are affected. The spinothalamic tract is spared.

BRAIN STEM INJURY

Injuries to the brain stem usually involve one or more of the cranial nerves and their nuclei. Cranial nerve deficits are very important in localizing and assessing the extent of the damage (see Chapter 19).

The *basilar artery* and its branches are the major blood supply to the ventral portion of the pontine brain stem. With occlusion of the basilar artery, somatosensory losses are limited to the bilateral tactile and proprioceptive losses associated with the medial lemniscus. Often, these are incomplete (see Fig. 9–13). Thrombus of the *posterior inferior cerebellar artery* is a more common clinical problem. The somatosensory deficits involve the spinothalamic tract (contralateral loss of pain and temperature sense) and the descending nucleus and tract of V (ipsilateral loss of pain, temperature, and tactile sense to the face), with a sparing of tactile and proprioceptive senses from spinal levels (see Fig. 9–12).

INJURY TO THE SOMATOSENSORY CORTEX

Discrete lesions involving only the postcentral gyrus are rare. Thrombi of the *middle cerebral artery* or one or more of its branches are more common (see Fig. 9–11). Damage to *S-I* results in a contralateral loss of two-point discrimination, stereognosis, vibratory and position sense, and a loss of texture discrimination. Pain and temperature sense loss is minimal; however, the patient has an inability to localize the stimulus. If *S-II* is selectively damaged with a sparing of S-I, there is little detectable sensory loss. However, higher order somatosensory processing and memory storage of mechanoreceptive information are impaired. All deficits due to cortical damage are contralateral and usually accompanied with motor deficits owing to the close proximity of the motor cortex.

SUGGESTED READING

Fields, H. L. and J.-M. Besson (Editors) (1988). *Pain Modulation. Progress in Brain Research*, Vol. 77. Elsevier Publishing Company, Amsterdam.

A current account of the modulation of nociceptive systems, in particular the pathways and their neurochemical properties. In addition, this volume contains assessments of some clinical approaches to pain control.

Kaas, J. H. (1990). The somatosensory system. In *The Human Nervous System*. G. Paxinos (Editor). Academic Press, New York.

An excellent review of somatosensory systems in humans by one of the leaders in the field. This chapter contains an in-depth discussion of thalamic and cortical components. Emphasis is on the mechanoreceptive systems.

Willis, W. D., Jr. (1985). *The Pain System: The Neural Basis of Nociceptive Transmission in the Mammalian Nervous System*. P. L. Gildenberg (Editor). *Pain and Headache Series*, Volumne 8. S. Karger, Basel.

This monograph, by one of the foremost researchers in the field, is an overview of nociceptive transmission systems. Pain, and in particular chronic pain, is a poorly understood sensory modality. In this monograph, developments of the last 15 to 20 years are compiled and the state of knowledge is assessed. An excellent background for the rational treatment of both chronic and acute pain.

Chapter

11

Visual Pathways

THE EYE
INFORMATION PROCESSING IN THE NEURAL RETINA
RETINOGENICULOCALCARINE TRACT
VISUAL CORTEX
INFORMATION PROCESSING IN THE VISUAL CORTEX
TECTAL AND PRETECTAL CONNECTIONS
VISUAL REFLEXES
CLINICAL CORRELATIONS

The visual system is one of three sensory systems designated *special somatic afferent* (*SSA*), a special sensory system innervating structures of somatic origin. The receptor organ, the *eye*, is both an optical instrument designed to focus an image of the visual world on a "screen" of sensitive photoreceptors, and an information processing station within the central nervous system (CNS). Some of these very sensitive receptors can respond to stimuli as small as a *single* photon of light.

In the *retina*, stimulation from light activates the *rods* and *cones* with the production of electrical signals. These signals are further processed or integrated by other cells of the retina. Axons from *retinal ganglion cells* relay these signals as action potentials via the *optic nerves* and *optic tracts* to the brain stem, principally to the *lateral geniculate nuclei*, the *superior colliculi*, and the *pretectal area*. Although we traditionally call the optic nerve a "nerve," in reality, it is a tract within the CNS (Fig. 11–1).

The *lateral geniculate nuclei*, part of the dorsal thalamus, project visual information to the *primary visual cortex* (*V-1*)—also called the *calcarine cortex, striate cortex*, or *Brodmann's area 17*. The visual pathways maintain a very high degree of topography from the retina to the cortex. Although the cortical representation of the visual field is not linear, i.e., the central or foveal area of the retina has a greater representation than the periphery, the brain perceives these signals as the *visual image* of the surrounding environment with which we are all familiar. Additional visual signals from the retina by-pass the lateral geniculate nucleus, terminating in the superior colliculus for *somatic reflexes* and in the pretectal area for *autonomic reflexes* (see Fig. 11–1).

The visual pathways extend the entire anteroposterior length of the brain, from the retina of the eye to the primary visual cortex at the occipital pole of the cerebrum. An understanding of the visual system and of the specific deficits resulting from damage to selected portions of this system can be important to the localization of neurological damage.

224

FIGURE 11-1

The visual pathways are superimposed on the ventral surface of the cerebrum. The principal pathways from the retina to the primary visual cortex and from the retina to the tectum of the midbrain are illustrated. (- - - - -), Fibers carrying visual information from the right visual hemifield; (_____), fibers carrying visual information from the left visual hemifield. Note the anteroposterior extent of the visual pathway, from the retina (eye) to the primary visual cortex at the occipital pole of the cerebrum. See text for discussion.

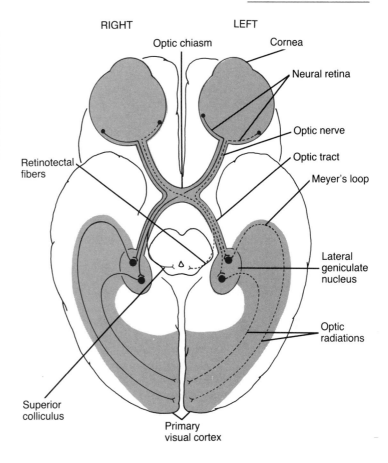

RIGHT   LEFT

Optic chiasm — Cornea

Neural retina

Retinotectal fibers

Optic nerve

Optic tract

Meyer's loop

Lateral geniculate nucleus

Optic radiations

Superior colliculus

Primary visual cortex

The Eye

ANATOMY

Anatomically, the eye resembles a spherical camera with an autofocus lens, a diaphragm (iris), and a light-sensitive film (neural retina). The *retina* develops from the *optic vesicle*, an outgrowth of the diencephalon, and is part of the CNS. The *lens* develops from *ectoderm* overlying the optic vesicle (see Chapter 1 and Fig. 1–24).

The receptors (*rods* and *cones*) and the other neuronal elements of the retina (*bipolar cells, horizontal cells, amacrine cells,* and *retinal ganglion cells*) differentiate from the inner or *neural portion* the retina, and the *pigmented layer* differentiates from the outer retinal layer. During the formation of the meninges, the mesoderm surrounding the optic stalk and optic vesicle differentiates into the *sclera* and *choroid layers* of the eye. In the anterior portion of the eye, the sclera becomes the clear, transparent *cornea* and, more peripherally, the choroid layer thickens to form the *ciliary body*. A cavity filled with clear

fluid forms between the cornea and lens, the *anterior (aqueous) chamber of the eye.* The central cavity of the optic cup becomes filled with a thick, gelatinous, but clear, material known as the *vitreous humor* (Fig. 11–2).

The *pupillary membrane* differentiates from the mesoderm over the anterior surface of the lens. In later development, the anterior portion of the early retina grows over the inner surface of the pupillary membrane. Together this combination of retinal neuroectoderm and mesoderm forms the *iris*. A series of circumferentially arrayed fibers suspend the lens from the ciliary body, the *zonula ciliaris,* or simply, the *suspensory ligaments* (see Fig. 11–2).

Changes in tension on the suspensory ligaments alter the thickness of the lens, providing a mechanism for focusing the eye on objects at varying distances. Smooth muscles differentiate in the ciliary body near the origin of the suspensory ligaments. When these muscles contract (most are circumferential), easing tension on the suspensory ligaments, the lens rounds up because of its inherent elasticity. This increase in convex-

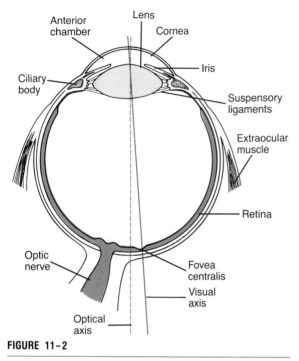

FIGURE 11-2

A horizontal section through the human eye at the level of the optic nerve. Both the optical and the visual axes are indicated. See text for discussion.

ity focuses the eye on nearer objects. When the ciliary muscles relax, increasing tension on the suspensory ligaments, the lens becomes less convex, focusing the eye on distant objects.

With further development, circumferential and radial smooth muscles extend into the pupillary membrane (the *iris*) and control the diameter of the *pupil*. The iris functions much as the diaphragm of a camera lens, adapting the eye to conditions of increased or decreased light, through pupillary constriction and pupillary dilatation, respectively. The diameter of the pupil also affects the depth of field much like the diaphragm of a camera lens. The larger the diameter is, the shorter the depth of field; the smaller, the greater the depth of field. Under bright conditions and a constricted pupil, the depth of field is greater than under darker conditions and a dilated pupil.

The *extraocular muscles* differentiate from the mesoderm surrounding the eye. *Cranial nerves III, IV,* and *VI* (the *oculomotor, trochlear,* and *abducens nerves*) innervate these six striated muscles attached to the sclera. The extraocular muscles move the eye through complex saccadic and tracking movements. The *eyelids* differentiate

from the mesoderm and ectoderm overlying the cornea.

OPTICS: VISUAL FIELDS AND RETINAL FIELDS

A line drawn through the center of the cornea to the posterior portion of the retina, marking the central axis of the eye, represents the *optical axis* (*anatomical axis*). A line drawn through the center of the pupil to the *fovea centralis* of the *macula* (the region of greatest visual acuity) represents the *visual axis*.

Two terms utilized in reference to vision are *visual field* and *retinal field*. The *visual field* is what is observed, the outside world, whereas the *retinal field* is the optical image of the outside world as projected on the retina. These distinctions are important, and their significance will become clear. The optics of the eye, as we have said, are much like a camera. The eye reverses and inverts the visual image projected on the retina, and the *retinal image* is the reverse of the *visual image*. What appears in the upper right quadrant of the visual field will be in the lower left quadrant of the retinal field (Fig. 11-3). In Figure 11-3, it is noted that humans have binocular vision. Most of the visual field projects to the retinae of both eyes. However, the peripheral (lateral) portions of the visual field project only to the retina of one eye. The peripheral portions of the visual field seen only by one eye are the *monocular zones*; the more central portion of the visual field seen by both eyes is the *binocular zone* (see Fig. 11-3).

NEURAL RETINA

The neural retina contains five principal types of neurons: the *photoreceptor cells* (*rods* and *cones*), *bipolar cells, horizontal cells, amacrine cells,* and *retinal ganglion cells.* Each group can be further subdivided on the basis of morphological or functional differences. Although some workers recognize six principal types (the sixth being an *interplexiform amacrine cell*), the traditional classification with five cell types is sufficient. Major subdivisions within the cell types are discussed where appropriate.

The *photoreceptors* transduce light stimuli into electrical signals that are relayed to the *bipolar cells* and then to the *retinal ganglion cells.* Axons of retinal ganglion cells then relay this information to other areas of the CNS, the *lateral genic-*

FIGURE 11–3

The relation of visual fields to retinal fields. The visual field is divided into four cross-hatched quadrants (top of illustration). The retinal field (the image of the visual field projected on each retina) is illustrated in the lower portion of the diagram for both left and right eyes. The foveal area is represented by the circle.

The shaded area of the visual field is the area of binocular vision; the unshaded area is the area of monocular vision. Note the complete reversal of the visual field on the retina. The optics are similar to those of a camera. See text for discussion.

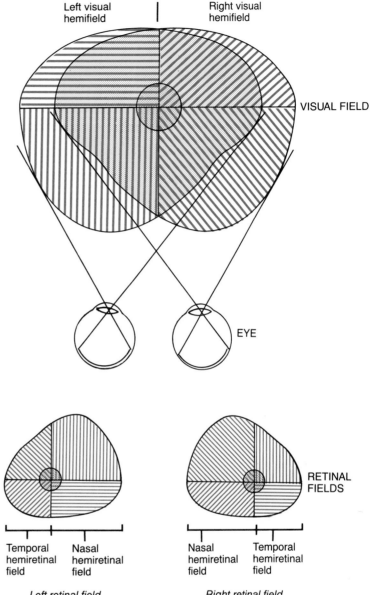

Left retinal field   Right retinal field

---

ulate nucleus of the diencephalon and the *superior colliculus* of the midbrain, via the *optic nerve*.

However, as part of the CNS, the retina is more than a relay station for visual stimuli. It functions as a miniature "brain." Here, the analogy between the eye and the camera ends. *Horizontal cells* and *amacrine cells* function as interneurons, modulating and integrating the activity of photoreceptors, bipolar cells, and ganglion cells. The resultant pattern of signals from the ganglion cells represents a complicated array of visual information, very much transformed from the initial excitation signal of the photoreceptor. These signals leave the retina in the optic nerve as parallel streams of information. Often, many ganglion cells carry signals that represent different receptive field properties derived from the excitation of the same photoreceptor.

A photomicrograph of the human retina illustrates the laminar organization of the neural elements (Fig. 11–4). The outer layer is the *photoreceptor layer*, containing the outer and inner segments of the rods and cones. This layer is separated from the *outer nuclear layer*, which

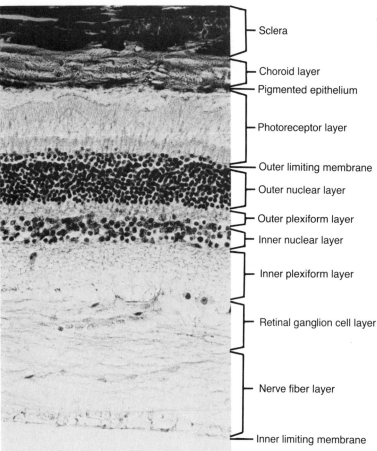

Sclera

Choroid layer

Pigmented epithelium

Photoreceptor layer

Outer limiting membrane

Outer nuclear layer

Outer plexiform layer

Inner nuclear layer

Inner plexiform layer

Retinal ganglion cell layer

Nerve fiber layer

Inner limiting membrane

FIGURE 11-4

Photomicrograph of the human retina illustrating the principal layers.

contains the nuclei and cell bodies of the rods and cones, by the *outer limiting membrane* (a glial membrane, see subsequent discussion). Immediately beneath the outer nuclear layer is a lamina of neuropil, the *outer plexiform layer*, containing synaptic connections principally between photoreceptor, bipolar, and horizontal cells. The *inner nuclear layer* contains the nuclei and cell bodies of bipolar, horizontal, and amacrine cells. The *inner plexiform layer*, another lamina of neuropil, contains synaptic connections between bipolar, amacrine, and retinal ganglion cells. The *ganglion cell layer* contains the cell bodies of the multipolar retinal ganglion cells, and the *nerve fiber layer* contains the axons of the retinal ganglion cells that form the optic nerve. The innermost layer of the neural retina is the *internal limiting membrane*, a glial membrane separating the neural retina from the vitreous humor.

In addition to neurons, the neural retina also contains glia. The *Müller cells* are glial elements unique to the retina. Processes from these cells form the inner and outer limiting membranes, comparable to the glial membrane covering the surface of the rest of the brain beneath the pia mater. The long, slender Müller cells span the neural retina. Their terminal processes spread out and contact the processes of other Müller cells to form the inner and outer limiting membranes (Fig. 11–5). In addition to the Müller cell, the retina also contains astrocytes.

Axons of retinal ganglion cells in the nerve fiber layer pass along the inner surface of the retina toward the *optic disc*, where they exit to form the *optic nerve (cranial nerve II)*. No photoreceptors are found at the optic disc, producing a *blind spot* just to the nasal side of the fovea (see Fig. 11–2). Because the blind spot is in the binocular field of vision, one normally is not aware of it.

In order for light to excite the outer segment of

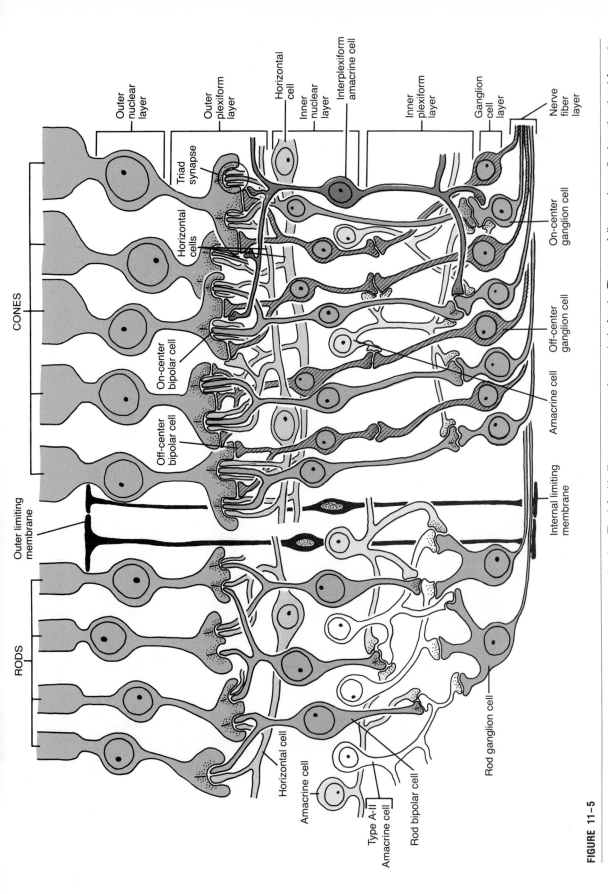

FIGURE 11-5

Some of the principal cell types and connections in the neural retina. The left side illustrates connections typical of rods. The type A-II amacrine cell relays the signal from the rod bipolar cell to the retinal ganglion cell. In general, the circuitry for the rod system is convergent. Müller cells (in black), specialized glial cells found in the retina, have processes that form the inner and outer limiting membranes.

In the outer plexiform layer, cones form invaginated triad synapses with processes of on-center bipolar and horizontal cells and surface synapses with off-center bipolar cells. In separate laminae of the inner plexiform layer, on-center and off-center bipolar cells synapse with on-center and off-center ganglion cells as well as with amacrine cells. Interplexiform amacrine cells synapse in both the inner and outer plexiform layers.

Axons from retinal ganglion cells form the nerve fiber layer as they converge on the optic disc to form the optic nerve. See text for details.

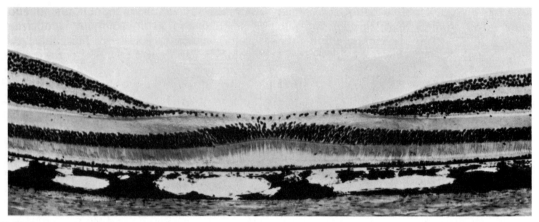

FIGURE 11-6

Photomicrograph of the fovea of a macaque retina showing the marked reduction in thickness in this area of maximal visual acuity. (Courtesy of H. Mizoguchi. Reproduced with permission from D. W. Fawcett, *A Textbook of Histology*, 11th Edition. W. B. Saunders Co., Philadelphia, 1986.)

a photoreceptor, it must pass through all layers of the retina—from the inner limiting membrane through the outer limiting membrane—to the light-sensitive photoreceptor layer. The central area of the retina, the *macula*, is an area of greater visual acuity and color vision and is suited for light-adapted or *photopic vision*. Within the macula, the *fovea centralis* is the area of

maximum visual acuity. At the fovea, the inner layers of the retina are displaced peripherally and light reaches the photoreceptors directly, without passing through other retinal cells and blood vessels (Fig. 11-6). Rods from peripheral portions of the retina *converge* on retinal ganglion cells, whereas cones from the macula do not. Therefore, peripheral portions of the retina are

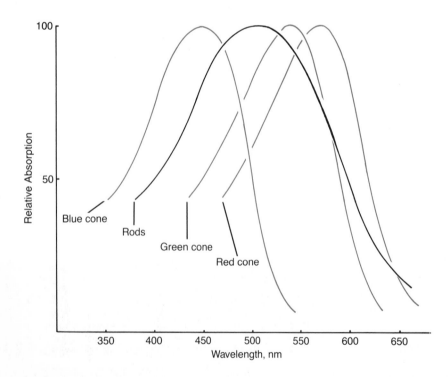

FIGURE 11-7

Curves for the absorption spectra for rods and three types of cones found in the human retina. Rods have a maximum sensitivity at 496 nm; blue-sensitive cones, at 420 nm; green-sensitive cones, at 531 nm; and red-sensitive cones, at 558 nm. All four curves are normalized to a maximum absorption value of 100. Note that spectra for cones = red; rods = black.

more sensitive to light but lack high visual acuity. This area is more suited for dark-adapted or *scotopic vision.*

Photoreceptors

The human retina contains two basic types of photoreceptors: *rods* and *cones.* A broad band of electromagnetic radiation, wavelengths from 390 to 770 nm and a peak at 496 nm, excites the rods (Fig. 11–7). Wavelength sensitivity is due to the physical properties of the photopigment, *rhodopsin.* Cones, in comparison, contain one of three different visual pigments called *opsins.* The opsins have maximum wavelength sensitivities of 420, 531, or 558 nm. The absorption properties of the three opsin proteins impart the spectral sensitivity to the particular cone cells (see Fig.

11–7). Thus, we can refer to the rods as *monochromatic,* containing one type of photopigment, and the cones collectively as *trichromatic,* each containing one of three types of photopigment. In the retina, there are over 100 million rods and nearly 10 million cones. Cones concentrate in but are not limited to the fovea of the retina; rods are absent from the fovea.

The outer segment of the rod is longer than that of the cone and contains a higher concentration of photopigment, rendering it more efficient at capturing light. The rods, in general, converge on the bipolar cells. This convergent circuitry increases the number of rods driving a single bipolar cell, thereby increasing the response of the bipolar cell during low levels of light. This increased sensitivity is at the expense of visual acuity—the loss of acuity is directly proportional

FIGURE 11–8

The fine structure of the rod and cone. Each rod and cone photoreceptor has four divisions: (1) outer segment, (2) inner segment, (3) cell body, and (4) synaptic terminal. Both the outer and inner segments of the photoreceptor are situated outside the outer limiting membrane of the retina.

The *outer segment* is the sensory transducer and contains numerous membranous discs with the molecular machinery for phototransduction. The discs in the rods become separated from the outer cell membrane and float free within the outer segment, whereas those of the cone do not.

The *inner segment* contains numerous mitochondria and the biosynthetic systems. The inner segment of the cone is thicker and contains many more mitochondria than that of the rod. The outer segment is connected to the inner segment at the neck, containing a characteristic cilium, and one or more cytoplasmic bridges.

The *cell body* is located in the outer nuclear layer and contains the nucleus and other cell organelles.

The *synaptic terminals,* located in the outer plexiform layer, make contact with bipolar and horizontal cells.

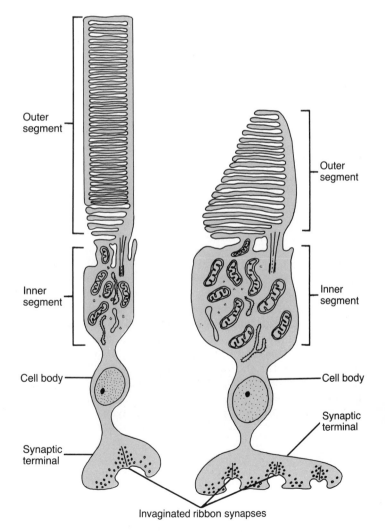

Outer segment

Outer segment

Inner segment

Inner segment

Cell body

Cell body

Synaptic terminal

Synaptic terminal

Invaginated ribbon synapses

to the number of rods converging on the bipolar cell.

The very regular array of stacked discs in the outer segments of both photoreceptors contains the appropriate photopigment. These discs form from an infolding of the cell membrane at the basal portion of the outer segment. A continuous turnover of these discs takes place, with new ones constantly formed and old ones sloughed from the distal part of the distal segment. Characteristic of the rods is a total separation of the disc from the external cell membrane, in the more distal portions of the outer segment. The discs in the cones always remain as an invagination of the cell membrane (Fig. 11–8). The adjacent pigmented epithelium is phagocytic and removes the discs sloughed by the photoreceptors. Cell bodies and nuclei of both types of photoreceptors are in the outer nuclear layer. The central process of the photoreceptor extends into the outer plexiform layer, where it makes synaptic contact with bipolar and horizontal cells. Characteristic of photoreceptors are the invaginated synaptic terminals and the "ribbon" synapse (see Fig. 11–8).

SENSORY TRANSDUCTION

Unlike many other receptors and neurons, the rods, when not stimulated by light (dark adapted), are in a constant state of excitation (*partially depolarized* or *hypopolarized*, with a resting potential near -30 mV). Cation channels, principally Na^+ channels, are in a constant state of activation. A continuous influx of Na^+ ions, in combination with the Na^+ pump, produces a constant Na^+ current (Fig. 11–9). The energy of a single photon will trigger the *cis-trans* photoisomerization of the *retinal* contained in a single molecule of the visual pigment, *rhodopsin*. This effect, through a sequence of molecular events, leads to the closure of hundreds of Na^+ channels, blocking the influx of more than 10^6 ions of Na^+. Closing these channels *hyperpolarizes* the membrane and increases the internal negativity of the receptor. At saturating levels of light, the resting potential may approach -90 mV, near the equilibrium potential for K^+.

The photoisomerization of retinal activates a second messenger system through a specific *G-protein*, *transducin*, in the plasma membrane of discs in the rod's outer segment. The activation of *transducin* is similar to the activation of other G-proteins discussed in Chapter 5. The *photoexcited rhodopsin* catalyzes the *guanosine triphosphate-guanosine diphosphate* (*GTP-GDP*)

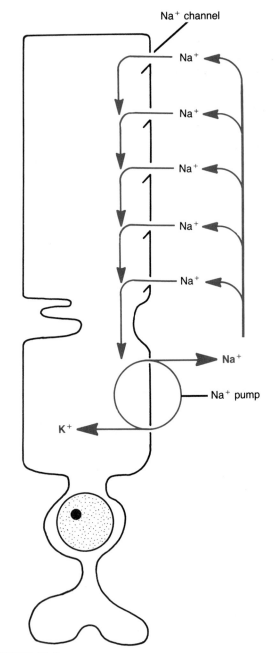

FIGURE 11-9

The dark-adapted photoreceptor is partially depolarized. Open sodium channels in the outer segment allow sodium to flow into the cell, along its electrochemical gradient. The active, ATP-dependent, sodium pumps in the inner segment move the sodium out of the cell and provide the driving force for the sodium current. When photoactivated, the sodium channels of the outer segment close, reducing the sodium current and hyperpolarizing the cell.

exchange in transducin, forming the active α-subunit, *transducin_α-GTP*. Transducin_α-GTP, in turn, activates *cyclic guanosine monophosphate (cGMP)-phosphodiesterase*, leading to the rapid hydrolysis of *cGMP* and the closure of the Na+ channels. The intrinsic *GTPase* activity of the transducin α-subunit converts transducin_α-GTP to the inactive transducin_α-GDP. The latter immediately binds with the *β-* and *γ-subunits*, reforming *transducin-GDP* (Fig. 11–10). Without activated cGMP-phosphodiesterase, cGMP levels increase, reactivating the Na+ channels and restoring the receptor to the "resting" state of depolarization. Although not studied as extensively, the molecular mechanism for sensory transduction in cones appears similar to that in rods.

Information Processing in the Neural Retina

RECEPTIVE FIELDS OF VISUAL SYSTEM NEURONS

The term *receptive field* describes a physiological property of individual neurons. For the visual system, *the receptive field of an individual neuron, at any level of the system, is that area of the retina which, when stimulated by light, leads to a change in the electrical properties of that neuron.* For neurons capable of generating action potentials, this is an increase (excitation) or a decrease (inhibition) in the firing rate; for neurons that do not generate an action potential (photoreceptors

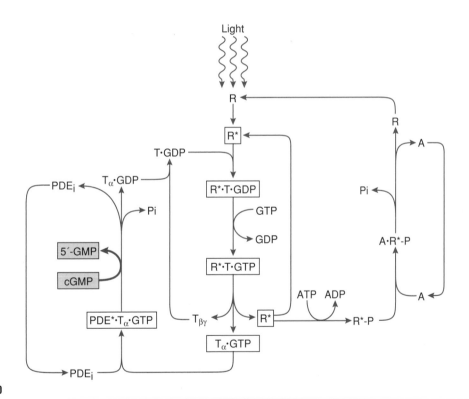

FIGURE 11–10

The molecular cycle for photoactivation of cyclic guanosine monophosphate (cGMP)-phosphodiesterase through the G-protein, *transducin-guanosine diphosphate* (T · GDP). Light striking the *rhodopsin (R)* converts it to the active form, *R**. Photoactivated rhodopsin binds to *transducin-GDP* (T · GDP), forming the *R* · T · GDP* complex. Guanosine triphosphate (GTP) rapidly displaces the GDP bound to the complex forming *R* · T · GTP*. This short-lived complex forms the inactive transducin subunit complex (T_{β,γ}), *R** (free to bind with another T · GDP), and the active α-subunit of this G-protein, T_α · GTP.

T_α · GTP, in combination with the inactive, cGMP phosphodiesterase (PDE_i), forms the enzymatically active *PDE* · T_α · GTP* complex. This active form of the diesterase converts *cGMP* to the inactive *5'-GMP*, which rapidly reduces the level of the active messenger for sodium channel activation, *cGMP*.

The intrinsic GTPase of T_α inactivates *PDE* · T_α · GTP*, with the formation of *PDE_i* and T_α · GDP. The last rapidly combines with T_{β,γ} re-forming T · GDP.

Rhodopsin kinase and subsequent binding of a capping protein, arrestin (A), lead to the inactivation of *R**.

and bipolar, horizontal, and amacrine cells), this is an increase or a decrease in the membrane potential.

OUTER PLEXIFORM LAYER AND CENTER-SURROUND ANTAGONISM

The direct flow of visual information in the retina is from the photoreceptor to the bipolar cell and to the retinal ganglion cell. However, these streams or channels of signals do not operate in isolation. The activity of one channel is continually modulated by the activity of neighboring or surrounding channels, a modulation known as *center-surround antagonism*. In the processing of visual information, the first site of

this modulation is the outer plexiform layer. This involves the *photoreceptors*, *bipolar cells*, and *horizontal cells*.

When a single photoreceptor is stimulated, the signal travels both *transversely*, through the retina via the bipolar cell, and *laterally*, in a radial fashion, via horizontal cells. The horizontal cells interact with neighboring photoreceptors and their associated bipolar cells. This interaction alters their subsequent response to photostimulation. Briefly, stimulation of a photoreceptor modulates the transmission of visual information in surrounding channels. Similarly, stimulation of surrounding photoreceptors modulates the response of the central photoreceptor. A very simplified schematic illustrates this precept (Fig. 11–11).

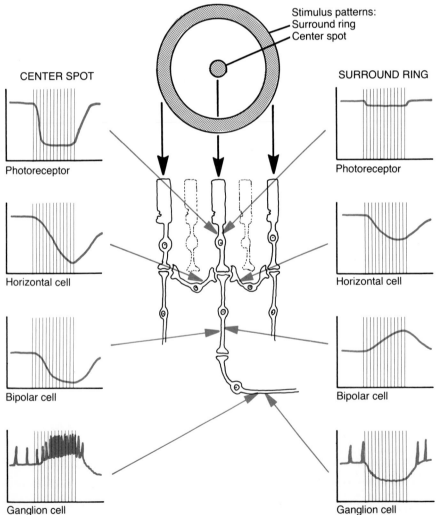

CENTER SPOT

Photoreceptor

Horizontal cell

Bipolar cell

Ganglion cell

Stimulus patterns:
Surround ring
Center spot

SURROUND RING

Photoreceptor

Horizontal cell

Bipolar cell

Ganglion cell

FIGURE 11–11

The mechanism for center-surround antagonism. This simplified diagram illustrates the interactions among photoreceptors, horizontal cells, bipolar cells, and ganglion cells. At the top is an illustration of the two light patterns used as stimuli, a center spot and a surround ring or annulus. Charts at the left are the changes in membrane potentials during a center spot stimulus to the central photoreceptor.

On the right are charts from the same cells during a surround ring stimulus. Shaded areas on the charts indicate periods of stimulation. Note that only the ganglion cell generates action potentials. See text for details.

When a test spot of light stimulates a single photoreceptor and the surrounding area of the retina is dark, the photoreceptor, bipolar cell, and horizontal cell all become hyperpolarized. The retinal ganglion cell responds with a burst of action potentials (Fig. 11–11, *left*). If, however, an annulus or ring of light stimulates the surrounding photoreceptors, and the center photoreceptor remains in the dark, the response of the horizontal cells—synapsing with both center and surround photoreceptors—is attenuated and the bipolar cell is depolarized. This effect leads to an inhibition of the retinal ganglion cell and a movement of the membrane potential away from the threshold for firing (Fig. 11–11, *right*). This *center-surround antagonism* results from the interaction of *horizontal cells*, *bipolar cells*, and *photoreceptors* in the *outer plexiform layer*.

Real visual space does not contain artificial points of light stimulating single photoreceptors nor rings of light selectively stimulating their surround; however, these laboratory findings provide needed insight into the nature of signal modulation at the level of the outer plexiform layer. Horizontal cells are constantly modulating the sensitivity of all retinal photoreceptors and their associated bipolar cells.

When using a camera, we adjust the exposure settings to the sensitivity of the film. In the eye, horizontal cells continually adjust the response range and sensitivity of the photoreceptors and bipolar cells to the overall light intensity in their part of the visual field. This "fine tunes" individual photoreceptors, viewing different areas of the visual scene, to local luminance conditions. Thus, *center-surround antagonism* optimizes contrast and resolution and dynamically adjusts the sensitivity range of the individual photoreceptors. These modulations of the visual signal are important for the detection of boundaries and edges.

ON-CENTER AND OFF-CENTER BIPOLAR CELLS

Each cone synapses with a pair of bipolar cells that respond in opposite directions to the release of the same neurotransmitter by the photoreceptor. *On-center bipolar cells* are *inhibited* by transmitter release and *off-center bipolar cells* are *excited* by the transmitter. *Remember, excitation of the photoreceptor by light hyperpolarizes the cell, causing it to release less neurotransmitter.* Thus, cones stimulated by light release less neurotransmitter, resulting in the *dis-inhibition of on-center cells* and the *de-facilitation of off-center cells*. The

result is that cones have a dual system of bipolar cells, transmitting parallel but opposite signals to their respective ganglion cells, the *on-center ganglion cells* and *off-center ganglion cells* (see Fig. 11–5).

No on-center and off-center bipolar cells exist for the rods. Characteristically, one rod bipolar cell receives synaptic input from more than one rod, a convergent pattern that increases sensitivity at the expense of acuity. Another difference between the rod and cone systems is the lack of a direct synapse between rod bipolar cells and retinal ganglion cells. The rod system utilizes a specific type of *amacrine cell* (*type A-II*) as an interneuron between bipolar and ganglion cells (see Fig. 11–5).

PHOTORECEPTOR SYNAPSES

The presynaptic terminals of the cone photoreceptors have one or more invaginated *ribbon synapses*. Each invagination usually contains three postsynaptic processes (the *triad*), two from horizontal cells and one from an on-center bipolar cell. The flat surfaces of cone presynaptic terminals make synaptic contact with the postsynaptic elements of off-center bipolar cells (see Fig. 11–5). Occasionally, ribbon synapses are found in the inner plexiform layer between bipolar presynaptic elements and postsynaptic terminals of ganglion and amacrine cells. The synaptic junctions between rod photoreceptors and bipolar and horizontal cells are similar to the invaginated synaptic junctions of the cone (see Fig. 11–5).

The mechanism of neurotransmitter release by photoreceptors differs from the traditional chemical transmission discussed in Chapters 4 and 5. No action potentials and no threshold potentials exist for the release of transmitter. Neurotransmitter is constantly being released, maximally by the dark-adapted photoreceptor and minimally by the light-saturated photoreceptor. Very small changes in the membrane potential of the photoreceptor alter the amount of transmitter released. Horizontal, bipolar, and amacrine cells behave in a similar fashion. Retinal ganglion cells, however, generate an action potential.

INNER PLEXIFORM LAYER

The *inner plexiform layer* is the final stage of visual information processing in the retina. Here, too, information flows both *transversely*, from bipolar cells to the retinal ganglion cells, and *laterally* (radially), via *amacrine cells*, the interneuron of the inner plexiform layer.

Based on anatomical and physiological criteria and neurotransmitter localization, at least 20 distinct populations of amacrine cells exist. Amacrine cells probably are the single most important cell type in processing and modulating visual information. Although the circuitry of the inner plexiform layer is much more complex than that of the outer plexiform layer, several generalizations can be made about amacrine cell function.

Most amacrine cells modulate the flow of information between bipolar cells and retinal ganglion cells. The basic pattern of radial organization, with *center-surround interactions*, described for the horizontal cells applies to many amacrine cell functions. However, instead of center-surround antagonism, one population of amacrine cells has a role in movement detection and directional selectivity. Others, organized in a similar center-surround pattern, are important in the processing of color information, especially color contrast.

Amacrine cells containing inhibitory neurotransmitters, either *gamma-aminobutyric acid* (*GABA*) or *glycine*, are essential in mediating ganglion cell responses that involve color contrast, movement detection, and selectivity for direction or size. In contrast, *cholinergic* amacrine cells increase the overall level of retinal ganglion cell excitability and counter the GABA-mediated and glycine-mediated responses.

Several suborders of organization exist within the inner plexiform layer. For example, off-center bipolar cells synapse with off-center ganglion cells in the outer portion of the inner plexiform layer, *sublamina A*; on-center bipolar cells synapse with on-center ganglion cells in the inner portion, *sublamina B*. Additional anatomical and neurochemical properties are employed to subdivide the inner plexiform layer into as many as five strata.

A special class of amacrine cell (*type A-II*) functions as an interneuron between rod bipolar cells and retinal ganglion cells (see Fig. 11–5). Other amacrine cells containing the monoamines, *dopamine* or *serotonin* (*5-HT*), also are associated with the *rod system*. Dopaminergic amacrine cells further modulate center-surround antagonism and adapt the retina to overall lighter or darker conditions. Rod stimulation drives at least three distinct serotoninergic amacrine cells that appear to increase the signal-to-noise ratio in these pathways. Many of these effects are not direct. At least two receptors for each monoamine are known to exist in the inner plexiform layer, each with opposite, antagonistic postsynaptic responses (e.g., D_1 and D_2 dopamine receptors and 5-HT_{1A} and 5-HT_2 serotonin receptors).

In addition, *interplexiform amacrine cells* project back to the outer plexiform layer, synapsing on both horizontal and bipolar cells. These specialized amacrine cells modulate the horizontal cells' contribution to center-surround antagonism. Dopamine is also the neurotransmitter for these interplexiform amacrine cells (see Fig. 11–5).

RETINAL GANGLION CELLS

Early physiological studies of the cat retina identified three classes of retinal ganglion cell: *X-cells*, *Y-cells*, and *W-cells*, each with different physiological properties and each transmitting different types of visual information to the brain stem. Each class of ganglion cell has a specific morphological correlate and a specific site of termination in the brain stem. A similar pattern exists in primates, including humans.

The *X-cells* have small dendritic fields and medium-size cell bodies and are associated with the transmission of information associated with high acuity vision. Their slow conducting axons terminate principally in laminae 3, 4, 5, and 6 of the lateral geniculate nucleus. Other X-cells project to the pretectal area and are involved in pupillary reflexes.

Y-cells have very large dendritic fields and large cell bodies and are important in the initial analysis of crude form and moving stimuli. Their large diameter, fast conducting axons terminate principally in laminae 1 and 2 of the lateral geniculate nucleus. Either collateral branches of these Y-cells or a separate population of Y-cells project to the superior colliculus.

W-cells, although they have large, expansive dendritic trees, are the smallest of the retinal ganglion cells. W-cells project principally to the superior colliculus and are involved in eye and head movements in response to visual stimuli. These ganglion cells have small diameter, very slow conducting axons.

The retinal ganglion cells are the only neurons of the retina to generate an action potential: the excitation and inhibition of all other neuronal elements of the retina spread passively. Although early physiological and morphological descriptions of retinal ganglion cells identified three classes of ganglion cells, further studies have identified at least 16 distinct types of ganglion cells. Each sends a different type of visual information to the brain stem for further processing.

The stimulation of a photoreceptor can trigger the firing of retinal ganglion cells in direct response to a visual stimulus. However, the parallel processing and integration of these signals in both the outer and inner plexiform layers result in a large number of ganglion cells transmitting different bits of information, in parallel, about the complex properties of the visual scene.

Retinogeniculocalcarine Tract

OPTIC NERVE, CHIASM, AND TRACTS

The axons of retinal ganglion cells (Y-, X-, and W-cells) leave the retina at the *optic disc* and become myelinated, as they form the *optic nerve.* Optic nerve fibers are organized roughly in a retinotopic fashion. Fibers from the superior temporal retinal quadrant are located in the superior lateral quadrant of a cross section of the nerve; inferior nasal quadrant fibers, in the inferior medial quadrant of the nerve. Macular fibers occupy a central position. At the *optic chiasm,* fibers from the nasal quadrants of each retina cross the midline, joining the uncrossed temporal fibers of the opposite side to form the *optic tract.* After crossing in the optic chiasm, fibers from the inferior nasal quadrant turn anteriorly into the optic nerve of the opposite side and then immediately turn back to enter the optic tract (Fig. 11–12). The *optic tracts* now contain fibers from the *contralateral visual hemifield*—i.e., the left optic tract contains fibers from the temporal quadrants of the left retina and from the nasal quadrants of the right retina.

Fibers within the optic tract retain a retinotopic organization as the tract swings laterally and posteriorly around the diencephalon to terminate principally in the *lateral geniculate nucleus* (*LGN*). Some fibers by-pass the LGN and end in the *superior colliculus* or the *pretectal area* of the midbrain. A few bifurcate and end in both the LGN and the midbrain.

LATERAL GENICULATE NUCLEUS (LGN)

The presence of the *LGN* produces an elevation on the posterolateral surface of the dorsal thalamus (see Figs. 7–3 and 7–4). The LGN contains six layers or laminae (seen best in horizontal section); each layer contains a *visuotopic map* of the contralateral visual hemifield (Fig. 11–13).

As the fibers of the optic tract terminate in the LGN, they segregate according to retina of origin. Each of the six layers receives fibers from only the contralateral or ipsilateral eye and not from both. Axons from retinal ganglion cells of the contralateral eye terminate in LGN layers 1, 4, and 6; those from the ipsilateral eye terminate in layers 2, 3, and 5. Because LGN neurons of layers 1 and 2 are large and those of layers 3 through 6 are relatively small, layers 1 and 2 are the *magnocellular layers* and layers 3 through 6, the *parvocellular layers* (see Fig. 11–13). Although not cut in a horizontal plane, the laminated nature of the LGN is apparent in Weigert-stained sections of the human brain stem (see Figs. 7–18 and 7–19).

If the six layers of the LGN were flattened, like a stack of pancakes, the visuotopic maps would be in vertical register. Identical points in the retinal hemifield are stacked one on top of the other (see Fig. 11–13). Of the three types of retinal ganglion cells, the Y-cells and the X-cells both project to the LGN. Y-cells have large dendritic fields in the retina and correspondingly large axonal terminal arbors in the LGN. These fibers end principally in the magnocellular layers. X-cells have small dendritic fields in the retina and have small, well-defined axonal terminal arbors in the LGN. These axons end in the parvocellular layers.

More retinal ganglion cells arise from the central or macular area of the retina than from the more peripheral areas. The *visuotopic maps* of the LGN reflect this differential representation; hence, the macular area occupies a much greater portion of the map than do the peripheral areas of the retina.

Neurons from both the parvocellular and magnocellular layers of the LGN relay visual information to the *primary visual cortex (V-1).* Although the primary function of the LGN is the accurate transmission of visual information from the retina to the primary visual cortex, a second and equally important function is the regulation of the flow of visual information to V-1. A combination of feed-forward and feedback inhibitory circuits, along with extensive corticogeniculate projections, regulate this flow of information.

In the *feed-forward inhibition,* collaterals of retinogeniculate fibers synapse on GABA interneurons that, in turn, inhibit the LGN relay neurons (see Fig. 4–10*B*). In the *feedback inhibition,* collaterals from LGN relay neurons synapse with inhibitory (GABA) neurons in the reticular nucleus of the thalamus that, in turn, project

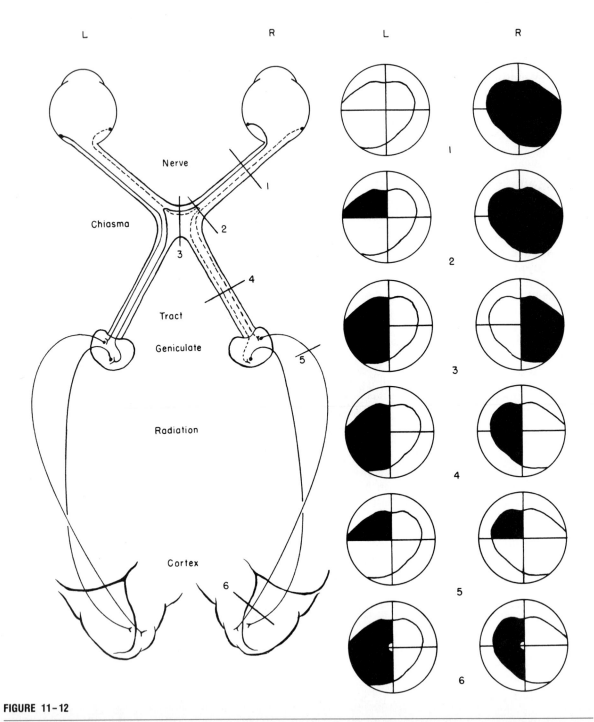

FIGURE 11-12

Visual field defects with interruptions of visual pathways at various levels. Corresponding numbers are used at the site of the lesion and on the field defect. In the lesion at 5, only the most ventral (in temporal lobe) fibers have been severed. See text for details. (Reproduced with permission from T. L. Peele, *The Neuroanatomical Basis for Clinical Neurology*, 3rd Edition. McGraw-Hill, New York, 1977.)

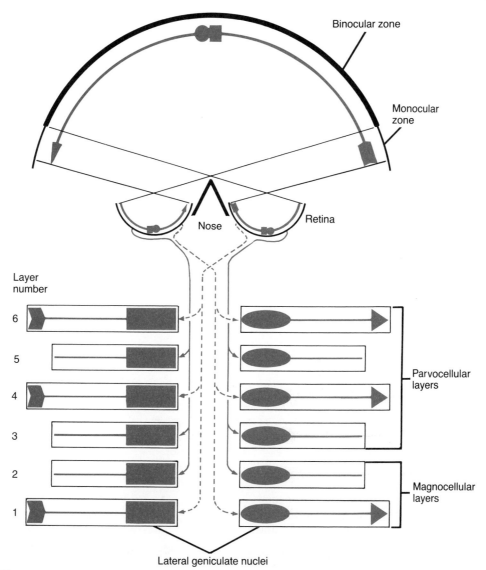

FIGURE 11-13

Highly schematic representation of the projections from the retinae to the lateral geniculate nuclei. Fibers crossing in the optic chiasm are represented by the dashed line. Noncrossing fibers are shown as solid. Uncrossed retinal fibers terminate in layers 2, 3, and 5 of the lateral geniculate nucleus (LGN); crossed fibers terminate in layers 1, 4, and 6.

The binocular zone of the visual field is represented in all six layers; the monocular zone is represented only in layers 2, 3, and 5. The foveal region of the visual field has a greater representation in the LGN layers. Each layer contains a precise visuotopic map of the visual field. All maps are in vertical register with those above and below. See text for details.

back to the LGN (see Fig. 4–10*A*). The role of the reticular nucleus of the thalamus in the regulation of thalamocortical signals is discussed in Chapter 20. The general principles of feed-forward and feedback inhibition are discussed in Chapter 4.

The *corticogeniculate projections*, from visual cortical areas, are the largest group of afferents to the LGN, exceeding in number the retinogeniculate projections. These cortical projections may have an important role in *arousal*, in regulating the level of *visual attention*, and in *modulating the flow of information* from the LGN to V-1. Together, these circuits regulate the signal threshold of LGN relay neurons and modulate the strength of the visual signal that ultimately reaches V-1.

Visual Cortex

Visual cortical areas are regions of the cerebral cortex containing a visuotopic map of some portion of the visual field. Neurons in these areas, in general, are responsive to some form of visual stimuli, be it motion, color, stereopsis, or some combination of visual stimuli.

At least 24 separate representations of the visual field, or portions thereof, are present in the posterior half of the cerebral hemisphere in primates other than humans. Clinical studies suggest that a similar pattern of representations is present in the human brain. Most of these areas are selectively sensitive to a specific parameter or a combination of parameters of visual stimuli (e.g., orientation, movement, contour discrimination, brightness, color, high resolution, and stereopsis).

The *primary visual cortex, V-1,* is the principal target for the cortical projections from the LGN of the dorsal thalamus. The *secondary visual cortex, V-2,* in turn, receives projections from V-1; processes the information; and relays it to a number of *tertiary visual areas,* such as *V-3* and *V-4* and the *middle temporal area (MT).*

PRIMARY VISUAL CORTEX, V-1

The *primary visual cortex (V-1)* is on the medial and posterior surfaces of the occipital lobe. The horizontal *calcarine fissure* divides *V-1* into the *cuneus (cuneate gyrus)* above and the *lingual gyrus* below (see Figs. 8–4 and 8–6). Although primarily confined to the medial surface of the occipital lobe, portions of both gyri extend onto the posterolateral surface of the occipital cortex. The cuneus and lingual gyrus together form *Brodmann's area 17* (see Fig. 21–3). When the tissue is Weigert-stained, a prominent band of myelinated fibers is visible in layer IVB, the *stripe of Gennari.* This is why V-1 is also called the *striate cortex.* Geniculocortical projections enter layer IVA and IVC of V-1.

Optic radiations are the projection fibers from the LGN to *V-1* via the internal capsule, in particular, the *retrolenticular* portion of the internal capsule. All of the fibers sweep around the lateral wall of the lateral ventricle and course toward the medial and posterior portion of the occipital cortex (see Fig. 11–1). En route to the

cortex, fibers from the upper quadrant of the visual field sweep in an anterior direction, then laterally and finally posteriorly. They form a fiber bundle near the anterior tip of the temporal horn of the lateral ventricle known as *Meyer's loop* (see Figs. 11–1 and 11–12). These fibers are of clinical importance in the diagnosis of certain temporal lobe tumors (see following section).

Projections from the LGN to V-1 retain a precise visuotopic organization: the lingual gyrus receives projections representing the upper contralateral quadrant of the visual field and the cuneate gyrus, the lower contralateral quadrant of the visual field. The anterior most portion of V-1, on the medial surface of the occipital lobe, represents the peripheral portion of the visual field. Conversely, the central or macular region is at the occipital pole. The central or macular portion of the visual field occupies a larger area of V-1 than does the periphery, a representation similar to, although somewhat larger than, that in the LGN (Fig. 11–14).

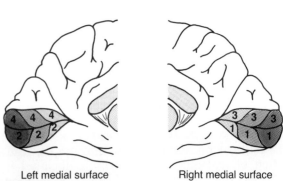

FIGURE 11–14

The proportional representation of the visual field at the level of the primary visual cortex (V-1).

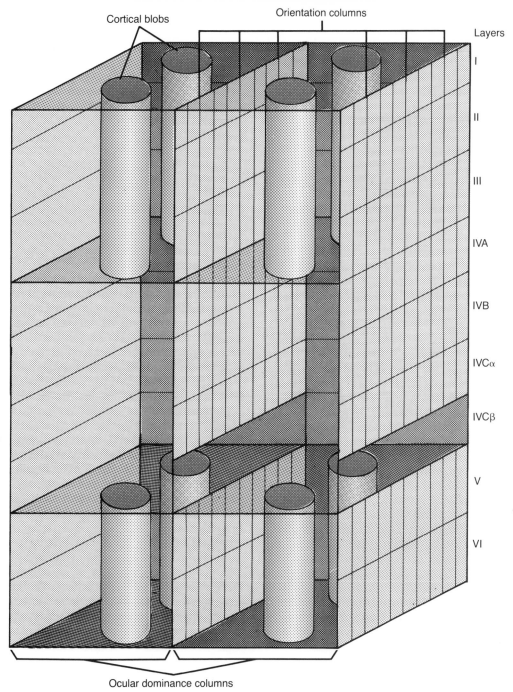

Cortical blobs

Orientation columns

Layers

I

II

III

IVA

IVB

IVCα

IVCβ

V

VI

Ocular dominance columns

FIGURE 11-15

The cortical module is the basic building block of V-1 and represents a single point in visual space. The modules are composed of two ocular dominance columns, one for each eye. Each ocular dominance column contains the information processing subdivisions, *blobs*, *interblobs*, and *layer IVB*.

Parvocellular signals from the lateral geniculate nucleus (LGN) are relayed to both the blobs and interblob areas. Magnocellular information is processed in layer IVB. *Blob* neurons respond to color and brightness. Those in *layer IVB* are most sensitive to the movement and the orientation of objects in visual space. *Interblobs* contain orientation columns, small vertically organized columns of cortical tissue in which the neurons are sensitive to bars or lines of visual stimuli, with a specific angular orientation in space.

Although the orientation columns are represented as vertical stripes on the side of each ocular dominance column, they extend into the substance of each column. Unlike the blobs, orientation columns include all of layer IV except IVCβ. The interblob areas are associated with shape analysis and high visual acuity. See text for details.

241

The visuotopic representation in V-1 is a mosaic of *cortical modules*, much like the pixels of a video screen, with each module or "pixel" representing a single point in visual space. Each module forms from two vertically orientated *ocular dominance columns*, subunits that receive visual information from the separate eyes. LGN projections from the contralateral eye (laminae 1, 4, and 6.) terminate in one ocular dominance column, and those from the ipsilateral eye (laminae 2, 3, and 5.), in an adjacent ocular dominance column. Together, the two ocular dominance columns form the cortical module (Fig. 11–15). The detailed organization of the module is discussed subsequently. Thus, V-1 retains the anatomical separation of the visual signals from the two eyes found in the LGN.

PRESTRIATE VISUAL AREAS, V-2, V-3, AND V-4

The *prestriate visual areas* are located in *Brodmann's areas 18* and *19*, specifically areas *V-2*, *V-3*, and *V-4* (see Fig. 21–3). The demarcation between areas 18 and 19 is not distinct. Although V-2, immediately adjacent to V-1, is entirely within area 18, portions of V-3 and V-4 may extend into area 19.

MIDDLE TEMPORAL VISUAL AREA (MT)

All visually responsive areas of cerebral cortex do not correspond to specific Brodmann's areas. However, Brodmann's classification is widely used. Therefore, this classification is helpful in approximating the location of physiologically responsive areas. The *middle temporal visual area (MT)* is anterior to area 19 on the lateral surface of the hemisphere along the boundary between occipital and temporal lobes and includes portions of *area 39* (see Fig. 21–3). MT is important for the detection of motion. Visual signals processed in MT have a very fast response time and an equally rapid response decay—even with continued stimulation. These properties are especially suited for the detection of moving objects.

OTHER VISUAL AREAS

Several other cortical areas with special visual significance are the *inferotemporal area (IT)* (portions of *Brodmann's areas 20* and *21*), the *posterior parietal visual area* (posterior portion of *area 7*) and the *frontal eye fields* (a portion of *area 8* in the frontal lobe) (see Fig. 21–3). The frontal eye fields are anterior to the premotor areas and coordinate movements of the eye and visual tracking.

Information Processing in the Visual Cortex

HIERARCHICAL AND PARALLEL INFORMATION PROCESSING

A number of separate channels or streams of visual information project from the retina to the LGN and from the LGN to V-1. As these streams of information are processed at the cortical level, many continue to remain separate pathways. Individual neurons at higher levels within a pathway respond to more complex patterns of visual stimuli than those at lower levels. As a reflection of this increasing complexity, visually sensitive cortical neurons have been classified as *simple cells*, *complex cells*, or *hypercomplex cells*. This pattern of increasing complexity is *hierarchical information processing*. At the same time, individual streams of visual information, each carrying unique bits of information or combinations of bits, are processed separately. This pattern is *parallel information processing*. The visual system processes information through a combination of both. There is a hierarchical processing of information within parallel streams. Each parallel stream processes a different dimension or dimensions of the very complex visual field.

ANATOMICAL ORGANIZATION OF V-1 AND V-2

Details of cortical organization at the cellular level are presented in Chapter 21. Of these, certain features are important to the visual system. The cortex has six layers, each with its characteristic histology, numbered (from the surface inward) layers I, II, III, IV, V, and VI. In V-1, layer IV is further subdivided from the surface inward, into layers IVA, IVB, IVCα, and IVCβ (Fig. 11–16). Geniculocalcarine projections from the *magnocellular layers of the LGN terminate in layer IVCα*, whereas those from the *parvocellular layers of the LGN terminate principally in layer IVCβ with some in layer IVA*. Both magnocellular and parvocellular projections send collaterals to layer VI. No geniculate projections terminate in layer IVB. However, layer IVB is an important information processing station. In this chapter, layers I, II, and III are denoted simply as the

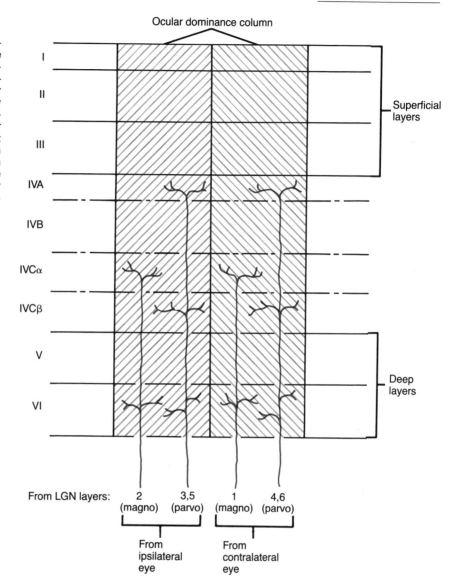

The principal geniculostriate terminations in layer IV of V-1. Note the different pattern of termination for magnocellular and parvocellular projections. Magnocellular projections terminate principally in layer IVCα, whereas parvocellular projections terminate in layer iVCβ, with a smaller component terminating in layer IVA. Both have collateral terminations in layer VI. Projections from the separate eyes are limited to their specific ocular dominance column. See text for details.

Ocular dominance column

I

II

III

IVA

IVB

IVCα

IVCβ

V

VI

Superficial layers

Deep layers

From LGN layers: 2 (magno) 3,5 (parvo) 1 (magno) 4,6 (parvo)

From ipsilateral eye

From contralateral eye

"superficial layers" and layers V and VI as the "deep layers" (see Fig. 11–16).

Histochemical staining of cortical areas V-1 and V-2 for the activity of cytochrome oxidase (a mitochondrial enzyme) revealed two very characteristic patterns. *V-1* had a mosaic pattern of densely staining, small *blobs* (ovoid areas approximately 0.2 mm in diameter) surrounded by paler staining *interblob* areas. The blobs are present in both superficial and deep layers but absent from layer IV (see Fig. 11–15). The histochemical staining pattern in *V-2* is one of irregular, parallel stripes—intense-staining *thick stripes* and intense-staining *thin stripes* separated by lighter staining stripes or *interstripe areas*. All are orien-

tated at right angles to the boundary between V-1 and V-2. In addition to providing anatomical landmarks, these staining patterns reflect differences in the processing of visual information.

Functional Organization of V-1

The *cortical module* is the functional building block of V-1. Although the ocular dominance columns (one from each eye representing the same point in visual space) are the major subdivisions of the module, each column contains a number of functional subunits (see Fig. 11–15). Color processing occurs in the cytochrome oxidase–positive *blobs*. Neurons in the blobs are wavelength sensitive, responding to color and to brightness. Surrounding the blobs are *interblob areas*, each containing *orientation columns*. Orientation columns are small, vertically organized columns of cortical tissue in which the neurons are sensitive to bars or lines of visual stimuli with a specific angular orientation in space. As one moves from one orientation column to an adjacent one, the orientation sensitivity of the responding neurons shifts approximately 10 to 15 degrees. Unlike the blobs, orientation columns include all of layer IV except IVCβ. *Parvocellular* signals from the LGN are processed both by the *blobs* and *interblob areas* of the superficial and deep layers of the cortex. Information carried by the *magnocellular* projections is processed in *layer IVB*. Neurons in layer IVB are most sensitive to movement and to the orientation of objects in visual space.

Functional Organization of V-2

In the next stage of information processing, specific components of the V-1 module project to specific areas of V-2. The orientation and movement cues remain separate as neurons from *layer IVB* project visuotopically to the cytochrome oxidase–positive *thick stripes* of *V-2*. Color segregation continues as the *blobs* project selectively to the cytochrome oxidase–positive *thin stripes* of *V-2*. The *interstripe areas*, important in shape analysis and high visual acuity, receive projections principally from the *interblob areas* of *V-1*. Thus, *V-2* continues the compartmentalization of specific combinations of visual information: color in the thin stripes, high resolution and shape analysis in the interstripes, and movement and orientation in the thick stripes.

MULTIPLE PROCESSING STREAMS

The parallel streams of visual information remain separate, as the signals project to tertiary visual areas in the parietal and temporal lobes. Three of these streams, documented for many primates and supported by clinical studies in humans, are good examples of parallel information processing. The first stream addresses *where it is*; the second stream addresses *what it is*; and the third carries information about *color*.

Magnocellular Stream (M)

The magnocellular stream (*M*) actually begins with the large *Y-cells* of the retinal ganglion cell layer that project to the *magnocellular layers* of

the *LGN*. The magnocellular layers of the LGN, in turn, project to *V-1*. The initial cortical processing occurs in *layer IVB*. Several substreams link *layer IVB* with the *thick stripes* of *V-2*, and subsequently with the *middle temporal area, MT*. Additional parallel information may reach *MT* from *V-1* by way of *V-3* or directly from *layer IVB* of *V-1* (Fig. 11–17). One of several streams leaving MT projects to the *posterior parietal visual area*. Most cortical neurons in the M stream respond to movement, orientation, and high contrast. These neurons do not respond to color. Most have relatively large receptive fields and a correspondingly poor visual acuity. The M stream processes those elements of information necessary to locate rapidly a moving object in visual space, i.e., it tells the individual *where it is*. The image is similar to a series of very high speed black and white photographs, with high contrast and low resolution.

Parvocellular-Interblob Stream (P-IB)

Visual information carried by the smaller, slow responding *X-cells* of the retinal ganglion cell layer projects to the *parvocellular layers* of the LGN. *Parvocellular neurons* project to V-1, and specific components of this projection are relayed to the *interblob areas*. From the interblob areas of V-1, the P-IB stream projects to the *interstripe areas* of *V-2*; from there to *V-4*; and, finally, to the *inferotemporal area* (*IT*). An additional substream, from *layer IVB* (of *V-1*) to *V-3* and then to *V-4*, combines some of the visual information of the M stream with that of P-IB (see Fig. 11–17). The P-IB stream is a high acuity pathway for shape analysis, with a strong orientation component. Objects are seen in fine detail, but not in color per se. The P-IB stream utilizes wavelength sensitivity to differentiate boundaries between colors of equal luminance as varied shades of gray—a feature lacking in the M stream. This detailed shape analysis with a high level of acuity in the P-IB stream tells the individual *what it is*.

Parvocellular-Blob Stream (P-B)

Parvocellular LGN projections to the *blobs* of V-1 represent the initial step in the perception of wavelength differences as color. As information processing continues in the *P-B* stream, the *blobs* of V-1 project to the *thin stripes* of V-2, then to area V-4, and finally to the *inferotemporal area* (*IT*). Both the P-B stream and the P-IB stream project to V-4 and IT; however, these streams

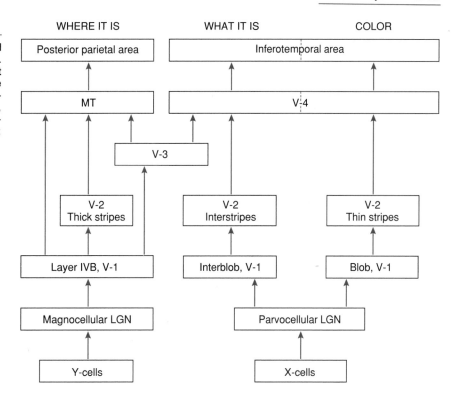

remain separate and utilize different regions within these cortical areas (Fig. 11-17). Nearly all cortical cells in the P-B stream have a high degree of wavelength selectivity but a lower level of acuity than the P-IB stream. This wavelength sensitivity of neurons in the P-B stream reflects their role in *color perception*.

Cross-Talk Between Streams

Of these three examples, only the P-B stream carries one primary type of visual cue, color. P-IB utilizes wavelength information but for finer resolution of boundaries and not for color perception. Both the P-IB stream and the M stream use orientation cues. However, P-IB utilizes these for fine detail discrimination, whereas M utilizes similar information for a low acuity orientation of moving objects in visual space. The same basic visual information, when processed by different streams, can provide a different "picture" or dimension of visual space.

Tectal and Pretectal Connections

SUPERIOR COLLICULUS

The *superior colliculus* is in the *tectum* or roof of the midbrain, posterior and medial to the LGN.

In those lower vertebrates lacking a cerebral cortex, the superior colliculus is the principal visual center, known as the optic tectum. In higher vertebrates, including humans, the superior colliculus is a reflex center for somatic motor reflexes in response to visual, auditory, and somatosensory stimuli.

Visual signals reach the superior colliculus either directly from the retina or indirectly from the visual cortex. *Retinotectal fibers*, axons from *W-cells*, and either collateral branches of axons from *Y-cells* or a separate population of *Y-cells*, by-pass the LGN and reach the superior colliculus by way of the *brachium of the superior colliculus* (see Figs. 7-3 and 7-4). The exact route of the *corticotectal fibers* is unknown.

Although not apparent from the Weigert-stained section (see Fig. 7-17), the superior colliculus is a laminated structure with seven layers. Visual fibers terminate in the three superficial layers, laminae 1 to 3. In contrast, laminae 4 to 7 receive somatosensory and auditory signals and contain efferent neurons related to head and eye movements.

Retinotectal projections form a visuotopic map of the contralateral visual hemifield in the superficial layers of each colliculus. The foveal portion of the hemifield is at the posterior pole of the colliculus, and the most peripheral portion of the

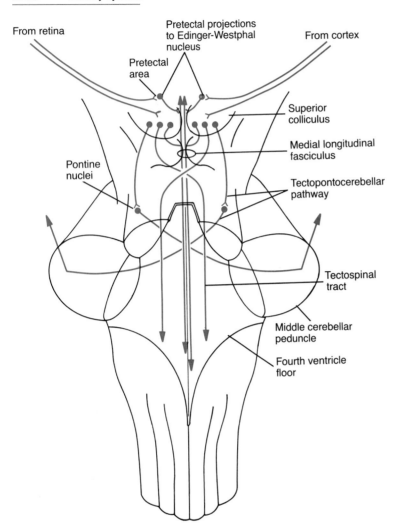

From retina

Pretectal projections
to Edinger-Westphal
nucleus

Pretectal
area

From cortex

Superior
colliculus

Medial longitudinal
fasciculus

Pontine
nuclei

Tectopontocerebellar
pathway

Tectospinal
tract

Middle cerebellar
peduncle

Fourth ventricle
floor

FIGURE 11–18

The principal afferent and efferent connections in the superior colliculus and pretectal
area that are related to the visual system.
See text for details.

visual hemifield is at the anterior pole. The upper
visual quadrant maps on the medial half of the
colliculus and the inferior visual quadrant, on the
lateral half.

The superior colliculus contains superficial and
deep subdivisions. The superficial layers receive
visual signals and have a major projection system
to the dorsal thalamus. The deeper layers, receiving auditory and somatosensory systems, contain
the principal efferents to lower brain stem structures. The latter include the crossed *tectospinal
tract*, important in the reflex movement of the
head and neck in response to sensory stimuli and
contributions to the *medial longitudinal fasciculus* (*MLF*), which supply the motor nuclei of
the cranial nerves innervating the extraocular
muscles—the *oculomotor* (*III*), *trochlear* (*IV*),
and *abducens* (*VI*). An intact superior colliculus
is essential for rapid eye movements. One of the
principal efferents from the superior colliculus is

the *tectopontocerebellar tract*, a fiber tract leaving
the superior colliculus and descending to the
pontine nuclei. From there, it enters the cerebellum via the *middle cerebellar peduncle* (Fig. 11–
18).

PRETECTAL AREA

The *pretectal area* lies immediately rostral to the
superior colliculus and posteroinferior to the dorsal thalamus (see Fig. 7–18). This area, composed of five separate nuclei, is associated with
autonomic visual reflexes, in particular, pupillary
light reflexes and the accommodation reflex (see
following discussion). A population of the slow
conducting *X-cells* from the retina projects to the
pretectum via the optic nerve, the optic tract, and
the brachium of the superior colliculus, leaving
the brachium before reaching the superior colliculus. These retinopretectal neurons are sensitive

to changes in the overall luminance of the visual field. Neurons from the pretectal area project bilaterally to the *preganglionic, parasympathetic Edinger-Westphal nucleus* of the oculomotor (cranial nerve III) complex (see Fig. 11–18). Preganglionic fibers from the Edinger-Westphal nucleus exit the brain stem with the somatic motor fibers of the *oculomotor nerve* and synapse with the *postganglionic, parasympathetic neurons* in the *ciliary ganglion*. These postganglionic fibers innervate the *pupillary constrictor muscles* (see Fig. 18–6).

Visual Reflexes

PUPILLARY LIGHT REFLEX

The pupil of the eye dilates and constricts in response to changes in the overall brightness of the visual field. The greater the light, the more constricted the pupil; the less the light, the more dilated the pupil. The parasympathetic component of the oculomotor nerve innervates the pupillary constrictors. Because the outflow from the pretectum to the Edinger-Westphal nuclei is bilateral, bright light in either eye produces a constriction of both pupils. When a light stimulates one eye, the pupillary response in the stimulated eye is the *direct response*. The pupillary response in the nonstimulated eye is the *consensual response*.

With optic nerve damage, both direct and consensual responses are absent following stimulation of the damaged eye. However, light shown in the undamaged eye will elicit both direct (intact eye) and consensual (damaged eye) pupillary responses, provided the oculomotor nerves are intact. When the optic nerve is intact but the efferent part of the reflex loop (oculomotor nerve) to the stimulated eye damaged, the individual perceives the stimulus but there is no direct pupillary response. The consensual response remains intact following unilateral damage to the oculomotor nerve. However, both direct and consensual responses are lost if the damage is bilateral.

ACCOMMODATION REFLEX

The *accommodation reflex* is a combined somatic and visceral motor reflex. This reflex is elicited when the focus of the eyes moves from a distant object to a near one. During this shift in focus, three motor events occur:

1. The eyes converge. This is a somatic motor response of the extraocular muscles, driven by a corticotectal pathway.

2. The circumferential muscles of the ciliary body contract, reducing tension on the suspensory ligaments and allowing the lens to become more convex for focus on a close object. The visceromotor (parasympathetic) component of the oculomotor nerve mediates this part of the reflex, and cortical projections to the pretectal area drive it.

3. The pupils constrict, also a parasympathetic reflex mediated by the oculomotor nerve.

The entire course of the reflex loop is not understood. However, visual stimuli must reach the visual cortex and cortical signals must reach the tectum (somatic motor component) and the pretectal area (visceral motor components). Details of other volitional and reflex movements of the eyes are presented in the oculomotor section of Chapter 19.

Clinical Correlations

RETINAL INJURY

A variety of conditions—genetic diseases, trauma, and infections—can lead to a loss of vision in the affected eye. Focal damage to the retina produces areas of impaired vision called *scotomas*. Damage can be focal or massive and the visual deficit correspondingly small or large. Patients often are unaware of small deficits, especially those in the binocular field of vision, just as most are unaware of the blind spot in each eye produced by the formation of the optic nerve. An ophthalmoscope can help to identify many of these insults, because they often are accompanied by changes in the appearance of the retina.

Most forms of *color blindness* involve the selective loss of one of the three types of cones. Although rare, more than one type of cone may be lost. The spectral sensitivities of the photopigments for each of the three cones overlap considerably (see Fig. 11–7). The perception of a specific color by the visual system results from the integration of the signals from all three cones. For example, stimulation with monochromatic light of 500 nm activates all three cones, but the sensitivity of each cone type to that wavelength determines the degree of activation. The ratios of these three signals ultimately determine the specific color perceived.

If red cones are absent, *protanopia*, only the green cones can respond to light at wavelengths longer than 530 nm see (Fig. 11–7). Above 530 nm, the *ratio* of red to green cone signals does not change, because red signals are absent and all colors in that part of the visual spectrum appear identical. *Protanopes* are unable to differentiate among red, orange, yellow, and green. They also have a shortened visual spectrum, due to the rapid decrease in green cone sensitivity at wavelengths longer than 580 nm and to the total absence of cones sensitive to longer wavelengths (see Fig. 11–7).

Deuteranopia is the selective loss of green sensitive cones. As with protanopes, *deuteranopes* cannot differentiate among red, orange, yellow, and green. However, they possess the red cone and therefore do not have a shortened visual spectrum (see Fig. 11–7)

Tritanopia is a loss of the blue cone and is a rare condition.

The genes for red and green cone vision are sex-linked recessives carried on the X-chromosome. Thus, red-green color blindness is rare in women. However, approximately 6% of men are deuteranopes and another 2% are protanopes. The blue gene deficit, however, is a rare autosomal recessive abnormality. When it does occur, the incidence is the same for men and women.

DAMAGE TO RETINOGENICULOCALCARINE TRACT

Visual deficits are generally described by visual field losses rather than by anatomical structures injured or damaged (see Fig. 11–3). The suffix *-anopsia* means a loss of vision; hence, *hemianopsia* and *quadrantanopsia* are losses of vision in one hemifield and one quadrant of the visual field, respectively. When describing visual field defects, two other terms are employed often, *heteronymous* and *homonymous*. Heteronymous indicates the visual field losses are not the same for the two eyes, homonymous indicates they are the same. For example, loss of the upper left quadrant of the visual field in both eyes would be a case of *left superior homonymous quadrantanopsia*; loss of the peripheral (temporal) half of the visual field in each eye would be a case of *bitemporal heteronymous hemianopsia*. The last is "tunnel vision," i.e., a loss of the left half of the visual field in the left eye and the right half of the visual field in the right eye. Most of the terminology, after a brief "dissection," gives one a precise description of the deficit.

Any injury or damage to the retina or the optic nerve, anterior to the optic chiasm, produces *homolateral* deficits, deficits confined to a single eye. These may be partial or, in the extreme, involve the entire optic nerve, as in example 1 of Figure 11–12. However, with severance of the right optic nerve immediately anterior to the optic chiasm, as in example 2, there is a total loss of vision in the homolateral eye and a loss of vision in the contralateral superior left quadrant of the visual field. (Fibers from the inferior nasal quadrants of the retina loop into the optic nerve before entering the optic tract.)

Damage to the optic chiasm, from a pituitary tumor for example, affects the crossing fibers, from the nasal halves of both retinae. This type of damage produces the classic tunnel vision symptomatology, or *bitemporal heteronymous hemianopsia*. Posterior to the optic chiasm and throughout the remainder of the visual pathway, including the LGN, optic radiations, and the V-1, any damage produces a *homonymous* deficit. The visual pathway at this level carries visual information from only the contralateral visual hemifield. Thus, total severance of the optic tract or the rare loss of the LGN results in a *contralateral homonymous hemianopsia* (see example 4 of Fig. 11–12). Involvement of only part of the pathway, as is the case with a temporal lobe tumor impinging on Meyer's loop, results in *left superior homonymous quadrantanopsia* (see example 5 of Fig. 11–12).

Insults to the occipital cortex and V-1 often result in a *homonymous hemianopsia* with *macular sparing*. Damage limited to either the lingual gyrus or the cuneus produces a *homonymous quadrantanopsia*, also with macular sparing. The vascular supply to V-1 provides the best explanation for the macular sparing phenomenon, because many of the cortical deficits are the result of vascular spasms or thromboses. The posterior cerebral artery is the major arterial supply to V-1. However, the posterior and posterolateral portions of V-1, containing the macular projections, can receive an anastomotic arterial supply from the middle cerebral artery.

INJURY TO SECONDARY VISUAL CORTICAL AREAS

Visual agnosias are visual deficits resulting from injury to secondary visual cortical areas. A person with a visual agnosia is not blind but has problems perceiving specific aspects of the visual scene. Often, agnosias are the result of small, discrete lesions to areas of the parietal and temporal cortex.

Prosopagnosia, the inability to recognize familiar faces and to learn new ones, results from bilateral lesions to the *inferotemporal visual area.* Patients with this disorder can recognize individuals through other cues, such as voice, gait, posture, and attire. Often they retain the ability to recognize familiar objects. More extensive damage to the inferotemporal area produces *visual object agnosia,* the inability to name or recognize familiar objects or to learn new ones.

Visual movement agnosia is an inability to discern moving objects and involves damage to the *middle temporal visual area. Visual color agnosia,* or *achromatopsia,* is the inability to recognize colors. This form of cortical color blindness results from lesions to portions of the prestriate cortex, presumably including all or part of V-4. Occasionally, it occurs in combination with prosopagnosia or visual object agnosia. Both visual movement agnosia and *achromatopsia* occur following either bilateral or unilateral damage. When the damage is confined to one hemisphere, the agnosia is confined to the contralateral visual hemifield.

Following unilateral injury to the *frontal eye field (area 8),* the two eyes deviate toward the side of the lesion. An inability to turn the eyes toward the opposite side on command exists. These losses usually are transitory, and eye movement improves within a few days. One explanation for the transient nature of the unilateral deficit is that the contralateral frontal eye field takes over the function of both eye fields. This occurrence may be related to the crossed and uncrossed corticobulbar projections to the oculomotor nuclei from the motor cortex. With bilateral damage to the frontal eye fields, patients cannot move the eyes on command. However, if they fixate on an object and the object is moved slowly across the visual field, their eyes will track the object. Oculomotor responses to vestibular stimulation remain intact.

STRABISMIC AMBLYOPIA

Normal infants, as young as 3 months, have stereoscopic vision. However, if the visual axes of the two eyes are not parallel *(strabismus)* the infant suppresses foveal vision in the nondominant eye to avoid *diplopia* (double vision) and the visual confusion resulting from two nonsuperimposed visual images. This suppression occurs at the cortical level, resulting in *strabismic amblyopia.* This condition is reversible if the *strabismus* is corrected during the first 6 months of postnatal development. Stereoscopic vision will not develop if the strabismus is corrected after the visual cortices have matured. In the latter case, the child will alternate the use of one eye or the other or will continue to suppress the central or foveal vision from the nondominant eye. Although the perception of depth from stereoscopic vision is absent, these individuals learn to perceive depth of field through many other visual cues.

SUGGESTED READING

Casagrande, V. A., and T. T. Norton (1990). Lateral geniculate nucleus: A review of its physiology and function. In *The Neural Basis of Visual Function,* A. Leventhal (Editor). Macmillan Press, London, pp. 41–84.

This chapter is a current review of the mammalian LGN by two of the leading authorities on the subject. The chapter is not limited to higher primates but utilizes cross species comparisons to shed light on the role of the LGN in visual information processing.

DeYoe, E. A., and D. C. Van Essen (1988). Concurrent processing streams in monkey visual cortex. Trends Neurosci, 11: 219–226.

In this review, the authors develop the present concept of multiple processing streams for visual information. Their work suggests that many aspects of visual perception involve significant overlap and "cross talk" between pathways and areas involved in these streams.

Dow, N. W., W. J. Brunken, and D. Parkinson (1989). The function of synaptic transmitters in the retina. Ann. Rev. Neurosci., 12: 205–225.

In this review, the authors consider our state of knowledge of neurotransmitters and relate these to function, in an area of the CNS in which the circuitry is fairly well understood, the retina. In the rapidly growing field of neurochemistry, they make generalizations about the functions of specific transmitter systems, relating these to known physiological functions.

Dowling, J. E. (1987). *The Retina.* Harvard University Press, Cambridge, Massachusetts, 282 pp.

This monograph surveys the vast literature on the physiology and anatomy of the vertebrate retina. Much of the literature surveyed represents Professor Dowling's own contributions. This volume is a valuable reference for those interested in visual mechanisms and in the retina in particular.

Stone, J. (1983). *Parallel Processing in the Visual System.* Plenum Press, New York, 438 pp.

This monograph succinctly develops the concept of parallel information processing, specifically as it applies to the visual system. These general features of parallel processing are applicable to most sensory systems.

Werblin, F. S. (1973). The control of sensitivity in the retina. Scientific American, 228: 70–79.

This article contains one of the clearest and most succinct presentations of the concept of center-surround antagonism, both in the enhancement of contrast and in the detection of movement. In this review, Werblin considers the role of the various retinal cell types in center-surround and illustrates the manner in which the retina is able to optimize its sensitivity over a wide range of stimulus intensities.

Chapter

12

Auditory and Vestibular Pathways

The *special somatic afferent* (*SSA*) classification includes the *auditory* and *vestibular systems*, in addition to the visual system (see Chapter 11). All three are special sensory systems innervating structures of somatic origin. Both the auditory receptor organ (the *cochlear duct*) and the vestibular receptor organs (the *semicircular canals*, the *saccule*, and the *utricle*) develop from an embryonic ectodermal vesicle, the *otocyst* (Fig. 12–1 and Fig. 1–24). Collectively, these auditory and vestibular receptor organs compose the *membranous labyrinth*. With subsequent development and differentiation, the membranous labyrinth becomes surrounded by the bone of the developing skull, the petrous portion of the temporal bone. This process thereby results in a membranous labyrinth containing the receptors, filled with *endolymph*, situated within a *bony labyrinth*, filled with *perilymph*. Together, they form the *inner ear* (*auris interna*) (see Fig. 12–1).

Phylogenetically, in lower forms, the inner ear was concerned only with equilibration—a function retained by the mammalian vestibular system. Higher vertebrates developed specializations of the inner ear that allowed the perception of sound or, at least, vibratory signals from an aqueous environment. Later, land-dwelling vertebrates showed additional specializations that allowed the auditory receptors to respond to sound vibrations of the air. In mammals, such specializations are the *external* and *middle ears* (*auris externa* and *auris media*).

The *auricula* (*pinna*) of the external ear channels sound vibrations carried by the air into the *external auditory canal*, where they vibrate the *tympanic membrane* (*eardrum*), a membranous wall separating the external auditory canal from the middle ear. Three small bones of the air-filled middle ear, the *auditory ossicles* (*malleus*, *incus*, and *stapes*), then relay the mechanical vibrations

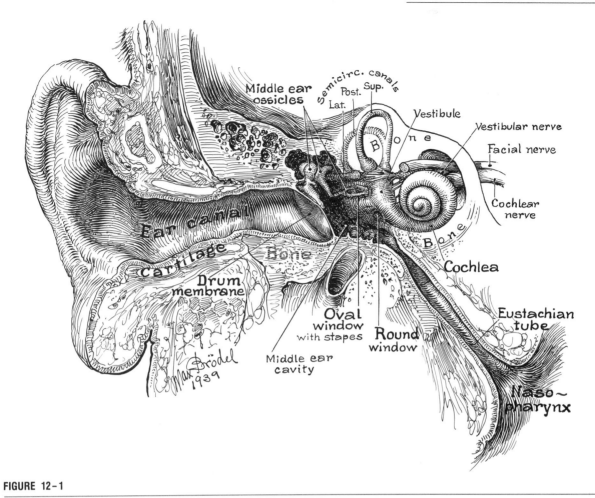

FIGURE 12-1

A schematic representation of the anatomical relations of the various parts of the human ear. (After M. Brödel. In Malone, Guild, and Crowe, *Three Unpublished Drawings of the Human Ear*. W. B. Saunders Co., Philadelphia, 1946.)

of the tympanic membrane to the perilymph of the inner ear. The *cochlea*, in turn, transduces the fluid vibrations of the perilymph into neuronal signals, action potentials.

In the vestibular system, the sensory signals arise from the movement and position of the head in space. These signals reach the sensory receptors without the aid of elaborate appendages. Fluid movement of the endolymph within the *semicircular canals* provides the signals for the detection of angular acceleration of the head. The *saccule* and *utricle* respond to linear acceleration and gravitational pull.

In the embryo, immediately rostral and medial to the otocyst, a cluster of neural crest cells forms the *vestibuloacoustic ganglion* or, simply, the *acoustic ganglion* (see Fig. 1-24). With further differentiation, and in parallel with the differen-

tiation of the membranous labyrinth, this ganglion separates into the *vestibular ganglion* and the *cochlear ganglion* (*spiral ganglion*). Both ganglia contain bipolar neurons with peripheral processes that innervate their respective receptor organs. Their central processes together form *cranial nerve VIII* (the *vestibulocochlear* or *statoacoustic nerve*). Although this is a single cranial nerve, the fibers of the two divisions remain physically separate. A cross section of the nerve resembles a figure 8, with one part vestibular and the other cochlear.

Cranial nerve VIII joins the brain stem at the medullopontine angle, where it separates into cochlear and vestibular divisions (see Figs. 7-3 and 7-10). Fibers of the *cochlear division* terminate in the *dorsal* and *ventral cochlear nuclei*. The *vestibular division* enters the brain stem deep to the restiform body, and its fibers terminate in the *vestibular nuclei* of the upper medulla and pons.

Sound

FREQUENCY

A pure sound of a single frequency travels through air as a series of waves of condensation and rarefaction. When the sound pressure is plotted as a function of time, the curve is sinusoidal (Fig. 12–2). The pitch of a tone reflects the frequency of the wave, measured in cycles per second or *Hertz* (Hz). The lower the frequency, the lower the pitch; the higher the frequency, the higher the pitch. *Optimal frequencies* for the human ear range from 1000 to 3000 Hz or 1 to 3 kHz. Young individuals normally have a *hearing frequency range* from 20 to 20,000 Hz. However, with maturation and aging, this range decreases to 50 to 8000 Hz or less, in some cases. In both cases, however, perception of sounds at frequencies above and below the optimal range requires an increase in volume (Fig. 12–3).

VOLUME

The volume of a tone is the amplitude of the sound pressure waves and is expressed on a spe-

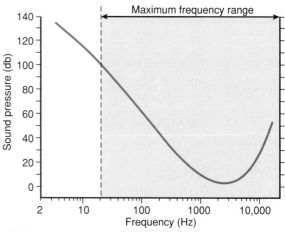

FIGURE 12-3

A diagram of the hearing threshold, in decibels (db), as a function of the logarithm of the sound frequency in Hz. The normal hearing range for a young human is 20 to 20,000 Hz (shaded area). Note the lowest threshold is for sound of approximately 2000 Hz. The human ear is most sensitive to sounds in this frequency range (see text for details).

cial logarithmic scale, the *decibel scale* (*dB*). Audiologists use a pressure value of 0.0002 dynes/cm² as a zero reference, or zero decibels (0 dB), the approximate threshold for a 1- to 3-kHz tone. All other sound pressures are measured as a logarithmic function of the ratio of the test sound to the reference sound:

$$\text{Sound pressure (dB)} = 20 \log_{10} P_t/P_r$$

where P_r is the reference pressure of 0.0002 dynes/cm², and P_t is the pressure of the test sound. Hence, a 20-dB sound would have 10 times the reference pressure, and a 40-dB sound would have 100 times the pressure. Sound levels in excess of 100 dB (100,000 times the reference pressure) can be heard without discomfort. Prolonged exposure to sounds of this volume can damage the inner ear permanently.

External and Middle Ear

EXTERNAL EAR

The *auricula* or *pinna* of the external ear acts as a funnel, channeling the airborne sound vibrations into the *external auditory canal*. The size of the auricula effects the sound-capturing efficiency of the ear. The cupping of one's hand behind the ear while facing a sound effectively increases the size of the "funnel" and increases one's sensitiv-

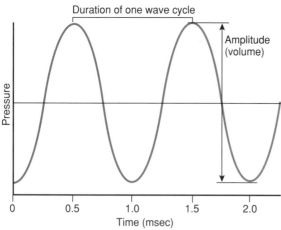

FIGURE 12-2

Diagram of the sinusoidal curve produced by a pure tone of 1000 Hz. The duration of one wave cycle in this example is 1.0 msec. The tone frequency is the reciprocal of the duration, in this example, 1000 cycles per sec, or 1000 Hz. The peaks represent waves of air compression, the troughs rarefaction, both relative to "quiet" air (horizontal line). The amplitude of the wave, in pressure units, is a measure of the loudness or volume.

ity to the sound. The airborne sound passes through the external auditory canal and strikes the *tympanic membrane* causing it to vibrate.

MIDDLE EAR ANATOMY

Embryonically, the middle ear develops from the *tuberotympanic recess*, an outgrowth of the first branchial pouch. In the adult, the original connection between the pharynx and the middle ear remains as the *eustachian tube*. This serves to equalize the air pressure on the inner and outer surfaces of the tympanic membrane and to provide an avenue for fluid drainage from the middle ear into the nasopharynx. With development, the entodermal-lined recess enlarges in the direction of the external auditory canal. In addition, the auditory ossicles differentiate from the cartilage of adjacent branchial arches.

The *incus* appears as a condensation in the dorsal end of the cartilage in the first arch. Later, the *malleus* separates from the same cartilage. The *stapes* differentiates from the dorsal end of the cartilage of the second branchial arch (Figs. 12–4 and 12–5). The medial portion or *footplate* of the stapes, differentiating adjacent to the otocyst, becomes surrounded by the cartilaginous matrix forming around the lateral wall of the otocyst. This gap in the cartilage is the precursor

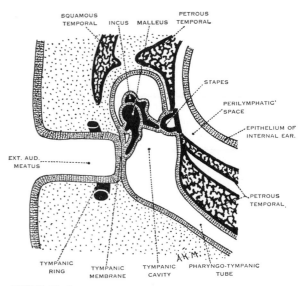

FIGURE 12-5

A final stage in the development of the middle ear cavity. Note the tuberotympanic recess, now the tympanic cavity, has enlarged and totally surrounds the auditory ossicles, leaving them vested with a layer of entoderm. (Reproduced with permission from W. J. Hamilton and H. W. Mossman, *Human Embryology*, 4th Edition. Williams & Wilkins Co., Baltimore, 1972.)

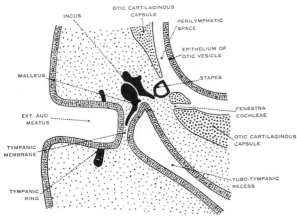

FIGURE 12-4

An early stage in the development of the middle ear. Note the early formation of the tympanic membrane between the external auditory canal (meatus) and the tuberotympanic recess and the trapping of the manubrium of the malleus between the layers of this membrane. The footplate of the early stapes is positioned in a gap, later to become the oval window, in the cartilaginous capsule forming around the otocyst. (Reproduced with permission from W. J. Hamilton and H. W. Mossman, *Human Embryology*, 4th Edition. Williams & Wilkins Co., Baltimore, 1972.)

of the *oval window*. A cartilaginous process of the malleus, the manubrium, becomes sandwiched between the ectoderm of the external auditory canal and the entoderm of the middle ear, firmly anchoring the developing ossicle to the tympanic membrane (see Figs. 12–4 and 12–5). With the later enlargement of the tuberotympanic recess, a thin layer of entoderm surrounds the auditory ossicles, leaving the articulating ossicles suspended in the cavity of the middle ear but anchored at each end—laterally at the tympanic membrane and medially at the oval window of the inner ear.

Two very small muscles also develop in the middle ear—the *tensor tympani* and the *stapedius*. The tensor tympani, a derivative of the first branchial arch, has its origin in the floor of the middle ear and inserts on the manubrium of the malleus (the process anchored to the tympanic membrane). The stapedius muscle, a derivative of the second branchial arch, has its origin near the roof of the middle ear and inserts on the neck of the stapes. A branch of the facial nerve (cranial nerve VII) innervates the stapedius muscle, a derivative of the second branchial arch. A branch of the mandibular division of the trigeminal nerve (cranial nerve V) innervates the tensor tympani muscle, a derivative of the first branchial arch (see Chapters 1 and 19).

MIDDLE EAR FUNCTION

The function of the middle ear is to convert sound waves of the air into waves in the fluid medium of the inner ear. Without the structure of the middle ear, the coupling of sound waves to fluid waves in the scala vestibuli of the cochlea would be very inefficient. If airborne sound waves struck the oval window directly, only about 3% of the sound would enter the inner ear, the equivalent to a 15-dB hearing loss.

The mechanism for the conversion of air waves to fluid waves by the middle ear is illustrated in Figure 12–6. Both the tympanic membrane and the footplate of the stapes act as pistons. Sound waves traveling through the air cause the tympanic membrane to move in and out. This motion moves the footplate of the stapes, via the articulations of the ossicles. The footplate of the stapes then moves in and out against the oval window, producing waves of pressure in the fluid-filled inner ear. The middle ear amplifies the pressure transmitted to the oval window in two ways: the tympanic membrane is much larger than the membrane of the oval window

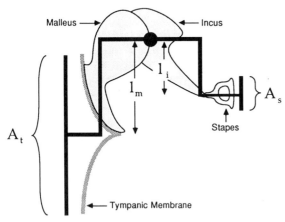

FIGURE 12–6

A seesaw model of the middle ear superimposed on a diagram of the tympanic membrane and the auditory ossicles. A_t and A_s represent the areas of the tympanic membrane and the footplate of the stapes at the oval window, respectively. l_m and l_i are the lever arms associated with the manubrium of the malleus and the long arm of the incus, respectively. (Reproduced with permission from E. M. Relkin, Introduction to the analysis of middle-ear function. In A. F. Jahn and J. Santos-Sacchi (Editors), *Physiology of the Ear*. Raven Press, New York, 1988.)

and the "lever arms" of the malleus and incus provide an additional mechanical advantage (see Fig. 12–6). At its peak of efficiency, i.e., 1000 Hz, the middle ear converts about 40% of the air pressure waves to fluid pressure waves. This efficiency falls to about 10% at 100 Hz and, at higher frequencies, to about 0.6% at 40,000 Hz.

The two muscles of the middle ear regulate the amount of sound energy transmitted from the air to the fluid of the inner ear. Contraction of the tensor tympani reduces the amount of movement, hence, sensitivity, of the tympanic membrane. Contraction of the stapedius muscle restricts the movement of the footplate of the stapes against the oval window (Fig. 12–7). These two muscles, in concert, dampen loud noises and protect the ear from damage.

Inner Ear and Sensory Transduction

COCHLEAR ANATOMY

The *cochlea* is the auditory portion of the inner ear. Deriving its name from the Greek word for a spiral-shelled snail, *kochlias*, the cochlea is a spiral-shaped, compound canal that winds 2½ times around a central bony axis, the *modiolus* (Figs. 12–1, 12–7, and 12–8). Spiraling around the inner margin of the cochlea, within the bony modiolus, is the *cochlear (spiral) ganglion* (Figs. 12–8 and 12–9). The peripheral processes of these bipolar neurons innervate the receptors. The central processes enter the core of the modiolus, where they form the *cochlear nerve* or, more properly, the *cochlear division of cranial nerve VIII* (see Fig. 12–8).

The membranous portion of the cochlea, the *cochlear partition*, containing the *cochlear duct* or *scala media*, develops from the otocyst and is part of the membranous labyrinth. The cochlear partition spans the bony labyrinth dividing it into two separate canals. When seen in cross section, the cochlear partition is triangular and divides the bony labyrinth into the *scala vestibuli* and the *scala tympani* (see Figs. 12–8 and 12–9). Two membranes of the cochlear partition, the *vestibular membrane (Reissner's membrane)* and the *basilar membrane*, separate the endolymph-filled cochlear duct from the perilymph-filled scala vestibuli and scala tympani. The lateral wall of the cochlear partition, lining a portion of the bony labyrinth, is the highly vascular *stria vascularis*, an important structure for maintaining the

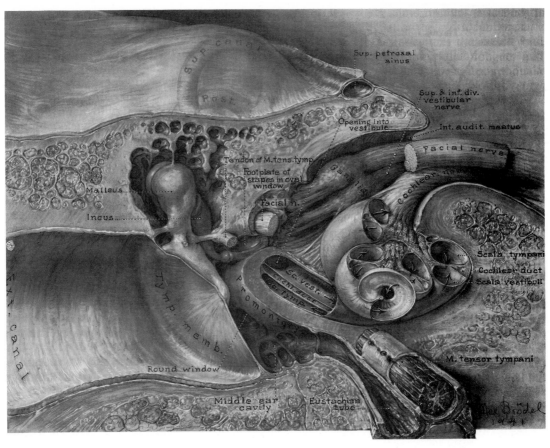

FIGURE 12-7

A drawing of some of the anatomical features of the external, middle, and inner ear. (After M. Brödel. In Malone, Guild, and Crowe, *Three Unpublished Drawings of the Human Ear.* W. B. Saunders Co., Philadelphia, 1946.)

unique ionic composition of the endolymph (see subsequent discussion) (see Fig. 12–9).

The cochlear partition does not extend to the apex or *cupula* of the cochlea but leaves a small aperture of communication between the scala vestibuli and scala tympani at the apex, the *helicotrema* (see Fig. 12–8). At the base of the cochlea, the membranes of the *oval window* and *round window* separate the scala vestibuli and the scala tympani, respectively, from the middle ear cavity (Fig. 12–10).

The *basilar membrane* is about 34 mm in length, extending from the bony wall between the round and oval windows to the helicotrema. During its spiral course, the width of the basilar membrane increases five-fold. At the base, its width is about 100 μm; at the helicotrema, it is 500 μm. In addition, the tension (degree of "tightness") on the basilar membrane decreases, with membrane tension greatest at the base and

least at the helicotrema. Both of these features are important to the *tonotopic responsiveness* of the basilar membrane. The basal portions are more sensitive to high frequency sounds, the apical portions to lower frequency sounds.

SOUND CONDUCTION

The middle ear converts airborne sound into fluid-borne compression waves. The perilymph-filled scala vestibuli and scala tympani are a closed system. Because the fluid is noncompressible, oscillatory movements of the stapes against the oval window result in equal but opposite movements of the round window (see Fig. 12–10). The endolymph-filled cochlear partition also is a closed system and separates the two perilymphatic channels except at the helicotrema. Hence, fluid vibrations traveling in the perilymphatic channels produce oscillatory or vibratory move-

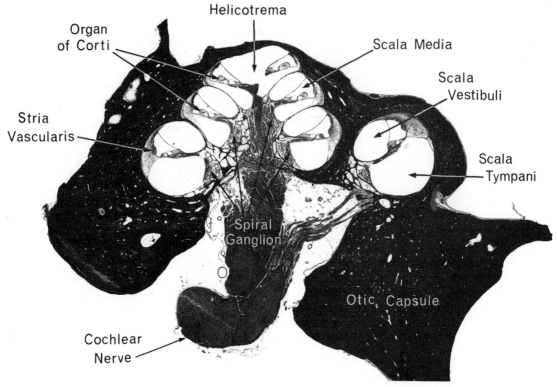

FIGURE 12-8

Photomicrograph of a section through the center of the modiolus of the cochlea of a rhesus monkey illustrating the spiral ganglion and the cochlear nerve. (Reproduced with permission from D. W. Fawcett, *A Textbook of Histology*, 11th Edition. W. B. Saunders Co., Philadelphia, 1986.)

ments of the cochlear partition, including the basilar membrane. These movements of the basilar membrane stimulate the hair cells of the organ of Corti, leading to the generation of action potentials in the neurons of the spiral ganglion (see subsequent discussion).

ENDOLYMPH AND PERILYMPH ELECTROLYTES

The electrolyte composition of perilymph is similar to that of other extracellular fluids. However, the endolymph has high K^+ and low Na^+ concentrations, resembling an intracellular fluid (Table 12-1). This difference is due principally to the activity of Na^+/K^+ pumps in the stria vascularis pumping Na^+ out and K^+ into the endolymph. In addition, an electrical potential difference of 160 mV exists between the endolymph and the inside of the hair cell. This potential difference is the driving force for the depolarization of the hair cells during sensory transduction.

ORGAN OF CORTI

Running longitudinally along the entire length of the basilar membrane and within the cochlear duct is the *organ of Corti* (Figs. 12-9 and 12-11). The organ of Corti is the sound-transducing organ of the inner ear and contains the sensory

TABLE 12-1

Comparison of Cochlear Fluids and Hair Cells with Other Fluids and Neurons

	Na^+	K^+	Cl^-	mV*
Perilymph	150.0	4.0	125.0	0
Endolymph	1.0	160.0	130.0	+85
Hair Cells†	5.0	130.0	40.0	-75
Neurons†	15.0	138.0	6.6	
CSF	149.0	3.0	125.0	
Serum	141.0	4.5	102.0	

* Potential relative to perilymph.
† Intracellular values.

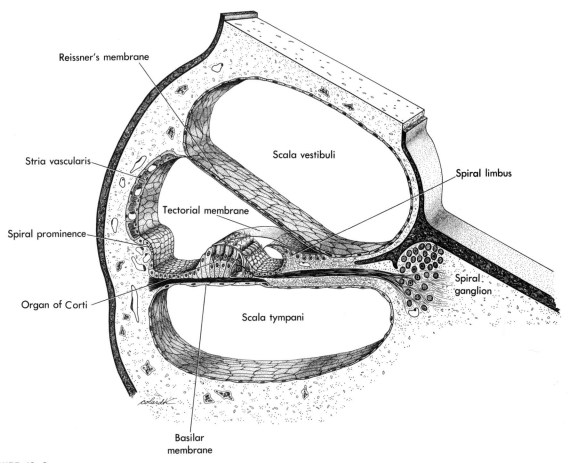

FIGURE 12-9

Schematic representation of a section through one of the turns of the cochlea. (Drawn by Sylvia Colard Keene. Reproduced with permission from D. W. Fawcett, *A Textbook of Histology*, 11th Edition. W. B. Saunders Co., Philadelphia, 1986.)

FIGURE 12-10

Displacement of the cochlear partition and round window following the inward movement of the stapes and oval window. The cochlea, in this diagrammatic illustration, is represented as a straight canal rather than a coiled canal. The scala vestibuli and scala tympani are separated by the cochlear partition except at the helicotrema.

Sound frequency determines the region of the cochlear partition that is displaced (dotted lines). Depression of the oval window leads to depression of the partition and the round window as indicated. For frequencies below hearing range, the cochlear partition is not displaced and the pressure is transmitted from the scala vestibuli to the scala tympani at the helicotrema.

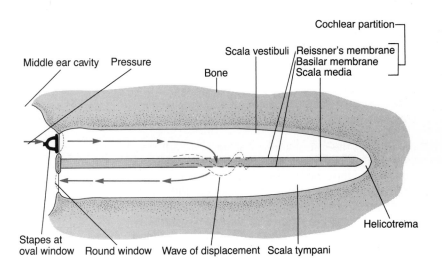

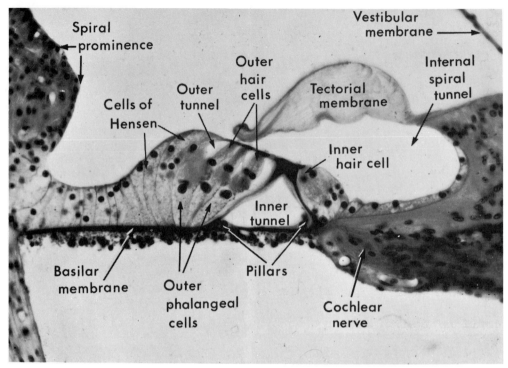

FIGURE 12-11

Photomicrograph of the organ of Corti of a cat. The tectorial membrane has been lifted away from the inner hair cells in specimen preparation. (Courtesy of H. Engström. Reproduced with permission from D. W. Fawcett, *A Textbook of Histology*, 11th Edition. W. B. Saunders Co., Philadelphia, 1986.)

receptors, the *hair cells*. These figures of the organ of Corti are of cross-sectional views. The entire organ of Corti actually extends the full length of the *basilar membrane*. Two types of hair cells are present in the human cochlea, *inner hair cells* and *outer hair cells*. Both have an elaborate arrangement of hairs or *stereocilia* projecting from their apical surfaces (Figs. 12–12 and 12–13).

An elaborate structure of supporting epithelial cells anchors the hair cells in position. Among these are the *pillar cells* and *phalangeal cells*. *Outer phalangeal cells* (*Deiters's cells*) invest the lower third of the outer hair cells and the nerve terminals around the base of the hair cell. In addition, they have a phalangeal process extending toward the apical surface of the hair cell that flattens into a plate. This plate forms tight junctions with the apical rims of adjacent hair cells and neighboring phalangeal plates (see Figs. 12–12 and 12–13). The *inner phalangeal cells* lack the phalangeal process and completely surround most of the inner hair cell and its nerve terminals. Apical processes of the *inner* and *outer*

pillar cells form tight junctions with each other and with adjacent hair cells. The network of tight junctions between apical processes of the phalangeal and pillar cells and with apical edges of both inner and outer hair cells, known as the *reticular lamina*, effectively isolates the hair cell body from the endolymph of the scala media (see Fig. 12–12).

Above the hair cells and extending from the inner margin of the organ of Corti is the *tectorial membrane*. This acellular structure, composed of mucopolysaccharides embedded in a collagen matrix, arches over the hair cells. The tips of the stereocilia of the outer hair cells embed in the substance of the tectorial membrane. Movement of the basilar membrane relative to the tectorial membrane displaces these cilia along their axes of symmetry, at right angles to the long axis of the basilar membrane. This mechanical distortion of the surface of the hair cell leads to an alteration in the membrane potential of the hair cell (see the following discussion). Inner hair cells are not attached to the tectorial membrane and are probably displaced by movement of the endolymph.

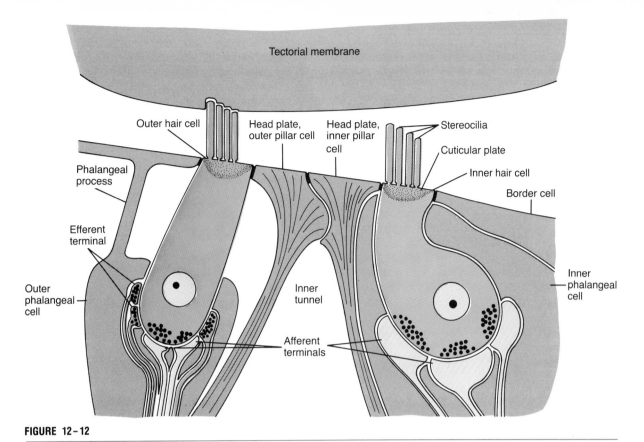

FIGURE 12-12

A portion of the organ of Corti. Inner hair cells and their afferent fiber terminals are surrounded by inner phalangeal cells. Outer hair cells receive efferent as well as afferent terminals. Relatively few efferents end in relation to the inner hair cells. These are not illustrated (see text).

The basal third of the outer hair cell is invested by the outer phalangeal cell. Processes from the outer phalangeal cells form tight junctions with the apical edge of the outer hair cells and other phalangeal processes. Processes from the inner and outer pillar cells line the inner tunnel and form head plates. See text for details.

FIGURE 12-13

Scanning electron micrograph of the organ of Corti from the guinea pig. The lowest row of cells are outer phalangeal cells (Deiters's cells, Dc), and continuous with them are the outer hair cells (ohc). Outer phalangeal cells have rod-like phalangeal processes that attach to the cuticular plates of neighboring outer hair cells along the organ of Corti. Note the V of the W-shaped outer hair cell's stereocilia bundles. The inner hair cells lie under the tectorial membrane (tm) behind the two rows of pillar cells (pc). Scale × 700. (Courtesy of Dr. Andrew Forge. Reproduced with permission from Holley, M. C., Semin. Neurosci., 2: 41–48, 1990.)

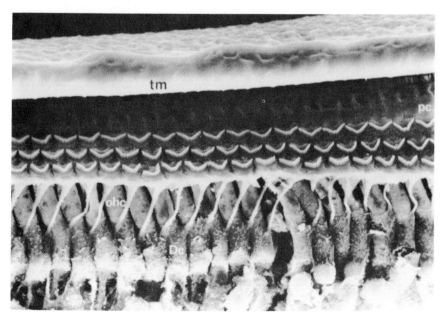

HAIR CELL STRUCTURE

The human cochlea contains 30,000 to 35,000 hair cells. A typical hair cell has up to 100 *stereocilia* and a single *kinocilium* organized in a symmetrical V- or W-shaped pattern when viewed from the surface (see Fig. 12–13). This arrangement imparts a plane of symmetry to the hair cell that is at right angles to the long axis of the organ of Corti. The anatomical symmetry, imparted by the arrangement of the cilia, reflects a physiological symmetry in its responsiveness. Hair cells are thereby sensitive only to movement of the cilia in this plane. The laterally placed kinocilium at the base of the V is longer than the stereocilia. The stereocilia become progressively shorter from the lateral (away from the modiolus) to the medial margins of the hair cell (see Fig. 12–12).

Inner hair cells are arranged in a single, longitudinal row; the *outer hair cells* in three to five, parallel, longitudinal rows (see Figs. 12–9, 12–11, and 12–13). Both types of hair cells extend the entire length of the basilar membrane; however, they have different physiological roles in sound transduction.

HAIR CELL INNERVATION

Distal processes of the primary afferent neurons in the spiral ganglion innervate the hair cells, forming postsynaptic terminals around the basal portion of the hair cells (see Fig. 12–12). The afferent innervation of the inner hair cells is much denser than that of the outer hair cells. Of the 28,000 to 35,000 spiral ganglion cells, up to 95% are large cells and innervate the roughly 3500 inner hair cells with up to 20 afferent fibers ending on each inner hair cell. The processes from the remaining smaller ganglion cells branch profusely with each neuron supplying 30 to 50 outer hair cells. The central processes of both ganglion cell types enter the central core of the modiolus, where they form the cochlear division of cranial nerve VIII. To date, all recordings of sound-induced action potentials from fibers in cranial nerve VIII have been associated with the innervation of inner hair cells. The cochlea also receives an efferent innervation, the *olivocochlear efferent*, that synapses on the outer hair cells (see subsequent discussion).

HAIR CELLS AS SENSORY TRANSDUCERS

The *hair cell* is the basic sensory transducer of the organ of Corti (Figs. 12–12 and 12–14).

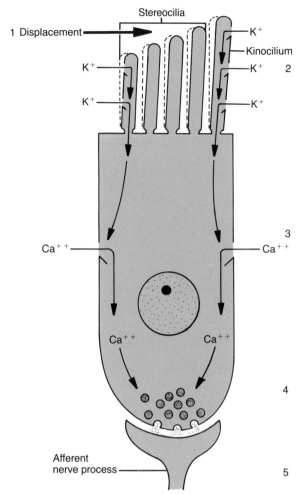

FIGURE 12–14

Molecular events in hair cell transduction. The mechanical displacement of the stereocilia opens cation channels ①. K⁺ ions are driven into the hair cell as a result of the electrical potential difference ②. This cation influx depolarizes the hair cell, opening voltage-sensitive Ca⁺⁺ channels ③. The calcium influx, in turn, triggers the release of neurotransmitter ④. The release of sufficient neurotransmitter then triggers an action potential in the afferent nerve process ⑤.

Because the basilar membrane is permeable to the perilymph of the scala tympani, the main body of the hair cell is surrounded by a fluid similar to the perilymph and the cilia are surrounded by endolymph (see Table 12–1). When physically displaced, the cilia bend at their base. Displacements as small as 0.1 nm alter the conductance of the cation channels. When conductance increases, the electrical gradient of 160 mV between the endolymph and the inside of the hair cells drives K⁺ ions into the hair cell (see Table 12–1; Fig. 12–14). At "rest," there is a small but steady K^+ current. This current increases as the cilia are displaced laterally (increasing channel conductance and depolarizing the hair cell) and decreases as the cilia are displaced medially (decreasing channel conductance and hyperpolarizing the hair cell).

Depolarization of the hair cell, in turn, triggers voltage-sensitive Ca^{++} channels. The subsequent influx of Ca^{++} activates the release of neurotransmitters through mechanisms similar to those in neurons (see Fig. 12–14). Hair cells are capable of responding up to 20,000 times per second. Glutamate, or a glutamate-like compound, is a prime candidate for the neurotransmitter at the synapse between the hair cells and the afferent fibers of the spiral ganglion.

TONOTOPIC DISTRIBUTION OF RECEPTORS

Portions of the basilar membrane move in response to sounds of specific frequencies. This movement stimulates selected populations of hair cells. In addition to this *tonotopic* distribution of responding receptors, there are anatomical differences between hair cells. Hair cells sensitive to high frequencies at the lower end of the basilar membrane have shorter, stiffer cilia. Those sensitive to low frequencies, at the apical portion of the basilar membrane, have longer and more flaccid cilia.

Electrophysiological measurements from single mammalian ganglion cells indicate maximal responses to sounds of a specific frequency. As with most neurons, the ganglion cells generate action potentials and each has a basal rate of firing in the nonstimulated state. When stimulated by the frequency to which they are most sensitive, individual neurons increase the firing rate immediately and then fall to a less than maximal rate for the duration of the stimulus. With discontinuation of the stimulus, the firing rate falls below the basal level for a few milliseconds, before returning to the original level.

The mechanism of interaction between inner and outer hair cells remains unknown. Stimulation of cochlear efferents dampens the frequency sensitivity of inner hair cells even though the outer hair cells receive most of the efferent innervation. No evidence exists of either synaptic or electrical coupling between the two hair cell types. Because cochlear efferent stimulation is known to contract the cilia of the outer hair cells, one proposed explanation is that this contraction adjusts the fine-tuning properties of the basilar membrane and the organ of Corti.

Central Pathways and Information Processing

The ascending central pathways of the auditory system form a bilateral, multisynaptic system with a large number of relay nuclei. The central nervous system (CNS) pathways contribute to the detection, localization, and interpretation of auditory stimuli. Parallel processing of the auditory information, as in other sensory systems, is a prominent feature. However, more "cross talk" occurs between parallel pathways of the auditory system than between other sensory pathways.

A consequence of this organization is that damage to the central pathways or the primary auditory cortex produces a diminished capacity for hearing in both ears and not a total loss in either. However, the inability to localize sound in the contralateral half of acoustic space does occur with unilateral damage to the primary auditory cortex or central pathways above the level of the pons.

In the auditory system, a strict *tonotopic representation* occurs throughout. Few, if any, connections exist between neurons that are not sensitive to the same auditory frequency, i.e., they are in *tonotopic register*. If a projection fiber arises from a neuron sensitive to 3-kHz sound, it will terminate in the 3-kHz lamina or subdivision of its target. Similarly with binaural cells (cells receiving input from both ears), each receives input from neurons responding to the same frequency.

Nuclei such as the cochlear nuclei, the central nucleus of the inferior colliculus, and the medial geniculate nucleus have well-defined *isofrequency laminae*. All neurons in an isofrequency lamina respond to auditory stimuli of a single or preferred frequency. However, the number of neurons in an isofrequency lamina reflects the number of receptors sensitive to that frequency. Although the laminar organization in other nuclei and subnuclei within the auditory system is not as distinct, they also have at least one complete tonotopic representation.

As fibers of the *cochlear nerve* leave the modiolus, they join the vestibulocochlear nerve and enter the posterior cranial fossa through the *internal auditory meatus* and, from there, enter the brain stem. When the vestibulocochlear nerve reaches the medullopontine angle of the brain stem, the nerve splits and the vestibular nerve fibers enter the medulla deep to the restiform body. Cochlear nerve fibers enter the *cochlear nuclei* on the dorsolateral surface of the restiform body (Fig. 12–15 and Figs. 7–3, 7–4, and 7–10).

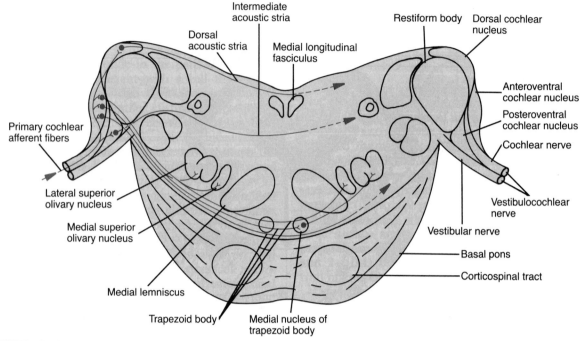

FIGURE 12-15

The principal projections from the cochlear nuclei. The dorsal aspect of the section is through the cochlear nuclei; ventral aspect is through the caudal portion of the basal pons. Dashed lines indicate fibers ascending out of the plane of the diagram. Ipsilateral projections to the lateral lemniscus are omitted. See text for details.

COCHLEAR NUCLEI

Two principal *cochlear nuclei* are evident on each side of the brain stem, the *dorsal cochlear nucleus* and the *ventral cochlear nucleus* (see Figs. 7-4, 7-10, and Fig. 12-15). As axons of the cochlear nerve enter the ventral cochlear nucleus, they form a band of fibers that divides the ventral nucleus into an *anteroventral cochlear nucleus* and a *posteroventral cochlear nucleus*. In the human, the anteroventral cochlear nucleus is the principal nucleus; the dorsal cochlear nucleus is small; and the function of the posteroventral nucleus is poorly understood.

Once in the ventral nucleus, the fibers bifurcate and send branches into both the dorsal and ventral cochlear nuclei. This divergent pattern of cochlear nerve terminations, however, is organized *tonotopically* within the nuclei. Fibers from the basal portion of the cochlea, responding to sounds of high frequency, run to the deepest part of the nucleus before bifurcating. In contrast, those from the apical portion of the cochlea, responding to sounds of low frequency, bifurcate and terminate in superficial layers of the nuclei. Within this *isofrequency laminar organization* of

the cochlear nuclei, fibers responding to the highest frequencies end in the deepest layers and those responding to the lower frequencies end in more superficial layers, with the lowest frequencies at the surface.

Although signals entering the cochlear nuclei via the primary afferent fibers code principally for intensity (firing rate) and sound frequency (origin in the organ of Corti), the output of the cochlear nuclei is more complex. Because of the information processing at the level of the cochlear nuclei, the afferent signals relayed to higher centers contain a variety of complex response and temporal patterns in addition to intensity and frequency. Thus at this level of the auditory system, there already are a number of parallel pathways.

Second-order ascending fibers leave the cochlear nuclei and ascend on the ipsilateral side of the brain stem or cross the midline in one of three pathways. The most prominent of these is the *trapezoid body*. These auditory fibers, principally from the anteroventral cochlear nucleus, cross the brain stem in the ventral portion of the pontine tegmentum, immediately dorsal to the basal pons (see Fig. 12-15). This pattern of crossing myelinated fibers can be visualized in Weigert-stained brain stem sections as a dark area in the shape of a trapezoid (see Fig. 7–11). The two lesser pathways are the *dorsal acoustic stria*, crossing immediately below the floor of the fourth ventricle and containing fibers from the dorsal cochlear nucleus, and the *intermediate acoustic stria*, crossing the brain stem immediately ventral to the medial longitudinal fasciculus and containing fibers from the posteroventral cochlear nucleus (see Fig. 12–15).

SUPERIOR OLIVARY NUCLEI

Many secondary auditory fibers, both crossed and uncrossed, terminate in nuclei of the *superior olivary complex* (Figs. 12–15 and 12–16 and Fig. 7–13). The two most prominent of these nuclei are the *medial* and *lateral superior olivary nuclei.* Neurons in both nuclei are *binaural*; they receive input from both ears. Functionally, the convergence of binaural, isofrequency auditory information on single neurons of these nuclei permits the localization of sound in acoustic space.

Projections from the anteroventral cochlear nuclei terminate bilaterally in the *medial superior olivary nuclei* (see Figs. 12–15 and 12–16). This nucleus utilizes differences in signal arrival time to localize the sound. Sound signals reach the ears at different times, unless originating at a point equidistant from each ear. These binaural neurons have two prominent dendrites, one oriented medially that receives afferents from the contralateral ear and the other oriented laterally that receives afferents from the ipsilateral ear. The firing patterns of these neurons are governed

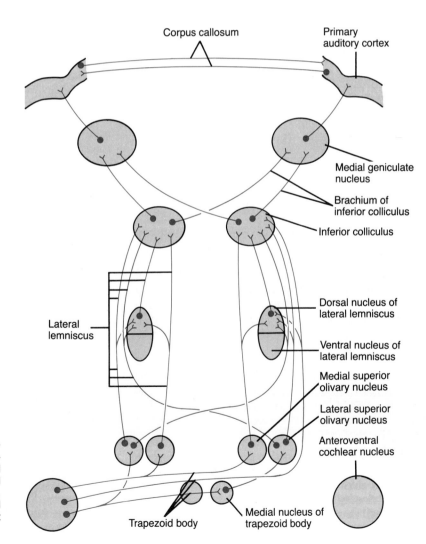

FIGURE 12-16

The major ascending auditory pathways arising from the anteroventral cochlear nucleus. Both ipsilateral and contralateral pathways are binaural. Pathways from the left anteroventral nucleus only are indicated. See text for details.

by the differences in arrival times of the afferent signals from the two ears. These neurons are sensitive to time differences as small as 400 μsec. As with all auditory system nuclei, the medial superior olivary nucleus is organized tonotopically.

The binaural neurons of the *lateral superior olivary nucleus*, in contrast, utilize differences in sound intensity to localize sound. These neurons are excited by signals from the ipsilateral anteroventral cochlear nucleus and inhibited by signals from the contralateral nucleus. The inhibition is by way of interneurons in the *medial nucleus of the trapezoid body* (see Figs. 12–15 and 12–16). A tonotopic organization exists within the lateral superior olivary nucleus.

LATERAL LEMNISCUS

Fibers from the superior olivary complex, along with both crossed and uncrossed second-order fibers from cochlear nuclei (ones that by-pass the superior olivary complex), combine to form the *lateral lemniscus*. Those from the *medial superior olivary nucleus* ascend in the ipsilateral lateral lemniscus, and those from the *lateral superior olivary nucleus* ascend in both the ipsilateral and contralateral lateral lemnisci (see Fig. 12–16). The lateral lemniscus ends in the inferior colliculus.

Nuclei of the Lateral Lemniscus

Within the lateral lemniscus are small groups of neurons, collectively known as the *nuclei of the lateral lemniscus* (Figs. 12–16 and 12–17 and Fig. 7–14). Some of the fibers of the lateral lemniscus synapse with these relay neurons and others do not. Ascending neurons from the superior olivary complex and the anteroventral cochlear nucleus may synapse on the binaural-responding cells of the *dorsal nucleus of the lateral lemniscus*. Fibers from the posteroventral and dorsal cochlear nuclei may synapse with the monaural-responding cells of the *ventral nucleus of the lateral lemniscus* (see Figs. 12–16 and 12–17).

INFERIOR COLLICULUS

Fibers of the lateral lemniscus, now containing relay projections from the three cochlear nuclei, the superior olivary complex, and the nuclei of the lateral lemniscus, ascend to the *inferior colliculus* (see Figs. 12–16 and 12–17). The infe-

rior colliculus is primarily a relay and information processing station in the ascending auditory pathway.

Ascending auditory fibers converge on the *inferior colliculus* and end in the appropriate *isofrequency lamina*. The most dorsal laminae receive signals from neurons that respond to low frequencies. In contrast, the more ventral layers receive higher frequency information. Within an isofrequency layer, the distribution of terminals is not uniform. For example, fibers from the dorsal cochlear nucleus terminate in the more ventral and caudal portions of the layer. However, the segregation of brain stem nuclear projections within the isofrequency laminae is not clear-cut —considerable overlap occurs. Within these layers, response properties of many of the individual neurons to sound stimuli are more complex than those leaving the cochlear nuclei.

MEDIAL GENICULATE NUCLEUS

Relay fibers from the inferior colliculus form the *brachium of the inferior colliculus*, as they ascend toward the *medial geniculate nucleus (MGN)*, which is the thalamic relay nucleus of the auditory system (see Fig. 12–16 and Figs. 7–4, 7–16, and 7–17). These fibers in the brachium of the inferior colliculus end in the appropriate isofrequency lamina of the MGN. Thalamocortical projections from the MGN enter the sublenticular portion of the internal capsule and project to the *primary auditory cortex* (see Figs. 12–16 and 12–17).

The MGN contains three subdivisions: *ventral (MGNv)*, *medial (MGNm)*, and *dorsal (MGNd)*. *MGNv* is the principal cortical relay nucleus and contains a very precise tonotopic representation. This nucleus relays accurate information on sound intensity and sound frequency and the binaural properties of the sound stimulus.

MGNd is less well defined, and the tonotopic organization is not as precise as MGNv. It receives afferent projections from the inferior colliculus and some nonauditory areas of the brain stem. The response properties of these neurons are complex. The tonotopic organization of *MGNm* is not precise, and the nucleus receives projections from both auditory and nonauditory neurons of the brain stem, with a major contribution from the superior olivary complex. Those neurons responding to auditory stimuli reflect the intensity and duration of the auditory signal rather than its precise frequency, although it is still a frequency-organized and frequency-responsive system.

FIGURE 12-17

The major ascending auditory pathways arising from the posteroventral and dorsal cochlear nuclei. The minor ipsilateral projections from the dorsal cochlear nucleus are omitted. Pathways from the left posteroventral nucleus and the right dorsal cochlear nucleus only are illustrated. See text for details.

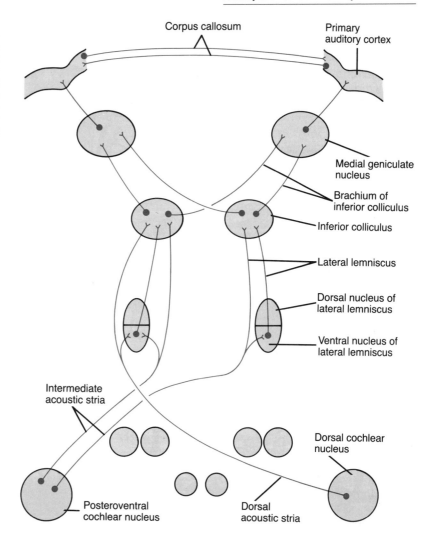

Corpus callosum

Primary auditory cortex

Medial geniculate nucleus

Brachium of inferior colliculus

Inferior colliculus

Lateral lemniscus

Dorsal nucleus of lateral lemniscus

Ventral nucleus of lateral lemniscus

Intermediate acoustic stria

Dorsal cochlear nucleus

Posteroventral cochlear nucleus

Dorsal acoustic stria

As with all thalamocortical interconnections, the flow of information between the thalamus and cortex is modulated by both *feed-forward* and *feedback inhibitory loops.* Colliculogeniculate collaterals synapse with inhibitory interneurons gamma-aminobutyric acid (GABA) within the MGN that inhibit MGN cortical relay neurons, forming a feed-forward inhibitory loop (see Fig. 4–10B). Collaterals from the cortical projection fibers of the MGN synapse with inhibitory (GABA) neurons of the reticular nucleus of the thalamus. These, in turn, feed back to the MGN, forming a feedback inhibitory loop (see Fig. 4–10A; Chapters 4 and 20).

AUDITORY CORTEX

The *primary auditory cortex* (*A-1* or *Brodmann's areas 41* and *42*) lies in the depths of the lateral

fissure, in the transverse temporal gyri of Heschl (see Fig. 21–3). Within A-1 are several complete tonotopic representations, an organization similar to that of other primary sensory cortices, such as S-1. The projections from the MGN terminate in layer IV, with some in layer III. On reaching A-1, the tonotopic organization of the auditory pathway changes from one of isofrequency layers to one of *isofrequency bands.* Within each cortical isofrequency band, all the neurons (from layer I to VI) are in frequency register.

A suborganization of columns is superimposed on the system of isofrequency bands within A-1, *summation* and *suppression columns.* In the summation columns, binaural responses are greater than either monaural response alone. In the suppression columns, the monaural response dominates, being greater than the binaural response.

Two other suborganizations have been proposed within A-1. One hypothesis suggests a cortical map of the contralateral acoustic hemifield. Central pathways on each side of the brain stem, rostral to the superior olivary complex, process auditory spatial information only for the contralateral acoustic hemifield. Hence, information on one side of the brain, above the superior olivary complex, is independently capable of localizing sounds only from the contralateral hemifield. This localization is accomplished over frequency-specific pathways, and at the cortical level may be represented as a map of acoustic space. Another hypothesis is the presence of a subfield of cells, within each isofrequency band, that is spatially arranged, according a preferred amplitude of sound or a preferred signal-to-noise ratio.

A-1 has numerous connections both with other cortical areas and with lower brain stem centers. Extensive corticothalamic and corticocollicular projections exist, and many of the corticothalamic projections are reciprocal with the same area of the MGN. As with other primary sensory cortical areas, many reciprocal connections exist between A-1 and secondary auditory areas.

The *corpus callosum* carries abundant projections from A-1 of one side to A-1 of the other side. Callosal terminations are not uniform but end in irregular stripes or blotches, alternating with areas receiving no callosal projections, all within the appropriate isofrequency band.

The auditory system operates under similar principles, in the processing of auditory information, as those of other sensory systems. Parallel processing is apparent at the level of the cochlear nuclei. However, at higher levels within the auditory system, the response properties of neurons become increasingly complex, indicating the superimposition of hierarchical processing on the parallel streams.

SECONDARY AUDITORY AREAS

The auditory system has many secondary cortical areas; however, they are not as well defined as those for the somatosensory and visual systems. In general, secondary auditory areas surround A-1 and connect, reciprocally, with A-1. Many other areas of the cortex contain cells that are sensitive to acoustic stimuli. These areas probably represent higher integrative centers, because other cells in the same areas respond to other sensory modalities. One area with important connections to both A-1 and secondary auditory areas is *Wernicke's area* (*Brodmann's area 22*). These connections are important to the interpretation of the spoken word (see Chapter 21).

DESCENDING AUDITORY PATHWAYS

The flow of information in the auditory system is modulated by an extensive system of descending, feedback pathways—more extensive than previously described for any other sensory systems. A-1 has extensive descending projections to both the MGN and the inferior colliculus. The inferior colliculus, in turn, has extensive descending projections to both the superior olivary complex and to the cochlear nuclei. The descending projections to the superior olivary complex are important in modulating the cochlear efferents (see following discussion).

Auditory Reflexes

OLIVOCOCHLEAR EFFERENTS

Small, binaural efferent neurons in the *lateral superior olivary nucleus* give rise to the *uncrossed olivocochlear bundle*. These cochlear efferents join the ipsilateral cochlear nerve and innervate both inner and outer hair cells of the cochlea. Most efferent fibers to the inner hair cells synapse on the primary afferent fiber from the cochlear ganglion and not on the hair cell directly. Large efferent neurons, organized in small *satellite nuclei* surrounding the medial and lateral superior olivary nuclei, receive bilateral auditory afferent signals from neurons of both ventral cochlear nuclei. Axons from these efferents of the olivary complex cross the midline, forming the *crossed olivocochlear bundle* (Fig. 12–18). These neurons innervate only the outer hair cells of the contralateral cochlea.

The reflex activation of both the crossed and uncrossed olivocochlear efferents is important to auditory sensitivity and selective tuning of the cochlea. In mammals, these efferent fibers regulate the response characteristics of hair cells, possibly through contractile mechanisms associated with the actin fibers in the cilia. In addition, olivocochlear efferents may have a role in the cortically initiated mechanism of "focusing" on specific auditory stimuli and "ignoring" others.

Acetylcholine is the principal excitatory efferent neurotransmitter to both the inner and outer hair cells. A few efferents are inhibitory with *GABA* as the neurotransmitter. Most of the cholinergic efferents have a co-transmitter. The opioid peptides, *dynorphin* and *met-enkephalin*, co-release at one population of efferent terminals; the *excitatory amino acids*, glutamate and aspartate, co-release at other terminals. Those terminals in which the peptides are co-released have both fast

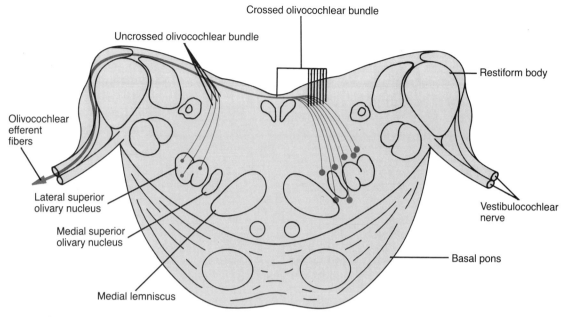

FIGURE 12-18

The olivocochlear efferent pathways. Axons from small efferent neurons in the lateral superior olivary nucleus form the uncrossed olivocochlear bundle. Axons from larger efferent neurons surrounding the superior olivary complex form the larger, crossed olivocochlear bundle. Both efferent bundles join the afferent fibers of the cochlear nerve. Only olivocochlear efferents to the left cochlear nerve are illustrated. See text for details.

and slow components to the postsynaptic potential; a response compatible with the two-phase inhibition by olivocochlear efferents. In contrast, postsynaptic excitation following the co-release of the excitatory amino acids has a rapid onset and a short duration.

SOMATIC MOTOR

Loud sounds stimulate the rapid contraction of both the tensor tympani and stapedius muscles. Acetylcholine is the neuromuscular transmitter. This results in a reduction of signal transmission through the middle ear and an indirect reduction of the sensitivity of the receptors. The sound threshold generally accepted for this reflex is 80 dB; however, many workers believe it to be much lower. This reflex is most effective for sounds of low frequencies. An increase in tension on the tympanic membrane and the stapes may facilitate middle ear transmission of high frequency sound.

Startle responses and rapid head movement in response to sound stimuli are other examples of somatic motor reflexes, some of which are mediated at the level of the inferior colliculus. Others are less well defined; however, the superior colliculus has a significant auditory represen-

tation in the deeper layers. These layers contain the efferent neurons of the tectospinal tract (see Chapter 11) and may be involved in these somatic motor reflexes.

Vestibular System

The sensory organs of the vestibular system, located within the *vestibular labyrinth* of the inner ear, respond to movement and position of the head in space. The central connections of the vestibular system are principally reflexive to motor centers and relate to the orientation of the body and head in space, the body's equilibrium, and the maintenance of muscle tone. Central pathways include extensive connections with (1) *the motor nuclei innervating the extraocular muscles*, (2) *the cerebellum*, (3) *the motor reticular formation of the pons and medulla*, and (4) *the spinal motor neurons*. Unlike the auditory, visual, and somatosensory systems, the vestibular system has little cortical representation. However, some projections go to the cerebral hemispheres by way of the dorsal thalamus, and these account for our perception of motion and the position of the head in space. Chapters 14 and 19 consider the role of the vestibular system in the coordination of motor function in greater detail.

Vestibular Labyrinth

The receptor organs of the vestibular system reside in the *vestibular portion of the membranous labyrinth* of the inner ear or simply, the *vestibular labyrinth* (Figs. 12–19 and 12–20). The vestibular labyrinth, continuous with the cochlea at the *ductus reuniens*, contains two ovoid sac-like structures, the *saccule* and *utricle*, and three *semicircular canals*, the *lateral, superior,* and *posterior* (see Figs. 12–19 and 12–20). As with the cochlea, the endolymph-filled membranous labyrinth of the vestibular system is enclosed within a *bony labyrinth*, all within the petrous portion of the temporal bone. The vestibular membranous labyrinth, however, is not firmly attached to the bone. Instead, it is suspended in the perilymph-containing bony labyrinth by a reticulum of periotic fibers arising from the periosteum and inserting in the thin, connective tissue layer enveloping the membranous labyrinth.

SACCULE

The *ductus reuniens* connects the saccule with the vestibule of the cochlea. The saccule, in turn, connects with the utricle via the *utriculosaccular duct.* A branch from the utriculosaccular duct, the *endolymphatic duct*, passes through the petrous bone and enlarges between the layers of the dura, within the cranial vault, forming the *endolymphatic sac* (see Figs. 12–19 and 12–20). This sac is the probable site for endolymph absorption (see Fig. 12–20).

The sensory organ within the saccule is the *macula of the saccule (macula sacculi)*, a small, thickened area of ectoderm containing supporting cells and *hair cell* receptors (see Fig. 12–20).

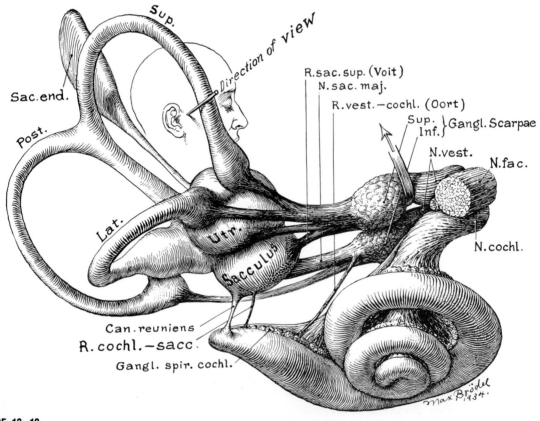

FIGURE 12–19

A semidiagrammatic presentation of the innervation of the membranous labyrinth as seen from a lateral view (see inset and compare with Fig. 12–20). Note the orthogonal orientation of the semicircular canals. (Reproduced with permission from M. Hardy, Anat. Rec., 59: 412, 1934.)

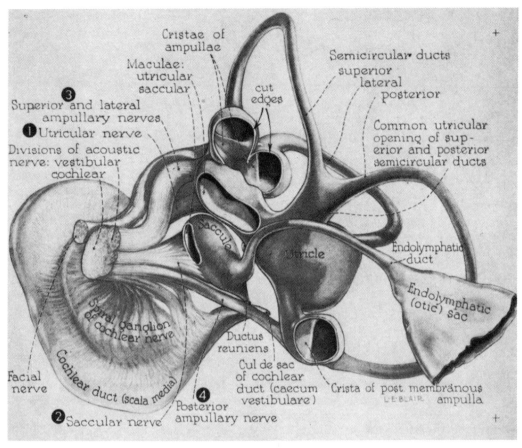

FIGURE 12-20

A reconstruction of the membranous labyrinth as seen from a medial view (compare with Fig. 12-19) in a newborn infant. Note the cutaway views illustrating the cristae ampullaris and maculae. (Reproduced with permission from Anson, B. J., Harper, D. G. and Winch, T. R., Arch. Otolaryng., 85: 499, 1967. Copyright 1967, American Medical Association.)

Superimposed on the cilia of the hair cells is an *otolithic membrane*, a gelatinous plate containing calcium carbonate crystals, *otoliths* (*statoconia*) (Fig. 12-21). The presence of the otoliths gives this membrane a specific gravity nearly three times that of the surrounding endolymph.

UTRICLE

The *utricle* is the largest of the chambers in the vestibular labyrinth, and all three semicircular canals originate and terminate in the utricle (see Fig. 12-20). The sensory organ of the utricle is the *macula of the utricle* (*macula utriculi*), a small, thickened area of ectoderm in the antero-lateral wall of the chamber containing hair cell receptors and an otolithic membrane, similar in structure to the macula of the saccule (see Fig. 12-21). When the head is in the anatomical

position (upright), the macula of the utricle is nearly horizontal, whereas the macula of the saccule is close to the vertical sagittal plane (see Figs. 12-20 and 12-22).

SEMICIRCULAR CANALS

Both ends of all three *semicircular canals* are continuous with the utricle. At one end of each canal is a dilation, the *ampulla*. Within the ampulla, the ectoderm of the wall and the underlying connective tissue form a ridge or crest, perpendicular to the long axis of the canal and partially blocking it, the *crista ampullaris* (Figs. 12-20 and 12-23). The ectodermal ridge of the crista contains the receptor hair cells and the supporting cells. The hair cells of the crista embed in a gelatinous cap, the *cupula*, that extends from the surface of the hair cells to the

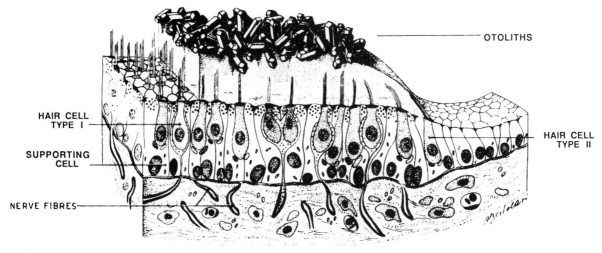

FIGURE 12-21

A macula. The cilia of hair cells, type I and type II, are embedded in the gelatinous matrix of the otolithic membrane. The more superficial part of the membrane is impregnated with carbonate crystals, or otoliths. (Reproduced with permission from S. Iurato, *Submicroscopic Structure of the Inner Ear*. Pergamon Press PLC, Oxford, 1967.)

opposite wall of the ampulla, effectively forming a barrier in the endolymph-filled canal (see Fig. 12-23).

The *lateral canals* are close to horizontal. Tilting the head forward 25 degrees will place both lateral canals in the horizontal plane. When the lateral canals are horizontal, the *posterior* and *superior canals* are vertical but at right angles to each other (see Figs. 12-19, 12-20, and 12-22).

The plane of each superior canal has an anterolateral orientation to the midsagittal plane of 41 degrees. Each posterior canal has a posterolateral orientation to the midsagittal plane of 56 degrees. Because of the orthogonal arrangement of the three canals, the superior canal of one side is in the same plane as the posterior canal of the opposite side, and the two lateral canals are in the same plane (see Fig. 12-22).

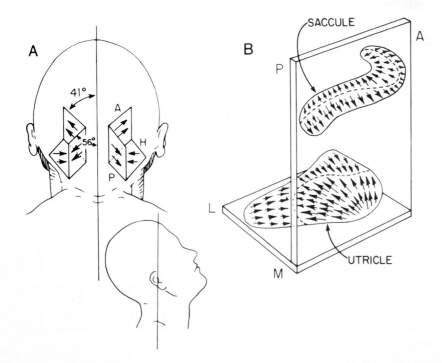

FIGURE 12-22

Preferred stimulus directions for hair cells in the semicircular canals (*A*) and in the maculae of the utricle and saccule (*B*). On the sensory epithelium, the arrows point from the smallest stereocilium toward the kinocilium of a representative cell at that location.

A, The head is tilted slightly backward for a better view of the canal planes.

B, P, posterior; A, anterior; L, lateral; and M, medial. (Reproduced with permission from A. F. Fuchs, The vestibular system. In H. D. Patton, A. F. Fuchs, B. Hille, A. M. Scher, and R. Steiner (Editors), *Textbook of Physiology*, Volume 1, 21st Edition. W. B. Saunders Co., Philadelphia, 1989.)

FIGURE 12-23

The crista ampullaris and cupula within the ampulla of a semicircular canal. Cilia of the hair cells insert into the gelatinous matrix of the cupula. Displacement of the cupula (dotted lines) occurs in response to movement of the endolymph. In this illustration, the displacement of the cupula is *utriculopetal*, bending hair cell cilia in the excitatory direction along their axis of polarity.

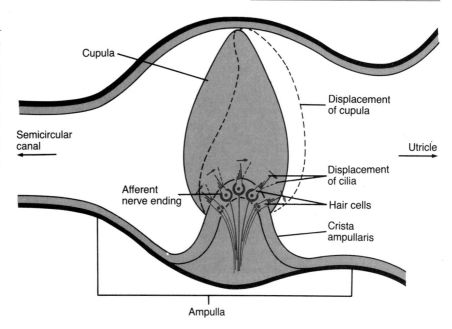

Vestibular Receptors and Sensory Transduction

HAIR CELLS

The *hair cell* is the primary receptor for the vestibular system. Structurally, vestibular hair cells are similar to those of the cochlea (Figs. 12-12 and 12-24). A large, chalice-like ending of a primary afferent neuron from the vestibular ganglion surrounds the goblet-shaped *type I hair cells*. Vestibular efferents end on the afferent chalice-like ending but not on the hair cell directly. *Type II hair cells* are somewhat smaller and more cylindrical, with numerous, small afferent and efferent endings around their bases (see Fig. 12-24).

A large number of stereocilia and a single kinocilium cover the apical surface of both types of hair cells. The kinocilium is always near one edge of the cell. Those stereocilia adjacent to the kinocilium are the longest; those farthest away are the shortest (see Fig. 12-24). This anatomical polarity reflects a physiological polarity. Displacement of stereocilia in the direction of the kinocilium excites the receptor cell; displacement of the stereocilia away from the kinocilium inhibits the cell.

The apical edges of the hair cells form tight junctions with the surrounding supporting cells, effectively isolating the main body of the hair cell from the endolymph. As with cochlear hair cells, the cilia are bathed by endolymph containing a high concentration of K^+. The body of the hair cell is bathed by an extracellular fluid, with a composition closer to that of perilymph (see Table 12-1). Also, a large electrical potential difference exists between the endolymph and the inside of the hair cell.

When the cilia are displaced toward the kino-

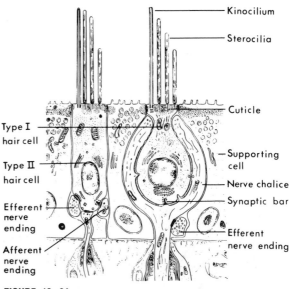

FIGURE 12-24

The two types of sensory hair cells in the mammalian labyrinth showing the fine structure organization of the type I and type II sensory cells and their innervation. (Reproduced with permission from J. Wersäll, and D. Bagger-Sjöbäck, Morphology of the vestibular sense organ. In H. H. Kornhuber (Editor), *Handbook of Sensory Physiology*, Volume VI, Part 1. Springer-Verlag, Berlin, 1974.)

cilium, cation channels open and the potential difference drives K+ ions from the endolymph through the cilia and into the hair cell. This process depolarizes the hair cell, activating voltage-sensitive Ca++ channels. The resultant Ca++ influx leads to an increase in the rate of neurotransmitter release (see Fig. 12–14).

Resting vestibular hair cells are partially depolarized, owing due to a small, but constant influx of K+ ions through a small population of open cation channels. When the cilia are displaced away from the kinocilium, these channels close and the cell hyperpolarizes. Hence, vestibular hair cells respond with either an increase or a decrease in the rate of neurotransmitter release, depending on the direction of cilia displacement. This results in a constant or tonic rate of firing of the vestibular afferent neurons—a rate of firing that increases or decreases in response to appropriate stimuli.

MACULAE

The cilia of the hair cells of the maculae are embedded in the otolithic membrane, and any displacement of the membrane bends the cilia. However, all of the hair cells do not respond because the functional polarity of the hair cells is not the same in all areas of a macula (see Fig. 12–22). The maculae of the two ears are mirror images of each other. The macula of the saccule is approximately at right angles to the macula of the utricle. Hence, with no head movement, the gravitational pull on the otoliths always stimulates some hair cells and inhibits others, regardless of the position of the head in space. The spatial pattern of afferent signals generated by this *static response* codes for the orientation of the head in space.

Linear acceleration or *linear deceleration* of the head also displaces the otolithic membrane. During acceleration, an initial displacement of the membrane away from the direction of movement takes place. When acceleration ceases, the momentum displaces the otolithic membrane in the opposite direction. The spatial patterns of excited and inhibited hair cells code the direction of the linear acceleration.

CRISTA AMPULLARIS

The polarity of all hair cells in a crista ampullaris is identical—at right angles to the crista and in the direction of the adjacent utricle. Thus, when displacement of the cupula is toward the utricle,

all hair cells are excited. When displacement is away from the utricle, all are inhibited.

Because each canal is in the shape of a large arc, increasing or decreasing the rate of *rotation* of the head in the plane of that arc produces maximal movement of the endolymph within that canal. This rotational movement of the head is *angular acceleration* and *angular deceleration*. When the head is rotated, there is an inertial lag in the movement of the endolymph in the semicircular canal, thus bending the cupula in the direction opposite that of the rotation (Fig. 12–25). If the rate of rotation decreases (angular deceleration), the momentum of the endolymph bends the cupula in the direction of the move-

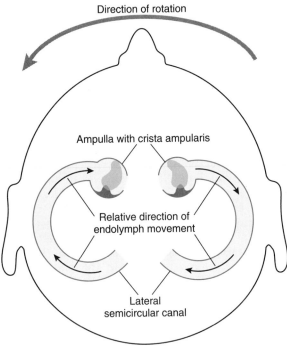

FIGURE 12-25

The two lateral semicircular canals during angular acceleration of the head (large arrow) as viewed from above. Assume the head is tilted slightly forward so that both canals are in the horizontal plane. Both the membranous semicircular canals and the endolymph are rotating in the direction of the head but during acceleration the endolymph moves slower because of inertia. A relative movement of the endolymph occurs in the opposite direction as indicated by the arrows in the canals.

The movement of the endolymph in the left canal is along the excitatory axis of the hair cells (utriculopetal); hence, afferent fibers from the left crista ampullaris increase their firing rate. Movement of the endolymph and the cupula in the right canal is along the inhibitory axis of the hair cells (utriculofugal), and afferents from the right crista ampullaris decrease their firing rate. The reverse is true for angular deceleration. See text for details.

ment, i.e., in the direction of the angular deceleration.

Consider the following illustration. An individual is sitting in a swivel chair and the head is tilted forward 25 degrees, so that the lateral semicircular canals are in the horizontal plane. The chair is spun to the individual's left. Viewing the canals from above, both lateral canals are rotating in a counter-clockwise direction (see Fig. 12–25). The two canals are mirror images of each other, and when one is stimulated, the other is inhibited (see Fig. 12–19). With the initial acceleration, the cupula of the left semicircular canal bends toward the utricle. The hair cells of the crista ampullaris are excited, whereas the cupula of the right semicircular canal bends away from the utricle and its hair cells are inhibited. Remember, the inertia of the endolymph causes it to lag behind the membranous labyrinth in its movement during acceleration. When acceleration ceases and the speed of rotation is constant, the endolymph "catches up" with the membranous labyrinth. No displacement of the cupula occurs, and the hair cells from both cristae release neurotransmitter at the same "resting" rate. However, if the rotation slows (deceleration), the reverse occurs and the hair cells of the left canal are inhibited and those of the right canal are excited.

This basic principle applies to all three pairs of semicircular canals for any rotatory or angular movement of the head. Most movements are not in the plane of a single pair of semicircular canals. However, the endolymph movement will be greatest in the pair of canals in the plane closest to the actual plane of head movement and least in the pair most removed from that plane. The central connections of the afferent fibers integrate these signals and "calculate" the actual plane of movement.

Central Pathways

The central pathways of the vestibular system are principally motor reflex connections to nuclei innervating the extraocular muscles, the motor reticular formation, the spinal motor neurons, and the cerebellum. The conscious appreciation of motion and position of the head are associated with modest projections to the cerebral hemispheres by way of the dorsal thalamus.

Although not studied as extensively as other sensory systems, it is apparent that the central connections of the vestibular system are complex.

The role of the vestibular system in the regulation of posture, muscle tone, and eye movement is not an isolated one. The CNS integrates information from three primary sensory systems for the maintenance of the position of the body in space—vestibular, visual, and proprioceptive (somatosensory). In addition, the cerebellum plays a major role in the integration of the sensory and motor information. Major connections exist between the vestibular nuclei and the cerebellum.

VESTIBULAR NUCLEI

The *vestibular nuclei* reside in the rostral medulla and caudal pons, immediately adjacent to the fourth ventricle and medial to the inferior and middle cerebellar peduncles. Traditionally, there are four nuclei: the *superior, medial, lateral* (*Deiters's nucleus*), and *inferior* (*spinal* or *descending*) *vestibular nuclei* (*SVN, MVN, LVN,* and *IVN*) (Fig. 12–26 and Figs. 7–10, 7–11, and 7–12). Cytoarchitecturally, these four nuclei are distinct and regional differences are found within each nucleus. The organization of these nuclei is more complex than that of most sensory relay nuclei. Within the structure of these nuclei, many bits of sensory information, in addition to those from the primary vestibular afferents, are integrated. Some of the efferents from these nuclei elicit direct motor reflexive responses.

Several satellite nuclear groups, known as the *cell groups f, x, y,* and *z,* are functionally related to the vestibular system, most through motor reflex circuits. Except for *cell group y,* these nuclei do not receive primary afferent fibers and, therefore, are not primary vestibular nuclei. Afferent fibers from the receptor organs within the vestibular labyrinth do not end uniformly within the vestibular nuclear complex; however, several generalizations can be made.

Primary Afferent Fibers to Vestibular Nuclei

The primary afferent neurons of the vestibular system reside in the *vestibular (Scarpa's) ganglion.* Although considered a single ganglion, the vestibular ganglion is actually two ganglia (see Fig. 12–19) with the central processes from both the superior and inferior ganglia uniting to form the vestibular division of the *vestibulocochlear nerve.* In the brain stem, afferents from the *cristae ampullaris* end in the more rostral nuclei, specifically, *SVN* and the rostral portion of *MVN. Utricular afferents* end in the ventral portion of

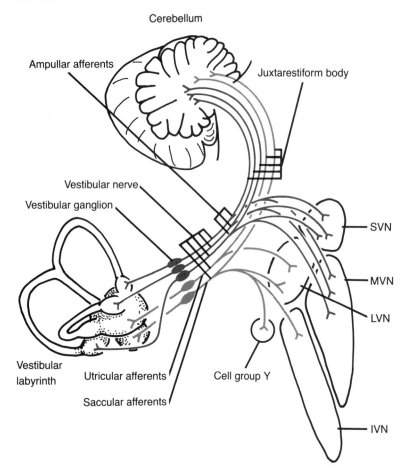

Cerebellum

Ampullar afferents

Juxtarestiform body

Vestibular nerve

Vestibular ganglion

SVN

MVN

LVN

Vestibular labyrinth

Utricular afferents

Cell group Y

Saccular afferents

IVN

FIGURE 12-26

The distribution of primary afferent fibers from the vestibular labyrinth. Afferents from the crista ampullaris terminate in the superior vestibular nucleus (SVN) and the rostral portion of the medial vestibular nucleus (MVN). Afferents from the utricle terminate in the lateral vestibular nucleus (LVN). Afferents from the saccule terminate in the lateral vestibular nucleus, in the rostral portion of the inferior vestibular nucleus (IVN), and in the cell group *y*. In addition, afferents project from all receptors to the vestibular portion of the cerebellum via the juxtarestiform body. See text for details.

the *LVN*, and those from the *saccule* end in the ventral portion of *LVN*, *cell group y* (a small cluster of neurons immediately dorsolateral to IVN), and in portions of *IVN* (see Fig. 12–26).

Thin afferent fibers synapse with the type II hair cells, which appear to be tonic receptors. The larger diameter afferent fibers synapse with the type I hair cells, which have more phasic properties. Both types of afferent fibers employ either *aspartate* or *glutamate* as the primary neurotransmitter. The postsynaptic receptors of neurons in the vestibular nuclei receiving primary afferent terminals respond to either excitatory amino acid.

Commissural Vestibulovestibular Fibers

Extensive *commissural connections* exist between the vestibular nuclei, especially involving MVN and SVN. These are of two types, reciprocal connections between like areas of the same nucleus and connections between different nuclei.

Some of these, especially those transmitting excitatory signals from the contralateral otolithic receptors, relay in the medullary reticular formation and do not project directly from one vestibular nucleus to another. Most of the commissural projections are inhibitory; some utilize GABA as the neurotransmitter and others utilize glycine.

Ascending Vestibular Projections to the Brain Stem

Most of the ascending brain stem projections of the vestibular nuclei are from the more rostral nuclei. Fibers from the *SVN* enter the *medial longitudinal fasciculus* (*MLF*) and project bilaterally to the *trochlear nucleus* and the nuclei of the *oculomotor nuclear complex*. Fibers from the *MVN* ascend in the *MLF* and project to the extraocular motor nuclei and the *interstitial nucleus of Cajal*, a nucleus of large neurons at the rostral end of the MLF, above the oculomotor complex and ventral to the periaqueductal gray. This nucleus coordinates eye movements through its projections to the extraocular motor nuclei and projections to the spinal cord via the MLF. These are important for the coordination of neck and trunk rotation with eye movements. Projections to the *abducens* and *oculomotor complex* are bilateral; those to the *trochlear nucleus* and *interstitial nucleus of Cajal* are contralateral. The *IVN* has diverse projections. Its ascending fibers arise primarily from the rostral end of the nucleus and enter the *MLF* bilaterally to end in the *trochlear* and the *oculomotor nuclei* (Fig. 12–27).

Descending Vestibular Projection Fibers

Fibers from the *LVN* form the heavily myelinated *lateral vestibulospinal tract* (*deiterospinal tract*), the principal ipsilateral, descending pathway from the vestibular nuclei. These fibers ini-

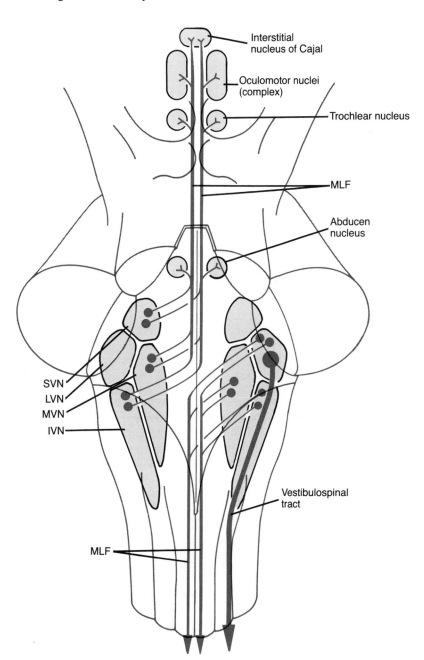

FIGURE 12-27

Principal ascending and descending pathways from the vestibular nuclei. The ascending pathways are illustrated for the left vestibular nuclei, the descending pathways for the right vestibular nuclei. See text for details. (MLF, median longitudinal fasciculus; SVN, superior vestibular nucleus; LVN, lateral vestibular nucleus; and IVN, inferior vestibular nucleus.)

Interstitial
nucleus of Cajal

Oculomotor nuclei
(complex)

Trochlear nucleus

MLF

Abducen
nucleus

SVN
LVN
MVN
IVN

Vestibulospinal
tract

MLF

tially descend through the substance of the *IVN*, giving it a characteristic speckled pattern because of the heavily myelinated fibers of the lateral vestibulospinal tract (see Fig. 7–10). On reaching the spinal cord, these fibers descend in the ventral quadrant of the cord, medial and ventral to the ventral spinocerebellar tract and ventral to the anterolateral system (ALS) (see Fig. 6–8).

Throughout its course in the brain stem, the lateral vestibulospinal tract gives off collaterals to the medullary reticular formation. In the spinal cord, its fibers synapse in the ventral horns, especially at cervical and lumbar levels. These synapses are both with interneurons and with the large, α-motor neurons of the ventral horn. Most of the descending vestibular fibers in the vestibulospinal tract are cholinergic, or they have acetylcholine as the primary transmitter and a peptide co-transmitter.

The *LVN* is organized somatotopically. Those fibers that descend to cervical levels and innervate forelimb musculature arise from the rostroventral half of LVN. Those to lumbar levels, innervating hindlimb musculature, arise from the caudodorsal half of LVN.

Other descending vestibular fibers arise from the *MVN* and the *IVN*. Those from the *MVN* descend bilaterally in the *MLF* and end in the cervical spinal cord. Those from the *IVN* are more diverse with projections to the *inferior olivary nucleus*, the *medullary reticular formation*, the *cerebellum*, and the *cervical spinal cord* via the *MLF*. The descending fibers in the MLF are frequently called the *medial vestibulospinal tract*.

In general, descending fibers in the lateral vestibulospinal tract end in lamina IX. Those fibers descending in the MLF usually end in laminae VII and VIII. Spinal motor activity mediated by the fibers of the vestibulospinal tract is excitatory and often through synapses directly with the large α-motor neurons. Spinal activity mediated by fibers in the MLF is usually via interneurons and may be either excitatory or inhibitory.

CEREBELLAR CONNECTIONS

The vestibular labyrinth is the only sensory organ to send primary afferent fibers directly to the cerebellum. Within the cerebellum, the *flocculus*, the *nodulus*, the *uvula*, and the *fastigial nucleus* are collectively known as the *vestibular cerebellum* (see Figs. 7–5 and 17–4). Cerebellar afferent fibers from the vestibular labyrinth enter the brain stem with the other primary vestibular afferents. However, some do not synapse in the vestibular nuclei but immediately enter the vestibular portion of the cerebellum via the *juxtarestiform body*. The juxtarestiform body lies along the inner surface of the inferior cerebellar peduncle and contains almost exclusively vestibulocerebellar and cerebellovestibular fibers (see Figs. 7–11 and 12–26).

The vestibular system also sends second-order afferent fibers to the cerebellum, principally from the *SVN*, *MVN*, and *IVN*. These vestibulocerebellar fibers, axons of neurons in the vestibular nuclei, enter the cerebellum via the juxtarestiform body and end in the vestibular portion of the cerebellum. Other vestibular afferents enter the cerebellum by a more indirect route. Some fibers from the IVN, for example, project to the inferior olivary nucleus (a cerebellar relay nucleus). The inferior olivary nucleus relays information to the cerebellum by way of the restiform body.

The cerebellum, in turn, has direct projections to the vestibular nuclei, some of which are reciprocal. Other projections from the cerebellum to the vestibular nuclei carry signals that represent an integration of sensory and motor information by the cerebellum. In general, fibers leaving the cerebellum exit via the superior cerebellar peduncle after a relay in the nuclei of the cerebellum (see Chapter 17). However, with the vestibular system, most of the cerebellar projections are axons from the *Purkinje cells* in the cerebellar cortex. These inhibitory, GABAergic axons leave the cerebellum via the *juxtarestiform body*, not the superior cerebellar peduncle, and end in the ipsilateral vestibular nuclei. These include projections from the *flocculus* to *SVN*, *MVN*, and *cell group y*; the *nodulus* and *uvula* to *MVN* and *IVN*; and a few, sparse projections from the *anterior lobe of the vermis* to *LVN*. In addition to the direct cortical projections, there are bilateral, excitatory projections from the *fastigial nucleus* of the cerebellum to *LVN* and *IVN*.

RETICULAR FORMATION

The ascending and descending pathways from the vestibular nuclei have many collaterals that end in various nuclei of the motor reticular formation of the medulla, pons, and midbrain. Two in particular are the *nucleus reticularis pontis caudalis* and the *nucleus reticularis gigantocellularis*. These two nuclei are considered by many workers as centers for the coordination of eyehead movements.

VESTIBULOCORTICAL PATHWAY

Vestibular stimulation produces a conscious appreciation of the sensations of movement and position of the head in space. However, the route by which vestibular information reaches the cerebral cortex is still open to debate.

One pathway involves ascending vestibular fibers from the rostral portion of the vestibular nuclear complex. Fibers from *LVN* and *SVN* ascend in both the ipsilateral and contralateral *MLF*. These fibers by-pass the oculomotor complex and the interstitial nucleus of Cajal to end in the *ventrobasal complex*, specifically the pars oralis of the *ventral posterolateral nucleus* (VPL_O) and the *ventral posteroinferior nucleus* (*VPI*) of

the dorsal thalamus. Thalamic relay fibers carrying vestibular information from VPL_O and *VPI* project to *area 3a* (Fig. 12–28).

Area 3a is immediately adjacent to the primary motor cortex (*area 4*), and connections between 3a and 4 involve the vestibular modulation of motor function at the cortical level. Additional studies implicate the *posterior complex* (*PO*) of the thalamus in the relay of vestibular information to the cortex, specifically to the vestibular field of *area 2v*. Area 2v is a subdivision of area 2 in S-I and lies in the inferolateral portion of the postcentral gyrus. Direct projections from the vestibular nuclei to PO are not defined, and the vestibular information reaching PO is probably indirect.

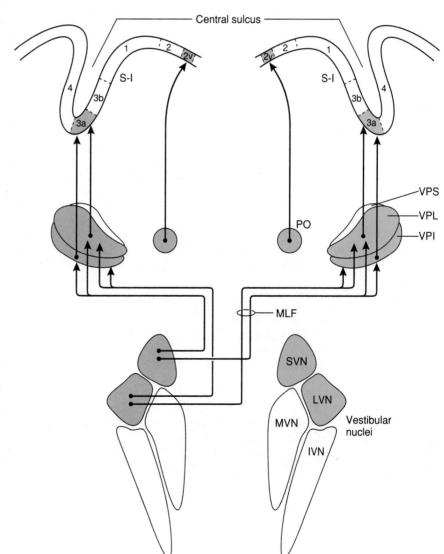

FIGURE 12-28

Vestibulocortical pathway. Ascending pathways for the left vestibular nuclei only are illustrated. The source of the vestibular signals to the posterior complex (PO) of the thalamus is unknown. See text for details. (VPS, ventral posterosuperior nucleus; VPL, ventral posterolateral nucleus; VPI, ventral posteroinferior nucleus; LVN, lateral vestibular nucleus; IVN, inferior vestibular nucleus; MVN, medial vestibular nucleus; MLF, median longitudinal fasciculus; and SVN, superior vestibular nucleus.)

VESTIBULAR EFFERENTS

The vestibular system has efferent projections from the brain stem to the vestibular labyrinth. These *vestibular efferents* are postulated to modulate the dynamic range of afferent signals to match the expected accelerations during head and body movement.

Vestibular Reflexes

Motor reflexes, especially those of the body and limbs initiated by centers in the brain stem and cerebellum, are complex. Most involve an integration of afferent information from three sensory systems: vestibular, proprioceptive, and visual. The vestibular system, however, has a dominant influence on several categories of motor reflex—those concerned with posture, maintaining balance, moving the eyes, and adjusting overall axial muscle tone. Although considered in an integrated fashion in other chapters, these categories are considered in this chapter with an emphasis on the vestibular component.

POSTURAL

The LVN is the source of the *lateral vestibulospinal tract*. The primary input to the LVN is from the *utricle* and the *saccule*. As a result of this strong macular afferent input, the LVN responds to movement of the head in space. When the head is tilted, some antigravity muscles are excited; others are inhibited, resulting in postural adjustments. *Antigravity muscles* include the lower limb extensors and upper limb flexors, in addition to the axial musculature. The muscle excitation by the lower motor neurons of the spinal cord is in direct response to the monosynaptic excitation by LVN neurons driven by macular afferents. The inhibition is the result of direct projections of the cerebellar Purkinje cells to the LVN. The cerebellum receives direct macular afferents via the juxtarestiform body. Much of the vestibular influence on the axial musculature is mediated through descending reticulospinal pathways. Both pontine and medullary reticular formations receive strong input from the vestibular nuclei. Other body and head movements, including angular and linear acceleration, use these same postural reflex pathways to maintain balance and appropriate axial muscle tone.

DECEREBRATE RIGIDITY

Higher motor centers (motor cortex and basal ganglia) have an overall inhibitory effect on lower motor neurons. Although the descending corticobulbar and corticospinal fibers are principally excitatory, glutaminergic neurons, they inhibit lower motor neurons by exciting local inhibitory interneurons. Thus, when the brain stem is severed above the pons, a condition known as *decerebrate rigidity* occurs. Essentially, the excitatory effects of the descending lateral vestibulospinal tract are unopposed except for cerebellar inhibition of LVN. The result is a rigidity of postural and antigravity muscles and exaggerated spinal reflexes. With the additional loss of the cerebellum, the degree of rigidity intensifies. This condition leaves the lower motor neurons in a chronic state of excitation—an excitation by neurons of the LVN that lack the normal inhibition of both the cerebellum and the higher motor centers.

REFLEX EYE MOVEMENT

The *SVN* and rostral portions of *MVN* and *IVN* project to the nuclei innervating the extraocular muscles: the oculomotor nuclear complex and the trochlear and abducens nuclei (see Fig. 12-27). Whenever the head moves, there are reflex adjustments to the extraocular muscles that tend to keep the eyes in a horizontal plane and fixed on an object. When the head turns, the eye movements are in the opposite direction, keeping the eye fixed on an object, even though the head is turning away. This reflex becomes more dramatic when the head and body are rotated. The eyes will fixate on an object until it is out of the field of vision (i.e., moving *slowly* in the direction *opposite to the rotatory movement*). Then, the eyes will snap back *rapidly in the direction of the rotatory movement* and fix on another object until it also is out of the field of vision. The sequence is repeated as long as the rotation occurs. This sequence of slow eye movement followed by rapid eye movement is the *vestibulooculomotor reflex* (*VOR*) or *nystagmus*. The slow component is driven by the vestibular nuclei via the MLF. The fast component, the *saccade*, is driven by the paramedian pontine reticular formation under the influence of the frontal eye fields.

Nystagmus is named for the direction of the *fast component*, or the saccade. For example, rotation of the head to the left will produce left nystagmus, or nystagmus with the rapid component to the left (in the direction of the rotation). When an individual is rotated to the left in a chair (see the previous example), the nystagmus will be to the left, in the direction of rotation. However, if the rotation is abruptly stopped (deceleration), the reverse occurs. This *postrotatory nystagmus* is in the direction opposite to the initial acceleration.

AUTONOMIC REFLEXES

The vestibular system also triggers autonomic reflexes, the most common of which is motion sickness. These pathways involve the vestibular projections to the pontine and medullary reticular formations and the subsequent stimulation of autonomic centers in the brain stem. In addition, damage to the vestibular system is often accompanied by nausea (see subsequent discussion).

Clinical Correlations

LOSS OF HEARING

Two types of hearing loss are possible: *conduction deafness* and *sensorineural deafness.* Conduction deficits involve pathology of the middle ear and the resultant loss of efficiency in the conversion of airborne sound waves to fluid waves in the inner ear. Sensorineural deficits usually involve the cochlea or the cochlear nerve and, less often, the central pathways.

Weber's test, a simple test involving a tuning fork, distinguishes between conduction and sensorineural deficits. When the base of a vibrating tuning fork is centered on the top of the head, a normal individual will hear the sound equally well in both ears. For individuals with *right ear conduction deafness*, the sound is loudest in the *right ear.* Intact neural mechanisms involving the cochlear efferents partially compensate for the loss. For a patient with *right ear sensorineural deafness*, the sound is loudest in the *left ear.*

Conduction Deafness

Conduction deafness due to *otosclerosis*, a bone overgrowth of the stapes that impedes normal movement of the ossicle, is a frequent cause of hearing loss in the elderly. Chronic *otitis media*, a long-term infection of the middle ear with accompanying fluid build up, also inhibits the vibration of the ossicles and decreases the con-

duction efficiency of the middle ear. A third cause of conduction deafness is damage to or disarticulation of the ossicles as a result of *trauma.*

Sensorineural Deafness

Sensorineural deafness may result from pathology of (a) the receptor organ, the cochlea; (b) the cochlear nerve; or (c) less often, central lesions involving the auditory pathways. Involvement of the *cochlea, cochlear nerve,* or *cochlear nuclei* produces an *ipsilateral hearing loss.* In contrast, damage at higher levels may result in a diminished sense of hearing in both ears. If damage to the cochlea is restricted, the loss may involve only the specific frequencies associated with the portion of the cochlea that has the damage.

Because of the bilateral nature of the ascending auditory pathways, deficits in the CNS at levels above the dorsal and intermediate acoustic stria and the trapezoid body produce only a bilateral diminution of hearing and not a total loss of hearing, in either ear (see Figs. 12–16 and 12–17). Damage to the *primary auditory cortex, A-1,* leads only to a minor loss in the ability to hear sound and discern frequency. However, damage to A-1 will lead to an *inability to localize sound* from the contralateral hemifield of acoustic space.

TINNITUS

Tinnitus, a condition of having a noise or a "ringing" in the ear, often occurs in association with hearing loss. The explanations for tinnitus are many and the pathophysiology is poorly understood. However, tinnitus often accompanies both auditory and vestibular deficits.

VERTIGO

The term *vertigo*, often misused to describe any form of dizziness, refers specifically to the sensation of turning or rotating, as if the external world were rotating around the individual, or as if the individual were turning in space. *Benign paroxysmal positional vertigo (BPPV)*, the most common form of vertigo in the elderly, is due to *cupulolithiasis* of the posterior semicircular canal. Cupulolithiasis is simply an accumulation of otolithic debris in the cupula of a semicircular canal. Debris sloughed from the otolithic membrane in the utricle can gravitate to the ampulla of the posterior semicircular canal situated immediately inferior to the utricle (see Fig. 12–20) and can become attached to the cupula. This increases the specific gravity of the cupula, thereby creating an overexcitability of the posterior canal to angular acceleration and possibly to positional changes that have a gravitational vector. *BPPV* produces attacks of *rotational vertigo* and *nystagmus* when the head is tilted laterally, toward the affected side. Frequently, there is spontaneous recovery. Often, therapy utilizing positional maneuvers of the head is effective in dislodging and dispersing the otolithic debris.

VESTIBULAR NEURITIS

An acute inflammation of the vestibular labyrinth, *vestibular neuritis*, can produce severe rotational vertigo, nystagmus, postural imbalance, and nausea. Hearing is not affected, unless the inflammation spreads to the cochlea. This neuritis is usually ipsilateral and characterized by a hyporesponsiveness of the vestibular labyrinth. At "rest," there is a tonic discharge from the normal vestibular receptors. Hence, depression of the responses from the labyrinth of one side leads to oculomotor and postural responses that are an exaggeration of the responses normally elicited by the intact side. Eyes are driven slowly toward the side of the inflammation, owing to unchecked (unopposed) input from the unaffected labyrinth, with the rapid, saccadic, movement toward the intact side. As the tonic balance between the two sides returns to normal, there is a gradual diminution of the symptoms.

TESTS FOR VESTIBULAR FUNCTION

The normal functioning of the semicircular canals is often demonstrated using a *Bárány chair*, a special rotating chair. In testing for normal function, pairs of semicircular canals are selectively stimulated by placing the head in an appropriate position, rotating the individual and observing the *postrotatory nystagmus*. Positioning of the head in a forward tilt of 25 degrees places both lateral canals in the horizontal plane; hence, spinning the chair will selectively stimulate this pair of canals. The posterior canal of one side is in the same plane as the superior canal of the opposite side, and appropriate positioning of the head places these pairs of canals in a horizontal plane. Normal postrotatory nystagmus lasts for 15 to 40 seconds, and exaggerated or diminished responses suggest abnormal labyrinthine functioning.

The *caloric test* allows one to check labyrinthine function, principally the lateral semicircular

canal, on each side independently. When the external auditory canal is flushed with warm water, the temperature differential causes the endolymph in the lateral canal of the treated side to move, resulting in nystagmus toward the treated ear. When cold water is applied, the endolymph moves in the opposite direction and the nystagmus is away from the treated ear. Deviations from the normal pattern suggest the presence of labyrinthine disease in one ear or the other.

COMBINED AUDITORY AND VESTIBULAR DISORDERS

Because of the proximity of the auditory and vestibular receptor organs, a disease that affects one often affects the other. *Menière's disease*, a disorder of unknown etiology, is characterized by a progressive loss or fluctuation in hearing and tinnitus and, later, by nystagmus, vertigo, and nausea. The problem is often bilateral and characterized by a swelling of the endolymphatic channels plus a concomitant loss of the cochlear hair cells. This pathology is due to an overproduction of endolymph, a blockage of the endolymphatic duct, or a problem in the reabsorption of the endolymph. In more advanced stages, there may be periodic rupturing of the membranous labyrinth with an extrusion of endolymph into the perilymph. When this occurs, the increased K^+ content in the perilymph, bathing the vestibular afferent fibers, results in a transient depolarization of the afferent fibers ("potassium palsy"), until the ionic balance is restored. With Menière's disease, a spontaneous remission rate of about 80% within 5 years is normal.

CNS deficits in auditory and vestibular functions are usually accompanied by deficits in other neural functions. One of the more common CNS deficits is *Wallenberg's syndrome*, resulting from an occlusion or a thrombus of the posterior inferior cerebellar or vertebral artery (see Fig. 9–12). This produces ipsilateral hearing loss, nystagmus, nausea, and ataxia toward the side of the lesion. The hearing loss is from the damage to the cochlear nuclei; the nystagmus and nausea, from the damage to the vestibular nuclei; and the ataxia, from the damage to both the vestibular system and the cerebellum. The nystagmus is apparent when the patient moves the eyes toward the side of the lesion. In addition, damage to the ALS results in a contralateral loss of pain and temperature sensation from the body. Damage to the spinal tract and nucleus of V produces an ipsilateral loss of pain and temperature from the face. Other deficits involve the motor systems (reviewed in other chapters) and include impairment of speech, swallowing, and autonomic dysfunctions (Horner's syndrome).

SUGGESTED READING

Carpenter, M. B. (1988). Vestibular nuclei: afferent and efferent projections. In *Progress in Brain Research*, Volume 76, O. Pompeiano and J.H.J. Allum (Editors). Elsevier Publishing Company, Amsterdam.

This well-documented review with many references presents late information on the afferent and efferent connections of the vestibular nuclei in the primate.

Edelman, G. M., W. E. Gall, and W. M. Cowan (Editors) (1988). *Auditory Function: Neurobiological Bases of Hearing.* John Wiley & Sons, New York, 817 pp.

This volume of collected chapters was written by workers active in the field. Organized in sections covering aspects of hearing ranging from development, the ear, and central processing of auditory information, to the perceptual aspects of hearing, the coverage is well balanced. Each chapter is well referenced and there is a common subject index for the book.

Fettiplace, R. (1990). Transduction and tuning in auditory hair cells. Semin. Neurosci., 2: 33–40.

A brief but well-referenced review of the physiology of sensory transduction by cochlear hair cells. Also discussed are theories of efferent modulation and frequency tuning of hair cells.

Holley, M. C. (1990). Cell biology of hair cells. Semin. Neurosci., 2: 41–48.

A brief review with good references of sensory transduction by hair cells of the inner ear. Emphasis is on the mechanics of the transduction at the cellular level.

Jahn, A. F. and J. Santos-Sacchi (Editors) (1988). *Physiology of the Ear.* Raven Press, New York, 539 pp.

This book is a well-balanced collection of chapters written by experts in the field. It is an excellent source of advanced-level information on the ear. Each of the 27 chapters has many references and there is a common subject index for the book.

Chapter

13

Taste and Olfactory Pathways

Chemical Senses

Both chemical senses, *taste* and *olfaction*, are *special visceral afferent* (*SVA*). The special sense of taste originates from receptors in *taste buds* located principally on the tongue. Olfactory receptors are in the *olfactory epithelium* (*olfactory mucosa*), a specialized region of the nasal mucosa in the superior recesses of the nasal cavity.

Phylogenetically the chemical senses are very old. Many lower animal forms rely on these senses for the basics of survival: feeding, escaping predators, and mating. In the brains of these forms, the olfactory structures are massive compared with other telencephalic structures. Humans do not rely on olfaction for survival, and the olfactory structures are relatively smaller and more rudimentary. Although both systems, taste (gustatory) and smell (olfactory), contain chemical detectors and utilize specialized molecules in the membranes of the receptor cells for sensory transduction, they have little else in common.

TASTE

Our normal *perception* of taste involves more than just the taste pathways from the oral cavity. The "taste" of food, beverages, and other substances, as we perceive it, actually is an integration of both gustatory and olfactory information. The *aroma* of a meal and the *bouquet* of a wine are dimensions of "taste" that the olfactory system provides. The taste of food and beverages often lacks these dimensions when our nasal passages are obstructed from the congestion of a head cold. However, this "flat taste" is closer to the "true taste" or the sensation evoked by the stimulation of only taste receptors, because the olfactory contribution to the perception is ineffective. *Taste, as used in this chapter, refers only to the gustatory information generated by taste bud receptors and the central taste pathways.*

OLFACTION

In the olfactory system, the primary afferent neurons differentiate from the epithelium of the olfactory placode (see Chapter 1). These neurons reside not in a ganglion but in the olfactory mucosa of the nasal cavities. Specialized ciliated processes from these afferent neurons spread over the mucosal surface and are the sensory transducing elements. Thus, in olfaction, sensory transduction is a direct depolarization of the primary afferent neuron. A number of attempts have been made to classify the vast spectrum of odoriferous sensations into a few basic elements, such as *floral, peppermint, ethereal, pungent, putrid, musk,* and *camphoraceous.* These are somewhat arbitrary categories and have been of little scientific value. Such a classification of olfaction, as with taste, appears to be an oversimplification.

The central processes of nearly 6 million primary afferent neurons collate and form the 100 or more individual "olfactory nerves" that enter the *olfactory bulbs.* These nerves collectively form the *olfactory nerve* (*cranial nerve I*). The olfactory bulbs are part of the telencephalon (see Figs. 1–16, 1–19, and 1–20). Hence, the olfactory nerve is the only nerve to enter the telencephalon directly. The areas of the telencephalon that receive projections of the olfactory bulb are parts of the *rhinencephalon* (literally translated as "nose brain").

Taste Buds and Sensory Transduction

The surface of the tongue is thrown into a series of irregular protrusions, the *lingual papillae,* most of which are the small filiform papillae (Fig. 13–1). Three other types of papillae, *fungiform, foliate,* and *circumvallate,* contain *taste buds,* the sensory organs of taste.

The newborn has numerous taste buds in the mucosa of the adjacent oral and pharyngeal cavities; however, most of these are lost with devel-

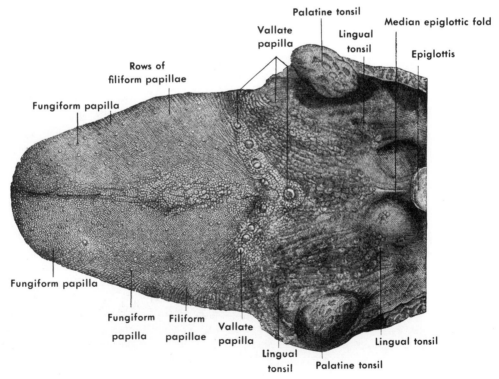

FIGURE 13–1

Dorsal surface and root of the human tongue (after Sappey). Note the V formed by the circumvallate papillae. Taste bud innervation anterior to the circumvallate papillae is by the facial nerve, posterior by the glossopharyngeal nerve. The vagus innervates residual taste buds of the epiglottis, if present. (Reproduced with permission from D. W. Fawcett, *A Textbook of Histology,* 11th Edition, W. B. Saunders Co., Philadelphia, 1986.)

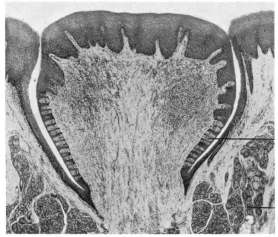

Stratified squamous epithelium

Lamina propria

Taste bud

Gland of v. Ebner

FIGURE 13-2

Section through a circumvallate papilla of *Macacus rhesus*. Photomicrograph, × 42.

Note the deep furrow surrounding the papilla and the numerous taste buds on the lateral surface of the papilla. (Reproduced with permission from D. W. Fawcett, *A Textbook of Histology*, 11th Edition, W. B. Saunders Co., Philadelphia, 1986.)

opment. In the adult, nearly all taste buds are on the tongue and its associated papillae, except for a few residual taste buds remaining in the epiglottis and adjacent areas of the pharynx (see Fig. 13–1).

PAPILLAE

The large *circumvallate papillae* form a V-shaped line, approximately parallel to the boundary between the anterior two thirds and posterior one

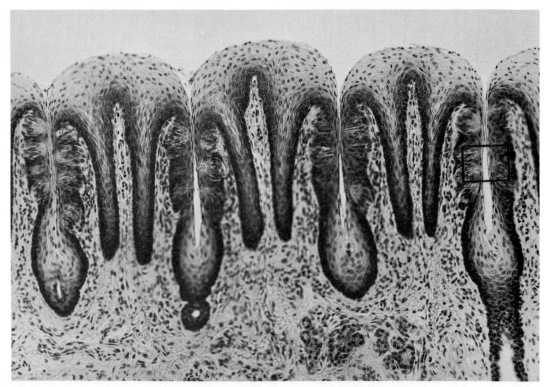

FIGURE 13-3

The foliate papillae of a rabbit, showing the alternating ridges and deep clefts with numerous taste buds on either side of the cleft. Photomicrograph, × 150.

An area such as that enclosed in the rectangle is shown at higher magnification in Figure 13–4. (Reproduced with permission from D. W. Fawcett, *A Textbook of Histology*, 11th Edition, W. B. Saunders Co., Philadelphia, 1986.)

third of the tongue (see Fig. 13–1). Each of the ten to 12 circumvallate papillae is surrounded by a deep furrow and recessed into the surface of the tongue. Lining the lateral margins of these giant papillae are numerous taste buds (Fig. 13–2).

The boundary between the anterior two thirds and posterior one third of the tongue marks a difference in the embryonic origin of the epithelium: the anterior two thirds from the first branchial arch and the posterior one third from the third arch. The innervation of these areas reflects this difference: general sensory innervation of the anterior two thirds from the trigeminal nerve and the posterior one third from the glossopharyngeal nerve (see Chapters 10 and 19). Similarly, the special afferent innervation of the anterior two thirds of the tongue is from the chorda tympani branch of the facial nerve and the posterior one third from the glossopharyngeal nerve (see following discussion).

The smaller *fungiform papillae* are scattered singly among the filiform papillae. They are most numerous at the tip of the tongue and along the lateral margins of the dorsal surface (see Fig. 13–1). The taste buds of the fungiform papillae are found on the surface of each papilla. *Foliate papillae* are found more on the dorsolateral aspect of the posterior portion of the tongue. The taste buds are located in clefts between the papillary ridges (Fig. 13–3).

TASTE BUDS

Taste buds appear as light-staining oval bodies embedded in the darker-staining epithelium of the tongue. A small opening in the epithelium immediately over the taste bud, the *taste pore*, allows fluids bathing the tongue to reach the apical surface of the receptor cells (Figs. 13–4 and 13–5). Four basic elements are in the taste bud: *receptor cells, supporting cells, basal cells,* and *afferent nerve endings.*

The *receptor cells* are the sensory transducing elements of the gustatory system, and the *basal* and *supporting cells* are but different stages in the production of new receptor cells. Unlike other sensory systems discussed thus far, receptor cells for taste have a life span of only 10 days. The *basal cells* are the early precursor cells, the proliferative elements. Daughter cells from basal cell proliferation become the *supporting cells.* These differentiate into the *receptor cells.* The basal portion of the receptor cells makes synaptic contact with the *afferent nerve terminals.* During the transition to new receptor cells, these nerve end-

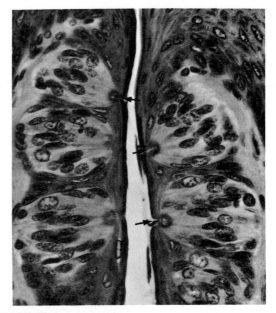

FIGURE 13–4

Taste buds from the foliate papillae of a rabbit. Photomicrograph, × 450. See Figure 13–3 for orientation. Arrows indicate the taste pores. (Reproduced with permission from D. W. Fawcett, *A Textbook of Histology,* 11th Edition, W. B. Saunders Co., Philadelphia, 1986.)

ings establish contact with the recently differentiated receptor cells (see Fig. 13–5). The afferent neurons sending these distal processes and terminals to the taste buds are in the peripheral ganglia of the facial, glossopharyngeal, and vagus nerves (see the following discussion).

TASTE SENSATIONS

In the gustatory system, *sweet, sour, bitter,* and *salty* are the traditional four basic elements of taste. This classification, however, may also be an oversimplification, because some studies indicate many "basic" elements of taste. These elements vary in different forms of animals. Cats, dogs, goats, and humans, for example, have unique combinations of different basic elements, each with a number and combination that reflect dietary habits. In some studies, as many as ten basic elements of taste are detectable in the human gustatory system, However, other studies indicate the number of basic "elements" is much smaller.

In either case, the production of a specific taste sensation represents an integration of signals gen-

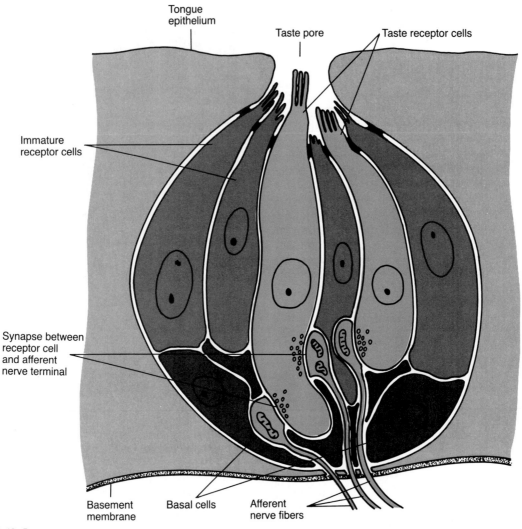

Tongue epithelium

Taste pore

Taste receptor cells

Immature receptor cells

Synapse between receptor cell and afferent nerve terminal

Basement membrane

Basal cells

Afferent nerve fibers

FIGURE 13-5

A taste bud. The receptor cells continually turn over. Basal cells produce new supporting cells, and these differentiate into new receptor cells. Terminals of the distal processes of the primary afferent nerves form synapses with the receptor cells. The taste pore allows salivary fluids to bathe the apical surface of the receptor cells.

erated by specific receptors responding to basic taste elements. The central pathways of the gustatory system, in turn, process the elemental information to give us the perception of a specific taste sensation. The elemental taste sensations evoked from the anterior two thirds of the tongue (facial nerve innervation) are different from those from the posterior one third (glossopharyngeal nerve innervation).

The *facial nerve* carries the four elemental *taste sensations*: *salty*, *sour*, *sweet*, and *bitter*. The *glossopharyngeal nerve* carries principally sweet and bitter sensations. Inorganic ions, especially Na^+ and Li^+, evoke the sensation of *salty*, and Brönsted acids, especially those with a proton-donating nitrogen such as histidine, evoke the sensation of *sour*. Low concentrations of some inorganic salts; sugars; amino acids, such as L-hydroxyproline and L-alanine; and the dihydrochalcones (dihydrobenzalacetophenone derivatives) produce the sensation of *sweet*. Hydrophobic amino acids; alkaloids; certain salts, such as $MgSO_4$; and some polyphenols produce the sensation of *bitter*.

SENSORY TRANSDUCTION

Microvilli cover the apical surface of the receptor cells. Salivary fluids of the oral cavity, containing the substances to be tasted, bathe the microvilli. The interaction of these substances with the appropriate receptor molecules in the unit membrane of the microvillus eventually leads to an excitation (depolarization) of the receptor cell. As with other receptor systems, the depolarization activates voltage sensitive Ca^{++} channels. This, in turn, leads to an increase in the rate of neurotransmitter release by the receptor cell at its synapse with the primary afferent nerve terminal (see Fig. 13–5).

The gustatory system also differs from other sensory systems in that the receptors, once stimulated by a ligand, use many varied mechanisms to depolarize the receptor cell. For example, the receptors for Na^+ and Li^+ ions are specific cation channels and the passive entry of the cation itself depolarizes the receptor cell. The sweet receptors are coupled to a G-protein system (G_s), with the resultant production of cAMP and an activation of a cation channel through a cAMP-dependent phosphorylation. This mechanism is similar to that of the β-adrenergic receptor. Other basic taste transduction mechanisms, still to be characterized, involve the utilization of the phosphatidylinositol system as a second messenger system. Thus, the gustatory system utilizes a variety of transduction mechanisms from the direct activation of an ion channel to a number of second messenger systems. In all, however, the result is the activation of voltage-sensitive Ca^{++} channels and an increase in release of neurotransmitter.

Some receptor cells respond to only one of the basic taste elements. However, others appear sensitive to more than one and probably have the receptors and transduction mechanisms for both basic taste elements. The messages sent to the central nervous system (CNS) appear to involve the activation of different subsets of taste receptor cell types, each sending information about one or several taste elements. At present, little is known about the mechanisms of processing this information in the CNS—a process that results in perceptions of a very broad spectrum of taste sensations in humans.

Peripheral Innervation of Taste Buds

The *facial nerve* (*cranial nerve VII*) innervates taste buds on the anterior two thirds of the tongue as well as some residual taste buds in the hard and soft palates; the *glossopharyngeal nerve* (*cranial nerve IX*) innervates those taste buds on the posterior one third of the tongue; and the *vagus* (*cranial nerve X*) innervates residual taste buds that may remain on the epiglottis.

FACIAL NERVE

The cell bodies of the unipolar, primary SVA neurons of the *facial nerve* are in the *geniculate ganglion*, at the genu of the facial nerve, within the petrous portion of the temporal bone. The distal processes of these sensory neurons continue with the facial nerve through the facial canal and, just before the facial nerve exits the cranium at the stylomastoid foramen, these fibers leave the main trunk of the facial nerve and enter the middle ear cavity as the *chorda tympani nerve* (Fig. 1–24 and Fig. 13–6). The chorda tympani crosses the lateral wall of the middle ear horizontally, along the inner surface of the tympanic membrane and over the manubrium of the malleus. Anteriorly, it exits the middle ear cavity; passes through the petrotympanic fissure; and leaves the skull, running along the medial surface of the spine of the sphenoid bone. From that position, the SVA fibers of the chorda tympani join the *lingual branch* of the *trigeminal nerve* (see Fig. 13–6 and Fig. 19–8) and distribute to the taste buds along the anterior two thirds of the tongue. The chorda tympani nerve also contains the preganglionic, parasympathetic fibers (general visceral efferents, GVE), from the facial nerve. However, these efferents leave the lingual nerve to end in the submandibular ganglion.

The central processes of these SVA neurons enter the brain stem as part of the *intermediate nerve*, immediately adjacent to the main trunk of the facial nerve at the medullopontine junction, just rostral to the inferior olive (see Figs. 7–2 and 7–3). These central afferent processes enter the ipsilateral *solitary tract* and terminate in the rostral portion of the *nucleus of the solitary tract* (*solitary nucleus*) (Fig. 13–7). The *gustatory nucleus* is another name for this region of the solitary nucleus.

GLOSSOPHARYNGEAL NERVE

The superior and inferior ganglia of the *glossopharyngeal nerve* are in the jugular foramen, at the point of exit of the nerve from the cranial vault. The *petrosal ganglion* (*inferior ganglion*) contains the visceral afferent neurons, both gen-

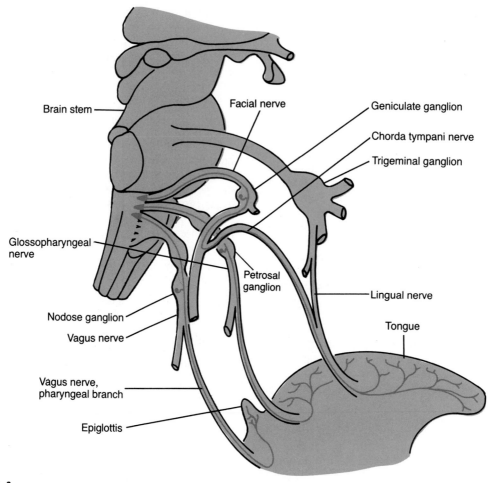

FIGURE 13-6

The peripheral innervation of the taste buds by the facial, glossopharyngeal, and vagus nerves. Special visceral afferent fibers innervating the taste buds are in red. See text for details.

eral visceral afferent (GVA) and SVA. The peripheral processes of the SVA fibers follow the course of the glossopharyngeal nerve, as it spirals down the stylopharyngeus muscle and enters the wall of the pharynx. At this point the nerve divides to form part of the pharyngeal plexus. The SVA fibers continue forward within the wall of the pharynx and distribute to the taste buds in the posterior third of the tongue and to a few rudimentary taste buds in the pharyngeal wall (see Fig. 13–6).

The central processes enter the brain stem with the other components of the glossopharyngeal nerve, dorsal to the inferior olive and immediately caudad to the medullopontine junction (see Figs. 7–2 and 7–3). These fibers follow the same central course as those of the facial nerve, ter-

minating in the rostral portion of the ipsilateral *solitary nucleus* (*gustatory nucleus*) (see Fig. 13–7).

VAGUS NERVE

In humans, the SVA component of the *vagus nerve* is very small and probably absent in most adults. Cell bodies of these afferent neurons are in the *nodose* (*inferior*) *ganglion* of the vagus, just below the jugular foramen where the vagus exits the cranial cavity. Distal processes of the SVA neurons descend with the main trunk of the vagus nerve and leave with the pharyngeal branch of the vagus to enter the posteroinferior portion of the pharyngeal plexus and terminate in the taste buds of the epiglottis (see Fig. 13–6). Cen-

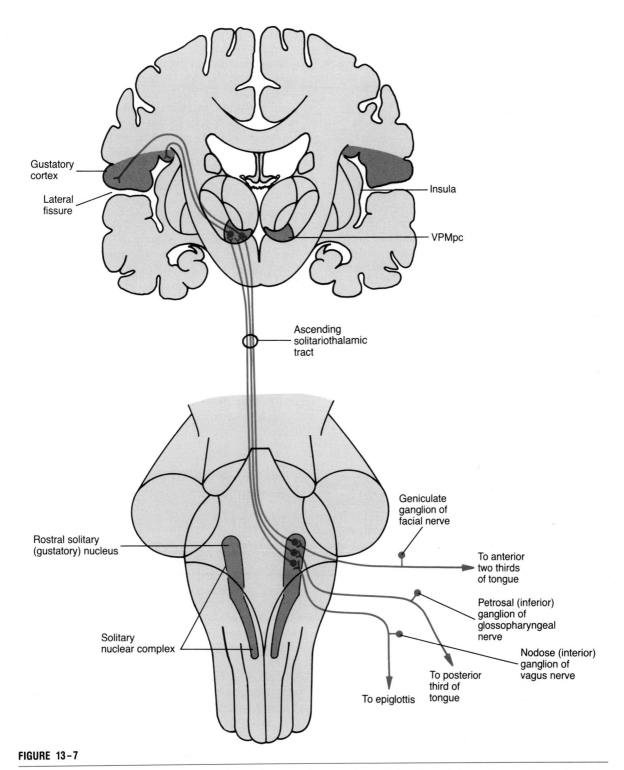

FIGURE 13–7

The central gustatory pathways. Primary afferent fibers terminate in the rostral portion of the solitary nucleus. Information ascends to the contralateral ventral posteromedial nucleus VPM_pc prior to relay to the primary gustatory cortex, Brodmann's area 43, and the adjacent parainsular cortex. See text for details.

tral processes enter the brain stem with the main portion of the vagus nerve (see Figs. 7–2 and 7–3) and terminate in the rostral portion of the ipsilateral *solitary nucleus (gustatory nucleus)* (see Fig. 13–7).

Central Pathways and Information Processing

The central pathways of the gustatory system are not as well defined as those of the other sensory systems. Adding to the difficulty is the fact that the course of these ascending pathways is different for different species, making the extrapolation to the human nervous system more difficult. The pathways described here, however, are consistent with clinical studies involving an impairment in taste.

SOLITARIOTHALAMIC PROJECTIONS

The primary afferent fibers carrying taste information via the facial, glossopharyngeal, and vagus nerves enter the *solitary tract*. These fibers ascend in the ipsilateral solitary tract and end in the rostral portion of the *solitary nucleus (gustatory nucleus)*. Neurons from the *gustatory nucleus* project to the dorsal thalamus with the fibers ascending near the *medial lemniscus*, adjacent to fibers carrying general sensory information from the tongue (see Fig. 13–7).

The thalamic termination of this pathway is the small, medially situated, parvocellular division of the *ventral posteromedial nucleus (VPM$_{pc}$)*. The termination of gustatory fibers is near but distinct from those relaying general sensory information from the surface of the tongue. Based on clinical evidence from unilateral lesions of the VPM$_{pc}$, the resultant *ageusia*, or loss of taste, is always contralateral to the lesion. This finding indicates a crossed solitariothalamic projection consistent with the other ascending sensory pathways (see Fig. 13–7).

PONTINE TASTE AREA

Another ascending pathway involves the *pontine taste area*, an area of the reticular formation in the rostral pons surrounding the brachium conjunctivum. This area may be analogous to the medial portion of the *parabrachial nucleus* of lower forms. Some studies suggest that the pontine taste area is an intermediate relay station for gustatory information ascending from the solitary

nucleus to VPM$_{pc}$ of the dorsal thalamus. This pathway may exist in some animals; however, definitive evidence is lacking in humans. Other gustatory-sensitive fibers from the pontine taste area ascend in the *central tegmental tract* and terminate in the *hypothalamus* and areas of the basal forebrain associated with the *limbic system*, including portions of the *amygdaloid complex*. These projections provide a link between gustatory information and the observed autonomic and behavioral responses associated with feeding activities (see Chapters 18 and 22).

CORTICAL REPRESENTATION

Fibers from VPM$_{pc}$ project to the *cortical taste area*, principally *Brodmann's area 43* (see Fig. 21–3) and the adjacent parainsular cortex. This site of termination places the cortical taste area just rostral to S-II and immediately below S-I, as illustrated in Figure 10–22. Destruction of the cortex in this area results in the anticipated loss of neurons in VPM$_{pc}$. Stimulation of this area in humans elicits taste sensations. This area is adjacent to, but separate from, sensory areas for the tongue and motor areas associated with chewing and tongue movement. Extensive reciprocal connections occur between these adjacent cortical areas.

Olfactory Mucosa and Sensory Transduction

OLFACTORY MUCOSA

The olfactory mucosa, containing the *bipolar primary olfactory neurons* and their *receptor processes*, lies in the superior recesses of the nasal cavity, immediately below the *cribriform* plate of the ethmoid bone of the skull (Fig. 13–8). The sense of smell is much less important to humans than to other animals, and the size of the olfactory mucosa and hence the number of primary olfactory neurons reflects this difference. Dogs can have as much as 100 cm² of olfactory mucosa, whereas humans have from 2 to 5 cm².

Histologically, the *olfactory mucosa* contains four types of cells: *supporting cells, basal cells, primary olfactory neurons*, and *immature, differentiating olfactory neurons* (Fig. 13–9). The primary olfactory neuron has a finite life span, from 30 to 60 days. These cells reproduce during the normal life time of the organism and are the only neurons known to proliferate during adult life.

FIGURE 13-8

Parasagittal section through the skull illustrating the nasal cavity, the location of the olfactory mucosa, the cribriform plate, and the olfactory bulb.

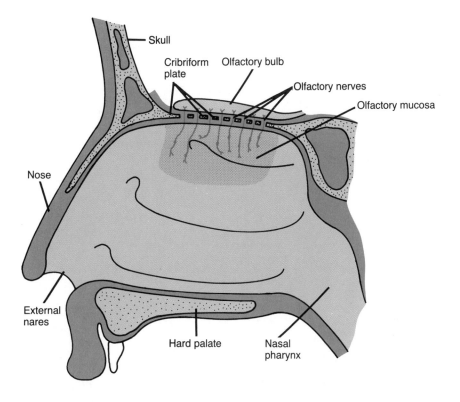

The *basal cells* are the proliferative elements, producing daughter cells that differentiate into the mature neurons. The daughter cells become *differentiating bipolar olfactory neurons* and send a distal process toward the surface of the mucosa. Near the surface of the mucosa, the distal process forms a bulb-like ending with ten to 20 modified cilia—the sensory transducing elements. These cilia spread out over the surface of the mucosa within the mucus layer. At the same time, the axon grows from the base of the differentiating bipolar cell (see Fig. 13-9). This growing nerve process follows the course of the axonal processes of fully mature olfactory neurons, through the cribriform plate and into the olfactory bulb, where it establishes the appropriate synaptic connections. The olfactory bulb is the first CNS information-processing station in the olfactory system.

SENSORY TRANSDUCTION

Some investigators propose a limited number (eight to ten) specific chemical receptors for olfaction. In this hypothesis, as that in taste, the sense of smell codes for a specific odorant in the pattern produced by the relative stimulation of many receptors.

However, no specific olfactory receptor molecule has been identified. This factor may be due to a very low binding affinity of odorants for the receptor molecules—an affinity too low for conventional techniques to detect. To date, we simply do not know how many classes of odorant receptor exist; however, we do know that some odorants act as antagonists to others. Individual receptor neurons respond to a large number of odorants, and a single odorant will stimulate, with differing levels of intensity, a large number of receptor neurons. Either each receptor neuron contains many different receptor molecules or the olfactory receptor molecules have a broad spectrum of sensitivity and are capable of responding to many odorants. The "profile" of odorant responsiveness appears to distinguish one receptor neuron from another, and this profile may reflect the coding of olfactory information. The receptor mechanism for olfaction is complex and differs from that of other chemoreceptors, i.e., taste.

The glands of the mucosa secrete a soluble, olfactory-specific protein, the *odorant binding protein* (*OBP*). OBP is in high concentration in the mucus layer bathing the ciliated receptor processes of the primary olfactory neurons. This protein has a high affinity for a large number of odorant molecules; however, its precise role in

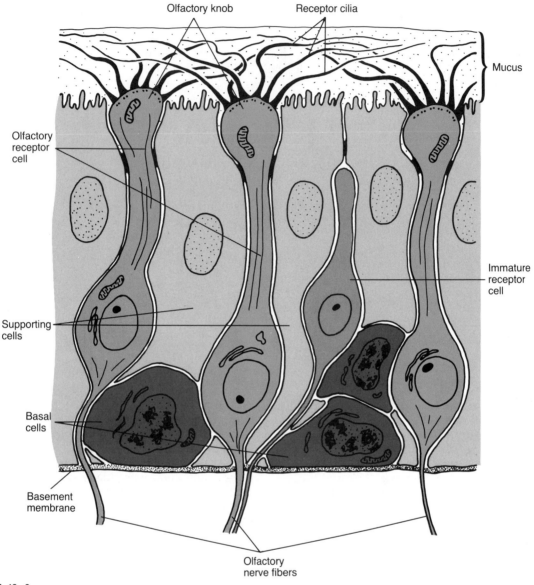

Olfactory knob   Receptor cilia

Mucus

Olfactory
receptor
cell

Supporting
cells

Immature
receptor
cell

Basal
cells

Basement
membrane

Olfactory
nerve fibers

FIGURE 13–9

The olfactory mucosa illustrating the principal cellular elements. Note the immature receptor cell. This developing neuron will send an axonal process centrally into the olfactory bulb, and the neuron will grow distally toward the surface of the mucosa and form the receptor-laden cilia. The trigeminal afferent fibers are not included. See text for details.

olfaction is unclear. It may function to concentrate the odorant near the receptor or as a carrier for odorants that by themselves are not soluble in the aqueous-based mucus. Alternatively, the OBP may function as a scavenger protein that removes odorants from solution in the mucosa, both in a routine "cleansing" capacity and as a protective agent against high concentrations of odorants or toxic substances.

In olfactory transduction, more is known about the second messenger systems than about the receptor mechanism per se. At least one population of receptors activates an adenyl cyclase through a G-protein designated G_o. This protein is similar to the adenyl cyclase–activating G_s, but it is specific to the olfactory mucosa and is absent from other parts of the respiratory system. Patients with a genetic deficiency in G_s also lack G_o.

Individuals with one form of pseudohypoparathyroidism (PHP) lack G_s and have olfactory deficits, and those with another form of PHP, in which the G-protein is unchanged, have normal olfactory function.

A number of odorants appear to stimulate cAMP formation in the cilia of the olfactory receptor cells, whereas others may not. Receptor activation of adenyl cyclase in the cilia of the olfactory neurons leads to the phosphorylation of a cation channel, a mechanism similar to that following stimulation of the β-adrenergic receptor. Some odorants activate another second messenger system, the phosphatidylinositol system. Thus, at least two different sensory transduction systems, probably responding to different broad classes of odorants, are present in the olfactory system.

The result, regardless of the second messenger system, is a depolarization of the bipolar olfactory neuron. When the passive spread of depolarization raises the trigger zone to the threshold, it generates an action potential through molecular mechanisms similar to other neurons. This signal travels to the olfactory bulb of the CNS, the first information processing station in the olfactory system.

TRIGEMINAL AFFERENTS AND AUTONOMIC INNERVATION

Beneath the epithelium of the olfactory mucosa is the lamina propria, the connective tissue layer. Within the lamina propria are *Bowman's glands* and other scattered glandular elements. These glands produce the OBP and the aqueous mucus that bathes and moistens the surface of the olfactory epithelium. The glands and small blood vessels of the lamina propria receive both *sympathetic* and *parasympathetic innervation*. Both the cholinergic parasympathetic fibers, with vasoactive intestinal peptide (VIP) as a peptide cotransmitter, and the β-adrenergic sympathetic fibers regulate the secretion of the acinar cells in Bowman's glands.

A branch of the *trigeminal nerve* also provides *afferent innervation* to the olfactory mucosa. Naked nerve endings from these fibers branch profusely in both the lamina propria and the sensory epithelium. Action potentials generated by these afferents stimulate glandular secretion through autonomic reflex centers in the brain stem. Noxious odorants also stimulate the naked nerve endings of the trigeminal nerve in the olfactory epithelium in addition to stimulating the olfactory receptor neurons. This stimulation of the trigeminal afferents produces (1) local release of substance P by the afferent fibers and (2) action potentials in the trigeminal afferents. The release of substance P modulates responsiveness of the olfactory receptor neurons and stimulates glandular secretion. The action potentials generated by the afferents elicit the secretomotor reflex. The trigeminal afferents do not contribute to the conscious perception of odors.

Olfactory Bulbs, Tracts, and Stria

STRUCTURE OF THE OLFACTORY BULB

The *olfactory bulbs* are a pair of small, highly laminar telencephalic structures, lying within the cranial vault, immediately above the cribriform plate (see Figs. 1–19, 13–8, and 8–7). Structurally, the olfactory bulb has five well-defined layers. From superficial to deep they are the *olfactory nerve layer, glomerular layer, external plexiform layer, mitral cell layer,* and *inner plexiform layer (granule cell layer)* (Fig. 13–10). These five layers surround a central core of white matter: the axons of the fibers leaving the olfactory bulb and those entering the bulb from other parts of the CNS. This central core continues posteriorly as the *olfactory tract.* The olfactory tract divides into the large *lateral* and smaller *medial* and *intermediate olfactory stria.*

Axons of the *olfactory nerves,* spread over the surface of the ipsilateral olfactory bulb and form the *olfactory nerve layer.* These primary afferent fibers terminate in small, spherical clusters of neuropil, the *glomeruli.* In the glomeruli, axons of the olfactory nerve synapse with both interneurons and with the principal relay neurons of the olfactory bulb (*mitral* and *tufted cells*) (see Fig. 13–10). The *glomerular layer* contains, in addition to the *glomeruli,* the cell bodies of *external tufted cells* and small interneurons, the *periglomerular cells.*

The *external plexiform layer* is a relatively thick layer of neuropil and contains the scattered cell bodies of *intermediate tufted cells.* The *mitral cell layer* is a deep, compact, but thin layer, containing the cell bodies of the *mitral cells.* Deep to the mitral cell layer is the *inner plexiform layer.* This is another layer of dense neuropil, containing the cell bodies of *granule cells.* The inner plexiform layer surrounds the central fiber core. This contains the axons of exiting tufted and mitral cells and the axons of entering

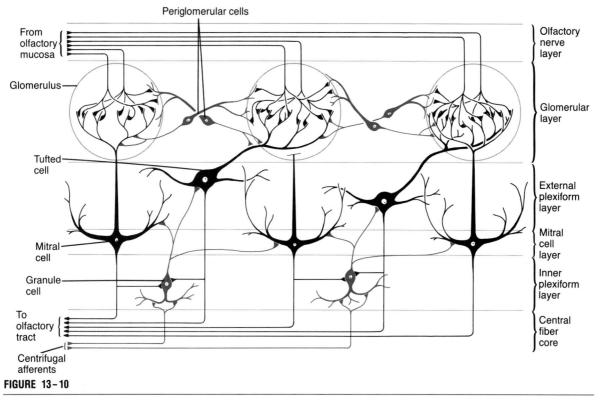

Periglomerular cells

From olfactory mucosa

Glomerulus

Tufted cell

Mitral cell

Granule cell

To olfactory tract

Centrifugal afferents

Olfactory nerve layer

Glomerular layer

External plexiform layer

Mitral cell layer

Inner plexiform layer

Central fiber core

FIGURE 13-10

The neuronal circuitry in the olfactory bulb illustrating the laminar organization and the major cell types and some of their principal connections. Interneurons (granule cells and periglomerular cells) and centrifugal afferents to the olfactory bulb are in red. See text for details.

centrifugal fibers from the contralateral olfactory bulb and other areas of the CNS. Collectively, these axonal processes form the *olfactory tract* (see Fig. 13-10).

INPUT TO THE OLFACTORY BULB

Olfactory neurons from the olfactory mucosa are the *primary afferent* projections to the olfactory bulb. These axons form peptidergic synapses (carnosine and possibly other peptides) on the dendrites of both mitral and tufted cells as well as periglomerular interneurons. The afferent input is highly convergent. Although numbers are not available for humans, in other animals as many as 1000 receptor cells will converge on a single mitral cell, with each glomerulus containing the dendritic arborizations from as many as 25 mitral cells.

Each olfactory bulb receives a large number of *centrifugal afferents*, axons of neurons from other areas of the CNS projecting to the olfactory bulb via the olfactory tract. These afferents include noradrenergic projections from the *locus ceruleus*,

serotoninergic projections from the *medial* and *dorsal raphe nuclei*, and cholinergic projections from both the *medial septal nucleus* and *nuclei of the diagonal band of Broca*. Many of the serotoninergic projections from the raphe system co-release substance P. In addition, each bulb receives projections from the contralateral olfactory bulb, relayed in the contralateral *anterior olfactory nucleus*.

OUTPUT FROM THE OLFACTORY BULB

Excitatory *mitral cells* are one of the principal efferent fibers from the olfactory bulb. Mitral cell projections include ipsilateral projections to the *olfactory cortex* (*piriform cortex*, the allocortex over the rostral half of the uncus), the *anterior olfactory nucleus* (a small nuclear group within the posterior portion of the olfactory bulb and rostral olfactory tract), the *nuclei of the lateral olfactory stria*, the *hypothalamus*, and portions of the *medial septal area* and *nuclei of the anterior perforated substance*. These excitatory projections have glutaminergic properties. The neurotransmitter is glutamate; aspartate; or the acetylated dimer, *N*-acetylaspartylglutamate.

Tufted cells are the other principal efferent projection from the olfactory bulb. Some of these excitatory neurons are heterogenous, and individual tufted cells utilize either a peptide or dopamine as the neurotransmitter. Substance P, cholecystokinin, and the enkephalins are the probable peptide neurotransmitters. Projections of the tufted cells vary with their location within the olfactory bulb. The *internal tufted cells* (immediately superficial to the mitral cell layer) have a pattern of projection similar to that of the mitral cells. The *middle* and many of the *external tufted cells* project principally to the *anterior olfactory nucleus*, the *olfactory cortex*, and the *olfactory tubercle*. The olfactory tubercle is a very small area of allocortex between the medial and lateral olfactory stria and receives fibers from the olfactory tract via the intermediate olfactory stria.

INFORMATION PROCESSING IN THE OLFACTORY BULB

The *primary afferent fibers* from the olfactory mucosa terminate topographically in the olfactory bulb, as if a map of the mucosa were wrapped around the bulb. Afferents from anterior and posterior areas of the mucosa end in glomeruli on the anterior and posterior portions of the bulb. Afferents from the inferolateral areas of the mucosa end in glomeruli on the superolateral portion of the bulb, and those from the inferomedial mucosa, on the superomedial part of the bulb. Afferents from the most superior portion of the mucosa end in glomeruli on the inferior surface of the bulb, immediately above the cribriform plate.

Different odors stimulate selected areas of the mucosa and, hence, selected regions of the bulb, suggesting that *specific odors code in a spatial pattern of responding neurons*. In comparison, higher levels of the olfactory system lack this patterned response. Lesions involving extensive portions of the olfactory bulbs or of the mucosa do not produce a selective loss in odor discrimination. This apparent dichotomy may be related to plasticity in the olfactory system. For example, prior experience can modify the response of the olfactory bulb to stimuli—changes often reflected in a modification of the spatial pattern.

Because olfactory neurons are in a constant state of turnover, processes normally associated with growth and differentiation (nerve sprouting, establishment of appropriate synaptic contacts,

and so forth) are permanent features in the olfactory bulb. This characteristic is reflected in the presence of many molecular markers normally associated with growth and differentiation. These unique features, no doubt, contribute to the plasticity observed in the olfactory system and its ability to adapt to changes, be they physical or behavioral.

Both *mitral* and *tufted cells* maintain a basal level of spontaneous activity. Responses to olfactory stimuli result in an increase or a decrease in this basal level or a sequential combination of both. The suppression of activity is the result of a combination of *lateral inhibition*, *feedback inhibition*, and *feed-forward inhibition* (see Fig. 4–10). The same chemical odorant at different concentrations may produce opposite responses. At a low concentration, it may excite a mitral cell but at a higher concentration it may inhibit it. Excitation of a mitral cell by a specific olfactory neuron inhibits surrounding mitral cells. However, as the level of excitation increases, more mitral cells are stimulated directly, including some that are inhibited at the lower concentration. This additional primary excitation leads to an increase in lateral inhibition and in feedback and feed-forward inhibition. The result is a brief burst of mitral cell activity followed by a prolonged suppression. As with the receptor cells, the specificity of the response patterns by both mitral and tufted cells is not very selective for particular odorants, and the overall specificity may be related to the sensitivity profile of many neurons.

Interneurons (*granule cells* and *periglomerular cells*) continually modulate the level of excitability of both projection neurons (mitral and tufted cells). Hence, these GABAergic interneurons play a major role in controlling the information flow from the olfactory bulb. These inhibitory neurons are driven by (1) incoming olfactory nerve signals, (2) collaterals from both the mitral and tufted cells, and (3) centrifugal afferents from other areas of the CNS and the contralateral olfactory bulb.

Other Central Pathways and Information Processing

NEOCORTICAL REPRESENTATION OF OLFACTION

The cortical representation of olfaction, homologous to the primary sensory areas of the other sensory systems, is the *neocortical* representation.

The olfactory system, unlike other sensory systems, initially projects to the primitive "smell brain" or rhinencephalon. These are principally allocortical areas, specifically paleocortex, areas of a very primitive cortex (see Chapters 21 and 22). These paleocortical areas relay information to the thalamus and hence to the neocortex.

Projections from the *olfactory bulb* enter the *intermediate olfactory stria* and terminate in the *olfactory tubercle*. The olfactory tubercle is a small area of paleocortical tissue at the base of the olfactory tract, situated between the medial and lateral olfactory stria, adjacent to the anterior perforated substance. In humans, the olfactory tubercle is very small and rudimentary. Fibers from the deep layer of the *olfactory tubercle* enter the *stria medullaris* (*stria medullaris thalami*) and terminate in the thalamus, specifically the *mediodorsal nucleus* (*MD*) (Figs. 13–11 and 13–13 and Fig. 7–21). Cortical projection fibers from *MD* terminate in the orbitofrontal cortex,

principally in the *orbital gyri* (see Fig. 8–7). This area of neocortex is essential for the conscious perception of odors.

LATERAL OLFACTORY STRIA

The largest bundle of fibers leaving the olfactory tract is the *lateral olfactory stria* (Figs. 13–12 and 13–13 and Fig. 8–7). Fibers of the lateral olfactory stria terminate principally in paleocortical structures and in the amygdaloid nuclei of the temporal lobe. Figure 1–19 illustrates the proximity of the developing olfactory tract and the amygdaloid complex.

A layer of paleocortex, the *nucleus of the lateral olfactory stria* (*lateral olfactory gyrus*), covers the lateral olfactory stria. Some of the fibers from the olfactory bulb terminate in this area. The majority of the fibers terminate in the *olfactory cortex* (*piriform cortex*), the cortical tissue forming the rostral half of the uncus (see Figs. 8–6

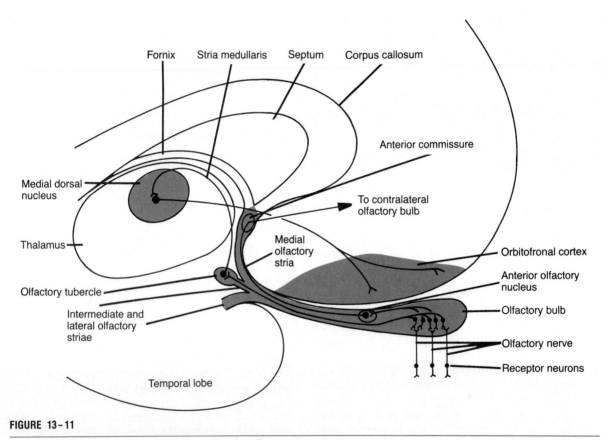

FIGURE 13–11

The central pathway from the olfactory bulb to the neocortical olfactory area and the projection from the anterior olfactory nucleus to the contralateral olfactory bulb are shown. See text for details.

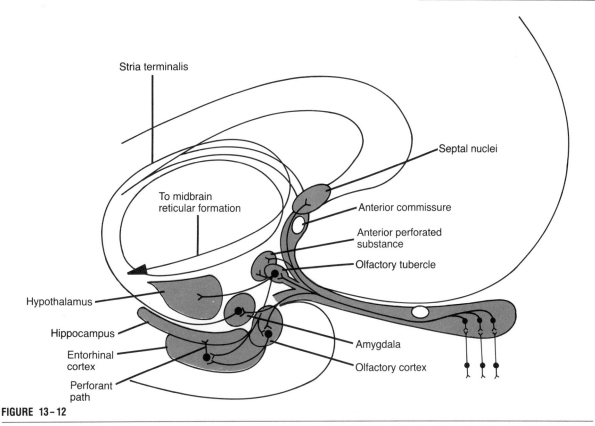

FIGURE 13-12

Some central projections of the olfactory system. See Figure 13–11; also, see text for details.

and 8–7). Other fibers from the olfactory bulb pass deep to the piriform cortex and terminate in the *amygdala*. Additional fibers of the lateral olfactory stria terminate in lateral regions of the *anterior perforated substance* (see Figs. 13–12 and 13–13).

In some classifications, the anterior perforated substance, olfactory tubercle, and lateral olfactory gyrus are paleocortex. In others, they are considered as basal forebrain structures. The important feature is that they are primitive structures and phylogenetically very old regions of the telencephalon associated with both the olfactory and limbic systems.

Secondary projections from the piriform cortex also terminate in the amygdala as well as the adjacent *entorhinal cortex*. The entorhinal neurons form the *perforant path*, a projection system to the adjacent *hippocampal formation*, a major limbic system structure. The *amygdala* has descending projections to the midbrain reticular formation via the *stria terminalis*, some of which are olfactory driven (see Figs. 13–12 and 13–13).

MEDIAL OLFACTORY STRIA

Most of the fibers of the medial olfactory stria arise from the *anterior olfactory nucleus* and project to the contralateral olfactory bulb by way of the *anterior commissure* (see Fig. 13–11). Those axons in the medial olfactory stria from mitral and tufted cells, however, terminate ipsilaterally in the medial portion of the *anterior perforated substance*, the *medial septal nucleus*, and the *bed nucleus of the stria terminalis* (see Figs. 13–12 and 13–13). A thin layer of paleocortex, the *nucleus of the medial olfactory stria (medial olfactory gyrus)*, also covers the medial olfactory stria.

INTERMEDIATE OLFACTORY STRIA

Most of the fibers in the intermediate olfactory stria terminate in the *olfactory tubercle*. In addition to projections to the MD nucleus of the dorsal thalamus, the olfactory tubercle projects to the *hypothalamus*, the *piriform cortex*, and the

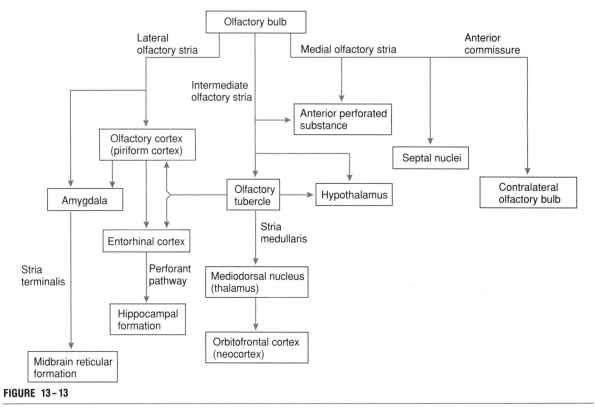

FIGURE 13-13

Flow chart summarizing some of the major central nervous system connections in the olfactory system. See text for details.

entorhinal cortex. Other fibers of the intermediate olfactory stria pass through the olfactory tubercle and end in the adjacent *anterior perforated substance* or project directly to the lateral portion of the *hypothalamus* (see Figs. 13–12 and 13–13).

INFORMATION PROCESSING

Detailed data concerning information processing in the olfactory system at higher levels (beyond the olfactory bulb) are lacking. Many of the secondary projections are *presumed* to have certain functions, based on the known functions of the target structure.

The orbitofrontal gyri, the neocortical area of olfactory representation, are of importance in the conscious perception of odors. Patients with lesions in this area of the cortex cannot discriminate between odorants.

The very extensive limbic system projections (entorhinal cortex, hippocampal formation, medial septal nuclei, and amygdala) may be important in the affective and emotional dimensions of olfactory perception. Other projections, direct and secondary, to the hypothalamus and to the midbrain reticular formation may be related to the modulation of autonomic function by the olfactory system.

Vomeronasal System

The *vomeronasal system,* if present in humans, is vestigial. In other mammals, including New World primates, this system is particularly sensitive to a number of odorants potentially involved in reproductive processes. The vomeronasal system has an accessory chemoreceptive organ, the *vomeronasal organ,* located in the nasal cavity with a sensory epithelium innervated by *vomeronasal nerves,* similar to the olfactory mucosa and the olfactory nerves. However, vomeronasal nerves travel separately and terminate in an *accessory olfactory bulb* that in turn projects to an area of the amygdaloid nuclei devoid of projections from the olfactory bulb.

Clinical Correlations

LOSS OF OLFACTORY FUNCTION

A total loss (*anosmia*) or a diminished (*hyposmia*) sense of smell frequently occurs following trauma to the head. A slight movement of the olfactory bulb, relative to the cribriform plate, has a shearing effect on the hundreds of small olfactory nerve fibers running from the olfactory mucosa to the olfactory bulb. Other more common but often temporary disruptions of olfaction occur from the physical obstruction of the nasal passages due to rhinitis or sinusitis. Similarly, any other damage to the olfactory mucosa, such as toxic industrial or environmental pollutants, can produce a temporary loss of the sense of smell. However, if the damage is severe, it may become permanent.

Following a severe cold or virus infection, patients often experience a variable period of hyposmia. During the infection, the rate of replacement of the primary olfactory nerves is slower than the rate of loss. Hence, there is a net reduction in the number of receptor neurons. Often in severe viral infections, especially in elderly individuals, there is a permanent loss in olfaction. Olfactory losses due to CNS disturbances are not as common, or they are accompanied by other more serious deficits in neural function and are overlooked.

Of particular interest are the observations that a very early sign in the onset of several neurological and psychological diseases (e.g., Alzheimer's disease, Parkinson's disease, cystic fibrosis, and Korsakoff's psychosis) is an impairment in olfaction. A convenient "scratch-'n-sniff" test kit is available to the medical practitioner for screening olfactory function.

LOSS OF GUSTATORY FUNCTION

Total ageusia is a total loss of all taste sensation, *partial ageusia* is a total loss of specific taste sensations, and *hypogeusia* is a diminished sense of all taste sensations. The loss of taste is less frequently encountered, clinically, than a loss of smell. With the bilateral innervation of the tongue by four cranial nerves (both facial and both glossopharyngeal nerves), a peripheral problem leading to a significant loss is an unlikely occurrence. As with olfaction, CNS problems involving taste usually are accompanied by more severe neurological deficits in other systems. In addition, for a significant taste deficit to occur from a CNS problem, it must be bilateral. Normally, a loss of taste sensation involving only one side is not apparent.

SUGGESTED READING

Boudreau, J. C. (1989). Analysis of mammalian peripheral taste systems. In *Sensory Processing in the Mammalian Brain*. J. S. Lund (Editor). Oxford University Press, New York, pp. 23–43.

This review challenges the adequacy of the classic concept of four basic taste elements. The author presents convincing evidence for a new approach to taste receptor classification. Evidence is provided for differences in the basic taste elements between animal forms, differences that reflect the normal diet of these animal forms.

Kinnamon, S. C. (1988). Taste transduction: a diversity of mechanisms. Trends Neurosci., 11: 491–496.

This brief review considers a variety of different transduction mechanisms utilized by gustatory receptors. The principal mechanisms discussed are sodium channels, voltage-sensitive potassium channels, and cAMP-dependent phosphorylation of ion channels.

Margolis, F. L. and T. V. Getchell (Editors) (1988). *Molecular Neurobiology of the Olfactory System*. Plenum Press, New York.

This volume concentrates on the application of molecular and cell biological techniques to basic problems associated with the chemical senses, taste and olfaction. This book contains good, "state-of-the-art" approaches to these problems and provides some insight into future directions.

Shirley, S. G. and K. C. Persaud (1990). The biochemistry of vertebrate olfaction and taste. Semin. in Neurosci., 2: 59–68.

This mini-review concentrates on the molecular biological aspects of our current concepts of sensory transduction in both the olfactory and gustatory systems.

Wilson, D. A. and M. Leon (1989). Information processing in the olfactory system. In *Sensory Processing in the Mammalian Brain*. J. S. Lund (Editor). Oxford University Press, New York, pp. 7–22.

A review of the olfactory pathways. Although many of the central pathways are mentioned, the emphasis is on receptor mechanisms and information processing in the olfactory bulb.

Part
V

MOTOR SYSTEMS

Chapter

14

Spinal Cord and Brain Stem Control of Motor Function

MOTOR UNIT
MUSCLE SPINDLES AND GOLGI TENDON ORGANS
FINAL COMMON PATH
SPINAL REFLEXES
CENTRAL PATTERN GENERATORS
MOTOR RETICULAR FORMATION
SUPRASPINAL SYSTEMS AND MOTOR CONTROL
CLINICAL CORRELATIONS

The two types of motor system are the *somatic motor system* and the *visceral motor system (autonomic nervous system)*. The somatic motor system innervates the striated musculature of the body. This system is the topic of this chapter and of Chapters 15, 16, and 17. Chapter 15 considers the motor cortex and descending pathways; Chapter 16, the basal ganglia; and Chapter 17, the cerebellum. The visceral motor system innervates the visceral organs and glands of the body and is discussed separately in Chapter 18.

The distinction between a *lower motor neuron* and an *upper motor neuron* is important in the understanding of motor systems. *Lower motor neurons* are the motor neurons with axons that leave the central nervous system (CNS) and *innervate the muscle effectors*. Lower motor neurons are the *final common path*, the last "link" between the CNS and the effector. *Upper motor neurons*, in constrast, are those cortical and brain stem neurons with axons that form the descend-

ing motor pathways that *drive the lower motor neurons either directly or indirectly, via spinal interneurons*. Important clinical differences exist between upper and lower motor neuron disorders.

The *somatic motor system* controls a multitude of bodily functions, from respiration and saccadic movements of the eye, to walking, reaching, standing, and chewing. Somatic motor activity leads to the contraction of skeletal or striated muscle, motor events that are initiated *voluntarily* or *modulated with intent*. To accomplish this, axons of the *lower motor neurons* leave the CNS and form a synapse-like junction, the *neuromuscular junction*, with striated muscle fibers, the *motor effectors*. The principal motor component of these volitional activities is *general somatic efferent (GSE)*.

Movements of specific parts of the body are the result of the controlled *contraction and relaxation* of selected muscles and muscle groups. The types and varieties of movements are diverse, from gross but coordinated body movements to delicate, finely controlled movements. Other motor activities represent learned sequences of motor commands—typing and playing a musical instrument. These involve the voluntary recall of learned motor sequences.

The somatic motor system has a very strong *reflex component*, and some motor activities operate almost exclusively in a reflex mode until intentionally altered or modulated. *Lower motor neurons* maintain a basal firing rate. This spontaneous firing is responsible for the maintenance of *muscle tone*. The firing rate, however, is under continuous modulation from both excitatory and inhibitory signals. These arise from local spinal afferents, spinal interneurons, and descending motor pathways from supraspinal levels of the brain stem or cerebral cortex.

Consider the "simple" act of pointing the index finger of one hand at a distant object. This voluntary act elicits a multitude of reflexes that produce the smooth and coordinated contraction and relaxation of many different muscle groups, muscle groups that we do not "consciously" activate, yet it is a "voluntary" motor activity. Moving the finger forward in space, along with the hand and arm, alters the body's center of gravity. As the finger and arm move forward, there is a continuous readjustment of the tone of postural muscles and limb muscles to compensate for the positional changes and to assure the smooth forward movement of the extremity and the maintenance of balance. In large measure, descending vestibular and motor reticular formation input to the spinal cord and indirect cerebellar input by way of higher motor centers are responsible for these associated motor actions.

Of equal importance is the somatosensory system and the precise information it continually provides the CNS about the position and rate of change in position of the body and its parts. The spinal cord, brain stem reticular formation, and cerebellum all use this afferent information to constantly readjust muscle tone. The important feature to note is that *somatic motor activity does not take place in a vacuum. The constant reflexive and coordinated readjustment of many muscle groups is an integral part of any intentional motor action.*

Some somatic motor activity is principally reflexive. Respiration is a good example. We breathe, without having to reinitiate the process with every breath; however, we can hold our breath or hyperventilate at will. The tendon-jerk reflex (the patellar or knee-jerk reflex) is an ex-

ample of a monosynaptic reflex, in which primary afferent fibers directly excite the motor neurons responsible for the muscle contraction. Yet, we can intentionally suppress, but not totally eliminate, the response if we anticipate it.

The various components of the somatic motor system do not act in isolation. They are discussed separately for convenience only. Intentional motor actions are a complex composite of cortically initiated actions, reflexes at the spinal cord and brain stem levels, and modulatory influences from the cerebellum and the basal ganglia. None of these components act alone. Reflexes and modulatory influences at all levels continually act in concert to maintain proper muscle tone and to permit a smooth, controlled voluntary movement. Damage or disease affecting any one of these components has repercussions on the overall motor performance. Observing and testing a patient's motor ability is an important diagnostic tool in the evaluation of neurological damage.

In addition to *general somatic efferent* (*GSE*) neurons, the *somatic motor system* also includes *special visceral efferent* (*SVE*) neurons. All are lower motor neurons innervating striated muscle. *GSE* neurons innervate striated muscle of embryonic somite and limb bud origin, whereas the *SVE* neurons, sometimes called *branchiomotor neurons*, innervate striated muscle of embryonic branchial (pharyngeal) arch origin. *Except for the embryonic origin of the muscle and some differences in the migratory patterns of the neuroblasts during CNS development, SVE neurons and the muscles they innervate are functionally indistinguishable from GSE neurons and the muscles they innervate.* All spinal nerves and four of the cranial nerves have a GSE component, whereas only five of the cranial nerves have SVE components (see subsequent discussion).

Motor Unit

DEFINITION AND PROPERTIES

Axons of the *lower motor neurons* leave the CNS and form the motor components of spinal and cranial nerves. In the spinal cord, axons of the *ventral horn cells* exit as the ventral root, which combines with the dorsal root to form the mixed *peripheral (spinal) nerve*. On reaching the target muscle, the axons of the motor neurons branch to form a terminal arborization, the telodendron. Each of the terminal branches of the axon then innervates a single muscle fiber (Fig. 14–1).

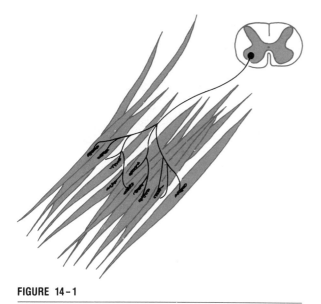

FIGURE 14-1

The motor unit. A single lower motor neuron and all the muscle fibers innervated by that neuron constitute the motor unit.

The definition of a *motor unit* is a *lower motor neuron* and all the *muscle fibers* that the lower motor neuron innervates (see Fig. 14-1). In the adult, each muscle fiber receives only one nerve terminal. The *neuromuscular junction* is the synapse-like contact between the nerve terminal and the muscle fiber. The axon terminal is the presynaptic component, and a modified area of the muscle membrane is the postsynaptic element (Figs. 14-2 and 14-3). A single action potential traveling down the axon of a motor neuron triggers the release of *acetylcholine* (*ACh*) at all terminal branches of that axon. Because of the all-or-nothing property of the neuromuscular junction, the release of ACh depolarizes the muscle membrane, triggering a contraction of the muscle fiber (see subsequent discussion). Thus, stimulation of a single motor neuron leads to the contraction of all muscle fibers in that motor unit.

In the axial muscles or the major limb flexor and extensor muscles, individual motor neurons innervate from 600 to several thousand individual muscle fibers. In the intrinsic muscles of the hand, the ratio is closer to 100 muscle fibers per neuron. In the extraocular muscles, the ratio approaches 10. The ratio is correspondingly lower for those muscles that require a finer and more precise level of motor control.

All motor units, however, do not have the same physiological properties, even those within the same muscle. By using the properties of the muscle fiber contraction (rate, tension generated, and fatigue characteristics), motor units can be grouped into three or four categories. *Type S* (slow) motor units are slow contracting, generate relatively low tension, but are very fatigue resistant. *Type FR* (fast and resistant to fatigue) motor units contract rapidly, generate good tension, and are relatively resistant to fatigue. *Type FF* (fast and fatigable) motor units also contract rapidly, generate the highest tension, but are the least resistant to fatigue. Different muscles contain different proportions of these motor unit subtypes. Consequently, each muscle has a combination of fiber types that best suit the normal physiological function of that muscle.

The motor neurons also show differences in physiological properties, such as conduction velocity, repolarization time, and membrane time constant. During development, it is the motor neuron, and apparently its physiological properties, that determines the properties of the muscle fibers it innervates.

LOWER MOTOR NEURONS

The two basic types of lower motor neurons are the *alpha motor neurons* and the *gamma motor neurons*. Skeletal muscles contain two types of contractile element: the *extrafusal fibers* and the *intrafusal fibers*. Alpha motor neurons innervate the extrafusal fibers, the principal contractile elements of the muscle. Gamma motor neurons innervate the intrafusal fibers, the contractile elements of the *muscle spindle*, an elaborate sensory organ within the mass of the muscle (see the following section).

Alpha motor neurons are large, multipolar neurons with dense, coarse Nissl bodies in the perikaryon and an extensive dendritic tree (see Figs. 2-6 and 2-8). These are among the largest and fastest conducting neurons of the CNS. Their large axons (9 to 20 μm in diameter) are heavily myelinated, fast conducting, type-Aα fibers, with conduction velocities of 50 to 100 m/sec. *Gamma motor neurons* are smaller and have axons of 3 to 7 μm diameter. However, these axons are well-myelinated and relatively fast conducting, type-Aγ fibers, with conduction velocities of 15 to 50 m/sec (see Fig. 10-3).

SPINAL CORD GSE NEURONS

The lower motor neurons of the spinal cord reside in the ventral or anterior horns, lamina IX

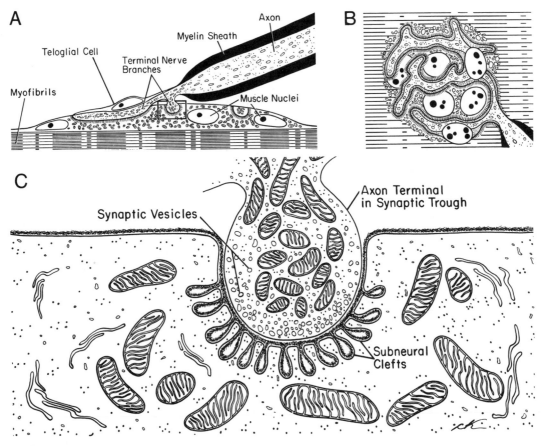

FIGURE 14-2

The neuromuscular junction.

A, Neuromuscular junction as seen in histological sections in the long axis of the muscle fiber.

B, As seen in a surface view with the light microscope.

C, As seen in an electron micrograph of an area such as that in the rectangle on *A*. (Reproduced with permission from D. W. Fawcett, *A Textbook of Histology*, 11th Edition, W. B. Saunders Co., Philadelphia, 1986.)

of Rexed. The *medial motor columns (nuclei)* extend the entire length of the spinal cord and contain motor neurons to the axial musculature. The larger *lateral motor columns (nuclei)* of the cervical and lumbosacral enlargements contain neurons to the musculature of the upper and lower extremities, respectively. In general, the alpha motor neurons of the lateral motor nuclei are somewhat larger than those of the medial motor nuclei.

The motor neurons in the spinal cord cluster in groups according to the specific muscle innervated. Similarly, there is a topographic organization in which those neurons innervating the extensor muscles are ventral (anterior) to those innervating the flexor muscles (Fig. 14-4). In addition, neurons innervating the most proximal muscles are medial, and those innervating pro-

gressively more distal muscles are more lateral (see Fig. 14-4). The primary dendritic branches of the motor neurons run longitudinally within the motor columns of the spinal cord. Some of these dendrites extend for several spinal segments in a rostrocaudal direction.

BRAIN STEM GSE NEURONS

In the brain stem, the *oculomotor, trochlear,* and *abducens nuclei* contain lower motor neurons that innervate the extraocular muscles (via *cranial nerves III, IV,* and *VI*). The *hypoglossal nucleus* contains the motor neurons that innervate the intrinsic musculature of the tongue via *cranial nerve XII*. All of these nuclei contain both alpha and gamma motor neurons, and all are GSE.

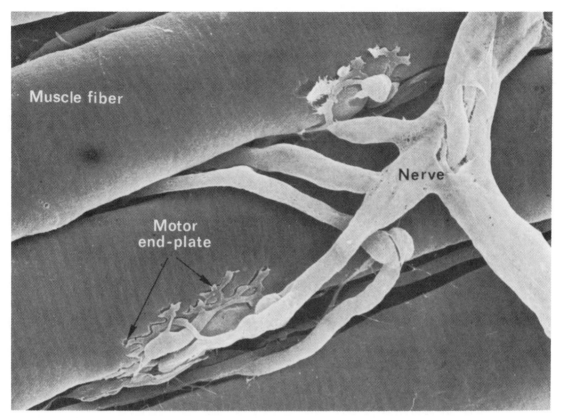

FIGURE 14-3

Scanning micrograph of a motor nerve and two motor end plates (neuromuscular junctions) on adjacent muscle fibers. (Reproduced with permission from J. Desaki, and Y. Uehara, J. Neurocytol., 10: 107, 1981.)

FIGURE 14-4

The organization of the lower motor neurons in the ventral horn of the spinal cord at cervical levels. Motor neurons cluster in small groups, according to the muscle they innervate.

Neurons innervating extensor muscles are ventral to those innervating flexors. Neurons to the axial and limb girdle musculature are medial to those innervating muscles in more distal parts of the extremity.

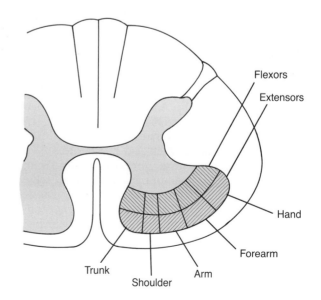

BRAIN STEM SVE NEURONS

The *motor nucleus of the trigeminal nerve* (*motor nucleus of V*) and the large *facial nucleus* contain motor neurons that innervate the muscles of mastication (via the *motor root of cranial nerve V*) and the muscles of facial expression (via *cranial nerve VII*). The *nucleus ambiguus* contains motor neurons that innervate muscles of the pharynx and the intrinsic musculature of the larynx, via *cranial nerve IX* to the stylopharyngeus muscle and via *cranial nerve X* to the remainder. The *spinal accessory nucleus* contains motor neurons that supply portions of the sternomastoid and trapezius muscles via *cranial nerve XI*. As with the brain stem GSE nuclei, all contain alpha and gamma motor neurons.

NEUROMUSCULAR JUNCTION

The *neuromuscular junction* in skeletal muscle is often 100 to 500 μm in diameter (see Figs. 14–2 and 14–3). Each muscle fiber, although many centimeters long, normally has only one neuromuscular junction in a central region of the fiber. The presynaptic portion, the nerve terminal, contains numerous clear, round synaptic vesicles filled with ACh and the appropriate enzymes for the rapid synthesis and storage of the neurotransmitter. When the action potential reaches the nerve terminal, the depolarization activates voltage-sensitive Ca^{++} channels, leading to the exocytotic release of ACh into the synaptic cleft, much like cholinergic synapses in the CNS.

The postsynaptic membrane, the specialized area of the muscle membrane underlying the nerve terminal, is thrown into a series of subjunctional folds or subneural clefts, increasing the effective surface area of the postsynaptic membrane. The postsynaptic membrane is densely packed with *nicotinic acetylcholine receptors* (*N-AChR*). These receptors are of the N_1-AChR subtype, activated by the agonist phenyl trimethylammonium, reversibly blocked by D-tubocurarine and irreversibly blocked by the snake venom α-toxins, such as α-bungarotoxin.

A basal lamina, with a composition similar to that of a basement membrane, totally invests the muscle fiber and extends between the presynaptic and postsynaptic membranes, following the contour of the muscle fiber membrane (see Fig. 14–2). At the neuromuscular junction, *acetylcholinesterase* (*AChE*) is extracellular, within the cleft, and anchored to the collagen matrix of the basal lamina. AChE inactivates the neurotrans-

mitter by hydrolyzing the ACh to acetate and choline.

Interaction of ACh with the N-AChRs triggers an excitatory postsynaptic potential (EPSP), the AChR being a ligand-gated sodium channel. Depolarization of the postsynaptic membrane at the neuromuscular junction activates voltage-sensitive Na^+ and K^+ channels in the surrounding muscle fiber membrane. This activation, in turn, produces a wave of depolarization that spreads the length of the muscle fiber. The molecular mechanisms for the depolarization of the muscle fiber membrane are similar to those for the generation and propagation of a neuronal action potential. The resultant depolarization of the muscle fiber initiates contractile mechanisms within the muscle fiber.

Muscle Spindles and Golgi Tendon Organs

In the performance of smooth and coordinated motor tasks, the afferent signals from specific mechanoreceptors are as important as the efferent signals to the muscles. Intimately involved with the somatic efferent system are two mechanoreceptors, the *muscle spindle* and the *Golgi tendon organ*. Together, these receptors continuously provide information about the current state of muscle contraction and the rates of change in muscle length and tension.

MUSCLE SPINDLE ANATOMY

The muscle spindle is a long, slender fusiform-shaped mechanoreceptor that responds to stretch and tension and to rates of change in these properties (Fig. 14–5). Located within the body of the striated muscle, these receptors contain from three to 12, miniature muscle fibers, *intrafusal fibers*, within a collagenous, fusiform sheath. This sheath is anchored to the connective tissue matrix of the muscle proper and is parallel to the large *extrafusal fibers* that make up the main body of the muscle.

The central or equatorial portion of each intrafusal fiber is devoid of contractile elements and functions as a specialized stretch receptor. The end regions of the intrafusal fibers contain actin and myosin filaments and have contractile properties. The two types of intrafusal fibers are the *nuclear bag fibers* and the *nuclear chain fibers*. The nuclei of the nuclear bag fibers cluster to-

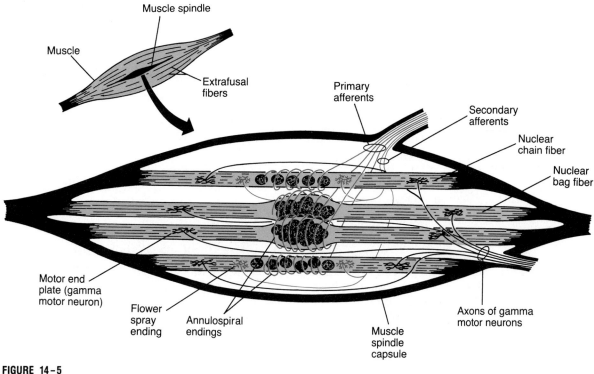

FIGURE 14-5

Diagram of a muscle spindle receptor organ illustrating the major components. See text for details.

gether in an enlarged central region, and the nuclei of the nuclear chain fibers line up in a row or chain with no enlargement of the central region (see Fig. 14-5). The relative number of the longer (8 to 10 mm) nuclear bag fibers and the shorter (4 to 5 mm) nuclear chain fibers varies from spindle to spindle.

Each muscle spindle receives both *primary* and *secondary afferent fibers*. Primary afferent fibers innervate the equatorial region of *each* intrafusal fiber, with the afferent terminal spiraling around the central region of the fiber, forming an *annulospiral ending*. These afferent nerve fibers are large, fast conducting, type-Aα fibers. Secondary afferent fibers, smaller type-Aβ afferent fibers, branch and form *flower spray endings* on either side of the equatorial region but primarily on the nuclear chain fibers. Both afferent terminals, annulospiral endings, and flower spray endings respond to changes in muscle length. Because the spindle is parallel to the extrafusal fibers of the muscle, changes in the total length of the muscle produce corresponding changes in the length of the muscle spindle.

Gamma motor neurons innervate the contractile ends of each intrafusal fiber (see Fig. 14-5).

The cell bodies of the gamma motor neurons are located in between the larger alpha motor neurons that innervate extrafusal fibers of the same muscle. Signals from gamma motor neurons contract the intrafusal fibers, shortening their length and effectively increasing the amount of stretch or tension on the central, noncontractile region of the fiber (see subsequent discussion).

MUSCLE SPINDLE FUNCTION

Stretching or tension on the central region of an intrafusal fiber produces a mechanical distortion of the afferent endings. This distortion activates cation channels in the afferent terminals, resulting in a depolarization of the terminal and the generation of a receptor potential. The afferent fiber then generates an action potential when the trigger zone of the afferent terminal reaches threshold.

The responses of these afferent terminals to stretch are nonlinear, especially for the primary afferent endings. The increase in rate of firing is greater, per unit of tension, with relatively small amounts of stretch. At greater tension, the total firing rate, although greater, is less per unit tension, a situation similar to that of the pacinian corpuscle discussed in Chapter 10.

Stretching the total muscle also involves stretching the spindle, with a concomitant increase in the afferent discharge. Contraction of the muscle (extrafusal fibers) shortens the muscle, reducing the stretch on the spindle. This results in a decrease in the rate of afferent nerve firing.

Contraction of the intrafusal fibers, through gamma motor neuron stimulation, shortens the length of the intrafusal fiber. This increases the amount of stretch on the central portion of the fiber, the area of the annulospiral endings. Thus, gamma efferent stimulation increases the rate of spindle afferent firing.

Although contraction of the extrafusal fibers reduces the tension on the spindle, the simultaneous stimulation of the gamma efferents shortens the intrafusal fibers, thereby maintaining tension on the central region of the spindle fiber. The simultaneous stimulation of the gamma efferents provides a mechanism for dynamically readjusting the tension on the spindles so that they can operate in an optimal range of sensitivity, regardless of the length of the muscle. Muscle spindles normally discharge through the entire range of movement of a muscle, suggesting that CNS mechanisms often co-activate both the alpha and gamma efferents to the same muscle. In addition, for spindle firing patterns to provide meaningful information, the CNS must correlate the spindle afferent signals with the gamma efferent firing patterns, to correct for the degree of spindle contraction.

GOLGI TENDON ORGAN

The *Golgi tendon organ* is an encapsulated stretch receptor situated at the junction between the muscle and its tendon. Normally ten to 12 individual muscle fibers, usually from different motor units, insert on the capsule of the Golgi tendon organ. The afferent fibers to the encapsulated receptor organ are large, fast conducting type-Aα fibers. Golgi tendon organs are in *series* with the large extrafusal fibers of the muscle and respond to total muscle tension. This is much like a spring balance that stretches with increasing weight only to rebound to the original position with the removal of the weight. The Golgi tendon organ does not differentiate between tension produced by stretch and that produced by contraction of the muscle. This tendon organ does not have an efferent component.

COMPARISON OF GOLGI TENDON ORGANS AND MUSCLE SPINDLES

Golgi tendon organs are in series with the extrafusal muscle fibers, whereas muscle spindles are in parallel with the fibers. Therefore, the Golgi tendon organ monitors *overall tension* on the muscle, tension produced both by stretch and contraction. In contrast, the muscle spindle monitors *relative length and rate of change in length* of the muscle. Both receptors generate afferent signals that are important for spinal cord reflexes, supraspinal reflexes, and cerebellar function.

Final Common Path

MOTOR NEURON AS INTEGRATOR

The lower motor neuron is the *final common path* between the complex circuitry of the CNS and the muscle effector. When the lower motor neuron transmits an action potential, all muscle fibers composing its motor unit contract in an all-or-nothing manner. However, in order to fire, the motor neuron must integrate thousands of incoming excitatory and inhibitory signals. Estimates indicate as many as 10,000 synaptic terminals from over 1000 different neurons converge on each alpha motor neuron. The motor neuron then integrates these thousands of synaptic signals through the *temporal* and *spatial* summation of the EPSPs and inhibitory postsynaptic potential (IPSPs). When the membrane potential at the trigger zone near the axon hillock reaches or exceeds threshold, the motor neuron generates an action potential and all muscle fibers of that motor unit contract.

The excitatory and inhibitory stimuli come from a variety of sources: local spinal circuits (excitatory monosynaptic spinal afferents and inhibitory and excitatory spinal interneurons) and descending supraspinal pathways (vestibulospinal, reticulospinal, corticospinal, tectospinal, and rubrospinal). The excitatory and inhibitory spinal interneurons are more than simple relay neurons. They also integrate a considerable amount of information before relaying it to the motor neuron.

In general, synaptic terminals of monosynaptic afferents make contact with the soma or proximal dendrites of the motor neuron and those from descending supraspinal pathways contact more distal dendritic processes. Synapses associated with supraspinal reflexes (e.g., vestibulospinal fibers) are closer to the soma than those from the motor cortex (corticospinal fibers). Inhibitory synapses also are closer to the axon hillock than are the competing excitatory synapses. Postsynaptic potentials spread passively, and an inhibitory synapse is more effective if situated between the competing excitatory synapse and the trigger zone of the axon.

MOTOR UNIT RECRUITMENT
Graded Contractile Force

Although the individual motor unit functions in an all-or-nothing fashion, motor responses normally are smooth and graded. An individual motor neuron may innervate 100 individual muscle fibers, but most muscles contain 100 or more motor units. Two features responsible for the smooth and graded contraction are (1) the different physiological properties of the individual motor units (speed of contraction, tension generation, and resistance to fatigue, e.g., type S, type FR, are type FF) and (2) the different thresholds and firing rates of the motor units in the same muscle.

Lower motor neurons receive a constant bombardment of excitatory and inhibitory signals, principally from spinal and brain stem centers, and are continuously firing at a rate consistent with the signals they receive. This constant firing of motor neurons and constant "leak" of quantal units of ACh at the neuromuscular junction are responsible for maintaining muscle tone. Skeletal muscles are not totally flaccid when "at rest." A state of nonmovement is really a fine balance between the levels of excitation of motor units in antagonistic muscle groups. When this balance is upset, a "tremor at rest" is the result. However, damage to the lower motor neurons itself produces a totally flaccid paralysis (see the following discussion).

Spinal Reflexes

DEFINITION

A *spinal reflex* is simply *an efferent motor neuron discharge following a sufficient afferent stimulation.* Spinal reflexes are independent of supraspinal pathways, i.e., if the spinal cord is severed, spinal reflexes below the level of damage remain intact. In addition to other roles, supraspinal pathways modulate spinal reflexes. Without these

supraspinal influences, spinal reflexes usually are exaggerated—the *net* effect of the supraspinal influence usually is inhibitory. Characteristically, spinal reflexes are very reproducible and stereotypical. The following are a few of the better characterized spinal reflexes.

AFFERENTS

Spinal reflexes require afferent signals, *general somatic afferent* (*GSA*) signals from the periphery: muscles, tendons, joint capsules, skin, and fascia. More than two thirds of the fibers in the peripheral nerves innervating muscle are afferent (sensory) and less than one third are efferent or motor, a reflection of the importance of afferent signals to motor function.

Of the muscle afferents, over 60% are from free nerve endings. Of these, over half are nociceptive, principally chemical, mechanical, and thermal. The remainder respond to similar stimuli, which are not noxious. Most of these are type-C, small, nonmyelinated fibers; the remainder are small, myelinated type-Aδ fibers. Of the afferents, 25% are large, heavily myelinated type-Aα fibers. Of these, about two thirds are from annulospiral endings and the remainder from Golgi tendon organs. Fibers from spindle flower spray endings, Ruffini's corpuscles and Pacini's corpuscles, type-Aβ fibers, account for the remaining 15%.

On entering the spinal cord, the large type-Aα fibers bifurcate into an ascending and a descending branch. The ascending branch continues in the dorsal column, terminating in one of the dorsal column nuclei of the medulla. Both ascending and descending branches give off numerous, regularly spaced collaterals over a distance of several spinal segments. The collateral branches enter the spinal gray matter. They branch profusely, making numerous connections with spinal interneurons and some directly with lower motor neurons (see Fig. 14–6). The smaller diameter afferents also bifurcate and give off collateral branches; however, many of these synapse with thalamic relay neurons in the spinal cord.

Afferents from cutaneous areas and the joints of the extremity trigger some spinal motor reflexes. These afferents are principally type-Aβ, type-Aδ, and type-C fibers from mechanoreceptors, thermal and chemical receptors, and nociceptors. One feature all these afferents have in common is the polysynaptic excitation of ipsilateral flexor motor neurons. For this reason, these are often collectively called *flexor reflex afferents*

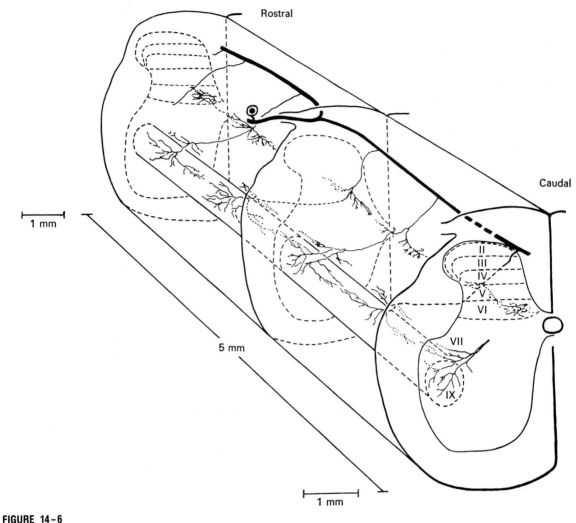

FIGURE 14-6

A type-Aα afferent fiber in the lumbosacral spinal cord illustrating the morphology of some of the collateral branches. The heavy line represents the primary afferent fiber along with its ascending and descending branches.

Note the regular arrangement of collateral branches, approximately every 1 mm, and their subsequent branching and distribution within the spinal gray matter. (Reproduced with permission from A. G. Brown and R. E. W. Fyffe, J. Physiol. (Lond.) 274: 123, 1978.)

(*FRAs*). The synapses between FRAs and the spinal interneurons occur in a large area of the spinal cord gray matter, laminae III through VII.

SPINAL INTERNEURONS

Spinal interneurons play a crucial role in somatic motor function and are as important an integrator of afferent and descending motor signals as the lower motor neurons themselves. A few function as simple relay neurons. Many are part of reflex circuits representing various levels of com-

plexity, and most are part of extensive neuronal networks known as central or spinal pattern generators (see the following section). The very extensive spinal interneuron network contains many different neurotransmitters; however, a few generalizations can be made. Inhibitory spinal interneurons are either glycinergic or GABAergic. Most of the GABAergic interneurons are in the laminae of the dorsal horn (laminae I, II, and III), whereas glycine-containing interneurons are in the more central and ventral locations. Excitatory spinal interneurons appear to utilize one of the excitatory amino acids (glutamate or aspartate) as the neurotransmitter. Although some of the interneurons have a peptide co-transmitter, most of the peptidergic activity is in the area of the intermediolateral cell column, the sympathetic preganglionic motor columns, or the descending serotoninergic projections from the raphe nuclei to the dorsal horns.

Of the spinal interneurons, the *Renshaw cell* is probably the best known. Renshaw cells are part of a recurrent inhibitory loop involving spinal motor neurons. Collaterals from spinal motor neurons form excitatory, cholinergic synapses on the Renshaw cells. These cells, in turn, form inhibitory, glycinergic synapses on the motor

neurons via a simple feedback inhibitory loop. However, Renshaw cells also produce IPSPs on many other neurons of the spinal cord, including other Renshaw cells, ventral spinocerebellar relay neurons, and many inhibitory interneurons including those driven by spindle afferent fibers. The greatest inhibitory effects of Renshaw cells are on the motor neurons that drive them, other homonymous motor neurons, and those innervating synergistic muscle groups. Motor neuron collaterals are not the only input to Renshaw cells. Many excitatory and inhibitory reflex afferents and supraspinal systems also drive these small, inhibitory interneurons.

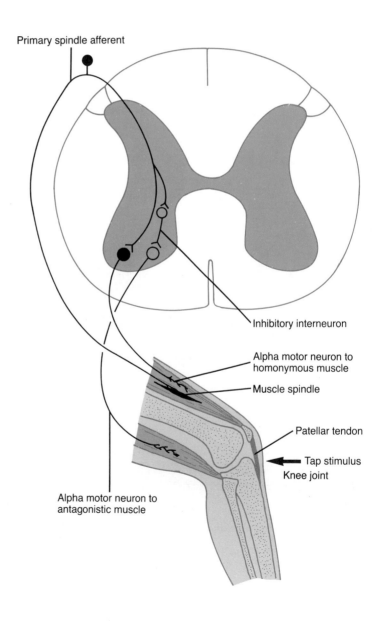

FIGURE 14–7

The tendon reflex. The inhibitory interneurons are open; the excitatory neurons and excited lower motor neurons are solid. See text for details.

TENDON REFLEX

The *knee jerk*, *myotatic*, or *patellar tendon reflex* is one of the best characterized *tendon reflexes*. A sharp tap to the patellar tendon transmits a quick but brief stretch to the quadriceps muscle, stimulating the primary spindle afferents (annulospiral endings). The large, fast conducting afferent fibers synapse directly on the alpha motor neurons innervating the homonymous muscle. If the temporal and spatial summation of the EPSPs reaches threshold, an action potential is generated and there is a twitch contraction of the quadriceps. The afferent signals also stimulate alpha motor neurons to synergistic muscles, however, these do not usually reach threshold. In parallel with the excitation of the homonymous motor neuron, the same spindle afferents excite interneurons that inhibit motor neurons to antagonistic muscles. Normally, there is a latency of about 5.5 msec between the tap (afferent stimulation) and the twitch response. This very rapid response is consistent with a monosynaptic or myotatic reflex, with 1.5 msec of synaptic delay and 4 msec of combined afferent and efferent conduction times (Fig. 14 – 7).

STRETCH REFLEX

The more one stretches a stiff coil spring, the stiffer it becomes. The *stretch reflex* works in much the same way. When a muscle is stretched, the extrafusal fibers contract in a graded response that increases with more stretching. As a result, the muscle becomes stiffer as the amount of stretch increases. The stretching stimulates both the primary and secondary spindle afferents (annulospiral endings and flower spray ending) and the Golgi tendon organs. During an increase in stretching, the muscle response becomes greater in proportion to the amount of stretch. However, when the stretch is maintained without a further increase in muscle length or tension, the contraction enters a tonic phase. A level of increased muscle tone remains as long as the muscle is in the stretched position. Although some of the afferent information terminates monosynaptically

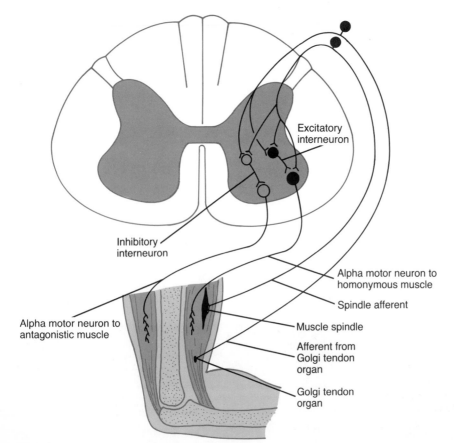

Excitatory interneuron

Inhibitory interneuron

Alpha motor neuron to antagonistic muscle

Alpha motor neuron to homonymous muscle

Spindle afferent

Muscle spindle

Afferent from Golgi tendon organ

Golgi tendon organ

FIGURE 14 – 8

The stretch reflex. The inhibitory interneurons and inhibited lower motor neurons are open; the excitatory neurons and interneurons and excited lower motor neurons are solid. See text for details.

on the alpha motor neurons, most is relayed by spinal interneurons (Fig. 14–8).

FLEXOR REFLEX

The flexion (withdrawal) of a limb from a noxious stimulus illustrates well the *flexor reflex* or the *withdrawal reflex*. The afferents for this reflex, the *flexor reflex afferents* (*FRAs*), are principally type-Aβ, type-Aδ, and type-C afferents (see previous discussion). All *flexor* reflexes are polysynaptic and involve one or more spinal interneurons. A very light stimulus to a cutaneous surface elicits a small but perceptible twitch-like contraction from underlying flexor muscles.

With an elevation in stimulus intensity, a more massive *excitation* of the *ipsilateral flexor motor neurons* and an *inhibition* of the *ipsilateral extensor motor neurons* occur. The combined effect of flexor excitation and extensor inhibition is the *limb withdrawal reflex*. We have all experienced this type of reflex—the rapid withdrawal of a hand from a hot surface or a bare foot from a sharp object (Fig. 14–9).

CROSSED EXTENSOR REFLEX

The *crossed extensor reflex* actually occurs in parallel with the flexor reflex, if the afferent stimulus is sufficient. *FRAs* send collaterals

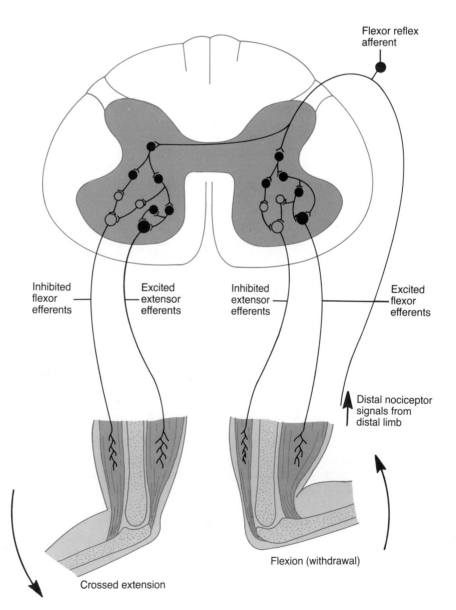

Flexor reflex afferent

Inhibited flexor efferents

Excited extensor efferents

Inhibited extensor efferents

Excited flexor efferents

Distal nociceptor signals from distal limb

Crossed extension

Flexion (withdrawal)

FIGURE 14–9

The flexor and crossed extensor reflexes. The inhibitory interneurons and inhibited lower motor neurons are open; the excitatory neurons and interneurons and excited lower motor neurons are solid. See text for details.

across the midline of the cord, into the dorsal horn of the contralateral half of the spinal cord, where they synapse with spinal interneurons. With an increased intensity in the noxious stimulus producing the flexor reflex, a concomitant *excitation* of the *contralateral extensor motor neurons* and an *inhibition* of the *contralateral flexor motor neurons* occur. The net effect of strong FRA stimulation is the flexion and withdrawal of the ipsilateral limb and the extension and protraction of the contralateral limb (see Fig. 14–9).

In both the flexion reflex and the crossed extensor reflex, the latency of response is much longer than that of the tendon reflex. Two factors contribute to this delay: first, the slower nerve conduction times of the FRAs and, second, the longer synaptic delay due to the polysynaptic nature of the reflex loop.

When the spinal cord is no longer under the influence of the higher centers, many reflexes become exaggerated, particularly the crossed extensor reflex. When the upper cervical spinal cord is severed, flexion and crossed extensor reflexes spread to the other pair of limbs but in a reversed pattern. For example, a stimulus that produces ipsilateral forelimb flexion and contralateral forelimb extension also produces ipsilateral hindlimb extension and contralateral hindlimb flexion. This pattern of spinal reflexive responses resembles a walking-type gait for a quadruped and may involve the spinal interneuron circuitry or "central pattern generator" associated with gait (see the following section).

CLASP-KNIFE REFLEX

A clasp knife is a hunting knife with a folding blade, much like a large pocket knife. To open a clasp knife, the blade is moved against the resistance of a flat spring, tending to keep the knife closed. At a certain point in unfolding the blade, the resistance suddenly disappears and the blade snaps open. The *clasp-knife reflex* is named for a similar action observed when a muscle is stretched to some critical point and suddenly all resistance disappears. The clasp-knife reflex is not demonstrable in the healthy human. It is present in patients with CNS damage to supraspinal motor pathways and is a common feature in spastic paralysis. When one attempts to straighten (extend) a spastic limb, stretching the extensor muscles meets with resistance. As the pressure is increased and some threshold point is reached, there is an immediate loss of resistance. Originally, this response was attributed to afferent signals from the Golgi tendon organs. It was

thought to function as a safety feature to protect the muscle against excessive stretching. We now know that the Golgi tendon organs are not involved. Clasp-knife reflex most likely involves afferent signals carried by type-Aβ and type-Aδ fibers.

Central Pattern Generators

Most motor functions involve a series of rapid, well-coordinated contractions and relaxations of specific motor units, muscles, and muscle groups. Activities such as walking involve synchronized arm-leg coordination. When we undertake these actions, we are not conscious of each coordinated movement but only of the general pattern of movement we wish to make. A conceptual model of spinal interneuron networks, known as spinal pattern generators, best explains the synchronization and coordination of this type of movement. Because these networks are in other parts of the CNS as well as the spinal cord, a more general and preferred term is *central pattern generators* (*CPGs*). Unlike the spinal reflexes, which are well understood, many of the specific components and organizational details of CPGs are still theoretical.

Activation of a CPG generates the essential neurological signals to drive and coordinate selected motor neurons in the proper temporal sequence, achieving the desired pattern of movement. Inhibition of selected motor units is of equal importance, because the relaxation of muscle is as essential to smooth movement as is contraction. CPGs are activated by, and subject to alteration and modulation by, descending motor systems, such as the corticospinal system. In addition, these neuronal networks are modulated by incoming afferent signals and by other descending motor systems, such as the reticulospinal and vestibulospinal systems.

Given the properties of excitatory and inhibitory spinal interneurons and some of their primary connections, theoretical models of CPGs for various patterned movements can be constructed. Although the circuit details are unknown, we do know, for example, that CPGs for gait reside in the spinal cord and those for the rhythmic motor patterns associated with respiration and mastication reside in the medulla.

Motor Reticular Formation

The *reticular formation* is the primitive, central core of brain stem gray matter. Extending from caudal medulla to rostral midbrain, it has roles in many neurological functions, ranging from the controlling and modulating of somatic motor function to the processing of sensory information, modulating autonomic nervous functions, and cortical arousal mechanisms. As the "newer" motor and sensory systems appear in higher vertebrates, they develop parallel with the systems already present in the reticular formation. In higher vertebrates, the reticular formation receives extensive modulation and regulation through collaterals from sensory and motor pathways and cerebellar efferent fibers as well as direct descending corticoreticular pathways.

The *corticoreticulospinal system* is a major descending somatic motor system involving the reticular formation. This system originates principally in the *premotor* and *secondary motor areas* of the cerebral cortex and projects to nuclei in the medial pontine and medullary regions of the reticular formation. These nuclei, in turn, give rise to the descending *medial* and *lateral reticulospinal tracts* (see subsequent discussion). A detailed discussion of the role of the corticoreticulospinal system in the control of motor function, and as a parallel system to the corticospinal system, is provided in the next chapter.

The descending serotoninergic fibers from the nucleus raphe magnus and nucleus gigantocellularis and the descending adrenergic pathways from the dorsolateral pontine reticular formation are important in the modulation of noxious stimuli (see Fig. 10–25). Because somatic motor function depends on primary afferent information at the spinal level, any alteration in the flow of this information affects motor function.

Within the reticular formation are many *CPGs*. For example, the CPGs that drive the rhythmic and patterned motor activities associated with respiration and mastication are in medullary centers of the reticular formation. The descending fibers that compose the motor *reticulospinal tracts* arise from large, multipolar neurons in principally two pontine and two medullary reticular nuclei (see the following discussion). These large diameter, heavily myelinated and fast conducting axons are principally motor in function. Their course is different from the descending reticular fibers associated with the modulation of pain.

Supraspinal Systems and Motor Control

Supraspinal motor systems are descending pathways and tracts that initiate, modulate, or in some way regulate somatic motor function. They include descending pathways from the cerebral cortex and from brain stem centers, such as the red nucleus, superior colliculus, and vestibular nuclei, and the pontine and medullary portions of the reticular formation. Most of these descending fibers synapse on spinal interneurons. Many activate or modulate spinal level CPGs, and some directly excite alpha and gamma motor neurons. Others form axoaxonal synapses on incoming primary afferent fibers (primary afferent depolarization) and influence motor function by modulating incoming afferent signals, information vital to the reflexive dimensions of motor function. The effects of most descending supraspinal systems are extensive and not limited simply to the excitation or inhibition of lower motor neurons.

CORTICOSPINAL TRACT

The *corticospinal* system originates in the sensorimotor cortex (*Brodmann's areas 4, 6, 3, 1, 2, and 5*). This includes the motor, premotor, primary somatosensory (S-I), and posterior parietal areas. These glutaminergic fibers descend through the internal capsule, the cerebral peduncles (crus cerebri), and the basal pons. They emerge to form the pyramids of the medulla. In the caudal medulla, most of the fibers cross to the opposite side and descend in the lateral funiculus of the spinal cord as the *lateral corticospinal tract*. A few fibers continue uncrossed as the *ventral corticospinal tract* (Fig. 14–10). Fibers of the corticospinal tracts end in laminae V through IX of the spinal cord and in greatest numbers in the cervical and lumbosacral enlargements. As the corticospinal tract courses through the brain stem, it gives off many collateral fibers that end in brain stem structures including the reticular formation. Other cortical motor fibers end in or near motor nuclei of the cranial nerves. These form the *corticobulbar system*.

The *corticospinal system* innervates lower motor neurons directly, or indirectly via spinal interneurons, that are associated with the distal limb musculature. This system is suited to the highly controlled, independent movement of the extremities or parts of the extremities. These are very precise, well-controlled movements. Activities controlled by the vestibular and reticular formation systems, in contrast, are the gross, but integrated and coordinated, motor functions associated with postural and antigravity body movement.

RUBROSPINAL TRACT

The *rubrospinal tract* arises from the caudal or magnocellular portion of the *red nucleus*; crosses

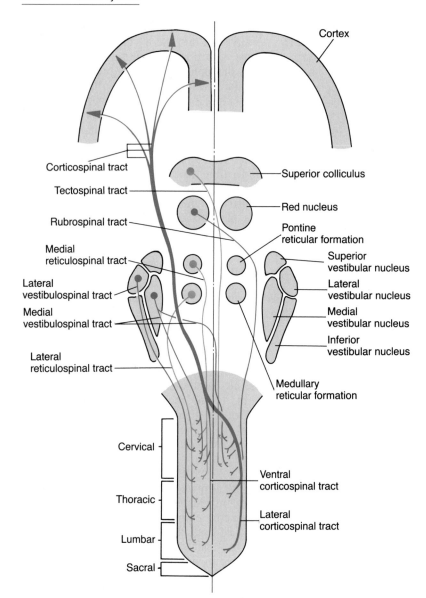

Cortex

Corticospinal tract

Tectospinal tract

Rubrospinal tract

Medial reticulospinal tract

Lateral vestibulospinal tract

Medial vestibulospinal tract

Lateral reticulospinal tract

Superior colliculus

Red nucleus

Pontine reticular formation

Superior vestibular nucleus

Lateral vestibular nucleus

Medial vestibular nucleus

Inferior vestibular nucleus

Medullary reticular formation

Cervical

Thoracic

Lumbar

Sacral

Ventral corticospinal tract

Lateral corticospinal tract

FIGURE 14-10

Summary of the principal supraspinal motor pathways. See text for details.

in the midbrain; and descends in the contralateral, ventrolateral brain stem to the spinal cord. In the spinal cord, the rubrospinal tract is adjacent to the corticospinal tract (see Fig. 14–10). The pattern of fiber termination is similar to that of the corticospinal tract. However, in the human nervous system, the rubrospinal system does not extend below cervical levels and may be of little clinical significance. The *rubrospinal system* also innervates lower motor neurons associated with the distal limb musculature, directly or indirectly via interneurons. As with the corticospinal system, these target muscles are involved in very precise, well-controlled movements.

VESTIBULOSPINAL PATHWAYS

The prominent *lateral vestibulospinal tract,* from the lateral vestibular nucleus, descends ipsilaterally in the ventral portion of the spinal cord (see Fig. 14–10). The fibers end throughout the length of the spinal cord in laminae VII, VIII, and IX. In general, these vestibulospinal fibers are excitatory, with some synapsing directly on alpha motor neurons. The primary targets for the lateral vestibulospinal tract are lower motor neurons and spinal interneurons concerned with the innervation of the axial and proximal limb musculature, especially the extensor muscles. The *lateral vestibulospinal tract*, in combination with the medial and lateral reticulospinal tracts (see subsequent discussion), plays an important role in postural adjustment and maintenance of balance. The lateral vestibular nucleus receives strong macular input and, as a result, responds well to the movement of the head in space. In general, the *vestibulospinal system excites lower limb extensors, upper limb flexors*, and *axial extensors*, whereas the *reticulospinal system excites lower limb flexors, upper limb extensors*, and *axial flexors*. Both systems are excitatory, either to the lower motor neurons directly or indirectly via spinal excitatory interneurons.

The less prominent *medial vestibulospinal tract* arises from the medial vestibular nucleus with contributions from lateral and inferior vestibular nuclei, and descends bilaterally, with fibers of the *medial longitudinal fasciculus* (*MLF*) (see Fig. 14–10). Most of these fibers end in the cervical region of the spinal cord, with some fibers reaching upper thoracic levels. Ending principally on interneurons of laminae VII and VIII, the *medial vestibulospinal tract* reflexly regulates head and trunk position in response to semicircular canal stimulation.

RETICULOSPINAL PATHWAYS

Fibers from the pontine reticular formation, especially the *nucleus pontis oralis* and the *nucleus pontis caudalis*, descend ipsilaterally in the ventral portion of the spinal cord as the *medial reticulospinal tract*. Fibers from the medullary nuclei, especially the *nucleus reticularis gigantocellularis* and the *nucleus reticularis ventralis*, descend ipsilaterally in the ventrolateral portion of the spinal cord as the *lateral reticulospinal tract* (see Fig. 14–10). Most fibers of the medial and lateral reticulospinal tracts end on spinal interneurons in laminae VII and VIII. Some reticulospinal fibers extend the length of the spinal cord, with collateral branches ending in the spinal gray matter of *both* the cervical and lumbosacral enlargements. Reticulospinal fibers, either directly or through spinal interneurons, excite lower motor neurons, predominantly those innervating flexor muscles of the upper and lower extremities and hip extensor muscles.

The *medial* and *lateral reticulospinal tracts* combine with the lateral vestibulospinal tract to play an important role in postural adjustment and maintenance of balance. The medullary reticular formation receives macular afferent information from the vestibular nuclei and responds to the movement of the head in space. In general,

the *reticulospinal system* excites lower limb flexors, upper limb extensors, and axial flexors, complementing the action of the vestibulospinal system. Descending reticulospinal fibers to the cervical cord, especially fibers from the *nucleus reticularis pontis caudalis* and *nucleus reticularis gigantocellularis* are involved in *eye-head coordination*. These reticular formation nuclei receive extensive sensory input from vestibular, visual, and auditory centers. In addition to these functions, the reticular formation is part of the extensive descending *corticoreticulospinal system* and has a major role in voluntary motor activity as discussed in Chapter 15.

TECTOSPINAL TRACT

In addition to its role in visual reflexes, the superior colliculus integrates sensory information from visual, somatosensory, and auditory systems and gives rise to a descending motor pathway, the *tectospinal tract*. The tectospinal tract crosses at the level of the midbrain and descends in the contralateral ventral portion of the spinal cord. Fibers of the tectospinal tract end in the upper cervical levels of the spinal cord and initiate reflexive movements of the head and neck in response to sensory stimuli, principally visual and auditory (see Fig. 14–10).

Clinical Correlations

UPPER VS. LOWER MOTOR NEURON DISORDERS

The distinction between upper and lower motor neuron disorders is important and straightforward; however, the mechanisms responsible for observed differences are complex. *Lower motor neuron disorders* affect the cell body of the lower motor neuron or the peripheral process of that motor neuron and produce a *flaccid paralysis* of the muscle. *Upper motor neuron disorders* affect any of the descending pathways that drive lower motor neurons directly or indirectly via spinal interneurons. These disorders produce *spastic paralysis*.

Damage to the *lower motor neuron*, the final common path, effectively denervates the muscle, eliminating the excitatory release of ACh at the neuromuscular junction. In the absence of neuronal stimulation, muscle becomes *flaccid* and, after a prolonged period of denervation, undergoes *atrophy*.

The production of *spasticity* as a result of

damage to *upper motor neuron systems* is more complex. If the damage to the brain stem occurs between the red nucleus of the midbrain and the vestibular nuclei of the upper medulla, the condition is *decerebrate rigidity*. Such a lesion releases the spinal cord and lower brain stem centers (reticular formation and vestibular nuclei) from cortical and upper brain stem control. This release results in exaggerated muscle tone and postural responses to somatosensory stimulation. Noxious stimuli to the trunk or head elicit gross axial and limb extension. The same stimuli to the distal limbs elicit both exaggerated flexor withdrawal and crossed extensor reflexes.

If the damage is unilateral, the effects are only on the ipsilateral side. If the damage is low enough to involve the lateral vestibular nucleus, the origin of the lateral vestibulospinal tract, the exaggerated extensor hypertonia is eliminated. This effect is due to the excitatory influence of the lateral vestibulospinal tract on lower motor neurons, especially those innervating the extensor and antigravity muscles.

The descending reticulospinal pathways have both excitatory and inhibitory influences on the spinal cord—influences that become exaggerated when released from cortical control. Part of the reticular formation's contribution to decerebrate rigidity is through the suppression of afferent signals from flexor muscles via *primary afferent depolarization* (*PAD*). This leads to an inhibition of flexors and an excitation of extensors provided the lateral vestibulospinal tract is intact.

With damage to the lower medulla or spinal cord, motor symptoms, below the level of the lesion, are typically those of spastic paralysis: exaggerated muscle tone and hyperactive reflexes. The overall effect of removing all supraspinal systems, cortical and brain stem, is to leave the spinal cord in a state of hypersensitivity to all somatosensory stimuli. Although there are both excitatory and inhibitory centers within the brain stem reticular formation, the net effect of removing all reticulospinal, vestibulospinal, and corticospinal input to the spinal cord is one of disinhibition, hence, the increased muscle tone and spasticity.

DISORDERS AFFECTING THE NEUROMUSCULAR JUNCTION

Myasthenia gravis is one of the more common disorders of the neuromuscular junction. Most forms of myasthenia gravis are of an autoimmune disease, in which the body produces anti-bodies against AChR. This increases the rate of receptor degradation at the neuromuscular junction, leading to a loss of efficiency at the synapse. Early signs of the disease are periodic muscle weakness followed by a more generalized weakness and loss of strength. Nerve function is intact, but the diminished number of receptors renders the neural message ineffective. Many forms of the disease are congenital, and some have a relatively late age of onset. Of the latter, one form selectively affects extraocular muscles, *ocular myasthenia gravis*. Later, however, the debilitating effects may spread to the rest of the body.

PERIPHERAL NERVE DAMAGE

Acute trauma, compression, or severing of the nerve produces either total paralysis or paresis, if the damage to the nerve is incomplete. With a motor nerve injury, or any injury affecting the lower motor neuron and its connection with the effector, the paralysis is always flaccid. The muscle is no longer stimulated.

When the disorder affects only one or two spinal segments, e.g., the ventral root compression from a herniated spinal disc, the motor deficit is often undetectable, except by electromyography. Most muscles receive innervation from nerve fibers arising from several spinal segments. The dermatomal pattern of sensory loss is often more apparent and useful in defining the precise level of involvement and the extent of injury.

Characteristic of peripheral nerve damage, or damage to lower motor neurons in general, is an initial weakness (paresis) in the muscle, a loss of tendon reflexes, and an eventual wasting of the muscle due to the loss of the trophic effect of normal innervation. An intact, functional motor nerve supply is essential for the maintenance of a muscle and the proper regulation of muscle metabolism. Without adequate innervation, the muscle fibers atrophy, the density of AChRs at the neuromuscular junction decreases, and "extrajunctional" AChRs appear over the surface of the muscle fiber. These AChRs have different properties from the normal junctional AChR. The appearance of extrajunctional AChRs results in microfibrillations of the muscle fibers; however, these are clinically detectable only with electromyography.

LOWER MOTOR NEURON DISEASES

Two of the more well-known diseases affecting lower motor neurons are *amyotrophic lateral sclerosis (ALS)* and *poliomyelitis.* In both diseases, there is a selective, irreversible loss of lower motor neurons. ALS is a chronic, progressive disorder of unknown etiology. The symptoms develop slowly, and the disease progresses slowly. Polio, however, is an acute viral disease, with rapid onset and symptom development. With immunization, polio is no longer the problem it once was.

Lower motor neuron loss is accompanied by flaccid paralysis or paresis, loss of tendon reflexes, and eventual wasting and atrophy of muscle fibers. During the progress of the diseases, fasciculation or twitching of the muscle is common. This symptom is due to the release of ACh following the spontaneous activation of one or more motor units. Many diseased motor neurons become hyperactive prior to degeneration: the action potential threshold drops, and the neurons fire spontaneously, producing the fasciculations. Fasciculation ends with the degeneration of the lower motor neuron.

ANTERIOR SPINAL ARTERY OCCLUSION

An occlusion of the *anterior spinal artery* limited to the cervical spinal cord (*central cord syndrome*) spares many of the ascending and descending motor and sensory pathways. However, there is bilateral damage to approximately two thirds of the spinal gray matter, including most of the ventral horn area (see Fig. 9–12). Involvement of C-4 impairs respiration, and involvement of lower cervical segments produces a bilateral flaccid paralysis of muscles in the upper extremity. Below the cervical level there are few problems from occlusion of the anterior spinal artery, because it is highly anastomotic with the segmental radicular arteries.

If the lesion produced by the occlusion extends rostrally, into the lower medulla, there is a bilateral involvement of both the corticospinal tracts and the medial lemnisci. This produces bilateral symptoms of paralysis and loss of tactile and proprioceptive sensation below the neck. The motor loss may be mixed: flaccid paralysis of muscles innervated by affected cervical segments

(loss of the lower motor neurons) and spastic paralysis at levels below the lesion due to the involvement of supraspinal motor pathways (see Fig. 9–12).

SPINAL CORD TRAUMA

The traditional example of this type of trauma is the *Brown-Séquard syndrome,* or *hemisection of the spinal cord.* Although rarely treated in the clinic, this condition helps illustrate the organization of both ascending and descending pathways in the spinal cord. The somatic motor deficit from this lesion is an ipsilateral spastic paralysis below the level of the lesion. The lower motor neurons are intact, except for a few at the site of the lesion, and the motor symptoms result from the severance of all descending supraspinal pathways, thus the spastic paralysis. The accompanying sensory deficits are a contralateral loss of pain and temperature and an ipsilateral loss of tactile and proprioceptive sensation, both below the level of the lesion.

SUGGESTED READING

Brooks, V. B. (1986). *The Neural Basis of Motor Control.* Oxford University Press, New York, 300 pp.

This monograph evolved from the author's courses on motor control. It contains a well-balanced synthesis of current concepts of motor function. The well-referenced chapters are excellent sources of material for the student interested in further information on the subject.

Loeb, G. L. (1987). Hard lessons in motor control from the mammalian spinal cord. Trends Neurosci., 10: 108–113.

This review questions the traditional concepts of spinal cord motor control. The author considers our knowledge of the increasing complexity of motor control at the spinal level that current research has established and suggests a reformulation of our basic operational hypotheses.

Patton, H. D., A. F. Fuchs, B. Hille, A. M. Scher, and R. Steiner (Editors) (1989). *Textbook of Physiology,* Volume 1, *Excitable Cells and Neurophysiology.* W. B. Saunders Company, Philadelphia.

Section V, Control of Movement, and especially Chapters 22 through 26 of this textbook provide an excellent, in-depth coverage of the physiology of the motor neuron and spinal and supraspinal reflexes.

Chapter

15

Motor Cortex and Descending Motor Pathways

MOTOR CORTICAL AREAS
PRIMARY MOTOR CORTEX (M-I)
SECONDARY MOTOR AREAS
CORTICOSPINAL PATHWAYS
CORTICOBULBAR PATHWAYS
CORTICORETICULOSPINAL SYSTEM
VOLUNTARY MOTOR ACTIVITY
RELATED DISORDERS

In Chapter 14, the emphasis is on the *lower motor neuron* and the motor unit; in this chapter, the emphasis is on the *upper motor neuron*. *Lower motor neurons* are the motor neurons with axons that leave the central nervous system (CNS) and innervate the muscle effectors. *Upper motor neurons*, in comparison, are those cortical and brain stem neurons that have axons which form the descending motor pathways. Upper motor neurons drive the lower motor neurons either directly or indirectly via spinal interneurons.

At least five cortical areas have a major role in motor function: the *primary motor cortex (M-I)* and four *secondary motor areas*—the *premotor cortex (PMC)*, the *supplementary motor area (SMA)*, the *frontal eye field (FEF)*, and the *posterior parietal motor area (PMA)*. All, except PMA, are in the frontal lobe. The PMA is in the

posterosuperior portion of the parietal lobe (Fig. 15–1). In addition to these motor areas, the *primary somatosensory cortex (S-I)*, in the postcentral gyrus, contributes fibers to the corticospinal tract. The S-I fibers project principally to sensory relay areas of the spinal cord, and their effect on motor function is principally through the modulation of incoming afferent information.

Electrical stimulation of motor cortical areas in the human brain elicits movement. Neurons in *M-I* have the lowest threshold and, when stimulated, produce simple, stereotypical muscle contractions or relaxations. These responses are involuntary. The patient cannot consciously alter the response produced by the stimulus. Thus, a primary function of *M-I* appears to be the *execution* of specific, well-defined motor responses.

Neurons in *secondary motor areas* have a higher threshold. When stimulated, they elicit

322

FIGURE 15-1

The primary and secondary motor cortical areas. M-I, primary motor cortex; SMA, supplementary motor area; PMC, premotor cortex; PMA, posterior parietal motor area; and FEF, frontal eye fields. Area numbers refer to Brodmann's areas (see Fig. 21–3).

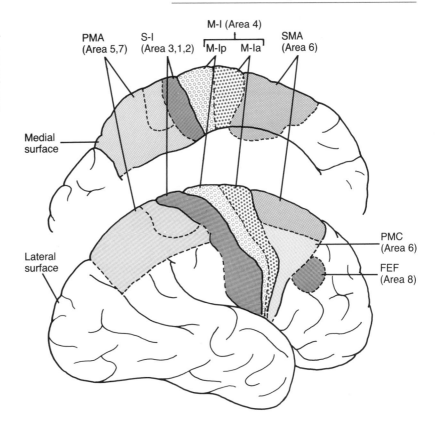

more complex motor responses, movements designed to attain a particular goal (e.g., coordinated limb movements, grasping, facial expressions, and vocalizations). Thus, the secondary motor areas appear to program the more complicated movements and to send this information to the primary motor area and directly to the spinal cord. Each secondary area is involved in a different dimension of the planning and initiation of motor activity.

Although secondary motor areas do drive M-I, the relationship is more complex. The interconnections between the primary and secondary areas are reciprocal, and both contribute extensively to the descending *corticospinal* and *corticobulbar systems*. Motor cortical areas also project to other brain stem centers that, in turn, give rise to descending motor pathways, such as the reticular formation, the tectum, and the red nucleus. Hence, in the *somatic motor system*, a combination of *hierarchical* and *parallel organization* exists. Ultimately, all of the descending streams of motor commands *converge* on the spinal interneurons and the *lower motor neuron*, the final common path (Fig. 15–2).

Defining descending motor systems as either *pyramidal* or *extrapyramidal* is no longer useful and is often confusing. Originally, the term *pyramidal system (tract)* referred to the motor pathway that occupied the medullary pyramids and was employed often as a synonym for the corticospinal tract. Because the pyramids have now been shown to contain corticobulbar and corticoreticular fibers as well as fibers en route from motor areas of the cortex to the inferior olivary nuclei and dorsal column nuclei, the term "pyramidal" is misleading.

The term *extrapyramidal system (tract)* originally referred to the descending motor pathways arising from the basal ganglia. Later, it became a "catch-all" term for any "nonpyramidal" descending motor system. Because the basal ganglia modulate motor function through the motor cortex, the term "extrapyramidal" is misleading. Unfortunately, the term "extrapyramidal" is still widely used to refer to a class of neurological disorders that affect the basal ganglia. In this text, the terms *pyramidal system (tract)* and *extrapyramidal system (tract)* are not employed in reference to motor pathways.

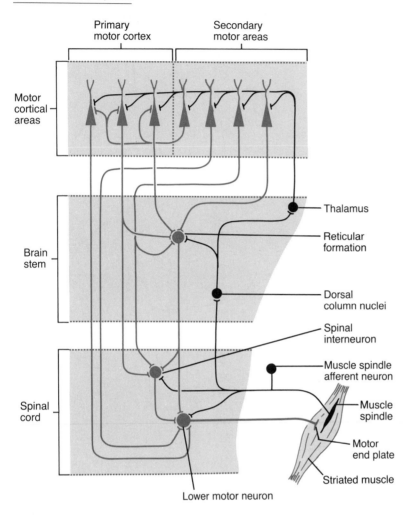

Primary motor cortex

Secondary motor areas

Motor cortical areas

Brain stem

Spinal cord

Thalamus

Reticular formation

Dorsal column nuclei

Spinal interneuron

Muscle spindle afferent neuron

Muscle spindle

Motor end plate

Striated muscle

Lower motor neuron

FIGURE 15-2

Some of the principal components of the somatic motor system. Note the combination of hierarchical and parallel organization of the pathways and their convergence on the final common path, the lower motor neuron. See text for details.

Motor Cortical Areas

HISTOLOGICAL ORGANIZATION

The *motor cortex* is principally an *efferent* structure, sending information rather than receiving it. This function is in contrast to that of the primary sensory cortices. The histological organization of the cortex reflects the difference. The *internal granular layer* (*layer IV*), the layer that receives thalamic projections, is especially prominent in the sensory cortices but nearly absent in the motor cortex. The main efferent layer, from the cerebral cortex to lower centers, is the *internal pyramidal layer* (*layer V*). This layer is especially prominent in the motor cortex and relatively thin in the primary sensory cortices. Because of these differences, the motor cortex is known as *agranular cortex* and the primary sensory area as *granular cortex* (Fig. 15-3).

The *pyramidal cells* are the principal efferent neurons of the cortex. Those projecting from the cortex to brain stem and spinal levels have their cell bodies in layer V, the *internal pyramidal layer*. Those projecting to the opposite hemisphere as callosal fibers are in layer III, the *external pyramidal layer*. In addition, small and medium-size pyramidal cells projecting to other cortical areas within the same hemisphere (corticocortical or cortical association fibers) reside in both layer II, the *external granular layer*, and in layer III. Layer VI, the *multiform layer*, contains small pyramidal cells that give rise to corticothalamic and additional corticocortical and callosal projections (see Fig. 15-3).

Nearly all neurons of the cerebral cortex are either *glutaminergic* or *GABAergic*. The 20 to 30% of the cortical neurons that use gamma aminobutyric acid (*GABA*) as a neurotransmitter represent a heterogenous population of cell types.

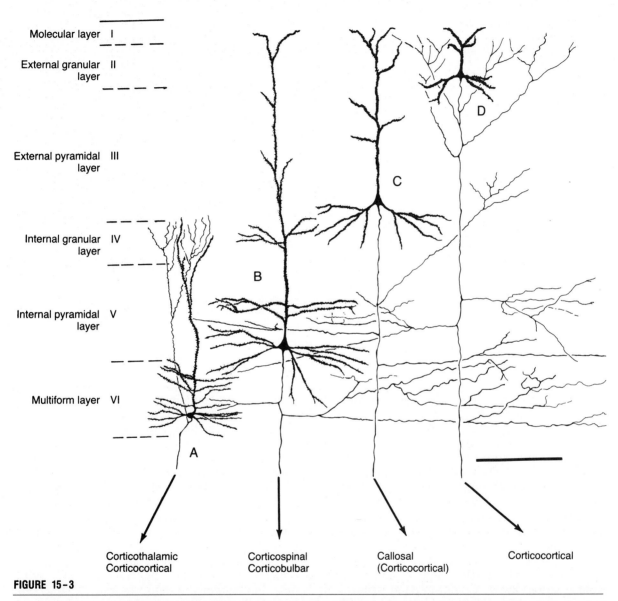

Molecular layer   I

External granular   II
layer

External pyramidal   III
layer

Internal granular   IV
layer

Internal pyramidal   V
layer

Multiform layer   VI

| Corticothalamic | Corticospinal | Callosal | Corticocortical |
| Corticocortical | Corticobulbar | (Corticocortical) | |

FIGURE 15-3

The laminar origins of efferent projections from the cerebral cortex. (Reproduced with permission from E. G. Jones, Laminar distribution of cortical efferent cells. In A. Peters and E. G. Jones (Editors), *Cerebral Cortex*, Volume 1, *Cellular Components of the Cerebral Cortex*, Plenum Press, New York, 1984.)

Nearly all, however, function as inhibitory interneurons. Of these, only one fifth are known to have a neuropeptide co-transmitter. Many other neurotransmitters are present in the cerebral cortex. However, these are in terminals of neurons that project to the cortex from subcortical centers, such as the basal forebrain, thalamus, and reticular formation.

The pyramidal cells are the efferent cells of the cerebral cortex, and all pyramidal cells use the excitatory neurotransmitter, *glutamate.* A few of these excitatory, glutaminergic corticospinal fibers end directly on spinal cord motor neurons. In these cases, the glutaminergic excitation of the lower motor neuron may produce a contraction of the muscle fibers innervated by the lower motor neuron. In most cases, however, these glutaminergic corticospinal fibers end on a spinal interneuron, which makes synaptic contact with a lower motor neuron. All of the corticospinal tract synapses in the spinal cord are glutaminergic and excitatory. The interneurons, however, can be either excitatory or inhibitory. Most of the inhibitory spinal interneurons utilize glycine as the primary neurotransmitter. Thus, *the major effect of the excitatory corticospinal fiber is to excite an interneuron that, in turn, either excites or inhibits the lower motor neuron.*

Primary Motor Cortex (M-I)

The *primary motor cortex (M-I)* is Brodmann's area 4 and occupies most of the *precentral gyrus* (see Fig. 15–1 and Fig. 21–3). M-I is widest at the dorsomedial surface of the hemisphere and tapers to a thin strip at the inferolateral margin of the precentral sulcus. Throughout the length of the precentral gyrus, much of M-I is hidden from view, buried deep in the central sulcus, forming the posterior margin of the precentral gyrus. M-I has a similar topographic organization as S-I and is classically depicted as a homunculus (Fig. 15–4). The topographic organization of the motor cortex is not as precise as that of the primary somatosensory areas. A point-to-point representation of the surface of the body does not exist. Instead, cortical neurons form colonies or clusters, with neurons in each cluster projecting to spinal motor neurons that innervate the same muscle. Similarly, clusters of cortical motor neurons that drive synergistic muscles are grouped together. Within the organization of M-I there are, as discussed further in this chapter, at least two parallel representations of the body.

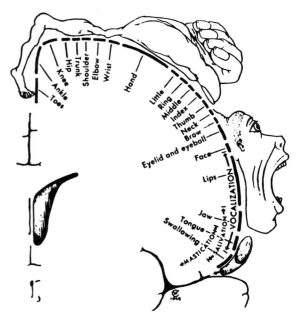

FIGURE 15–4

Motor homunculus. A schematic representation of the motor organization of the precentral gyrus in the human brain. The right side of the figure is laid upon a cross section of the left hemisphere. (Reproduced with permission from W. Penfield, and T. Rasmussen, *The Cerebral Cortex of Man,* Macmillan, New York, 1950.)

CORTICOSPINAL TRACT AND M-I

The largest single pathway arising from M-I is the *corticospinal tract,* axons of *layer V* pyramidal cells that descend from the motor cortex to the spinal cord. Stimulation of these pyramidal cells generates excitatory postsynaptic potentials (EPSPs) on lower motor neurons and on interneurons in the spinal cord. Of those generated on motor neurons, many have short latencies, suggesting direct synaptic contact between the pyramidal cell of the motor cortex and the lower motor neuron of the spinal cord. The EPSPs on those spinal motor neurons innervating distal limb muscles tend to be larger than those on spinal motor neurons innervating the more proximal musculature. As discussed in Chapter 14, the vestibulospinal and reticulospinal systems have their principal projections to the motor neurons innervating proximal and axial musculature, whereas the corticospinal and rubrospinal systems have their principal projections to the motor neurons innervating the more distal musculature.

The majority of the corticospinal projections from M-I, however, synapse with spinal interneurons that are either excitatory or inhibitory. These, in turn, generate postsynaptic potentials, either EPSPs or inhibitory postsynaptic potentials (IPSPs), on the lower motor neurons. As with monosynaptic excitation, these postsynaptic potentials are primarily on lower motor neurons that innervate the distal limb musculature. In the control of motor function, the generation of IPSPs is as important as the generation of EPSPs. Many descending fibers of the corticospinal tract form excitatory synapses on inhibitory spinal interneurons that, in turn, form inhibitory synapses on the lower motor neurons. These are the same inhibitory interneurons that receive synapses from the primary afferents of muscle spindles.

In addition to producing a contraction or relaxation of a single muscle, stimulation of M-I can generate specific patterns of movement, probably through the activation of specific brain stem and spinal cord *central pattern generators*. This topic is reviewed in greater detail in Chapter 14.

OTHER EFFERENTS FROM M-I

Other projections from *layer V* of *M-I* include *corticostriatal fibers* to the striatum, *corticorubral fibers* to the red nucleus, and projections to the medullary and pontine reticular formations. *Layer VI* is the origin of the *corticothalamic projections* from M-I, principally to the *ventral lateral nucleus* of the thalamus.

M-I has strong corticocortical projections as well. These include heavy reciprocal connections with the ipsilateral *supplementary motor area* and the *premotor cortex* of the frontal lobe and the *posterior parietal motor area* and *S-I* of the parietal lobe. Callosal connections, also reciprocal, are with M-I of the contralateral hemisphere. All of these corticocortical projections are in topographic register, i.e., to the same area of body representation, be they to motor or to somatosensory cortical areas.

AFFERENTS TO M-I

Except for corticocortical connections, all information reaching M-I must first pass through the *dorsal thalamus*. The *thalamocortical projections* to the motor areas relay information from the somatosensory system, vestibular system, cerebellum, and basal ganglia. These projections are quite specific, and different motor areas receive different combinations of thalamic information (Fig. 15–5). In all cases, this information is in topographic register with the motor cortical area, i.e., the appropriate thalamic nucleus relays somatosensory or cerebellar information related to the hand to the hand area of M-I.

At least two distinct body representations occur in M-I. These are reflected in the somatosensory projections to the primary motor area. The *anterior half* of M-I, *M-Ia* receives proprioceptive information via the *ventral posterosuperior nucleus (VPS)*; the *posterior half* of M-I, *M-Ip* receives cutaneous afferent information via the *ventral posterolateral nucleus (VPL)* (see Fig. 15–5). Somatosensory signals, especially those from the proprioceptors (spindle and joint afferents) reflexly activate cortical neurons. These cortical-level proprioceptive reflexes alter the discharge of cortical motor neurons to insure smooth, coordinated, and precise fine movements. The activity of the upper motor neurons is under continuous modulation by ascending sensory signals. Just as in the spinal cord, this modulation can produce either a facilitation or an inhibition of muscle contraction, but via the descending corticospinal system to the lower motor neuron.

The cerebellar information reaches M-I and PMC after relay in the posterior division of the *ventral lateral nucleus (VLp)* of the thalamus. Neurons in the anterior division of the *ventral lateral nucleus (VLa)* relay most of the information from the basal ganglia to SMA with only sparse projections to M-I. Both the cerebellum and the basal ganglia are somatotopically organized and this somatotopic organization is retained in the thalamic nuclei and in the cortical projections (see Fig. 15–5).

Secondary Motor Areas

SUPPLEMENTARY MOTOR AREA (SMA)

The *supplementary motor area (SMA)* occupies the medial and superolateral portion of *area 6* (see Fig. 15–1). SMA contains a topographic representation of the body, with the head located in the anterior portion of SMA and the legs and feet in the posterior part, adjacent to area 4.

The pyramidal cells in layer V of SMA give rise to *corticospinal fibers*. The smaller pyramidal cells of layer II have extensive projections to both *M-I* and to *PMC*; these projections are reciprocal. Callosal projections from SMA to its *contralateral* counterpart also are extensive and reciprocal.

Afferents to *SMA*, in addition to the reciprocal corticocortical connections, include a substantial input from the basal ganglia. These projections

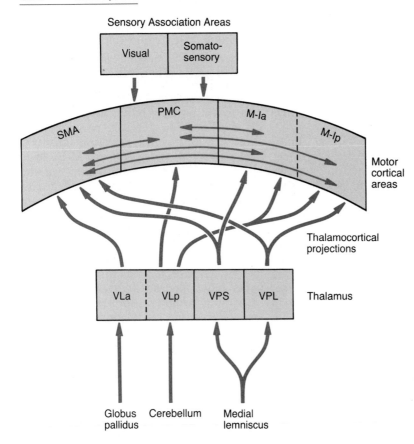

Sensory Association Areas

FIGURE 15-5

Some of the major projections to the motor cortical areas. See text for details and for explanations of abbreviations.

are from the efferent nucleus of the basal ganglia, the *globus pallidus,* and the *pars reticularis* of the *substantia nigra.* Both the *pallidothalamic* and *nigrothalamic projections* are to the anterior division of the *ventral lateral nucleus* (*VLa*) of the thalamus (see Fig. 15-5). In addition, SMA receives both proprioceptive and cutaneous afferents from *VPS* and *VPL*. The SMA does not receive cerebellar information relayed from the thalamus.

The *motor responses* elicited from cortical stimulation of *SMA* are more *complex* than those of M-I, and the thresholds for cortical neuron responses to electrical stimulation are greater. Stimulation of SMA in the human will produce vocalizations, facial expressions, and coordinated limb movements that are generally symmetrical, including bilateral opening and closing of the hands. Physiological data indicate that the corticospinal projections from SMA terminate principally on spinal interneurons and not directly on lower motor neurons. In addition, signals from SMA drive upper motor neurons in M-I.

PREMOTOR CORTEX (PMC)

The *premotor cortex* (*PMC*) occupies most of area 6 on the lateral surface of the hemisphere—the portion of area 6 not occupied by SMA (see Fig. 15-1). In the human brain, the size of this area is approximately six times that of M-I.

Efferents from *PMC* include extensive reciprocal projections to both SMA and M-I. The contributions to the corticospinal tract, however, are small in comparison with those of SMA and M-I.

Afferents to *PMC* include some thalamocortical projections from VPS and VPL (proprioceptive and cutaneous afferent information). However, *most* of the sensory information reaching the PMC is from cortical association areas. *Thalamocortical* projections from *VLp* carry cerebellar information to PMC. PMC also receives extensive visual information, primarily from secondary visual association areas, *area 19*, and the *middle temporal visual area*. PMC does not receive information from the basal ganglia via the thalamus (see Fig. 15-5).

Stimulation of *PMC* elicits complex motor responses, but like SMA, the threshold for stimulation is relatively high. Responses often involve coordinated movements of the limbs. These responses are often dominated by the visual context of the task. The spontaneous activity of PMC diminishes with the initiation of the motor task, consistent with a role in planning and setting the stage for the motor task.

POSTERIOR PARIETAL MOTOR AREA (PMA)

The *posterior parietal motor area* (*PMA*) is between the primary somatosensory cortex, S-I, and the secondary visual association area, area 19, in the posterior portion of the parietal lobe, Brodmann's *area 5* and *area 7* (see Fig. 15–1). This includes the *posterior parietal visual area* described in Chapter 11.

Efferent projections from *PMA* include a minor contribution to the corticospinal tract and major cortical projections to *M-I* and to both *SMA* and *PMC*. Most of the *afferent projections* to *PMA* are cortical association fibers from the adjacent *visual* and *somatosensory areas*.

The area 5 portion of PMA is associated with the tactile aspects of reaching and guiding movements; area 7, also known as the posterior parietal visual area, is associated with visually guided movements. Area 7 "tells" the individual where an object is in visual space. Damage to PMA often leads to a neglect of contralateral space (see subsequent discussion).

FRONTAL EYE FIELD (FEF)

The *frontal eye field* (*FEF*) is in the posteroinferior portion of *area 8*, on the lateral surface of the frontal lobe immediately anterior to the premotor cortex, area 6 (see Fig. 15–1). The FEF coordinates eye movements, especially those involved in visual tracking. Following unilateral damage to FEF, both eyes deviate toward the side of the lesion. An inability to turn the eyes in the opposite direction results. This loss is transitory, suggesting that the contralateral FEF can take over the function of both fields. The FEF appears to generate "volitional" saccadic eye movements. This ability provides a mechanism for a cortical override of the more rigidly controlled saccadic movements generated in the brain stem through optokinetic and vestibulo-ocular reflexes.

Corticospinal Pathways

The *lateral corticospinal tract* arises from pyramidal cells in layer V of the cortex and descends through the brain stem and into the spinal cord (Fig. 15–6). Of the axons making up the corticospinal tract, approximately two thirds arise from the frontal cortex. Half are from area 4 and the remainder from area 6, principally from SMA with a small contribution from PMC. The other third arises from parietal cortical areas, PMA, and somatosensory areas (S-I and S-II).

The internal pyramidal layer of M-I contains approximately 34,000 *giant pyramidal cells* (*Betz's cells*). These are huge cells with cross-sectional areas of 1000 to 4000 μm^2. These giant cells give rise to corticospinal fibers, most of which terminate in the lumbosacral enlargement of the spinal cord. Although the presence of these cells is a characteristic histological feature of M-I, they account for only 2% of the fiber population in the corticospinal pathway. *Most of the fibers of the corticospinal tract are very small: more than 90% have diameters of less than 4 μm and only about half of these are myelinated.* Hence, except for a few large, fast-conducting fibers, small, slow conducting axons are the predominant fiber population in the corticospinal tract.

Axons of the corticospinal tract descend through the *internal capsule* to the *crus cerebri* of the midbrain and from there enter the *basal pons*. As they pass through the internal capsule, corticospinal fibers occupy a position near the *genu of the internal capsule* and extend into the *posterior limb of the internal capsule* (see Fig. 8–3). The exact location and degree of compactness of the fibers of the corticospinal tract in the internal capsule of the human brain are variable. In the midbrain, corticospinal fibers occupy the middle third of the *crus cerebri*. This compact bundle of fibers, upon reaching the pons, divides into a number of smaller fascicles as the fibers continue their descent through the substance of the basal pons (see Fig. 15–6).

In the lower pons, fascicles of corticospinal fibers from each hemisphere begin to cluster together and emerge from the lower end of the basal pons as the *medullary pyramids*. The medullary pyramids form a pair of prominent, longitudinal elevations on the ventral surface of the medulla. At this level, the descending corticospinal tracts are still *ipsilateral* to their hemisphere of origin (see Fig. 15–6).

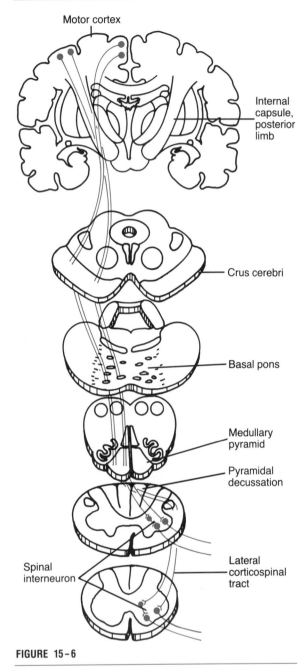

Motor cortex

Internal capsule, posterior limb

Crus cerebri

Basal pons

Medullary pyramid

Pyramidal decussation

Spinal interneuron

Lateral corticospinal tract

FIGURE 15-6

The course of the descending lateral corticospinal tract from the motor cortex to the cervical and lumbar levels of the spinal cord.

In the lower medulla and upper cervical spinal segments, the *corticospinal tract* decussates, or crosses to the opposite side. This is known as the *pyramidal decussation* (see Figs. 7-2 and 7-7). Following decussation, the fibers assume a position in the dorsal portion of the lateral funiculus

of the spinal cord as the *lateral corticospinal tract*. Once the fibers have decussated, the *lateral corticospinal tract* is *contralateral* to the cerebral hemisphere of origin. Some fibers of the corticospinal tract do not decussate but continue to descend on the *ipsilateral side*, in the ventral funiculus of the spinal cord. These fibers form the *ventral (anterior) corticospinal tract* (Fig. 15-7 and Fig. 6-8).

On reaching the spinal cord, corticospinal fibers from the frontal areas, M-I, SMA, and PMC, terminate in the ventral part of the spinal gray matter, principally laminae VII, VIII, and IX. In general, a greater density of terminals is

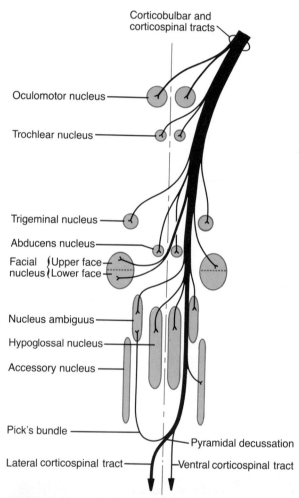

Corticobulbar and corticospinal tracts

Oculomotor nucleus

Trochlear nucleus

Trigeminal nucleus

Abducens nucleus

Facial {Upper face
nucleus {Lower face

Nucleus ambiguus

Hypoglossal nucleus

Accessory nucleus

Pick's bundle

Pyramidal decussation

Lateral corticospinal tract

Ventral corticospinal tract

FIGURE 15-7

The course of the principal corticobulbar pathways as they descend with the corticospinal tract through the brain stem to terminate in cranial nerve nuclei. Not illustrated are the corticobulbar endings on interneurons or neurons in the adjacent brain stem reticular formation. See text for details.

located near the lateral motor columns of the cervical and lumbosacral enlargements. Those corticospinal fibers from the parietal cortex terminate in the more dorsal areas of the cord, suggesting an involvement in the regulation of primary afferent signals through either presynaptic or postsynaptic modulation.

Corticobulbar Pathways

The *corticobulbar pathways* are analogous to the corticospinal tracts except that they project to motor nuclei of the cranial nerves. From the differing descriptions of the corticobulbar pathways in the human brain, the course of these fibers appears variable. Most travel in the company of corticospinal tract fibers until they approach the target nucleus, whereupon they leave the corticospinal tract and synapse with motor neurons in that nucleus or with interneurons in the nucleus or within the adjacent reticular formation (see Fig. 15–7).

Corticobulbar fibers leave the cortex and enter the internal capsule and the crus cerebri. At the level of the crus cerebri, corticobulbar fibers destined for the motor nuclei of extraocular muscles enter the midbrain tegmentum and bilaterally innervate the *GSE* motor nuclei of cranial nerves *III* (*oculomotor*), *IV* (*trochlear*), and *VI* (*abducens*). The trochlear and abducens nerves innervate the superior oblique and lateral rectus muscles respectively. The oculomotor nerve innervates the remaining four extraocular muscles and the levator palpebra superior (see Fig. 15–7; Chapter 19).

Corticobulbar fibers to the *special visceral efferent* (*SVE*) motor nuclei of the *trigeminal nerve* (*V*) leave the corticospinal tract near the boundary between the pons and the midbrain, enter the pontine tegmentum, and bilaterally innervate the motor nuclei of V. All lower motor neurons innervating the muscles of mastication receive bilateral projections from upper motor neurons except those neurons to the *external pterygoid muscles*. These muscles usually receive upper motor neuron innervation only from the *contralateral motor cortex* (see Fig. 15–7).

Corticobulbar fibers to the *SVE* motor nuclei of the *facial nerve* (*VII*) leave the corticospinal tract in the midpons, enter the pontine tegmentum, and innervate the motor nuclei of VII, the *facial nuclei*. The facial nerve supplies the muscles of facial expression. Those lower motor neurons innervating muscles in the *upper half of the face* receive *bilateral* projections from upper motor neurons; those to the *lower half of the face* usually receive upper motor neuron innervation only from the *contralateral* motor cortex (see Fig. 15–7).

The *nucleus ambiguus* is the *SVE* motor nucleus for the *glossopharyngeal* (*IX*) and *vagus* (*X*) *nerves*. These cranial nerves innervate the palatine, pharyngeal, and laryngeal musculature. Of these, the glossopharyngeal nerve innervates the stylopharyngeus muscle and the vagus nerve innervates the remainder. The *corticobulbar fibers* leave the corticospinal tract in the lower pons or upper medulla and project *bilaterally* to the lower motor neurons of the *nucleus ambiguus*. One consistently aberrant group of fibers to the nucleus ambiguous, *Pick's bundle*, continues with the corticospinal fibers until they reach the pyramidal decussation. At that point, the fibers decussate and loop back into the medulla, approaching the *contralateral nucleus ambiguus* from below (see Fig. 15–7).

The *accessory nucleus* provides *SVE* innervation to portions of the sternomastoid and trapezius muscles via the *spinal accessory nerve* (*XI*). These *corticobulbar fibers* leave the corticospinal tract in the mid medulla and project ipsilaterally to the accessory nucleus (see Fig. 15–7).

Corticobulbar fibers to the *GSE* motor nucleus of the *hypoglossal nerve* (*XII*) also leave the corticospinal tract in the medulla and pass through the medullary reticular formation to reach the *hypoglossal nuclei*. The hypoglossal nerve innervates both the extrinsic and intrinsic musculature of the tongue, and these lower motor neurons receive *bilateral upper motor neuron projections*, except for those neurons innervating the *genioglossus muscle*. Lower motor neurons innervating the genioglossus muscle usually receive upper motor neuron projections only from the *contralateral motor cortex* (see Fig. 15–7).

Corticoreticulospinal System

Chapter 14 discusses the motor reticular formation's role in the modulation of segmental and postural reflexes and in the regulation of muscle tone. In addition to these functions, *the brain stem reticular formation plays a prominent role in the control of voluntary motor activity.*

Corticoreticular fibers arise from both *PMC* and *SMA* and descend to nuclei of the pontine and medullary reticular formations. These descending cortical projections, in turn, drive or modulate the activity of many neurons that give rise to the reticulospinal tracts. The *corticoreticular fibers*, in combination with their target nuclei in the *reticular formation*, and the descending *reticulospinal tracts* form what is collectively known as the *corticoreticulospinal system.*

Many descending fibers in both the *medial* and *lateral reticulospinal tracts* are under cortical control. The significant difference between the corticoreticulospinal system and the reticulospinal system is the dimension of cortical modulation (see Chapter 14). From the brain stem to spinal cord, the pathway is the same. The corticoreticulospinal system is a motor system that descends in parallel with the corticospinal system.

Cortically driven reticular formation neurons whose axons descend in the *medial reticulospinal tract* are principally inhibitory. They inhibit both spinal interneurons and lower motor neurons. Others are inhibitory to lower motor neurons through the excitation of inhibitory spinal interneurons. In addition, some of these fibers form inhibitory, axoaxonal synapses on primary afferent terminals, thereby blocking the incoming afferent signals from muscle spindles by primary afferent depolarization. This inhibits stretch reflexes, allowing the smooth and rapid execution of voluntary motor tasks. Many others synapse with long propriospinal neurons. These spinal interneurons extend for many segments within the cord and synapse with large numbers of lower motor neurons that innervate axial and limb girdle muscles. These muscles are responsible for the axial and proximal limb movements required in conjunction with the more distal muscle contractions driven by the corticospinal system. Other cortically driven reticular formation neurons have axons that descend in the *lateral reticulospinal tract*. In general, these modulate the activity of lower motor neurons that innervate more distal limb muscles.

Together, descending reticulospinal components of the corticoreticulospinal system have roles complementary to the motor functions driven by the corticospinal system. The corticospinal system provides the signals for fine, delicate movements, principally of distal muscles. At the same time, the corticoreticulospinal system provides motor signals to other limb and trunk muscles required for the execution of the motor task and blocks segmental reflexes that might interfere with the smooth execution of the motor task.

Voluntary Motor Activity

Our knowledge of the human motor cortex and voluntary motor function is extrapolated from experimental primate studies and from clinical studies. Some of the clinical studies are of patients suffering from specific cortical lesions. Others are of patients whose motor areas were stimulated electrically during neurosurgical procedures. Positron emission tomography (PET) studies with normal volunteers demonstrate sequential changes in neuronal activity in different cortical and subcortical areas of the brain during the learning, initiation, and performing of specific motor tasks. However, the specific and sequential roles of the various cortical areas in voluntary motor function still remain unclear.

INITIATION AND PERFORMANCE OF A COMPLEX MOTOR TASK

Voluntary motor activity is a cortically initiated process. A patterned firing occurs of selected populations of motor neurons in M-I with each voluntary movement. The decision process, however, is at a higher level within the cortex. The primary and secondary motor areas respond to that command rapidly and in a semiautonomic fashion, adapting that command to current circumstances (e.g., environment, posture, and motor activities in progress).

When a subject "thinks" about a sequence of motor tasks, SMA increases in activity and in blood flow. This effect continues during the performance of the motor tasks as does the activity in the sensory cortex. During the "thinking" stage, the increased activity is limited to SMA.

The secondary areas, *SMA* and *PMC*, appear to "plan" specific but different parameters of the motor response. These areas then drive the primary motor cortex, M-I, the source of the final "command" signal. As activity accelerates in the primary motor cortex, activity correspondingly diminishes in the secondary motor areas. While driving M-I, the secondary areas also signal the corticoreticulospinal system and initiate the necessary complementary motor responses in axial, limb girdle, and proximal limb muscles.

During the entire process, the basal ganglia and the cerebellum are very active. These structures play important roles in the planning and performing of coordinated motor tasks. They specify such parameters as the pattern of muscles activated and the direction and amplitude of movement. These functions are discussed in greater detail in the following chapters.

Related Disorders

Paralysis, plegia, paresis, and *apraxia* are four terms frequently used to describe motor deficits. *Paralysis* is a *total loss of muscle function. Plegia* is another word for paralysis and most often is employed in a combined form, e.g., *hemiplegia. Paresis* is a *weakness* or partial loss of muscle function. *Apraxia,* however, is a disorder of motor activity that consists of an *inability to perform a purposeful movement,* in spite of the lack of paralysis or paresis.

MIDDLE CEREBRAL ARTERY OCCLUSION

The middle cerebral artery supplies most of the lateral surface of the cerebral hemisphere. The artery has deep penetrating branches that supply much of the striatum and internal capsule (see Figs. 9–11 and 9–15). With a massive infarct or thrombus of the entire *middle cerebral artery,* the damage is extensive. The patient has *contralateral hemiplegia* of the upper and lower extremities with *Babinski's sign.* Normally, stimulation of the foot pad produces a plantar flexion. However, following damage to the corticospinal tract or to M-I, hyperextension and fanning of the toes occur, along with an upward movement of the foot. This is *Babinski's sign* and is the classic clinical test for damage to the primary motor cortex or the corticospinal tract. A contralateral hemiplegia of the lower face also is noted. In addition, the tongue deviates toward the side of the lesion on protrusion.

These massive motor deficits are due to the loss of corticobulbar and corticospinal fibers, as they pass through the internal capsule. This area is supplied by *lateral striate arteries,* branches of the middle cerebral artery (see Fig. 9–15). The upper facial muscles are spared because of the bilateral corticobulbar projections to that portion of the facial nucleus.

Sensory losses also accompany motor deficits. The patient has contralateral hemianesthesia of the face, trunk, and upper and lower extremities due to involvement of the thalamocortical projections, as they traverse the internal capsule. Contralateral homonymous hemianopsia is experienced because of damage to the geniculocalcar-

ine fibers, as they pass through the temporal and parietal lobes. If the lesion involves the dominant hemisphere, the patient also will have various forms of agnosia, apraxia, agraphia, and acalculia (see Chapter 21).

A more restricted lesion, such as an occlusion of the *rolandic artery,* spares the internal capsule and the symptoms are less severe. Damage is limited principally to the somatosensory and motor cortical areas. The rolandic artery courses along the central sulcus and supplies much of the precentral and postcentral gyri, S-I and M-I. The symptoms of motor and somatosensory deficits are similar to the aforementioned, except that much of the contralateral foot and leg are spared, because the anterior cerebral artery supplies the medial and part of the superior surface of the hemisphere (see Figs. 9–10 and 9–11).

The more distal the branch or branches of the middle cerebral artery involved in the insult, the more restricted the damage. For example, an infarct involving only the distal portion of the rolandic artery would produce sensory and motor deficits in only the contralateral arm and trunk (see Figs. 9–11 and 15–4).

LESIONS RESTRICTED TO SPECIFIC MOTOR CORTICAL AREAS

If a lesion involves only the primary motor cortex, M-I, the *initial symptom* is a *contralateral flaccid paralysis* of the body areas involved. Following an acute phase of 1 to 2 weeks, the patient often regains movement, especially of the proximal portions of the limbs. Concomitant with the restoration of proximal mobility is a continued *contralateral paralysis* and an increased *spasticity of the distal musculature,* especially the wrist and finger extensors. The returning motor function lacks the normal independent, controlled movement. Instead, it often consists of synergistic contractions of similar muscles or muscle groups, i.e., all fingers of the hand will flex in concert. With this lesion, the reticulospinal, tectospinal, and vestibulospinal systems are intact as are the corticospinal and corticoreticulospinal projections from the secondary motor areas. When an M-I lesion involves the head area, the muscles of the upper face are spared, owing to bilateral upper motor neuron projections to that portion of the facial nucleus. Deficits in the pharynx and larynx are generally not observed, because of the bilateral upper motor neuron projections to the nucleus ambiguus. Tongue deviation toward the side of the lesion is due to the unopposed action of the ipsilateral genioglossus muscle. Corticobulbar fibers to that part of the hypoglossal nucleus are crossed.

With a lesion restricted to the *supplementary motor area, SMA,* there is a deficit in *bimanual coordination.* The patient is able to perform identical movements with the two hands. However, simultaneous but different movements are difficult, if not impossible. Often this *apraxic condition* is not apparent until the individual is instructed to perform different motor tasks, simultaneously, with the two hands. The SMA has strong callosal connections, and the intact SMA appears to take over the function of the damaged area and drive both M-Is. The patient cannot relearn motor tasks based on proprioceptive cues but has no problem when the cues are visual, as long as the PMC is intact.

A lesion involving only the *premotor cortex (PMC)* also produces an *apraxic condition,* with the patient unable to move the two arms simultaneously in a coordinated fashion. These lesions also produce a generalized weakness in the contralateral proximal limb musculature, making it difficult for the patient to elevate and abduct the arm. As with SMA, problems exist in relearning motor tasks. With a PMC lesion, visually cued tasks are problems, whereas proprioceptively cued tasks are not.

Lesions in the *posterior parietal motor area, PMA,* result in a *sensory neglect* of the contralateral hemifield of extrapersonal space, both visual and somatosensory. Accompanying this sensory neglect is an *apraxia,* an inability to initiate purposeful limb movements in the contralateral hemifield. Although there is some hypokinesia of the contralateral limbs, there is no paresis or paralysis. Questions remain, however, as to whether the apraxia is secondary to the lack of sensory and perceptual attention or whether it too is a primary deficit.

WEBER'S SYNDROME

Weber's syndrome may occur from an occlusion of either the bifurcation of the basilar artery or the short circumferential branches from the proximal portion of the posterior cerebral artery (see Fig. 9–14). Motor deficits include a contralateral hemiparesis or hemiplegia of the body and the lower half of the face due to interruption of corticospinal and corticobulbar fibers. Babinski's sign is evidenced. The degree of motor loss varies with the amount of the crus cerebri involved. If the lesion extends to the red nucleus, the patient may exhibit some ipsilateral tremor. An ipsilateral oculomotor paralysis (external strabismus, eyelid ptosis, dilated pupil, and absence of pupillary light reflexes) due to the involvement of the oculomotor nerve is observed.

SUGGESTED READING

Brinkman, C. (1984). Supplementary motor area of the monkey's cerebral cortex: Short- and long-term deficits after unilateral ablation and the effects of subsequent callosal section. J. Neurosci., 4: 918–929.

The results of these studies involving cortical lesions present convincing evidence for a role of SMA in the programming of complex movements, especially tasks requiring bimanual motor coordination. These data are related to the findings of clinical studies from patients with SMA and callosal lesions.

Brooks, V. B. (1986). *The Neural Basis of Motor Control.* Oxford University Press, New York, 330 pp.

This monograph evolved from the author's courses on motor control. It contains a well-balanced synthesis of current concepts of motor function. The chapters have many references and are an excellent source of material for the student interested in further information on this subject.

Evarts, E. V. (1986). Motor cortex output in primates. In E. G. Jones and A. Peters (Editors), *Cerebral Cortex,* Volume 5. *Sensory-Motor Areas and Aspects of Cortical Connectivity.* Plenum Press, New York, pp. 217–241.

This review presents a succinct description of descending motor pathways in the primate. In addition, the concept of transcortical reflexes, the reflex activation of cortical neurons by proprioceptive and cutaneous afferents, is discussed.

Jones, E. G. (1986). Connectivity of the primate sensory-motor cortex. In E. G. Jones and A. Peters (Editors), *Cerebral Cortex,* Volume 5. *Sensory-Motor Areas and Aspects of Cortical Connectivity.* Plenum Press, New York, pp. 113–183.

The interdependence of somatomotor and somatosensory cortical areas is stressed in this review. Evidence is presented for the continual afferent feedback to the cortical motor neurons during movement and postural adjustment.

Chapter

16

Basal Ganglia and Related Nuclei

NUCLEI OF THE BASAL GANGLIA
RELATED NUCLEI
BASIC CIRCUITS BETWEEN THE BASAL GANGLIA AND CORTEX
MODULATORY CIRCUITS
PARALLEL CIRCUITS: TERRITORIES AND COMPARTMENTS
ANATOMY OF THE PATHWAYS OF THE BASAL GANGLIA
MOTOR FUNCTIONS OF THE BASAL GANGLIA
THE BASAL GANGLIA AND DISORDERS OF MOTOR FUNCTION

The *basal ganglia* are a group of nuclei situated deep in the ventral telencephalon that *modulate* and *regulate specific cortical functions.* Neurons from nearly every area of the cerebral cortex send information to the basal ganglia. This information is processed and relayed back to discrete areas of the frontal cortex by way of specific thalamic nuclei. Although once thought to be principally motor in function, the basal ganglia have significant roles in the modulation of limbic and associational cortical activity and motor activity. Information processing once thought to be strictly cortical in nature involves circuits that include the basal ganglia.

The basal ganglia are an integral part of well-defined neuroanatomical circuits or loops that link these nuclei to at least five specific areas of the frontal lobe. This chapter includes the anatomical organization of the basal ganglia, the general properties of the "loop" circuits, and the role of the basal ganglia in somatic motor function. Only general references are made to the involvement of the basal ganglia in associational

and limbic functions. These are discussed in Chapters 21 and 22, respectively.

Nuclei of the Basal Ganglia

The *basal ganglia* develop from the ventral wall of the telencephalic vesicle (see Fig. 1–19). These telencephalic structures differentiate into the principal nuclei of the basal ganglia: the *caudate nucleus, putamen, globus pallidus* (*pallidum*), and *amygdala* (*amygdaloid nuclei*). Together the *caudate nucleus* and *putamen* form the *striatum* (*neostriatum*). In the adult brain, the internal capsule separates the caudate nucleus from the putamen and globus pallidus. Together the *putamen* and *globus pallidus* form the *lentiform nucleus* (*lenticular nucleus*) (Fig. 16–1*A*).

Occasionally, the term *basal ganglia* is used to include other functionally related nuclei, such as the *subthalamic nucleus* of the ventral thalamus and the *substantia nigra* of the midbrain and ventral thalamus (see the following discussion). In

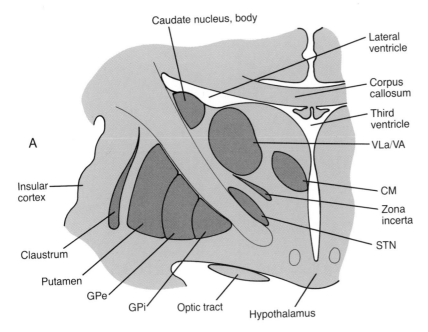

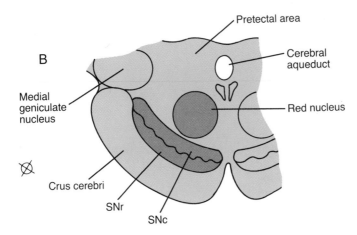

FIGURE 16-1

The basal ganglia and related nuclei. *A,* Transverse section through the diencephalon; the plane and level are similar to those in Figure 7–20.

B, Transverse section through the midbrain; the plane and level are similar to those in Figure 7–18. GPe, globus pallidus, external division; GPi, globus pallidus, internal division; CM, centromedian nucleus; VLa, ventral lateral nucleus, anterior division; VA, ventral anterior nucleus; STN, subthalamic nucleus; SNr, substantia nigra, pars reticulata; and SNc, substantia nigra, pars compacta.

this text, the term *basal ganglia* refers only to those nuclei differentiated from the ventral portion of the telencephalic vesicle: the *caudate nucleus,* the *putamen,* the *ventral striatum* (as subsequently defined), and the *globus pallidus* (Fig. 16–1).

STRIATUM

The *striatum* is the main receiving station for the basal ganglia. It receives massive projections from all areas of the cerebral cortex and from certain thalamic nuclei, the substantia nigra, and other brain stem nuclei. The *caudate nucleus* and the *putamen* are the largest of the nuclei composing the striatum. The *ventral striatum* consists of

ventral portions of the *caudate nucleus* and the *putamen,* the deep layers of the *olfactory tubercle,* the *nucleus accumbens,* and the *substantia innominata.* Although the nucleus accumbens and the substantia innominata are frequently referred to as part of the *basal forebrain* and the olfactory tubercle as a part of the *olfactory system,* the *ventral striatum,* including these nuclei, is an important functional part of the basal ganglia.

PALLIDUM

The *pallidum* or *globus pallidus* contains the principal efferent nuclei of the basal ganglia. The pallidum contains three subdivisions. An internal lamina of myelinated fibers divides the globus pallidus into *internal* (*GPi*) and *external* (*GPe*) *divisions* (see Fig. 16–1*A*). The *ventral division* (*GPv*) is in the anteroventral portion of the pallidum, ventral and adjacent to the anterior commissure. A ventral and lateral subdivision of the substantia nigra (SNr) has many of the same connections and functions as GPi but is not, for purposes of this book, considered part of the basal ganglia (Fig. 16–1*B*).

Weigert-stained sections of the human brain stem, illustrating the nuclei of the basal ganglia, are provided in Figures 7–20, 7–21, 7–22, 8–10, and 8–11.

Related Nuclei

The *subthalamic nucleus*, the *substantia nigra*, and several nuclei of the *dorsal thalamus* are integral parts of the basal ganglia circuitry. Specific thalamic nuclei relay information from the basal ganglia to selected areas of the frontal cortex, and other thalamic nuclei have extensive projections back to the striatum.

SUBTHALAMIC NUCLEUS

The almond-shaped *subthalamic nucleus* (*STN*) is one of four nuclei of the ventral thalamus. In transverse sections of the brain stem, STN lies dorsomedial to the junction between the crus cerebri and the internal capsule, lateral to the hypothalamus, and ventral to the zona incerta and dorsal thalamus (see Fig. 16–1*A*).

SUBSTANTIA NIGRA

The *substantia nigra* (*SN*) lies in the ventral midbrain and extends rostrally into the ventral thalamus. It is immediately caudal to STN and dorsomedial to the crus cerebri (see Fig. 16–1*B*). The SN has two subdivisions: the *pars reticulata* (*SNr*) and the *pars compacta* (*SNc*). The SNc contains *pigmented*, dopaminergic neurons that project to the striatum. In contrast, SNr receives efferent projections from the striatum and contains GABAergic neurons that project to the dorsal thalamus. The latter connections are similar to those of GPi.

NUCLEI OF THE DORSAL THALAMUS

In the dorsal thalamus, two nuclei relay information from the basal ganglia to the frontal cortex, specifically, the *anterior division* of the *ventral lateral nucleus* (*VLa*) and the *ventral anterior nucleus* (*VA*). These nuclei belong to the somatomotor system. In the human brain, and that of other primates, the very prominent *medial dorsal nucleus* is important in the relay of basal ganglia information to association and limbic areas of the frontal cortex. Two intralaminar nuclei, the large *centromedian nucleus* and the *parafascicular nucleus*, also are important in the circuitry of the basal ganglia, not as cortical relay centers, but in thalamostriate projections to all three areas of the striatum: the caudate nucleus, the putamen, and the ventral striatum (see Fig. 16–1*A*).

Weigert-stained sections of the human brain stem illustrating these nuclei are provided in Figures 7–17 through 7–22 and 7–25 through 7–27.

Basic Circuits Between the Basal Ganglia and Cortex

The human brain contains over 100 million *corticostriate fibers* in each cerebral hemisphere. These fibers arise from all areas of the cortex and terminate in a highly organized fashion within the caudate, putamen, and ventral striatum. Information leaving the basal ganglia projects to select areas of the frontal cortex via a relay through the dorsal thalamus.

Within the striatum, there is a segregation of information processed, according to function. The *putamen* processes *sensorimotor* information that ultimately projects to the *supplementary motor area* (*SMA*). The *caudate nucleus* processes information destined for the *dorsolateral prefrontal area*, the *lateral orbitofrontal area*, and the *frontal eye fields*; the *ventral striatum* processes *limbic system* information destined for the *anterior cingulate* and *medial orbitofrontal areas*. All striatal regions receive input from large areas of the cerebral cortex, although the most intense projections are from cortical areas related to the function of the striatal region, i.e., sensorimotor, associational, or limbic (Fig. 16–2). Territorial and compartmental details are discussed later in this chapter.

Two basic types of circuits, or loops, link the cortex and the basal ganglia. These loops are in parallel; however, they have opposite effects on the target cortical area. The first, the *direct loop*, *increases* the level of cortical activity through a *dis-inhibition* of thalamocortical projections. The term *dis-inhibition* simply refers to the *inhibition*

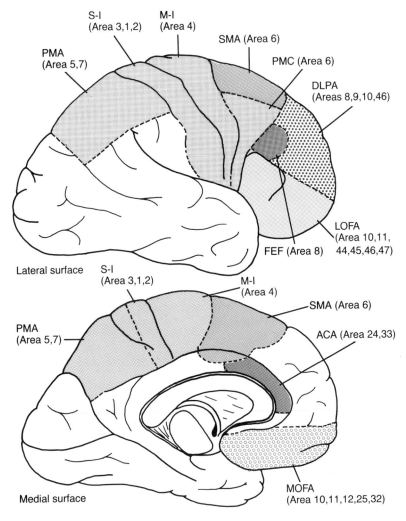

FIGURE 16–2

The principal frontal lobe areas receiving projections from the basal ganglia (illustrated in red): SMA, supplementary motor area; FEF, frontal eye fields; DLPA, dorsolateral prefrontal area; LOFA, lateral orbitofrontal area; ACA, anterior cingulate area; MOFA, medial orbitofrontal area. Also illustrated are the posterior parietal motor area (PMA), primary somatosensory area (S-I), primary motor cortex M-I), and premotor cortex (PMC). Numbers refer to Brodmann's areas (see Fig. 21–3). See text for details.

of inhibitory neurons. The second circuit, the indirect loop, reduces the level of cortical activity through an inhibition of the thalamocortical projections.

To understand how these loops work, it is important to realize that projections to the thalamus from both GPi and SNr have a high rate of spontaneous firing and inhibit the flow of information from the thalamus to the cortex. The direct loop inhibits the activity of these inhibitory neurons that project to the thalamus, hence, increasing the activity of thalamocortical projections; the indirect loop excites or increases the activity of these inhibitory neurons, hence, decreasing the activity of thalamocortical projections.

DIRECT LOOP

In the direct loop, cortical fibers project to the striatum and striatal efferent neurons project to GPi and SNr. Efferents from GPi and SNr project to the dorsal thalamus, and the thalamic neurons project to specific areas of the cerebral cortex (Fig. 16–3). Both the glutaminergic corticostriate projections and the thalamocortical projections are excitatory. However, the efferents from the striatum to GPi and SNr and their projections to the thalamus are all inhibitory (GABAergic).

The glutaminergic corticostriate fibers excite a select population of striatal efferent neurons that project to GPi and SNr. These striatal efferents (GABAergic with substance P or dynorphin as a

FIGURE 16-3

The *direct loop*. Excitatory neurons are in black; excitatory synapses (+). Inhibitory neurons are in red; inhibitory synapses (−). The size of the fiber indicates the relative rate of neuronal activity following loop stimulation. GPe, globus pallidus, pars externa; GPi, globus pallidus, pars interna; STN, subthalamic nucleus; SNr, substantia nigra, pars reticulata; and SNc, substantia nigra, pars compacta. See text for details.

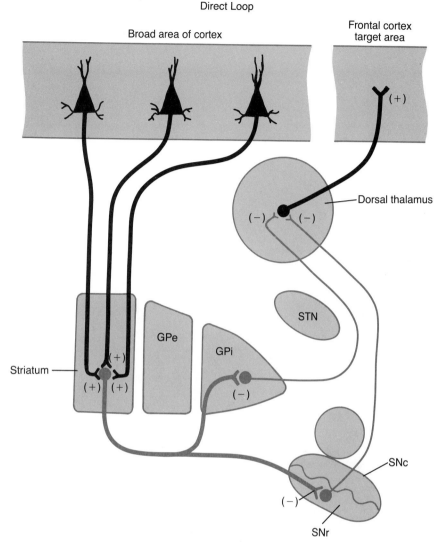

Direct Loop

Broad area of cortex

Frontal cortex target area

Dorsal thalamus

STN

GPe

GPi

Striatum

SNc

SNr

co-transmitter) *inhibit* the spontaneously firing *GPi* and *SNr* efferents to the *thalamus*. Both of these latter projections inhibit cortical relay neurons in *VLa*, *VA*, or *MD*. Inhibition of these inhibitory neurons, in GPi and SNr, leads to a dis-inhibition of the thalamocortical projections and a corresponding increase in cortical activity (see Fig. 16–3).

INDIRECT LOOP

In the *indirect loop*, *cortical fibers* project to the striatum; *striatal efferent neurons* project to *GPe*; and *efferents* from *GPe* project to *STN*. Neurons in *STN* project to both *GPi* and *SNr*. The remainder of the loop, from GPi and SNr to the cerebral cortex, is the same as the direct loop (Fig. 16–4).

The glutaminergic *corticostriate* fibers *excite* a specific population of *striatal efferent neurons* that projects to *GPe*. These striatal efferents are GABAergic, with enkephalin or neurotensin as a co-transmitter, and they *inhibit* neurons in *GPe*. The GPe projections to *STN* normally have a high rate of spontaneous firing and are inhibitory (GABAergic). *STN* neurons, in comparison, are excitatory (glutaminergic) and project to both *GPi* and *SNr* (see Fig. 16–4).

Because of the high spontaneous firing rate of the inhibitory neurons in GPe, the excitatory effects of STN on neurons in GPi and SNr normally are minimal. However, when the activ-

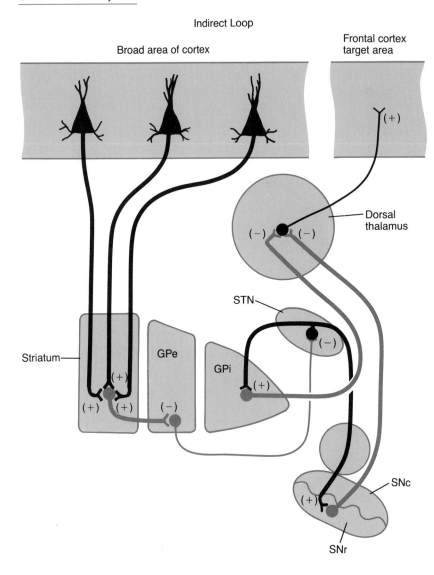

Indirect Loop

Broad area of cortex

Frontal cortex
target area

Dorsal
thalamus

STN

Striatum

GPe

GPi

SNc

SNr

FIGURE 16–4

The *indirect loop*. Excitatory neurons are in black; excitatory synapses (+). Inhibitory neurons are in red; inhibitory synapses (−). The size of the fiber indicates the relative rate of neuronal activity following loop stimulation. GPe, globus pallidus, pars externa; GPi, globus pallidus, pars interna; STN, subthalamic nucleus; SNr, substantia nigra, pars reticulata; and SNc, substantia nigra, pars compacta. See text for details.

ity of the *indirect loop* increases, *there is a dis-inhibition of STN* (see Fig. 16–4). The *increased rate of firing of STN neurons excites neurons in GPi and SNr. The excitation of neurons in GPi and SNr is inhibitory to thalamic relay neurons.* A corresponding decrease in the level of cortical activity occurs.

LIMBIC LOOPS

In the *limbic pathway*, the differentiation between the direct and indirect loops is not as clear. In addition, the *ventral pallidum* does not contain distinct subdivisions comparable with GPe and GPi. This lack of distinction probably reflects only our present level of resolution, because

physiological studies indicate a similar complement of direct and indirect loops for the limbic portion of the basal ganglia (see Chapter 22).

Modulatory Circuits

Several other pathways and "loops" modulate the function of the basal ganglia. These include extensive projections *to the striatum* from both the *pars compacta*, of the *substantia nigra (SNc)* via the *nigrostriatal pathway*, and the *intralaminar nuclei* of the *dorsal thalamus*, principally the *centromedian* and *parafascicular nuclei (CM-PF)* (Fig. 16–5). In addition, secondary loops between

FIGURE 16-5

Summary of the principal projections to the striatum. The dopaminergic, nigrostriatal pathway arises from both the substantia nigra (SNc) and the retrorubral nucleus. SNc projections are excitatory (black, (+)), whereas the retrorubral projections are inhibitory (red, (−)). The other projections are excitatory (black, (+)). Of these, the projections from subthalamic nucleus (STN) are the sparsest.

GPe, globus pallidus, pars externa; GPi, globus pallidus, pars interna; CM-PF, centromedian and parafascicular nuclei of the dorsal thalamus; STN, subthalamic nucleus; SNr, substantia nigra, pars reticulata; and SNc, substantia nigra, pars compacta. See text for details.

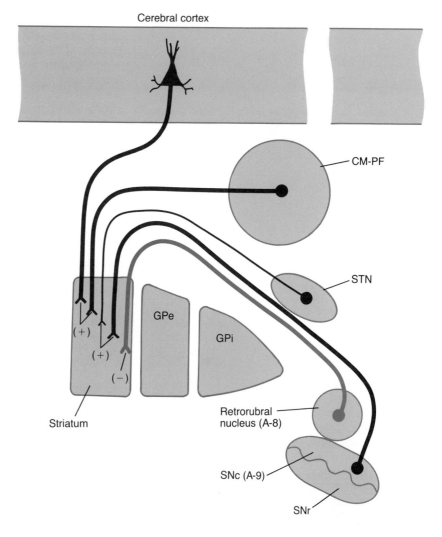

neurons of the *STN*, the *SNr*, and the *pedunculopontine tegmental nucleus* (*PPN*) influence the activity of both the direct and indirect loops (Fig. 16-6). The precise role for each of these pathways in motor activity is not known.

SNc AND THE NIGROSTRIATAL PATHWAY

The *SNc* contains large clusters of dopaminergic neurons that project to either the *association area of the striatum* (caudate nucleus) or the *sensorimotor striatum* (putamen). The neurons of any one cluster project either to the association area of the striatum or to the sensorimotor area of the striatum—never to both. The basal midbrain contains three identifiable groups of dopaminergic neurons, often called *A-8*, *A-9*, and *A-10*. *A-9* is *SNc*; *A-8* is immediately rostral to SNc and is part of the *retrorubral nucleus*; and *A-10* is in the

ventral midbrain tegmentum. Both *SNc* and the *retrorubral nucleus* have strong projections to the striatum and are functionally similar. The term *nigrostriatal pathway* often refers to the projections from both of these nuclei and not from SNc alone (see Fig. 16-5). The loss of *nigrostriatal neurons* and their terminals in the caudate and putamen is a prominent feature of Parkinson-like diseases.

The dopaminergic, nigrostriatal projections are both *excitatory* and *inhibitory*. Postsynaptic responses are properties of the receptor and not the transmitter. D_1 dopamine receptors activate adenyl cyclase, whereas D_2 receptors inhibit adenyl cyclase. The nigrostriatal projections from *SNc* (*A-9*) end principally on D_1 receptors and *excite* the GABA–substance P striatal neurons of the *direct loop*. Dopaminergic projections from the more rostral *retrorubral nucleus* (*A-8*) end on

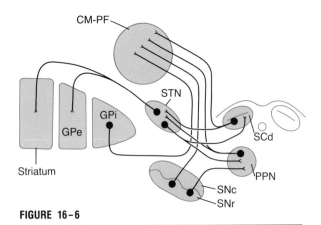

FIGURE 16-6

Several other "loops" and pathways that modulate the output of the basal ganglia.

CM-PF, centromedian and parafascicular nuclei of the dorsal thalamus; STN, subthalamic nucleus; GPe, globus pallidus, pars externa; GPi, globus pallidus, pars interna; SNc, substantia nigra, pars compacta; SNr, substantia nigra, pars reticulata; PPN, pedunculopontine tegmental nucleus; and SCd, superior colliculus, deep layers. See text for details.

D_2 receptors and *inhibit* the GABA-enkephalin striatal neurons of the *indirect loop* (see Fig. 16–5). The overall effect of the nigrostriatal system is one of reinforcing cortically initiated motor activity through a *facilitation of the direct loop and a suppression of the indirect loop.*

The vast number of large *cholinergic interneurons* within the striatum counterbalances the cortical reinforcing effect of the dopaminergic neurons. These interneurons preferentially *excite* the GABA-enkephalin striatal efferents of the *indirect loop* and thereby suppress the action of thalamocortical projections.

CENTROMEDIAN AND PARAFASCICULAR NUCLEI

The *intralaminar nuclei* of the dorsal thalamus, especially the *centromedian* and *parafascicular nuclei* (*CM-PF*) have extensive projections to the *striatum* and, to a lesser extent, to the GP and STN. Unlike VLa and VA, these intralaminar nuclei have sparse projections to the cerebral cortex. One dimension of the circuitry of the basal ganglia includes a loop from *GPi* and *SNr* to *CM-PF* and back to the *striatum* (see Figs. 16–5 and 16-6). The projections from CM-PF to the putamen have a pattern of termination that is similar to corticostriate projections—a pattern of somatotopically organized parallel

oblique bands. Besides GPi and SNr, CM-PF receives projections from many brain stem centers, the motor reticular formation, the PPN, and the deep layers of the superior colliculus and pretectum. Many limbic system structures project to CM-PF. However, these remain segregated from those related to the sensorimotor system, and the CM-PF projections from these areas terminate in the ventral striatum. Most of the sensorimotor-related projections involve the centromedian nucleus. The limbic-related projections involve the parafascicular nucleus, although some overlap occurs.

SECONDARY LOOPS

Besides the involvement of STN in the indirect loop with its projections to GPi and SNr (see Fig. 16–4), *STN* also has reciprocal projections with *GPe* and *PPN* and the deep layers of the *superior colliculus* (see Fig. 16–6). The *PPN*, in turn, receives projections from *SNr* and projects to *CM-PF* and *STN* (see Fig. 16–6).

Parallel Circuits: Territories and Compartments

MULTIPLE CIRCUITS

The direct and indirect loops, which link the basal ganglia with the cortex via the dorsal thalamus, and the modulatory circuits, which alter the activity of the loops, are general patterns or "wiring diagrams" for the principal circuits associated with the basal ganglia. At least *five* well-defined systems of circuits or loops are known; *motor, oculomotor, limbic, association-1,* and *association-2.* These categories are broad. Within each system are thousands of parallel, separate circuits, and each represents a small component of the total. For example, in the motor category one loop may respond to the directional rotation of the wrist; another, the knee; but, all use the same basic circuit pattern.

The five basic systems differ, however, in the specific nuclei or subdivisions of nuclei in the basal ganglia and dorsal thalamus that are part of their unique loops. In addition, although they all receive corticostriate fibers from a broad expanse of the cerebral cortex, the major areas from which corticostriate fibers originate differ for each system as does the specific cortical area targeted for the thalamocortical projections.

MOTOR CIRCUITS

Corticostriate fibers associated with the motor system arise from a broad area of the cortex but most heavily from the *premotor cortex (PMC)*, *primary motor cortex (M-I)*, *somatosensory area (S-I)*, and *posterior parietal motor area (PMA)* (see Fig. 16–2). These fibers end somatotopically in the *putamen*. Portions of the limbs and body are represented by oblique strips running the length of the putamen. Within the *globus pallidus*, the motor circuits reside in the ventrolateral two thirds of both *GPe* and *GPi* and remain separate from those of the other systems (associational, limbic, and oculomotor). A similar segregation exists in the *SNr* and the *STN*. Thalamic projections from GPi and SNr end in *VLa* and *VA* of the dorsal thalamus, and the thalamocortical projections end selectively in the *supplementary motor area (SMA)*. In each of the nuclei is a somatotopic representation of the body parts.

OCULOMOTOR CIRCUITS

The heaviest *corticostriate* projections in the oculomotor circuitry are from the *dorsolateral prefrontal cortex (DLPA)*, *PMA*, and the *middle temporal visual area (MT)*. These corticostriate fibers terminate in the *body* of the *caudate*. Pallidal connections segregate to the posterior, dorsomedial part of GPe and GPi. Thalamocortical fibers, arising from both the *mediodorsal nucleus (MD)* and *VA*, project to the *frontal eye fields (FEF)*, part of Brodmann's area 8 (see Fig. 16–2).

LIMBIC CIRCUITS

Most of the *corticostriate* fibers in the limbic circuitry arise from the *hippocampus*, the *entorhinal cortex*, and the *superior*, *middle*, and *inferior temporal gyri*. These corticostriate fibers project to the *ventral striatum*; the *ventral striatum*, in turn, projects to *GPv*. Thalamocortical projections arise from *MD* and terminate in the *anterior cingulate (ACA)* and *medial orbitofrontal areas (MOFA)* (see Fig. 16–2).

ASSOCIATION-1 CIRCUITS

The first of the association circuits contains *corticostriate fibers* originating in the *posterior parietal cortex* and *PMC* and terminating in the *head of the caudate*. Pallidal connections are in the dorsomedial third of *GPe* and *GPi*, and thalamocortical projections originate in *VA* and *MD* and terminate in the *dorsolateral prefrontal cortex (DLPA)* (see Fig. 16–2).

ASSOCIATION-2 CIRCUITS

In the other association circuit, *corticostriate* fibers arise from the *superior*, *middle*, and *inferior temporal gyri* and from the *anterior cingulate area (ACA)*. These cortical fibers also terminate in the *head of the caudate*. The pallidal and thalamic nuclei are similar to *association-1*, but the thalamocortical fibers project selectively to the *lateral orbitofrontal area (LOFA)* of the prefrontal lobe (see Fig. 16–2).

STRIATAL COMPARTMENTS

Although the *striatum* appears homogenous and without internal organization following routine histological staining (see Figs. 7–21 and 7–22), a definite heterogeneity is seen in the distribution of neurotransmitter systems. Initially defined on the basis of acetylcholinesterase-rich (AChE-rich) areas, the striatum can be divided into compartments. Small, irregular, AChE-rich regions, *striosomes*, are surrounded by extensive extrastriosomal areas known as the *matrix*. These irregular, three-dimensional compartments reflect differences in neurotransmitters and in striatal connections. The boundaries are not totally distinct, considerable overlap is noted, but several generalities can still be made. *Striosomes* account for only 15% of the striatal volume. They are rich in large cholinergic interneurons and have a high concentration of D_1 dopamine receptors. The *matrix* has few cholinergic interneurons and an abundance of D_2 dopamine receptors.

In the putamen, most of the striatal afferents related to sensorimotor processing end in the matrix. Those limbic system afferents to the putamen are split. Some limbic system structures, such as the amygdala, project to the striosome compartment. Fibers from the hippocampus end preferentially in the matrix. This partitioning of limbic afferents (amygdala to striosomes and hippocampus to matrix) is apparent in the ventral striatum as well, the area processing most of the limbic system circuitry.

The efferents from the striosome and matrix compartments are quite different. Matrix neurons give rise to all GABAergic, inhibitory projections to GPi, GPe, and SNr. Few if any axons from neurons in the striosomes project to the pallidum, most project directly to the dopaminergic nuclei in the midbrain, the retrorubral nucleus

(A-8), the SNc (A-9), and the midbrain tegmentum (A-10).

SIGNIFICANCE OF STRIATAL COMPARTMENTS AND PARALLEL CIRCUITS

The differences in connections and the relative partitioning of neurotransmitter systems between the compartments may reflect physiologically distinct information processing centers. This mosaic of miniprocessing centers is superimposed on the larger somatotopic pattern of movement-specific regions within the putamen. Identifying a pattern, analogous to the somatotopic pattern in the motor striatum (putamen), for those regions of the striatum associated with the limbic and association systems is not possible at this time. Because the boundaries between compartments, or miniprocessing centers, are not absolute, cross-compartment connections may integrate information in a neurochemically specific fashion.

Anatomy of the Pathways of the Basal Ganglia

Several of the fiber pathways associated with the basal ganglia are visible in Weigert-stained sec-

tions of the brain stem. Most of these are *palli-dofugal fibers* leaving the globus pallidus, destined principally for the dorsal thalamus.

ANSA LENTICULARIS

The *ansa lenticularis* contains fibers leaving the anterior portion of GPi. These fibers accumulate along the ventral surface of the nucleus and collate at the anteromedial margin of GPi. The ansa lenticularis swings anteriorly and ventromedially around the anterior margin of the internal capsule; after passing around the internal capsule, the ansa lenticularis swings caudad and enters the *prerubral field* (*H field of Forel*) (Fig. 16–7).

LENTICULAR FASCICULUS (H₂ FIELD OF FOREL)

The *lenticular fasciculus* (*H₂ field of Forel*) also is a collection of efferent fibers from GPi but from the more caudal portion of the nucleus. These fibers pass medially, in small fascicles, through the internal capsule. As they emerge on the medial side of the internal capsule, near the rostral end of the STN, the fibers accumulate as a dense band of myelinated axons immediately ventral to the zona incerta and dorsal to the STN. The fibers of the lenticular fasciculus course medially

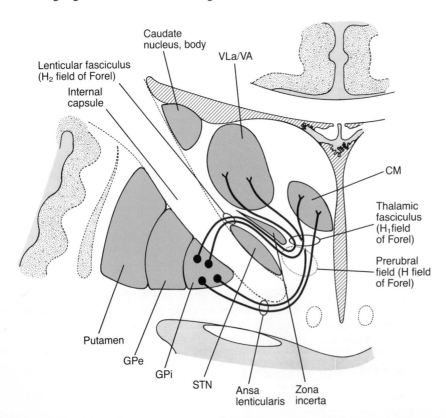

FIGURE 16–7

Principal pallidofugal fibers from the globus pallidus, pars interna (GPi) as seen in the transverse section of the diencephalon. The level and orientation of the section are the same as those in Figure 16–1.

Fibers of the *ansa lenticularis* leave the GPi along its ventral surface, swing around the anterior margin of the internal capsule, and enter the *prerubral field*. Fibers of the *lenticular fasciculus* pass through the internal capsule and over the dorsal surface of STN before joining fibers from the ansa lenticularis in the prerubral field. Fibers leave the prerubral field to enter the dorsal thalamus from the *thalamic fasciculus*. GPe, globus pallidus, pars externa; CM, centromedian nucleus; VLa, ventral lateral nucleus, pars anterior; VA, ventral anterior nucleus; and STN, subthalamic nucleus. See text for details.

to join those of the ansa lenticularis, forming the *prerubral field* (*H field of Forel*) (see Fig. 16–7).

THALAMIC FASCICULUS (H_1 FIELD OF FOREL)

Fibers passing through the *prerubral field* destined for the dorsal thalamus swing dorsolaterally, along the dorsomedial surface of the zona incerta and into the dorsal thalamus as the *thalamic fasciculus* (*H_1 field of Forel*). The fibers of the *thalamic fasciculus* end in VA, VLa, and MD and in the CM-PF complex of the dorsal thalamus (see Fig. 16–7).

The *prerubral field* and the *thalamic fasciculus*, although containing a large number of fibers from the pallidum, are not composed exclusively of efferent fibers from the basal ganglia. Fibers from the dentate, emboliform, and globose nuclei of the cerebellum enter the prerubral field and then the thalamic fasciculus *en route* to the dorsal thalamus. In addition, nigrothalamic fibers from SNr enter the prerubral field and the thalamic fasciculus and both striatonigral and nigrostriatal fibers pass through the prerubral field.

Motor Functions of the Basal Ganglia

Considerable information is known about the interconnections between the cerebral cortex and basal ganglia. Similarly, many of the chemical specificities of these pathways and their physiological properties are known. Little, however, is known of the cellular mechanisms within these circuits that modulate and regulate motor activity. However, these data are the bases of a number of hypotheses that attempt to define the role of the basal ganglia in motor function.

During motor activity, the activity of the neurons in the loops is initiated at the cortical level and rapidly spreads to the neurons in the basal ganglia. Neurons in both the motor cortical areas and in the basal ganglia also have simultaneous, movement-related discharges. This simultaneous activity occurs *both* during the *preparation* and the *planning* of the motor activity *and* during the actual *execution* of the motor activity.

With initiation of a motor activity, individual neurons in GPi, for example, show *either* a phasic decrease in activity *or* a phasic increase in activity but not both. The phasic decrease in activity dis-inhibits neurons in VLa, thereby facilitating the cortical activity. The phasic increase in activity has the opposite effect and suppresses

cortical activity. In one hypothesis, the direct loop would be responsible for the dis-inhibition, thereby reinforcing motor actions initiated at the cortical level. Similarly, the indirect loop would be responsible for the inhibition and possible suppression of conflicting patterns of movement at the cortical level.

A vast number of neurobehavioral variables integrate at the level of the basal ganglia; e.g., motivation, memory, target location, muscle contraction patterns, and limb movement patterns. These may represent separate but parallel loops that utilize different subcompartments of the basal ganglia. Each may have specifically defined, neurophysiological parameters, e.g., conditioned activity, anticipatory activity, sensorimotor activity and memory. Such an integration would require both the temporal and spatial summations of the vast array of information projecting to the basal ganglia.

Nearly every known neurotransmitter and putative neurotransmitter is present in the basal ganglia, alone and in various combinations. Although a massive array exists of parallel incoming signals to the basal ganglia, the neurochemical heterogeneity within the basal ganglia and the communication between the striatal microcompartments may work together to recombine, selectively, incoming information in a variety of ways. This integrated information would alter motor cortical activity through projections principally to SMA.

The Basal Ganglia and Disorders of Motor Function

The circuitry of the basal ganglia is complex. Many loops link the motor cortex with the basal ganglia as well as many well-defined modulating circuits. A number of these have been described earlier in this chapter. In addition, these pathways cover a large portion of the midbrain, diencephalon, and basal telencephalon. Hence, focal lesions can produce a variety of disorders, often with opposite symptomatology.

With the large number of neurotransmitter systems in the basal ganglia, diseases that selectively affect one system produce one type of problem, and diseases that affect another system may produce the opposite problem. Further, as a disease progresses, the loss or impairment of one chemically defined system can produce secondary effects in other, previously intact, systems.

Theoretically, an alteration as subtle as the loss of a single peptide could produce marked effects on basal ganglia function. Loss of Substance P, for example, would alter the direct loop with opposite effects to those from a loss of neurotensin or enkephalin in the indirect loop. As we unravel the complexities of the circuitry and chemistry of the basal ganglia, we will be able to define more clearly the precise deficits that produce the broad spectrum of clinical disorders of the basal ganglia. The selective treatment of these disorders will be a challenge to the neuropharmacologist.

Most movement disorders associated with basal ganglia pathology fall into one of two categories with opposite symptomatology. The first is characterized by *akinesia* (*lack of movement*) and *hypertonia* (*muscle rigidity*); the second, by *dyskinesia* (*abnormal movement*) and *hypotonia* (*muscle flaccidity*).

Akinesia is an inability to move, or in a milder from, *hypokinesia* is a limited or reduced ability to move. A related kinetic disorder is *bradykinesia*, a slowness of movement. Only the more advanced forms of basal ganglia disease show a total akinesia. Instead, varying degrees of hypokinesia and bradykinesia are observed.

Dyskinesia is the presence of abnormal, involuntary movements. Those associated with basal ganglia disease range from the tremor-at-rest or "pill-rolling" tremor, characteristic of parkinsonian diseases, to the unpredictable irregular choreiform and ballistic movements of Huntington's chorea or hemiballism. Some dystonic movement disorders, e.g., torsion dystonia and dystonia musculorum deformans, may be of a basal ganglia origin or at least have a basal ganglia component.

Hypertonia or *muscle rigidity* is a state of constant muscle contraction. This is most apparent as a resistance to the passive movement of a patient's limb by an examiner. Both agonist and antagonist muscles resist the passive flexion and extension of a limb throughout the range of joint movement. *Hypotonia* or *muscle flaccidity* is just the opposite—muscles lack normal tone and little or no resistance is present during the passive movement of a limb. The causes of rigidity or flaccidity are not clear but probably involve long-latency, tonic reflex mechanisms. *Hypertonia* may reflect a release of the brain stem reflex centers from the modulatory influences of the basal ganglia, and *hypotonia* may reflect a hyperactivity of the same modulatory mechanisms.

DISORDERS WITH AKINESIA AND HYPERTONIA

Parkinson's disease or, more correctly, the parkinsonian-like diseases are the best-documented and studied of the basal ganglia disorders. *Akinesia, rigidity, tremor-at-rest, stooped posture*, and *expressionless face* all are cardinal signs of Parkinson's disease. The *akinesia* is characterized by (1) *delay in the initiation* of movement (the patient takes longer than normal to respond to a stimulus); (2) *slowness in the execution* of the movement; and (3) a *difficulty in the performance* of complex movements, especially repetitive movements. The expressionless face reflects the akinesia of the facial muscles.

In Parkinson's disease, a selective loss of dopaminergic neurons in the SNc and a corresponding loss of dopaminergic fibers and terminals in the striatum occur. The administration of L-dopa, the immediate precursor of dopamine, elevates the striatal levels of dopamine and reduces some of the symptoms. However, as the disease progresses and as increasing numbers of nigrostriatal neurons disappear, L-dopa therapy becomes less effective.

As discussed earlier in this chapter, the intact nigrostriatal dopaminergic system reinforces cortically initiated motor activity. Thus, loss or damage to this modulatory pathway would suppress cortically initiated motor activity and thus explain the observed akinesia and hypertonia.

The tremor-at-rest or pill-rolling tremor is a form of dyskinesia, an involuntary movement. This tremor has a frequency of about 5 Hz and usually involves the fingers, hand, and forearm. The tremor is present during periods of inactivity but disappears during volitional activity. Lower motor neurons as well as neurons in VLa of the thalamus and in the motor cortex have discharge bursts that are in synchrony with the tremor. Patients with Parkinson's disease who lack a visible tremor have a similar pattern of bursting activity but only in VLa. This finding indicates that the thalamic firing pattern precedes the tremor and may eventually be the cause. Because dopamine antagonists elicit the tremor in akinetic primates, *dopamine projections to the striatum probably inhibit the thalamic bursting activity* in the normal brain. In patients with Parkinson's disease, the loss of the dopaminergic SNc projections may lead to a pattern of rhythmic bursting activity in the thalamus that, in turn, drives the motor cortex and produces the tremor.

DISORDERS WITH DYSKINESIA AND HYPOTONIA

Chorea and *ballismus* are two related forms of dyskinesia. Both show continual, unpredictable, and uncontrolled muscle contractions. Chorea involves only the distal musculature of a limb, whereas ballismus involves the more proximal limb and limb-girdle muscles, producing a wild and flailing movement of the entire limb. Both movement disorders are present when the patient is awake but absent when the patient is asleep. Unlike the akinetic disorders, *hypotonia* is a feature of both chorea and ballismus. The muscles are flaccid, and the limbs, when not moving involuntarily, are easily moved. The accompanying flaccidity tends to exaggerate the dyskinetic movements, because the antagonistic muscles offer little resistance.

Hemiballismus is one of the few disorders of the basal ganglia in which a focal lesion has been shown to be responsible for the observed symptoms. Focal destruction of the *subthalamic nucleus* (*STN*) leads to the ballistic movement of the contralateral limbs. Lesions involving only a portion of the nucleus may produce symptoms in only one limb, consistent with the somatotopic organization of the nucleus.

STN is an integral part of the indirect loop (see Fig. 16–4) and excites the GABAergic neurons in both GPi and SNr that project to the thalamus. Without the influence of STN, the level of excitation of GPi and SNr neurons is less. Hence, they have less of an inhibitory influence on the thalamocortical projections, i.e., thalamocortical activity increases. Removal of STN essentially ends the influence of the indirect loop, leaving the direct loop unopposed. The effect of the direct loop is facilitation of the thalamocortical projections (see Fig. 16–3).

Huntington's chorea is an inherited, autosomal dominant disease, but the clinical symptoms are not apparent until adulthood. Associated with this disease is a massive, bilateral loss of cells in the neostriatum. The clinical signs of bilateral choreiform movement are assumed to be asso-ciated with this destruction. Inconsistent with this assumption is the observation that unilateral damage to the neostriatum rarely produces hemichorea. In Huntington's disease, the damage to the CNS is massive. Although it seems reasonable to assume the motor component of the disease is striatal, the specific circuitry is unknown.

VASCULAR INFARCT

Infarct of the *anterior choroidal artery* or of the *lateral striate branches* of the *middle cerebral artery* (see Fig. 9–15) can produce a variety of motor disorders, some of which are caused by basal ganglia damage. Most, however, include damage to a portion of the internal capsule containing the corticospinal system. Consequently, pure striatal or pallidal lesions are rare.

SUGGESTED READING

Alexander, G. E., M. R. DeLong, and P. L. Strick (1986). Parallel organization of functionally segregated circuits linking basal ganglia and cortex. Ann. Rev. Neurosci., 9: 357–381

Basal Ganglia Research (1990). Special issue. Trends Neurosci., 13: 241–308.

This special issue includes some of the more exciting frontier-oriented studies on the basal ganglia. Included are excellent reviews of the functional, neurochemical, and morphological organization of the basal ganglia. Hypotheses on the mechanisms of basal ganglia disease are related to our new understanding of the organization of these structures. Of special interest are the following three articles:

Alexander, G. E. and M. D. Crutcher (1990). Functional architecture of basal ganglia: neural substrates of parallel processing. Trends Neurosci., 13: 266–271.

Graybiel, A. M. (1990). Neurotransmitters and neuromodulators in the basal ganglia. Trends Neurosci., 13: 244–254.

Parent, A. (1990). Extrinsic connections of the basal ganglia. Trends Neurosci., 13: 254–258.

Chapter

17

Cerebellum

ORGANIZATION
CEREBELLAR CORTEX
CEREBELLAR CIRCUITS
CONTROL OF MOVEMENT
MOTOR PLASTICITY AND LEARNING
DISORDERS OF MOTOR FUNCTION

The word *cerebellum* is the Latin diminutive form of *cerebrum* and means *little brain*. The cerebellum is a modulator and regulator of motor function. Unlike other portions of the motor system, damage to the cerebellum does not produce paralysis or paresis. Instead, cerebellar damage results in a diminution or loss of muscle synergy. The integrity of the cerebellum is important for the performance of smooth, accurate, and coordinated motor tasks; the maintenance of a stable posture, both static and dynamic; and the learning and modulation of complicated motor patterns.

Situated in the *posterior cranial fossa*, dorsal to the medulla and pons, the cerebellum is a highly convoluted cortical structure (Figs. 17–1 and 17–3). Three large fibers trunks, the *inferior cerebellar peduncle*, the *middle cerebellar peduncle*, and the *superior cerebellar peduncle* connect the cerebellum with the brain stem (Figs. 17–3 and 7–4).

The anatomical location of the cerebellum is ideal for the monitoring of descending motor signals and ascending sensory information from both the spinal cord (principally proprioceptive) and the vestibular system. In addition, massive inputs are sent to the cerebellum from the cerebral cortex, through the basal pons, for the relay of information essential to the execution and planning of movements.

The cerebellum decides how we perform a particular action (*planning*) via the cerebrocerebellar system. The cerebellum orchestrates the actual motor event by way of both the cerebrocerebellar and spinocerebellar systems (*coordination* and *execution*). In addition, the cerebellum helps to maintain the body's position and balance in space during the execution via the vestibulocerebellar system (*postural adjustment*). Another dimension to cerebellar function is *learning* motor tasks along with modulating and adjusting previously learned patterns in response to alterations in the immediate situation or environment.

Cardinal signs of *cerebellar dysfunction* include *postural instability* (vestibulocerebellum), *lack of motor control during the execution of motor activities* (spinocerebellum), and *loss of timing and appropriate planning of motor actions* (cerebrocerebellum). These dysfunctions can occur separately or in combination and reflect the particular region or regions of the cerebellum involved.

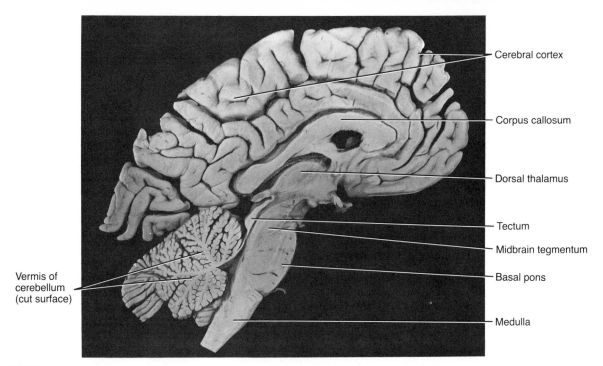

FIGURE 17-1

Midsagittal section through the human brain. Note the relative position of the cerebellum to the brain stem and the cerebral cortex. *In situ*, the cerebellum is separated from the cerebral cortex by the tentorium cerebelli. The cut surface of the cerebellum is through the vermis and illustrates the high degree of folding in the cerebellar cortex.

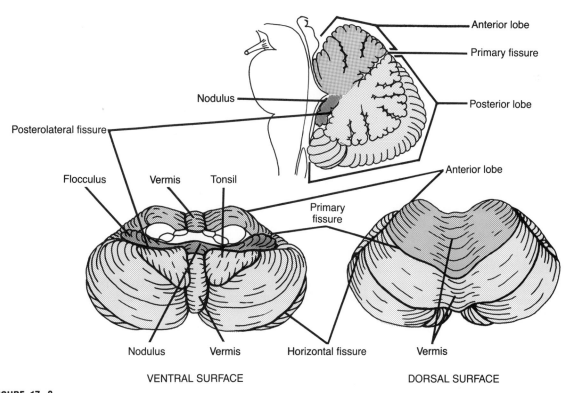

FIGURE 17-2

Midsagittal, dorsal, and ventral views of the cerebellum indicating the principal anatomical landmarks. See text for details.

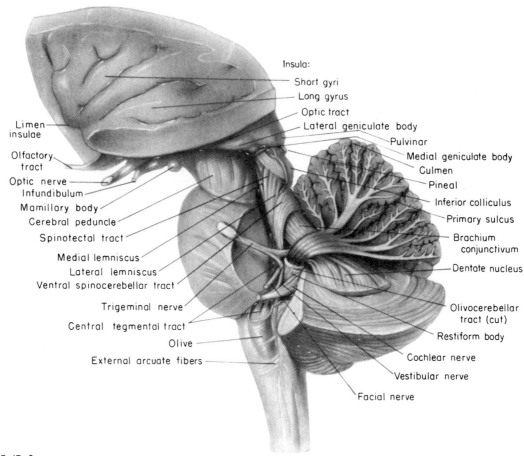

FIGURE 17-3

Lateral view of the human brain stem with dissection to show the internal structures. See text for details. (Modified from Büttner, Z. Anat. Entwicklungsgeschichte, 84: 536, 1927.)

Organization

DEVELOPMENT

The cerebellum develops from the rhombic lip of the mesencephalon, along the rostral margin of the fourth ventricle. As the rhombic lip enlarges and grows back over the fourth ventricle, differentiating neuroblasts migrate to the surface and begin to form the *cerebellar cortex*. Because the sheet-like cortex of the cerebellum grows at a much faster rate than the remainder of the structure, this throws the surface into a series of longitudinal folds (*folia*) that extend the width of the cerebellum. Small clusters of neuroblasts remain in the basal portion of the rhombic lip, where they proliferate and form the *nuclei of the cerebellum* (see Fig. 1–15). Because of this rapid

growth and folding, only about 15% of the cortical area is visible from the surface of the adult cerebellum (see Figs. 17–1 and 17–2).

CEREBELLAR CORTEX

A simple diagram, representing the entire surface of the cerebellum, is a useful tool when referring to specific areas of the cortex, especially for mapping different features of cerebellar connections or functions (Fig. 17–4). This figure represents the entire surface of the cortex; the center of the dorsal surface is the center of the diagram, and the more ventral portions of the cerebellar cortex are peripheral. Compare the labeled components in the diagram of Figure 17–4 with those in Figure 17–2.

FIGURE 17-4

Schematic representation of the cerebellar cortex in a single plane. In this diagram, the cortical surface seems "unrolled" from the cerebellum. The anteroventral portion of the cortex is represented superiorly, the posteroventral portions (floccular nodular lobe) inferiorly, and the dorsal surface centrally.

A, Compare the relative positions of the major lobes and fissures with those in Figure 17-2.

B, The cerebellar cortex is divided into vestibulocerebellum, spinocerebellum, and cerebrocerebellum. This division reflects the function, connections, and phylogenetic age of the areas. See text for details. (Adapted from O. Larsell, *Anatomy of the Nervous System,* 2nd Edition, Appleton-Century-Crofts, New York, 1951.)

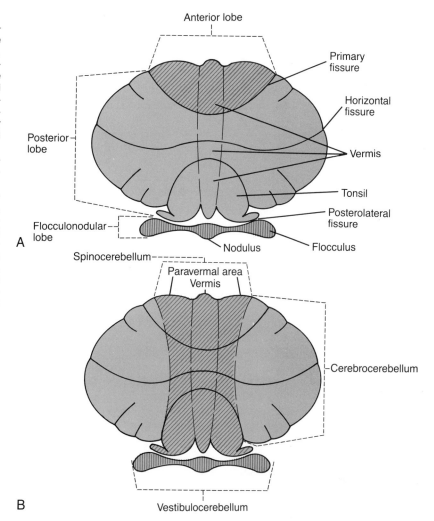

The cerebellar *cortex* is divided into three regions, based on both function and phylogenetic age. The *flocculonodular lobe* or *vestibulocerebellum* has extensive connections with the vestibular system and is the oldest phylogenetically (*archicerebellum*). The medial region of the cerebellum or *spinocerebellum* consists of the *vermis* located in the midline and the adjacent *paravermal region.* The spinocerebellum has extensive connections with the spinal cord and brain stem and is the second oldest part of the cerebellum (*paleocerebellum*). The largest portion of the cerebellum, the *cerebrocerebellum,* is composed of the prominent *cerebellar hemispheres* (except for the paravermal region). The cerebrocerebellum has extensive connections with the cerebral cortex, through relay stations in the cerebellar nuclei and the dorsal thalamus, and is the newest part of the cerebellum (*neocerebellum*) (see Fig. 17-4).

The folding of the cortex during development creates a number of fissures, some larger and more prominent than others. Prominent among these are the *primary fissure,* separating the *anterior lobe* from the *posterior lobe;* the *posterolateral fissure,* separating the posterior lobe from the *flocculonodular lobe;* and the *horizontal fissure,* dividing the posterior lobe in about half (see Figs. 17-2 and 17-4). All of these major fissures extend from one side of the cerebellum, through the central or *vermal portion,* to the opposite side.

The cerebellum also is subdivided into medial and lateral components; the central or midline *vermis* and the more lateral *cerebellar hemispheres.* This division is most apparent from the ventral and posterior views and less apparent from the dorsal surface. With this division, the vermis and the hemispheres include portions of both the anterior, posterior, and flocculonodular lobes (see Figs. 17–2 and 17–4). When the cerebellum is cut in the sagittal plane, the knife passes through the middle of the vermis (see Figs. 17–1 and 17–2).

CEREBELLAR PEDUNCLES

The cerebellum communicates with the brain stem through three pairs of cerebellar peduncles or fiber trunks: the *superior cerebellar peduncle* (*brachium conjunctivum*), the *middle cerebellar peduncle* (*brachium pontis*), and the *inferior cerebellar peduncle* (*restiform body* plus the *juxtarestiform body*). These structures contain all the fibers entering the cerebellum (*cerebellar afferents*) and all the fibers leaving the cerebellum (*cerebellar efferents*) (see Fig. 17–3).

The *superior cerebellar peduncle* contains most of the cerebellar efferent fibers and all those arising from three of the four pairs of cerebellar nuclei; the *dentate nucleus*, the *emboliform nucleus*, and the *globose nucleus* (Fig. 17–5 and Figs. 7–11 and 7–12). In addition, the superior cerebellar peduncle contains one cerebellar afferent pathway, the *ventral spinocerebellar tract*,

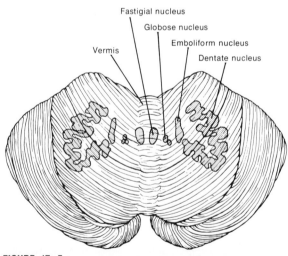

Fastigial nucleus
Globose nucleus
Emboliform nucleus
Dentate nucleus
Vermis

FIGURE 17–5

The dorsal surface of the cerebellum illustrating the relative position of the cerebellar nuclei. The nuclei are deep to the surface, located in the central white matter of the cerebellum. (Reproduced with permission from J. K. Werner, *Neuroscience: A Clinical Perspective*, W. B. Saunders Co., Philadelphia, 1980.)

carrying proprioceptive information to the cerebellum from the lower extremity and trunk.

Fibers of the *middle cerebellar peduncle* convey information that originates from the cerebral cortex. *Corticopontine fibers* synapse on neurons in the *basal pons*. Most axons from these pontine neurons cross in the basal pons and enter the middle cerebellar peduncle of the opposite side as *pontocerebellar fibers*. A small component of pontocerebellar fibers projects to the ipsilateral cerebellar cortex. Together, the corticopontine and pontocerebellar pathways make up the *corticopontocerebellar system*. The corticopontocerebellar system projects primarily to the cerebrocerebellum.

The *inferior cerebellar peduncle* has two components: the *restiform body* and the *juxtarestiform body*. The *restiform body* contains ascending spinal proprioceptive fibers from three of the *spinocerebellar tracts*: the dorsal spinocerebellar, rostral spinocerebellar, and cuneocerebellar tracts. Spinocerebellar pathways project primarily to the spinocerebellum. In addition, the restiform body contains *olivocerebellar fibers*, which are projections from the contralateral *inferior olivary nuclei* to the cerebellar cortex. The olivocerebellar fibers project to all areas of the cerebellar cortex. The *juxtarestiform body* contains both afferent and efferent fibers associated with the *vestibular system* (*vestibulocerebellar* and *cerebellovestibular fibers*). These fibers project principally to and from the vestibulocerebellum and the vermal portion of the spinocerebellum. In addition, significant reciprocal connections exist between the motor reticular formation and the spinocerebellum, most of which pass through the restiform body. *Reticulocerebellar fibers* arise from reticular nuclei in the medulla and pons and project to both the vestibulocerebellum and the spinocerebellum. In turn, most of the *cerebelloreticular fibers* arise from the fastigial nucleus.

CEREBELLAR NUCLEI

Embedded in the central core of white matter at the base of the cerebellum are four pairs of nuclei, the *cerebellar nuclei* (see Fig. 17–5 and Fig. 7–11). From medial to lateral, these are the *fastigial, globose, emboliform,* and *dentate nuclei*. These nuclei are the principal source of efferent fibers from the cerebellum, projecting to the dorsal thalamus as well as to the vestibular nuclei, the red nucleus, and the other brain stem nuclei. These nuclei receive information from three principal sources: (1) collaterals from most of the afferent fibers en route to the cerebellar cortex; (2) axons of Purkinje cells from the cerebellar cortex; and (3) for the fastigial nucleus, vestibulo-cerebellar fibers from the vestibular labyrinth and the vestibular nuclei.

The *dentate nucleus* receives projections from Purkinje cells in the *cerebrocerebellum*, collaterals from some of the *pontocerebellar fibers*; and other afferents to the *cerebrocerebellum*. Fibers from the dentate nucleus enter the *brachium conjunctivum*, cross to the *contralateral* side in the *decussation of the brachium conjunctivum*, and terminate in the posterior division of the contralateral *ventral lateral nucleus* (*VLp*) of the dorsal thalamus. *VLp*, in turn, projects to the cerebral cortex, principally the *premotor cortex*

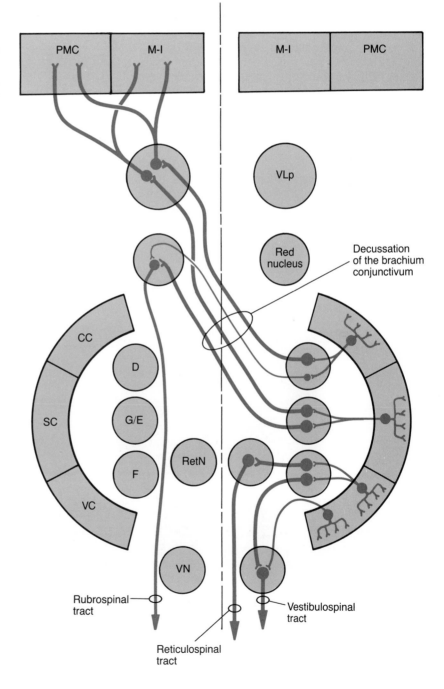

FIGURE 17-6

The principal efferent projections from the cerebellum. PMC, premotor cortex; M-I, primary motor cortex; VLp, posterior division of the ventral lateral nucleus of the thalamus; CC, cerebrocerebellum; SC, spinocerebellum; VC, vestibulocerebellum; D, dentate nucleus; G/E, globose and emboliform nuclei; F, fastigial nucleus; RetN, reticular nuclei; and VN, vestibular nuclei. See text for details.

(*PMC*) and the *primary motor cortex* (*M-I*). A small number of fibers from the dentate nucleus leave the cerebellum in the same manner but terminate in the *contralateral red nucleus* (Fig. 17–6).

The *globose* and *emboliform nuclei* receive projections from the Purkinje cells in the *spinocerebellum* and collaterals from the afferents entering the cerebellum via the *restiform body* and the *ventral spinocerebellar tract*. Fibers from the globose and emboliform nuclei also enter the *brachium conjunctivum*, decussate to the *contralateral side* and terminate in both the *VLp* and the *red nucleus* (see Fig. 17–6). In other vertebrates, the globose and emboliform nuclei are closely apposed to each other and frequently are called the *interposed nuclei* (*nuclei interpositus*). The anterior and posterior interposed nuclei are the homologues, respectively, of the emboliform and globose nuclei.

The *fastigial nucleus*, closely associated with the vestibular system, receives projections from the Purkinje cells in the *vestibulocerebellum* and afferent collaterals from the vestibular labyrinth and the vestibular nuclei. The fastigial nucleus projects primarily to the *lateral and inferior ves-*tibular nuclei (*fastigiovestibular fibers*) and to areas of the *pontine* and *medullary reticular formation* (*fastigioreticular fibers*) (see Fig. 17–6). Projections to the vestibular nuclei modulate the descending vestibulospinal system and those to the reticular formation modulate the activity of the corticoreticulospinal system. As discussed in Chapters 14 and 15, these motor pathways descend parallel to the corticospinal tract and regulate primarily postural and proximal limb movements.

Cerebellar Cortex

The cerebellar cortex has three distinct layers: an inner *granular layer*; an outer *molecular layer*; and between the two, the *Purkinje cell layer*. Deep to this cortical gray matter is a central core of *white matter*, containing axons that are entering and leaving the cortex (Fig. 17–7). Five types of neurons are in the cerebellar cortex: *Purkinje cells*, *granule cells*, *Golgi cells*, *basket cells*, and *stellate cells*. The *granular layer* contains billions of *granule cells* and a much smaller number of *Golgi cells*; the *molecular layer* contains the *stel-*

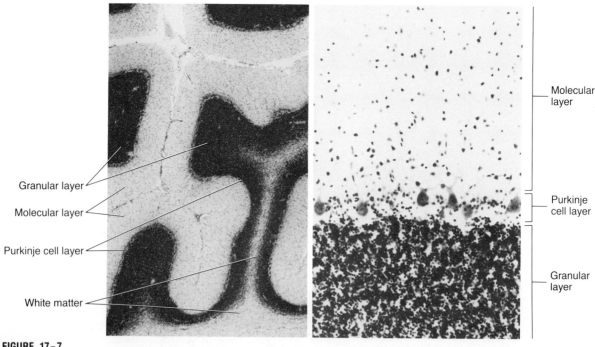

Granular layer

Molecular layer

Purkinje cell layer

White matter

Molecular layer

Purkinje cell layer

Granular layer

FIGURE 17–7

Nissl-stained section of the human cerebellar cortex. The prominent granular layer in (*A*) contains the dark staining and densely packed nuclei of the granule cells. At higher magnification (*B*), the large soma of the tetraploid Purkinje cell is evident.

late cells and *basket cells*; and the *Purkinje cell layer* contains the *perikarya (cell bodies) of the Purkinje cells.* Each of the five cell types has a characteristic morphology and a specific role in the basic circuitry of the cerebellum (Fig. 17–8).

Unlike the cerebrum, the histological organization of the cerebellar cortex is uniform. The basic cellular components and the circuits are similar for all areas. Distinct differences exist, however, in the localization of some neurotransmitter systems. This neurochemical heterogeneity may reflect parallel circuits with similar patterns but modulated by a different neurochemical transmitter, co-transmitter, or modulator.

PURKINJE CELLS

Purkinje cells are the largest and some of the most distinctive of the neurons in the central nervous system (CNS) (Fig. 17–9). The cell bodies of these large (60 to 90 μm in diameter), tetraploid neurons form a single-cell layer between the molecular and granular layers, the *Purkinje cell layer.* The massive dendritic tree of the Purkinje cell, with its characteristic branching and perfusion of dendritic spines, radiates through the molecular layer to the surface of the cortex (Figs. 17–8, 17–9 and 17–10). Unlike most neurons, the dendritic arbor is planar. These dendrites form a sheet of branches oriented in a plane transverse to the long axis of the folium, much like an espaliered fruit tree. The axons of the Purkinje cells project primarily to the cerebellar nuclei, although a few exit the cerebellum and terminate directly in the vestibular nuclei. The Purkinje cell axon is the only exit route for information leaving the cerebellar cortex (see Fig. 17–10). In addition, Purkinje cell axons usually have one or more collateral branches that re-enter the cortex. These are inhibitory to other cortical interneurons.

GRANULE CELLS

The *granular layer* of the cerebellum contains approximately 1×10^{11} *granule cells*—more neurons than in both cerebral hemispheres combined. The small, densely packed granule cells

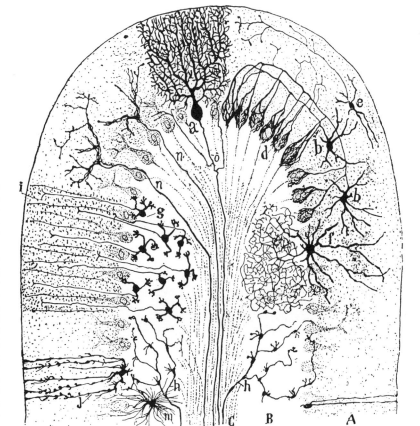

FIGURE 17–8

Semischematic diagram of a transverse section through a folium of the cerebellum illustrating the major neuronal elements. *A*, Molecular layer. *B*, Granular layer. *C*, White mater.

a, *Purkinje cell* with axon (*o*) with two recurrent collaterals. *b*, *Basket cells* in molecular layer, including axonal processes with terminal axonal arborizations (*d*) around the Purkinje cell soma. *e*, *Stellate cell*. *f*, *Golgi cell*. *g*, *Granule cells* in the granular layer with axons extending into the molecular layer and bifurcating (*i*). *h*, Mossy fibers. *n*, Climbing fibers. *j* and *m*, Neuroglia. (Reproduced with permission from S. Ramon y Cajal, *Histologie du Système Nerveux*, Tome II. Translated by L. Azoulay, Instituto Ramon y Cajal, Madrid, 1955.)

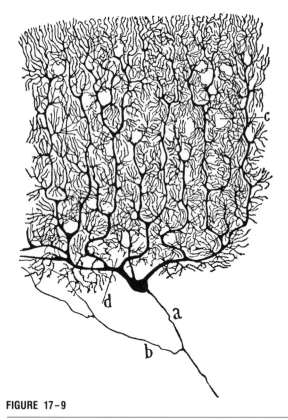

FIGURE 17-9

The Purkinje cell—adult human, Golgi method. *a*, Axon. *b*, Recurrent collateral. *c*, Capillary space. *d*, Space occupied by unstained basket cell. (Reproduced with permission from S. Ramon y Cajal, *Histologie du Système Nerveux*, Tome II. Translated by L. Azoulay, Instituto Ramon y Cajal, Madrid, 1955.)

have a very small perikaryon and a sparse dendritic tree, limited to three or four short branches within the granular layer (see Figs. 17–8 and 17–10). In Nissl-stained sections, the granular layer of the cerebellum is darkly stained and appears to contain little except densely packed nuclei of granule cells. This is a characteristic feature of cerebellar histology (see Fig. 17–7). The axon of the granule cell passes toward the surface of the folium, through the Purkinje cell layer, and into the molecular layer. In the molecular layer, it bifurcates and each branch runs *parallel* to the long axis of the folium (see Fig. 17–10). These very thin, unmyelinated *parallel fibers* are densely packed in the molecular layer (Fig. 17–11) and extend for distances of up to 1 mm, while making excitatory, glutaminergic synapses with the dendrites of numerous Purkinje

cells. Each Purkinje cell receives synaptic contact from about 200,000 parallel fibers. In the adult, the cerebellum contains more than 100,000 kilometers of parallel fibers—enough to encircle the earth nearly two and a half times.

GOLGI CELLS

The *Golgi cells* are inhibitory interneurons in which the soma are located in the granular layer. Golgi cells send extensive dendritic branches into the molecular layer, where they receive excitatory input from the parallel fibers and climbing fibers. They also receive excitatory input from mossy fibers in the granular layer. Golgi cell axons branch profusely in the granular layer and synapse with dendrites of a large number of granule cells, forming a negative feedback loop (see Figs. 17–8 and 17–10).

BASKET CELLS AND STELLATE CELLS

The *basket cells* and *stellate cells* are the only interneurons in the molecular layer, and both are inhibitory. Both have relatively large but planar dendritic trees that parallel those of the Purkinje cells, and both are excited by parallel fibers. *Basket cell* axons run transverse to the long axis of the folium and transverse to the parallel fibers. These axons form "basket-like" terminal arbors around the soma of the adjacent five to eight Purkinje cells. The axons of the *stellate cells* also run transverse to the long axis of the folium and parallel to the axons of the basket cells. The axon terminals of stellate cells form inhibitory synapses on the dendrites of the Purkinje cells (see Figs. 17–8 and 17–10).

Cerebellar Circuits

Afferent projections to the cerebellum fall into three general groups: *mossy fibers*, *climbing fibers*, and *monoaminergic fibers*. Both the mossy fibers and the climbing fibers *excite* neurons in the *cerebellar nuclei* and *excite* the *Purkinje cell*. Climbing fiber excitation of the Purkinje cell is direct. The mossy fiber excitation is indirect via the granule cells. The nature of the excitation of the Purkinje cells by these two systems (climbing fiber and mossy fiber) is quite different. Both responses are modulated by a network of inhibitory cortical interneurons.

The *axon* of the *Purkinje cell* is the only efferent fiber from the cerebellar cortex. Thus,

FIGURE 17-10

The cellular organization in a single folium of the cerebellar cortex. Surface on the left is in a plane transverse to the long axis of the folium; the surface on the right is in a plane parallel to the long axis of the folium.

BC, Basket cell. *CF,* Climbing fiber. *G,* Golgi cell. *Gl,* Glomerulus. *Gr,* Granule cell. *MF,* Mossy fiber. *PC,* Purkinje cell. *PF,* Parallel fiber. *SC,* Stellate cell.

Parallel fibers course through the dendrites of the Golgi, Purkinje, basket, and stellate cells along the length of the folium. Terminal branches of the climbing fibers are in the same plane as the Purkinje cells, as they wrap around the dendritic tree of the Purkinje cell. See text for details.

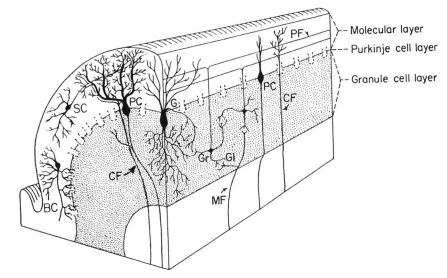

(Reproduced with permission from M. E. Anderson, The cerebellum. In *Textbook of Physiology*, Volume 1, 21st Edition. H. D. Patton, A. F. Fuchs, B. Hille, A. M. Scher, and R. Steiner, (Editors). W. B. Saunders Co. Philadelphia, 1989.)

the Purkinje cell is the final station for information processing at the level of the cerebellar cortex. This information passes to the cerebellar nuclei and, in the case of some Purkinje cells in the vestibulocerebellum, directly to vestibular nuclei. The principal *efferent system* of the cerebellum resides in the four pairs of *nuclei.*

MOSSY FIBER SYSTEM

The *mossy fiber projections* are, by far, the largest single type of input to the cerebellum. They account for all the input to the cerebellum except for the olivocerebellar climbing fibers. Mossy fibers carry information from a wide variety of sources: the *spinocerebellar pathways*, both the primary and secondary *vestibular afferents*; the brain stem *reticular formation*; and the pontocerebellar projections of the *cerebropontocerebellar system.*

Mossy fibers projecting to the vestibulocerebellum and the spinocerebellum immediately bifurcate and send one branch to the cerebellar nuclei. The other ascends to the granular layer of the cortex, where it branches profusely and synapses with the dendrites of 500 to 600 granule cells (see Figs. 17-8 and 17-10). Mossy fibers to the cerebrocerebellum, however, have only sparse projections to the cerebellar nuclei. Acetylcholine is the leading candidate for the primary neurotransmitter both at the excitatory synapses be-

tween the mossy fibers and the neurons in the cerebellar nuclei and at the excitatory mossy fiber–granule cell synapse. Because of the dense packing of granule cells in the granular layer, individual mossy fibers actually influence a very small area of the cortex.

Mossy fibers of different origins project to specific regions of the cerebellum. For example, *vestibular afferents project to the vestibulocerebellum and the fastigial nucleus, spinal afferents, to the spinocerebellum; and the globose and emboliform nuclei and the pontocerebellar fibers, to the cerebrocerebellum with sparse projections to the dentate nucleus.* Although nearly all mossy fibers synapsing with granule cells that project to the vestibulocerebellar and spinocerebellar areas send a branch to the cerebellar nuclei (the fastigial, globose, and emboliform nuclei), only a small number of those synapsing with granule cells that project to the cerebrocerebellum send a branch to the dentate nucleus.

Within each of these general categories is a well-organized pattern of projections. Although most vestibular afferents project to the vestibulocerebellum, a significant number terminate throughout the vermal or midline portion of the spinocerebellum. Within the *spinocerebellum*, several areas contain *somatotopic* representations of the *ipsilateral half of the body* (Fig. 17-12). The representations of these spinocerebellar afferents are not as discrete as the somatosensory

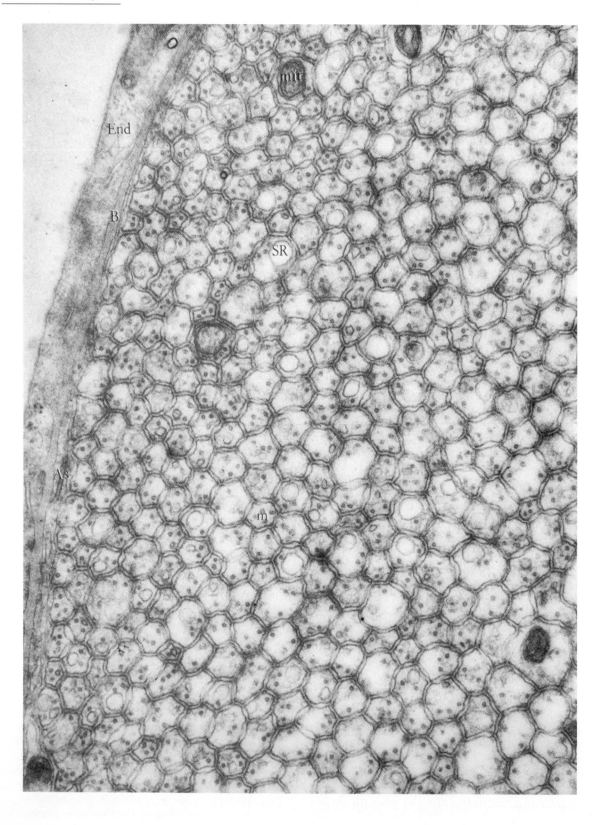

representations found in S-I. *Auditory afferents*, both from the cochlear nuclei and from A-1, terminate in a dorsal region of the vermis as do *visual afferents* from both the visual cortical areas and the superior colliculus (see Fig. 17–12). Purkinje cells responsive to either auditory or visual stimuli are most sensitive to information about the location and movement of the sound or object in space.

By far, the largest number of projections to the cerebellum are from the *cerebral cortex*, via the cerebropontocerebellar system. The greater representations are from the primary and secondary motor areas and the primary somatosensory area (Brodmann's areas 4 and 6 in the frontal lobe and areas 3, 1, 2, 5, and 7 in the parietal lobe). These cortical projections descend through the internal capsule and crus cerebri to the basal pons, where they synapse with pontine neurons that project to the contralateral cerebellar cortex, principally the *cerebrocerebellum*. Although generally considered to be a contralateral projection, there is a small ipsilateral pontocerebellar pathway.

CLIMBING FIBER SYSTEM

All *climbing fibers* are axons of neurons in the contralateral *inferior olivary nucleus* or nuclear complex, and all areas of the cerebellar cortex receive climbing fiber projections. A single climbing fiber may project to several adjacent lobules of the cerebellum; however, the projections are all within a very narrow parasagittal plane. In fact, *all the afferent systems that provide mossy fiber projections to the cerebellum (somatosensory, visual, auditory, vestibular, and corticopontocerebellar) also send afferents to the cerebellum by way of the inferior olivary nuclei and the climbing fiber system.* A precise topographic relation exists between parts of the inferior olivary nuclear complex and the cerebellar cortical area of termination of these *olivocerebellar climbing fibers*.

As climbing fibers enter the cerebellum, all except some projecting to the cerebrocerebellum give off a collateral branch to one of the cerebellar nuclei before entering the cortex where each climbing fiber divides into 10 to 15 terminal branches. *Each terminal branch then innervates a single Purkinje cell.* It branches, climbs, and wraps itself around the soma and dendrites of the Purkinje cell, much like a vine climbs a trellis. Each terminal branch often makes 300 to 500 individual synapses on a single Purkinje cell. *Each Purkinje cell, however, receives the input from only one climbing fiber* (Figs. 17–8, 17–10 and 17–13).

PURKINJE CELL EXCITATION BY PARALLEL AND CLIMBING FIBERS

Both the parallel fibers and the climbing fibers are excitatory. *Parallel fibers* (granule cell axons) use *glutamate* as their neurotransmitter. *Aspartate* is the most likely neurotransmitter candidate for the *climbing fibers* (axons of inferior olivary neurons). Stimulation of a parallel fiber produces a simple, monosynaptic, Na^+-dependent, excitatory postsynaptic potential (EPSP) on the Purkinje cell dendrite. This is a classic type of postsynaptic response, generating a small postsynaptic current that spreads passively. With the stimulation of additional parallel fibers, the post-synaptic potentials sum, spatially and temporally, resulting in the generation of a Purkinje cell action potential, *only* when the initial segment of the Purkinje cell axon reaches threshold.

The response of the Purkinje cell to climbing fiber stimulation is very different from the response to parallel fiber stimulation. Each single climbing fiber may have up to 500 individual synapses on the Purkinje cell. When the climbing fiber fires, there is a massive, synchronous depolarization of the Purkinje cell. This depolarization is sufficient to activate voltage-sensitive Ca^{++} channels in the dendritic membrane. *The channel activation generates an action potential in the*

FIGURE 17–11

An electron micrograph of parallel fibers in the molecular layer of the cerebellum ($\times$ 62,000). This field consists almost entirely of transversely sectioned axons of granule cells (parallel fibers). These axons are termed "parallel fibers" because of their remarkable regular arrangement.

This neuropil is unusual in that no neuroglial cell processes intervene between closely packed axons. Each axon contains a few microtubules (*m*), and some show profiles of smooth endoplasmic reticulum (*SR*). Where mitochondria (*mit*) occur, they almost fill the axon. Separating the axons from the endothelial cell (*End*) on the left are the neuroglial limiting membrane (*As*) and the basal lamina (*B*) that surround the parenchyma of the brain. (Reproduced with permission from A. Peters, S. L. Palay, and H. DeF. Webster, *The Fine Structure of the Nervous System*, 2nd Edition, W. B. Saunders Co., Philadelphia, 1976.)

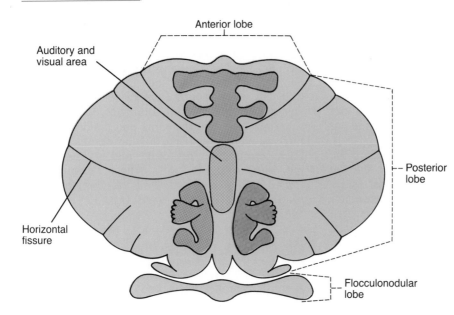

Auditory and visual area

Anterior lobe

Horizontal fissure

Posterior lobe

Flocculonodular lobe

FIGURE 17-12

Sensory representations in the cerebellar cortex. Auditory and visual afferents project to the central portion of the vermis, both rostral and caudal to the horizontal fissure.

Ipsilateral somatosensory information is present in two regions of the spinocerebellum. Representation in the anterior lobe spans both vermal and paravermal regions; representations in the posterior lobe are confined to the paravermal area. See text for details.

dendritic tree, an action potential that uses voltage-sensitive Ca^{++} channels for its propagation. The resultant depolarization of the Purkinje cell is large, attenuated, and complex. This attenuated depolarization from the dendritic-initiated action potential, in turn, generates a series of action potentials at the initial segment of the Purkinje cell axon. These initial-segment action potentials are the standard type of voltage-sensitive Na^+ channel–mediated action potentials.

Stimulation of the climbing fiber alters the responsiveness of the Purkinje cell to subsequent parallel fiber stimulation for periods of up to several hours. This alteration is a *depression* or reduction in Purkinje cell sensitivity to parallel fiber stimulation, an effect known as *long-term depression (LTD)*. Because the GABAergic Purkinje cells are inhibitory, the *LTD* of the Purkinje cells *dis-inhibits* neurons in the *cerebellar nuclei*, increasing their basal firing rate and rendering them more sensitive to other excitatory signals, i.e., collaterals from mossy fibers and climbing fibers.

The most significant consequence of the climbing fiber discharge is the entry of Ca^{++} into the Purkinje cell. This entry probably leads to a number of long-term responses, specifically ones produced by protein phosphorylation reactions. Ca^{++} influx stimulates, among other respones, calcium-calmodulin–dependent protein kinases, and it may trigger a cascade of second messenger –mediated molecular responses. Kinase activa-

tion and protein phosphorylation are leading candidates for the production of long-term changes in the behavior or sensitivity of the Purkinje cell during LTD.

MONOAMINERGIC AFFERENTS TO THE CEREBELLUM

The *monoaminergic projections* to the cerebellum originate from the *pontine raphe nuclei*, the *locus ceruleus*, and the *hypothalamus*. The raphe nuclei are the source of *serotoninergic* projections to both the granular and molecular layers. The *locus ceruleus* is the source of *noradrenergic* projections to all three layers of the cerebellar cortex. And the *dorsomedial nucleus* and the *dorsal* and *lateral areas* of the *hypothalamus* are the sources of *histaminergic* projections to all three layers of the cerebellar cortex.

All three monoaminergic projection systems are diffuse, with terminal axonal branches forming large plexuses within the cortex. The number of individual monoaminergic projections is relatively small, and a single fiber influences a large area of the cerebellar cortex. The serotoninergic and adrenergic projections probably modulate the overall level of cerebellar activity; however, the precise mechanisms are not understood. Both *noradrenergic* and *serotoninergic* fibers, for example, appear to inhibit Purkinje cells, suppressing their level of excitability to parallel fiber stimulation. However, other serotoninergic projections

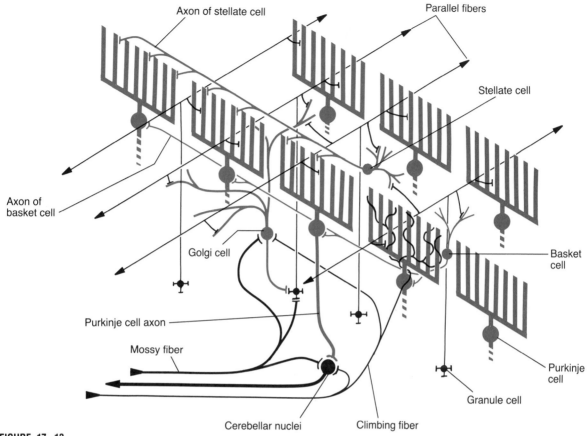

FIGURE 17–13

Some of the principal connections within the cerebellum. Excitatory neurons and their processes are in black; inhibitory neurons and their processes in red. Climbing fibers (olivocerebellar fibers) excite the Purkinje cells and send collaterals to the cerebellar nuclei and Golgi cells.

Mossy fibers both excite granule cells and send collaterals to the cerebellar nuclei and to the Golgi cells. Granule cells form parallel fibers and excite Purkinje cells. Granule cells are excited by mossy fibers and inhibited by Golgi cells. Golgi cells inhibit granule cells. Golgi cells are excited by climbing fibers, mossy fibers, and parallel fibers. Stellate cells and basket cells are excited by parallel fibers and inhibit Purkinje cells. See text for details.

facilitate the formation of complex spikes in Purkinje cells following climbing fiber stimulation. Because the hypothalamus is an important visceromotor center, the direct *histaminergic* projections from the hypothalamus may be associated with a coordination of somatomotor and visceromotor functions (see Chapter 18).

ROLE OF CEREBELLAR INTERNEURONS

All three of the cerebellar interneurons, *Golgi cells*, *basket cells*, and *stellate cells*, are inhibitory *GABAergic* neurons. However, some evidence exists that *taurine* may be the inhibitory neurotransmitter for some stellate cells. The *Golgi cells*

of the granular layer have an extensive dendritic tree that has processes in all three layers of the cortex. Incoming *mossy fibers* and *climbing fibers* as well as the *parallel fibers* of the molecular layer all have *excitatory synapses on the Golgi cell*. The *Golgi cell*, in turn, *inhibits granule cells*, thereby modulating neurotransmission in the mossy fiber–granule cell system (see Fig. 17–13).

Parallel fibers, in comparison, are the only excitatory input to both the *basket cells* and the *stellate cells*. Both cells are inhibitory to *Purkinje cells* and both have axonal processes that run transverse to the long axis of the folium, i.e., at right angles to the parallel fibers. The *basket cells* form axonal arbors or "baskets" around the soma and the initial axonal segment of Purkinje cells in the adjacent five to eight rows (see Figs. 17–8, 17–10 and 17–13). In contrast, the *stellate cells* form inhibitory synapses in the dendritic trees of the adjacent Purkinje cells (see Figs. 17–10 and 17–13). Because the inhibitory effect of both basket and stellate cells is principally lateral with reference to the parallel fibers, these interneurons may "sharpen" the signal generated by the Purkinje cells following their stimulation by a beam of parallel fibers. The same parallel fibers would simultaneously excite both the Purkinje cells and the inhibitory interneurons. The latter would then inhibit the Purkinje cells on either side of the row, an example of lateral inhibition. In addition, the inhibition of the Purkinje cells in the immediate vicinity of these interneurons is delayed by the duration of one synapse. Thus, the normal pattern of the Purkinje cell response to parallel fiber stimulation is an initial EPSP (monosynaptic excitation by parallel fibers) followed by an inhibitory postsynaptic potential (IPSP) (disynaptic inhibition by the interneurons) (see Fig. 17–13).

EFFERENT FIBERS FROM THE CEREBELLAR CORTEX

The Purkinje cells send inhibitory GABAergic projections to the *cerebellar nuclei*: the *fastigial, globose, emboliform,* and *dentate nuclei* (see Figs. 17–6 and 17–10). Some Purkinje cells in the vestibulocerebellum send axons directly to the vestibular nuclei, via the juxtarestiform body, completely bypassing the cerebellar nuclei. Except for these Purkinje cell axons, the principal efferent projections from the cerebellum to other areas of the CNS are from neurons in the *cerebellar nuclei.*

Although generally thought of as a homogeneous population of GABAergic neurons, the Purkinje cells may represent a very heterogenous population of cells. Many, if not all, Purkinje cells have a peptide co-transmitter. A large number of different peptides may be acting in this capacity. Neurochemical heterogeneity led to the discovery of functional diversities in the striatum, and the neurochemical heterogeneity within the cerebellum probably reflects a functional diversity yet to be defined.

Control of Movement

The principal connections between cells types in the cerebellar cortex is well defined as are the origins and terminations of the principal cerebellar afferents and efferents. Although we do not know how the cerebellum processes this information, several observations can be made about the functions of the cerebellum as a modulator of motor activity.

The *efferent pathways* from the cerebellum arise from the *cerebellar nuclei,* except for those direct projections from the Purkinje cells to the vestibular nuclei. In their "resting state," neurons of the cerebellar nuclei maintain a firing rate of about 20 to 30 action potentials per second. Cerebellar signals for the modulation of motor activity encode as changes in this firing rate.

Each of the three functional regions of the cerebellum influences a different parameter of motor function, and each uses different cerebellar nuclei. The *cerebrocerebellum* is involved in the *planning* and *initiation* of the motor action. These efferents exit from the *dentate nucleus* en route to the posterior division of the ventral lateral nucleus of the thalamus (VLp) and the cortical motor areas (see Fig. 17–6). The *spinocerebellum* oversees the actual *execution* and *coordination* of the motor event. These efferents exit from the *globose* and *emboliform nuclei* and project both to the motor cortex via VLp and to the red nucleus of the brain stem (see Fig. 17–6). The *vestibulocerebellum* functions during the execution of the motor activity to *maintain* and *adjust body posture.* These efferents arise from the *fastigial nucleus* and directly from the *Purkinje cells* in the cortex of the vestibulocerebellum. Efferents from the vestibulocerebellum project to both the vestibular nuclei and the motor nuclei of the brain stem reticular formation (see Fig. 17–6).

COORDINATED RESPONSE OF CEREBELLAR AREAS

A simple motor response to a command or signal, e.g., raising the arm and pointing the index finger of the hand toward a light bulb in response to the bulb being turned on is considered. As noted in Chapter 14, a "simple" motor act such as this triggers reflexes at all levels of the CNS, in addition to the primary motor signals traveling in the corticospinal tract. This motor task *also* involves all three areas of cerebellar function: (1) *initiation,* (2) *coordination,* and (3) *postural maintenance.*

From the point when the stimulus signal (the light) comes on until the motor act ends, there is a closely timed sequence of cerebellar events, especially apparent in the cerebellar nuclei. *Im-*

mediately following the light signal, a change occurs in the rate of firing of neurons in the *dentate nucleus*. This change is followed immediately by changes in the firing pattern of neurons in the premotor and motor cortical areas. All these changes occur *prior* to the actual motor event, the firing of lower motor neurons and muscle contraction. The maximal changes in firing patterns of neurons in the *globose* and *emboliform nuclei* are *coincident with the onset of muscle contraction* and continue until the termination of the motor action.

INITIATION AND PLANNING

This sequence of events supports the hypothesis that the *cerebrocerebellum* is the *initiator* of the motor response. Signals from cerebral cortical areas enter the cerebellum, are processed in the cerebrocerebellum, and exit the cerebellum through the dentate nucleus en route to VLp and the motor cortical areas. The cerebellar excitation of the motor cortical areas results in the onset of the actual motor event via the descending corticospinal system. Individuals with selective damage to cerebrocerebellar structures have problems initiating and terminating motor actions.

COORDINATION AND EXECUTION

The subsequent muscle activity and extremity movements generate afferent signals. Many of these enter the cerebellum via the spinocerebellar pathways and the mossy fiber system, projecting principally to the *spinocerebellum* and the *globose* and *emboliform nuclei*. These afferent signals trigger cerebellar efferents from the globose and emboliform nuclei that, acting through both the motor cortical areas and the red nucleus, modulate the motor activity *once it is initiated*, leading to a smooth *coordinated execution* of the motor task (see Fig. 17–6). Individuals with selective damage to spinocerebellar structures have poor motor coordination. Their movements are jerky, and pronounced kinetic (intention) tremor is evident (see subsequent discussion).

POSTURAL BALANCE AND EQUILIBRIUM

When the arm moves forward in space, the body's center of gravity changes. Afferents associated with these changes enter the *vestibulocerebellum*. The vestibulocerebellum sends efferents via the *fastigial nucleus* and directly from the *Purkinje cells* to the vestibular nuclei and the nuclei of the brain stem reticular formation.

These cerebellar efferents modulate the descending vestibulospinal and reticulospinal systems, two systems that are constantly *maintaining* and *adjusting body posture*.

Motor Plasticity and Learning

The *learning* of complex motor tasks and sequences along with *motor plasticity* are two functions that involve the *olivocerebellar climbing fiber system*. The word learning, as used here, refers to the ability to modify motor responses or sequences in order to adapt the responses to a new situation or changes in surrounding conditions. As discussed in the preceding chapters, much of somatic motor function is semiautomatic. We do not consciously "think" about all the motor movements involved when we reach for an object. Our only conscious, volitional decision is to reach for the object. The remaining details of the motor event are preprogrammed, i.e., we do not "consciously" extend each finger to grasp the object or consciously adjust the tone in postural muscles to maintain balance. Many of these are *reflex responses* and many are preprogrammed in *central pattern generators (CPGs)*. However, motor actions are normally very plastic and adaptable to change. If, for example, the object we are reaching for suddenly moves, we "automatically" and smoothly readjust our movements to the new situation.

A major component of this plasticity resides in the cerebellum and the *olivocerebellar climbing fiber system*. Selective damage to this system results both in a loss of the ability to modify a motor response and the ability to maintain or "store" a modified response.

The inferior olivary nuclei receive afferents from the motor cortical areas and project to the entire cerebellar cortex. Although firing at a slow rate, one to two action potentials per second, the resultant complex spikes generated in the Purkinje cells depress the sensitivity of the Purkinje cells to future parallel fiber stimulation. This depression of sensitivity, LTD, decreases the Purkinje cell inhibition of neurons in the cerebellar nuclei, i.e., it dis-inhibits neurons in the cerebellar nuclei.

Although the mechanisms responsible for adaptive motor behavior remain largely hypothetical and the site of "motor memory storage" is equally vague, it is clear that *the cerebellum and the climbing fiber system are essential for both the induction of changes and the later storage of these changes*. The molecular and cellular mechanisms associated with motor learning and motor plasticity probably reside in the Purkinje cell. Some hypotheses suggest that the Ca^{++} influx from complex spike generation triggers a chain of intracellular events, from short term modifications in receptor and/or ion channel sensitivity via protein phosphorylation to longer more permanent alterations in synaptic efficiency.

MODIFICATION OF THE STRETCH REFLEX

Adaptive changes in the stretch reflex are examples of motor plasticity. During the stretch of a muscle, signals from the primary and secondary afferents in the muscle spindles trigger an increase in muscle tone that is proportional to the amount of stretch, the stretch reflex. As with other reflexes, this is also subject to modulation by higher centers and the afferent signals project to both the cerebellum and the cerebrum. Cerebellar afferents enter the spinocerebellum as mossy fiber afferents from the spinocerebellar pathways. Afferents to the cerebrum travel in the medial lemniscus to the ventral posterosuperior nucleus (VPS) of the dorsal thalamus and from there to the cortex. Signals from the cerebral cortex, prompted by stretch reflex afferents, project to the cerebellum via the inferior olivary nuclei and the climbing fiber system. These are the signals responsible for the adaptive changes.

Dorsiflexion of the foot stretches both the gastrocnemius and soleus muscles. This dorsiflexion elicits a stretch reflex, with the increased tension of the two muscles tending to return the foot to the original position. For example, when an individual, standing upright with feet together, leans forward without bending at the waist, dorsiflexion of the feet and elicitation of a stretch reflex contraction of the gastrocnemius and soleus muscles occur. This reflex contraction tends to plantar flex the feet and is partially responsible for restoring the body to its original vertical position.

When the dorsiflexion is produced by tilting the floor and not the body, the reflex causes the individual to fall backward. If there is a repeated tilting of the floor, such as one would encounter on the deck of a ship in a rolling sea, there would be repeated sequences of dorsiflexion of the feet. With repeated stretching of the muscles, the stretch reflex response becomes diminished, i.e., it becomes altered to meet the current environmental circumstances (the repetitious rolling of the boat). Once the individual leaves the boat and steps on land, there is a period of minimal instability in balance until the stretch reflex re-adapts to the original environment. Individuals with cerebellar disorders do not exhibit this reflex plasticity. With continued exposure to a tilting deck, there is little or no adaptation of the stretch reflex response. This same principle applies to other reflexes as well.

Disorders of Motor Function

Damage to the cerebellum produces a variety of motor disturbances. Depending on the location and extent of the insult, these occur singly or in combination. Most cerebellar disorders lead to the abnormal performance of the motor task rather than to a loss of motor function or a paresis.

CLASSIC SIGNS OF CEREBELLAR DAMAGE

The symptoms of cerebellar damage can be grouped into six general categories. Depending on the extent of the cerebellar damage, individual patients may have one symptom or a combination of these symptoms. In all cases, symptoms from unilateral damage appear on the side ipsilateral to the cerebellar damage. Ascending spinocerebellar pathways are uncrossed, and descending corticopontocerebellar fibers are crossed. Thus, motor deficits from *cerebellar* damage are *ipsilateral* to the lesion, whereas motor deficits from damage to motor areas of the *cerebral cortex* are *contralateral* to the lesion.

The six categories of symptoms are (1) *postural instability*; (2) *delayed initiation and termination of motor actions*; (3) *inability to perform continuous, repetitive movements*; (4) *errors in the smoothness and direction of a movement*; (5) *lack of coordination or synergy of movement, especially complex movements*; and (6) *lack of motor plasticity or motor learning*.

Postural Instability

One symptom of cerebellar damage is *postural instability*, both *static* (while standing) and *dynamic* (during a movement such as walking). The postural instabilities indicate damage to the *vestibulocerebellum*. The patient is unable to maintain portions or all of the body (limbs, trunk, head, and eyes) in a stable, steady position. *Static postural instability* is most evident when the patient is asked to stand with the arm raised and eyes closed. With removal of the visual cues, the patient's body will sway and the arms will oscillate. *Dynamic postural instability* is apparent during walking. The patient will have a characteristic *cerebellar ataxia* consisting of a spread or broadened stance, with difficulty in walking a straight line. The individual staggers and has a very irregular gait, similar to that of someone who is drunk. Additional problems with gait occur if the involvement extends to the spinocerebellum and cerebrocerebellum (see the following discussion).

Delayed Initiation and Termination of Motor Actions

Both *initiation* and *termination of movement* utilize the same neurological mechanism, and in one sense both are "initiation" mechanisms. The first initiates the beginning of the motor task; the second initiates the conclusion of the motor task. Both initiation and termination of movement are problems when damage occurs in the lateral or *cerebrocerebellum*. On command, the patient is slow to initiate a movement and once a movement has begun, the patient is equally prone to overreach a target or to be otherwise tardy in the termination of the movement. This problem is often manifest in the gait. When asked to walk across the room, the patient is slow to respond (initiation). Once the walking has begun, the patient often has a problem stopping (termination). In the more severe case, the patient will continue to accelerate and has to be physically stopped.

Another example of the inability to terminate a movement is illustrated by having the patient extend the arm, with the forearm flexed at a right angle to the upper arm and parallel to the chest. The examiner then asks the patient to resist the examiner's efforts to straighten the forearm. When the examiner suddenly releases the forearm, it evokes an unchecked flexion of the forearm with the hand or wrist striking the patient's chest. This excessive overreach or *rebound* of the arm represents a lack of coordination between antagonistic muscles and an inability to terminate a motor action, i.e., applying resistance to the examiner's pressure on the forearm.

Inability to Perform Continuous, Repetitive Movements

The term *dysdiadochokinesis* describes the clinical condition in which a patient is unable to perform a series of rapid alternating movements.

The Greek word *diadoch* means taking turns or alternating; hence, the term, *dys-diadocho-kinesis* means a malfunction (*dys-*) of alternating (*diadocho*) movement (*-kinesis*). One test for this condition is to have the patient rapidly tap one hand with the other, while alternating the position of the palmar and dorsal surfaces of the hand being tapped. When there is damage to the cerebellar hemisphere, the individual will have difficulty performing this task rapidly. The pronation or supination is often incomplete, or the tapping may be asynchronous with the rotation of the hand. The longer the exercise continues, the worse the performance. *Dysrhythmokinesis* is a related condition in which the patient is unable to maintain a rhythmic pattern of alternating movements.

Errors in Smoothness And Direction of Movement

Related to cerebellar abnormalities in motor function are several forms of *dysmetria*, a patient's inability to "target" an object. When reaching for an object, the patient often *overreaches or underreaches the target*. A good test is to have the patient move the index finger from the tip of the nose to the extended index finger of the examiner and back to the nose again. As the finger approaches the target, there are oscillations and irregularities in the movement as the finger overreaches and underreaches the target. These movement oscillations become increasingly large as the finger nears the target, producing a *kinetic tremor* (*intention tremor*).

Lack of Coordination or Synergy of Movement

The lack of coordination of movement is most apparent during *complex movements*. Complex movements involve rotation, or movement of more than one joint. Reaching for an object is a complex movement because it involves motion at the shoulder, elbow, wrist, and metacarpal joints. Normally, such a sequence proceeds in a coordinated and synchronized manner resulting in a smooth, directed movement. With cerebellar lesions, the movements at the different joints become out of phase. They lack synergy and may take on a step-like pattern. *Decomposition of movement* is the descriptive term often applied to this asynchronous separation of complex movements into their components.

Lack of Motor Plasticity or Motor Learning

The *olivocerebellar climbing fiber system* is integral to motor plasticity and modification of motor responses, such as reflexes. Damage to either the inferior olivary nuclei or their projection fibers will result in a loss of ability to adapt to changing conditions. If we use the same example of the modification of the stretch reflex of the soleus and gastrocnemius muscles during the rolling of a boat, the patient with damage to this system will be unable to adapt to these changing conditions or will do so very slowly. This loss of plasticity also can result from brain stem damage involving the inferior olivary nuclei and not the cerebellum itself.

SUGGESTED READING

Ito, M. (1984). *The Cerebellum and Neural Control.* Raven Press, New York.

This comprehensive monograph reviews the role of the cerebellum in the modulation of motor activity. An extensive discussion is provided of the comparative anatomical and comparative physiological aspects of cerebellar function. A comprehensive bibliography is also included.

King, J. S. (Editor) (1987). *New Concepts in Cerebellar Neurobiology.* Alan R. Liss, Inc., New York.

Review articles are given that present a number of the more recent advances in the study of the cerebellum. Many of these articles represent presentations at a symposium of the Cajal Club organized by the editor of this volume.

Strata, P. (Editor) (1989). *The Olivocerebellar System in Motor Control.* Springer-Verlag, Berlin.

This volume of the Experimental Brain Research Series is devoted to the olivocerebellar system. Anatomical, physiological, biochemical, and behavioral studies are included. This system has captured the imagination of many neurobiologists, with its potential for the study of learning and memory mechanisms.

Chapter

18

Autonomic Nervous System and Hypothalamus

Definitions and General Organization

Motor components of the nervous system fall into two categories: the *somatic motor system* or *voluntary motor system* (Chapters 14 through 17) and the *autonomic nervous system* or *visceral motor system*. The word *autonomic* is from the Greek *autonomos*, meaning *independent*. The *autonomic nervous system* is the motor component that innervates the visceral organs, the glands, and the cardiovascular system. This part of the nervous system functions primarily in a reflex manner, i.e., it is *autonomous* or *independent* of voluntary control.

GENERAL VISCERAL EFFERENT (GVE)

The *general visceral efferent* (*GVE*) component of the spinal and cranial nerves represents the efferent outflow from the central nervous system (CNS) of the *autonomic nervous system*. The other visceral efferent component, the *special visceral efferent (SVE)*, innervates the striated muscle of branchial or pharyngeal arch origin and is part of the voluntary motor system and not of the autonomic nervous system.

Several distinct anatomical differences exist between the autonomic and somatic motor systems. In the *somatic motor system*, the target organs (striated muscles) receive direct innervation from *lower motor neurons* with cell bodies that lie *within the central nervous system (CNS)*. *In the autonomic nervous system*, the motor innervation of the target organs consists of a *two-neuron chain*, a *preganglionic neuron* with its cell body *within the CNS* and its axon projecting to a *peripheral ganglion* containing the *postganglionic neuron*. The axon of the *postganglionic neuron innervates the target organ* (Fig. 18–1).

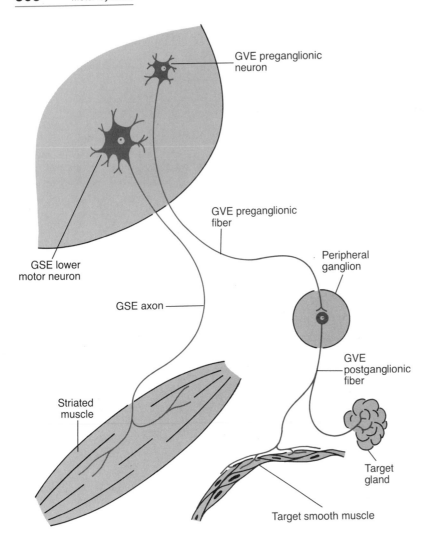

GVE preganglionic neuron

GSE lower motor neuron

GVE preganglionic fiber

GSE axon

Peripheral ganglion

GVE postganglionic fiber

Striated muscle

Target gland

Target smooth muscle

FIGURE 18-1

Basic differences between the visceromotor system (GVE) and the somatomotor system (GSE). The GSE's lower motor neurons in the central nervous system (CNS) innervate target striated muscle directly. GVE neurons in the CNS are preganglionic, exit the CNS, and synapse in a peripheral ganglion. Postganglionic fibers from neurons in the ganglion innervate the target tissue, usually smooth muscle or glandular. GVE, general visceral efferent; GSE, general somatic efferent.

TARGET ORGANS

In the somatic motor system, a specialized motor end plate is located on each striated muscle fiber. Each fiber contracts in response to the stimulation of only that end plate. In the visceral motor system, smooth and cardiac muscle fibers lack the specialization of a motor end plate and the individual muscle fibers often are coupled electrically. Hence, the stimulus applied to one smooth muscle fiber spreads to those adjacent fibers with which it is electrically coupled. This junction between smooth muscle fibers is a *nexus*. The direct electrical coupling between cardiac muscle fibers is an *intercalated disc*.

In the *heart*, for example, the conduction system is composed of modified cardiac muscle fibers, e.g., the nodes, the bundle of His, and the Purkinje fibers. These modified fibers couple directly to the contractile cardiac muscle fibers via tight junctions. The degree of "networking" of *smooth muscle cells* varies with the target organ. Other autonomic innervations are glandular, and the release of the neurotransmitter by the postganglionic neuron stimulates the secretory process. Sometimes, actual contractile elements (smooth muscle or myoepithelial cells) facilitate the glandular secretion. In others, changes in the blood flow (vasoconstriction or vasodilation) modulate the secretory state of the gland.

SYMPATHETIC AND PARASYMPATHETIC DIVISIONS

Two anatomically and neurochemically distinct divisions occur within the autonomic nervous system, the *sympathetic* and *parasympathetic divisions*. Also, when an organ or organ system receives innervation from both divisions, the physiological effects are antagonistic—sympathetic stimulation increases the heart rate, and parasympathetic stimulation decreases it.

In the sympathetic division, the *preganglionic sympathetic neurons* are in the *thoracic* and *lumbar* levels (T-1 through L-3) of the *spinal cord* and are the source of the GVE component in the thoracic and lumbar spinal nerves. Axons from these preganglionic neurons project to the *sympathetic ganglia*, which contain the *postganglionic sympathetic neurons*. Axons from the postganglionic neurons then innervate the target organs (Figs. 18–2 and 18–3). *Acetylcholine (ACh)* is the principal neurotransmitter for the preganglionic neurons, and *norepinephrine (NE)* is the neurotransmitter for *most* of the postganglionic neurons in the sympathetic division. Because of the location of the preganglionic neurons and the postganglionic neurotransmitter, the sympathetic division also is known as the *thoracolumbar division* or the *adrenergic division* of the autonomic nervous system.

In contrast, the *preganglionic parasympathetic neurons* are either in the *brain stem* or in the *sacral levels* of the *spinal cord*. They are the source of the GVE component in cranial and sacral nerves. The preganglionic neurons project to the *parasympathetic ganglia* that contain the *postganglionic parasympathetic neurons*. These ganglia lie adjacent to or within the substance of the target organ; hence, axons of the postganglionic parasympathetic neurons are relatively short (Fig. 18–4). *Acetylcholine (ACh)* is the principal neurotransmitter for *both* the preganglionic and postganglionic neurons of the parasympathetic division. Because of these features, the parasympathetic division also is known as the *craniosacral division* or the *cholinergic division*.

Both the parasympathetic and the sympathetic ganglia are more than simple relay stations. Many of these ganglia contain small interneurons, and most receive collaterals from visceral afferent signals that are en route to the spinal cord. One population of interneurons, the *small intensely fluorescent (SIF) cells*, are dopaminergic. When stimulated, they generate inhibitory postsynaptic potentials (IPSPs) on the postganglionic autonomic neuron. Hence, a significant

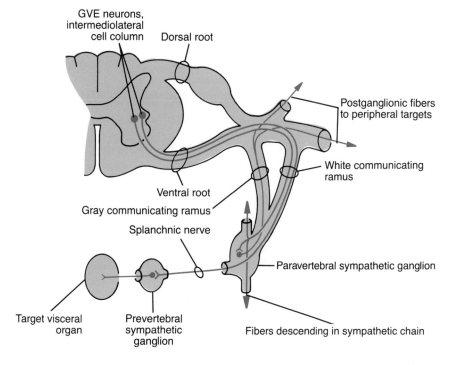

FIGURE 18–2

The thoracic spinal cord and the general visceral efferent (GVE) components. Preganglionic neurons from the intermediolateral cell column exit with the ventral root and form the white communicating ramus. Some of these preganglionic fibers synapse in a paravertebral ganglion. Others pass through the paravertebral ganglion and synapse in a prevertebral ganglion.

Postganglionic fibers from the paravertebral ganglion form the gray communicating ramus and distribute to peripheral targets as a component of the mixed spinal nerve. Postganglionic fibers from the prevertebral ganglion innervate visceral target organs.

GVE neurons, intermediolateral cell column

Dorsal root

Postganglionic fibers to peripheral targets

White communicating ramus

Ventral root

Gray communicating ramus

Splanchnic nerve

Paravertebral sympathetic ganglion

Target visceral organ

Prevertebral sympathetic ganglion

Fibers descending in sympathetic chain

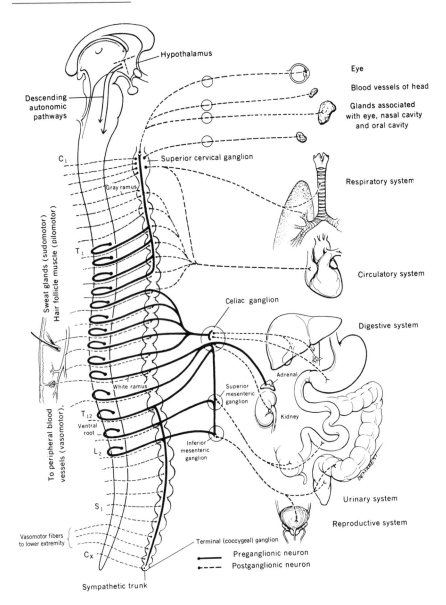

Hypothalamus

Descending
autonomic
pathways

C₁

Gray ramus

Sweat glands (sudomotor)
Hair follicle muscle (pilomotor),

T₁

Celiac ganglion

White ramus

Superior
mesenteric
ganglion

To peripheral blood
vessels (vasomotor),

T₁₂
Ventral
root

L₂

Inferior
mesenteric
ganglion

S₁

Vasomotor fibers
to lower extremity

Cₓ

Terminal (coccygeal) ganglion

Sympathetic trunk

Superior cervical ganglion

Adrenal

Kidney

Eye

Blood vessels of head

Glands associated
with eye, nasal cavity
and oral cavity

Respiratory system

Circulatory system

Digestive system

Urinary system

Reproductive system

———— Preganglionic neuron
- - - - - Postganglionic neuron

FIGURE 18-3

The sympathetic division of the autonomic nervous system. The preganglionic neurons are cholinergic; most of the postganglionic neurons are adrenergic.

The white communicating rami (preganglionic fibers) are limited to spinal levels T-1 through L-2 (illustrated) or L-3. The gray communicating rami (postganglionic fibers) are present at all spinal levels. (Reproduced with permission from C. R. Noback, and R. J. Demarest, *The Human Nervous System*, 3rd Edition, McGraw-Hill, New York, 1984.)

amount of modulation of neuronal activity occurs in the peripheral ganglia and plexuses of the autonomic nervous system.

Although *ACh* and *NE* are the primary neurotransmitters for *most* of the preganglionic and postganglionic neurons in the autonomic nervous system, they do *not* operate alone. Many different co-transmitters are present in these neurons, and some may utilize an alternate neurotransmitter as the primary transmitter. This factor is especially true for the innervation of the gastrointestinal tract by the enteric nervous system, in which

numerous peptides and other neurotransmitters are present.

ENTERIC NERVOUS SYSTEM

Another "subdivision" within the autonomic nervous system is the *enteric nervous system*—that portion of the autonomic nervous system innervating the gastrointestinal tract. *The enteric nervous system* (located within the substance of the gastrointestinal tract) *contains parasympathetic*

FIGURE 18-4

The parasympathetic division of the autonomic nervous system. The preganglionic neurons and the postganglionic neurons are cholinergic. Preganglionic fibers exit from the brain stem with cranial nerves III, VII, IX, and X and from the sacral levels of the spinal cord. (Reproduced with permission from C. R. Noback, and R. J. Demarest, *The Human Nervous System*, 3rd Edition, McGraw-Hill, New York, 1984.)

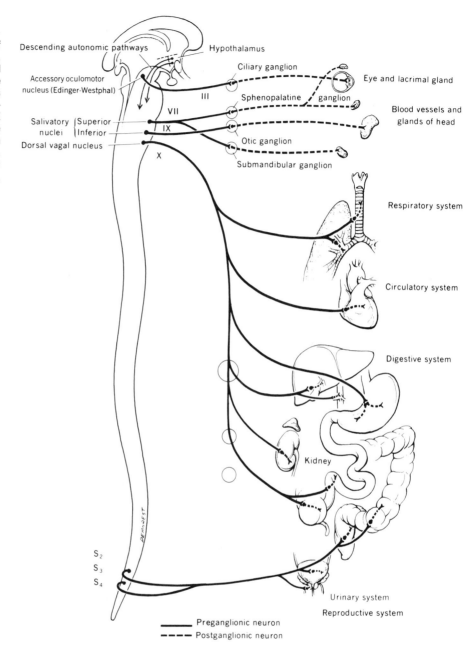

preganglionic fibers, sympathetic postganglionic fibers, and parasympathetic postganglionic neurons. In addition to these visceromotor components are many sensory neurons and interneurons.

The normal driving *efferent components* of the enteric nervous system are the *parasympathetic* and *sympathetic* neurons, and therefore it is a part of the *autonomic nervous system*. However, the enteric nervous system contains a large number of interneurons and visceral afferent neurons. Extensive interconnections occur between all the elements. The enteric nervous system has the capability of functioning by reflex, independent of its connections with the CNS. It therefore warrants separate consideration (see subsequent discussion).

SPINAL CORD AND BRAIN STEM REGULATION

A *hierarchy of regulation* exists within the autonomic nervous system. Nearly all autonomic functions respond to *spinal* and *lower brain stem reflexes*, in a manner similar to that of the somatic motor system. The *brain stem* contains the *centers* responsible for generating the rhythmic patterns of activity associated with visceral functions, such as heart beat. These centers are similar, conceptually, to the central pattern generators (CPGs) of the somatic motor system. The *hypothalamus*, however, is the principal integration center and regulator of autonomic function in the CNS. It is through the hypothalamus that the *limbic system* and the areas of the *neocortex* influence autonomic function. In addition to cortical and limbic afferents, the hypothalamus functions as a *sensory transducer*. Specific hypothalamic neurons are sensitive to changes in body temperature and serum osmolality. The hypothalamus also receives afferent information from the principal ascending sensory pathways.

Hypothalamic regulation of autonomic function occurs in two primary ways, *neuroanatomical* and *neurohumoral*. The hypothalamus is the origin of direct and indirect *descending pathways* to the autonomic centers and nuclei in the brain stem and spinal cord. The *neurohumoral regulation* is through the direct production and release of neurohormones (*oxytocin* and *vasopressin*) by the *magnocellular neurosecretory system*, and through the indirect regulation of the adenohypophysis via the production and release of *hypothalamic hypophysiotropic hormones* (*HHHs*) by the *parvocellular neurosecretory system*. Specific hypothalamic neurons produce and secrete HHHs in response to neuronal and humoral stimuli. The HHHs enter the hypothalamic hypophysial portal system (specialized vascular channels linking the hypothalamus and adenohypophysis). Once in the adenohypophysis, these humoral messengers selectively activate or inhibit the production of pituitary hormones.

Sympathetic Division

PREGANGLIONIC NEURONS

The cell bodies of the *preganglionic sympathetic neurons* are in the *intermediolateral cell column* of the *spinal cord*. The intermediolateral cell column usually extends from *T-1* through *L-3*, although some individual variation may occur (see Fig. 18–2 and Figs. 6–10 and 6–11). Axons from these preganglionic sympathetic neurons exit the spinal cord in the ventral root in the company of the somatic efferent neurons. These preganglionic fibers then leave the spinal nerve, form the *white communicating ramus* and enter the *paravertebral sympathetic chain*. They either synapse in the sympathetic chain or pass through the chain, forming a *splanchnic nerve* en route to one of the *prevertebral sympathetic ganglia* (see Figs. 18–2 and 18–3).

Immediately adjacent to the intermediolateral cell column and extending through the same spinal segments is a functionally related nuclear group, the *intermediomedial cell column*. Neurons in this column are essential for *visceromotor reflexes*; however, they are not the origin of preganglionic efferent fibers. These neurons function as interneurons that integrate visceral and somatic afferent signals and, in turn, modulate the responsiveness of preganglionic neurons in the intermediolateral cell column.

SYMPATHETIC GANGLIA

The two groups of sympathetic ganglia are the *paired paravertebral sympathetic chains* and the *prevertebral ganglia*. The paravertebral ganglia differentiate from the early neural crest, and initially there is a single pair of ganglia for each spinal segment. With later development a number of these fuse, especially in the cervical and sacral levels. Thus, the normal adult pattern consists of three cervical ganglia, 12 thoracic ganglia, four to five lumbar ganglia, and a variable number of sacral ganglia. The preganglionic fibers enter the chain via the white communicating rami from thoracic and lumbar levels only. Those from upper thoracic levels ascend to the cervical ganglia; those from lumbar levels descend to the sacral ganglia. Other preganglionic fibers ascend or descend one or more segments within the sympathetic chain before synapsing. These ascending and descending preganglionic fibers link the ganglia together into a chain-like structure that runs from the upper cervical regions to the coccyx (Fig. 18–5).

The *prevertebral ganglia* also differentiate from neural crest material. However, these differentiating neuroblasts migrate toward the developing mesentery and descending aorta in the embryonic abdominal cavity. Preganglionic fibers pass through the paravertebral sympathetic chain and enter the extensive plexuses formed around the

FIGURE 18-5

The paravertebral sympathetic chain and the principal prevertebral ganglia. Preganglionic fibers to the prevertebral ganglia (splanchnic nerves and branches from the lumbar ganglia) are illustrated. The extensive sympathetic and parasympathetic plexuses on the aorta, esophagus, and trachea are omitted.

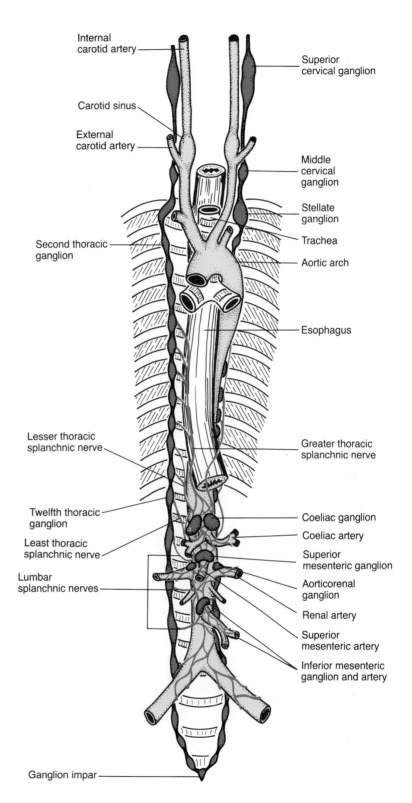

Internal carotid artery

Carotid sinus

External carotid artery

Second thoracic ganglion

Lesser thoracic splanchnic nerve

Twelfth thoracic ganglion

Least thoracic splanchnic nerve

Lumbar splanchnic nerves

Ganglion impar

Superior cervical ganglion

Middle cervical ganglion

Stellate ganglion

Trachea

Aortic arch

Esophagus

Greater thoracic splanchnic nerve

Coeliac ganglion

Coeliac artery

Superior mesenteric ganglion

Aorticorenal ganglion

Renal artery

Superior mesenteric artery

Inferior mesenteric ganglion and artery

abdominal aorta and its primary branches. Within these plexuses, developing neuroblasts aggregate and form the prevertebral ganglia. A number of these are readily identifiable. However, many small clusters of ganglionic neurons are spread throughout the extensive abdominal plexuses. Some of the more prominent ganglia found in the adult are the *celiac, aorticorenal, superior mesenteric,* and *inferior mesenteric ganglia* (see Figs. 18–3 and 18–5).

SYMPATHETIC CHAIN

The *superior cervical ganglion,* the largest and most rostral of the sympathetic ganglia, is at the level of the second and third cervical vertebrae, between the internal carotid artery and the internal jugular vein and in front of the prevertebral musculature. Postganglionic fibers from the superior cervical ganglion form the *internal* and *external carotid nerves.* These nerves form extensive plexuses over the surface of the internal and external carotid arteries, the *internal* and *external carotid plexuses.* These sympathetic nerve plexuses course with the arteries and their terminal branches throughout the head. Some of these postganglionic fibers reach their target organ or tissue with the arterial supply, others leave the blood vessel and join a distal branch of one of the cranial nerves (Fig. 18–6). Other fibers from the superior cervical ganglion form the small *superior cervical cardiac nerve.* Additional, but smaller, branches from this ganglion join the glossopharyngeal, vagus, and hypoglossal nerves. The superior cervical ganglion also gives off gray communicating rami to the uppermost two to four cervical spinal nerves (see Figs. 18–3 and 18–5).

The *middle cervical ganglion,* the smallest of the cervical sympathetic ganglia, is at the level of the cricoid cartilage. Postganglionic fibers innervate the cervical region, upper extremity, and heart. These innervations include several gray communicating rami to cervical nerves and the very small *middle cervical cardiac nerve* (see Figs. 18–3 and 18–5).

The *inferior cervical ganglion* is at the level of the seventh cervical vertebra and usually fuses with the first thoracic ganglion. The large ganglion, formed from the fusion, is the *stellate (cervicothoracic) ganglion.* Postganglionic fibers from the stellate ganglion also innervate the cervical region, head, heart, and upper extremity. These innervations include the *inferior cardiac nerve* and the gray communicating rami to the

lower cervical and upper thoracic spinal nerves (see Figs. 18–3 and 18–5).

All the *thoracic sympathetic ganglia* have both white and gray communicating rami. All receive preganglionic fibers from the thoracic spinal cord, and all contribute postganglionic fibers to each of the thoracic spinal nerves. Many of the preganglionic fibers entering the chain from the first two or three thoracic spinal levels ascend to the cervical ganglia, which in turn innervate the head, neck, and upper extremity.

Each thoracic ganglion forms a gray communicating ramus and provides sympathetic innervation to the area supplied by that spinal nerve. In addition, other postganglionic fibers contribute to the *cardiac plexus,* the *pulmonary plexus,* and the *esophageal plexus.* In all three plexuses, the postganglionic fibers mix with preganglionic parasympathetic fibers from the vagus nerve to provide the combined sympathetic and parasympathetic innervation of the viscera.

The *lumbar* and *sacral levels* of the sympathetic chain provide the sympathetic innervation to the pelvic viscera. The number of ganglia present varies owing to the fusion of some ganglia during development. At the first two or three lumbar levels, the sympathetic chain has both gray and white communicating rami. Lower lumbar and all sacral levels of the chain have only the gray communicating rami, the postganglionic fibers entering the spinal segmental nerves. As the two chains reach lower sacral levels, they merge into a common ganglion at the most caudal level of the sympathetic chain, the *ganglion impar* or the *coccygeal ganglion* (see Fig. 18–5).

SPLANCHNIC NERVES AND PREVERTEBRAL GANGLIA

A large number of thoracic preganglionic fibers pass through the sympathetic chain without synapsing and form the *thoracic splanchnic nerves.* Preganglionic contributions from T-5 through T-9 form the *greater thoracic splanchnic nerve.* The greater thoracic splanchnic nerve also contains some postganglionic fibers that leave the nerve in the chest cavity to innervate the esophagus, aorta, and thoracic duct. The remainder, principally preganglionic fibers, pass through the diaphragm en route to the pair of midline *celiac ganglia,* one on each side of the origin of the *celiac artery.* The *lesser thoracic splanchnic nerve,* arising from T-10 and T-11, and the *least thoracic splanchnic nerve,* from T-12, follow a similar course through the diaphragm, ending in the

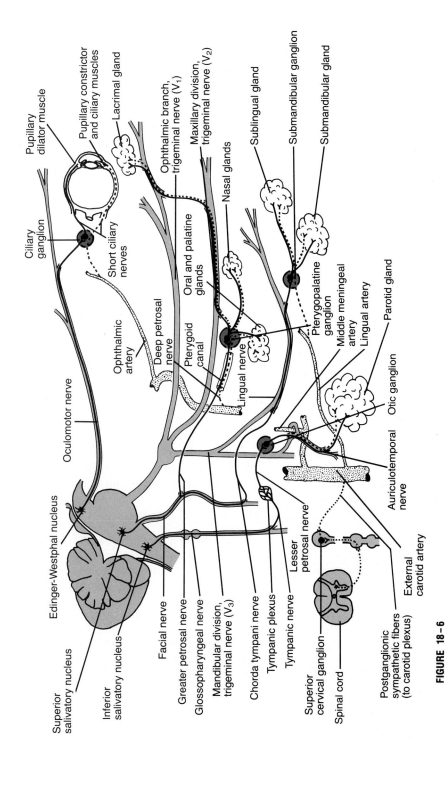

Superior salivatory nucleus

Inferior salivatory nucleus

Edinger-Westphal nucleus

Oculomotor nerve

Ciliary ganglion

Pupillary dilator muscle

Pupillary constrictor and ciliary muscles

Lacrimal gland

Short ciliary nerves

Ophthalmic branch, trigeminal nerve (V$_1$)

Maxillary division, trigeminal nerve (V$_2$)

Ophthalmic artery

Deep petrosal nerve

Pterygoid canal

Oral and palatine glands

Nasal glands

Lingual nerve

Sublingual gland

Submandibular ganglion

Submandibular gland

Pterygopalatine ganglion

Middle meningeal artery

Lingual artery

Parotid gland

Otic ganglion

Auriculotemporal nerve

External carotid artery

Facial nerve

Greater petrosal nerve

Glossopharyngeal nerve

Mandibular division, trigeminal nerve (V$_3$)

Chorda tympani nerve

Tympanic plexus

Tympanic nerve

Lesser petrosal nerve

Superior cervical ganglion

Spinal cord

Postganglionic sympathetic fibers (to carotid plexus)

FIGURE 18–6

The autonomic innervation of the head. Parasympathetic preganglionic fibers leave the brain stem via the oculomotor, facial, and glossopharyngeal nerves. Sympathetic postganglionic fibers enter the head as components of the carotid plexus and distribute to target organs either with the arterial supply or by joining a branch of one of the cranial nerves. Parasympathetic fibers are solid lines, sympathetic fibers are dashed. See text for details.

375

celiac ganglia, the *aorticorenal ganglia* (at the origin of the renal arteries), or the *superior mesenteric ganglion* (at the origin of the superior mesenteric artery) (see Figs. 18–3 and 18–5). Some of these preganglionic fibers also pass through the prevertebral ganglia and enter the adrenal medulla to synapse with adrenal chromaffin cells (see subsequent discussion).

At both lumbar and sacral levels, many preganglionic fibers pass through the sympathetic chain without synapsing and end in prevertebral ganglia of the abdomen and pelvis. These preganglionic fibers form the *lumbar* and *pelvic splanchnic nerves*. Most lumbar splanchnic nerves end in the *inferior mesenteric ganglion* or join the pelvic splanchnic nerves and end in one of the small pelvic sympathetic ganglia in the *hypogastric plexus*.

Parasympathetic Division

In contrast to the sympathetic division, *preganglionic neurons* of the *parasympathetic division* are in the *brain stem* nuclei or the *sacral spinal cord*. Those in brain stem nuclei exit the CNS as the GVE component of a cranial nerve, those in the sacral cord, as the GVE component of the sacral spinal nerves.

CRANIAL NERVES

Four cranial nerves contain the GVE, parasympathetic preganglionic component: the *oculomotor nerve* (*cranial nerve III*); the *facial nerve* (*cranial nerve VII*); the *glossopharyngeal nerve* (*cranial nerve IX*); and the *vagus nerve* (*cranial nerve X*). Of these four nerves, the oculomotor, facial, and glossopharyngeal nerves provide the parasympathetic innervation to the head, and the vagus nerve alone provides the parasympathetic innervation to the visceral contents of the entire thoracic cavity and most of the abdominal cavity.

The preganglionic fibers of the oculomotor nerve are in the *Edinger-Westphal nucleus* of the oculomotor complex in the midbrain. These preganglionic fibers exit the brain stem with the oculomotor nerve, enter the orbit, and synapse with the *postganglionic neurons* in the *ciliary ganglion*. Axons from the neurons in the ciliary ganglion form the short ciliary nerves and innervate the eye, specifically the ciliary muscle and the pupillary sphincter muscle (see Fig. 18–6).

The preganglionic fibers of the *facial nerve* are in the *superior salivatory nucleus*, just rostral to

the medullopontine junction. These preganglionic fibers exit the brain stem as a component of the *intermediate nerve* (a division of the *facial nerve*). The GVE preganglionic fibers subsequently leave the facial nerve as one of two branches, the *greater petrosal nerve* or the *chorda tympani nerve*.

Near the geniculate ganglion, the *greater petrosal nerve* leaves the facial nerve and canal, enters the cranial cavity through the hiatus of the facial canal, and runs toward the internal carotid artery. It joins the deep petrosal nerve (sympathetic fibers from the internal carotid plexus) to form the *nerve of the pterygoid canal* (*vidian nerve*). After passing through the pterygoid canal, this nerve enters the pterygopalatine fossa where it ends in the *pterygopalatine ganglion*. From there, postganglionic fibers provide parasympathetic innervation to the many *nasal*, *oral*, and *palatine glands* in addition to the *lacrimal gland*. Postganglionic fibers reach the lacrimal gland by first "hitching a ride" with the maxillary division of the trigeminal nerve and then with the lacrimal nerve, a terminal branch of the ophthalmic division of the trigeminal nerve (see Fig. 18–6).

The *chorda tympani nerve* leaves the facial nerve and canal, enters the *tympanic cavity*, crosses the cavity, and exits the skull via the *petrotympanic fissure*. Once outside the cranium, the chorda tympani nerve hitches a ride with the *lingual nerve*, a terminal branch of the mandibular division of the trigeminal nerve. These preganglionic fibers end in the *submandibular ganglion*. From there, postganglionic fibers provide parasympathetic innervation to the *submandibular* and *sublingual glands* and other neighboring, smaller salivary glands in the oral cavity (see Fig. 18–6).

The preganglionic neurons of the *glossopharyngeal nerve* are in the *inferior salivatory nucleus* of the medulla, immediately rostral to the large dorsal motor nucleus of the vagus nerve. Preganglionic fibers leave the main trunk of the glossopharyngeal nerve as the *tympanic nerve*, enter the tympanic cavity, and cross the tympanic membrane as a plexus of fibers, the *tympanic plexus*. The fibers re-collate within the cranial cavity as the *lesser petrosal nerve*; exit the cranium via the *sphenopetrosal fissure*; and end in the *otic ganglion*, immediately below the foramen ovale. Postganglionic fibers from the otic ganglion hitch a ride with the *auriculotemporal nerve*, a terminal branch of the mandibular division of the trigeminal nerve, and provide parasympathetic innervation to the *parotid gland* (see Fig. 18–6).

The preganglionic neurons of the *vagus nerve* are in the large *dorsal motor nucleus* of the *vagus nerve* (*dorsal nucleus of X*). These preganglionic fibers exit the brain stem and the cranium as part of the vagus nerve and descend to the thoracic cavity in the *carotid sheath*. As the vagus enters the thoracic cavity, it gives off many branches to the various plexuses associated with the visceral organs of the thorax and abdomen. These preganglionic fibers synapse with *postganglionic neurons* in small ganglionic patches, situated largely within the walls or supporting connective tissues of the target organs. The vagus supplies all parasympathetic innervation to *thoracic* and *abdominal viscera* except for the descending and sigmoid colon, rectum, and anus. These receive sacral parasympathetics (see Fig. 18–4).

SACRAL NERVES

The *sacral preganglionic parasympathetic neurons* are in the sacral spinal levels *S-2* through *S-4*. These neurons form a column of cells comparable in location with the intermediolateral cell column of the thoracic spinal cord. Preganglionic fibers exit the spinal cord, with the motor roots of the sacral nerves, and enter the nerve plexuses of the pelvis and lower abdominal region. These nerves provide parasympathetic innervation to all pelvic viscera and that portion of the intestinal tract not innervated by the vagus nerve (the descending and sigmoid colon, rectum, and anus). These preganglionic fibers synapse with the *postganglionic neurons*, in *small patches of ganglia* within the walls or surrounding the connective tissue of the target organs (see Fig. 18–4).

Sympathetic and Parasympathetic Innervation of Specific Organs

GENERAL FEATURES

The stimulation of the sympathetic and the parasympathetic innervations of a particular organ or organ system generally elicit opposite or *antagonistic* effects. Sympathetic stimulation increases heart rate; parasympathetic stimulation decreases it. Sometimes, the effects are not opposite, only different. For example, sympathetic stimulation of salivary glands produces a thick mucus secretion, whereas parasympathetic stimulation produces copious amounts of a clear, watery, serous secretion. Some targets, alternatively, receive innervation from only one of the divisions, e.g., sweat glands and erector pili muscles. No antagonistic or different effect is noted.

The functional state of an organ receiving the dual innervation often reflects a balance between the two. For example, parasympathetic stimulation leads to a constriction of the pupil, whereas sympathetic stimulation leads to dilation. However, at any moment, the size of the pupil is a function of the relative levels of activity of the two divisions. The application of eye drops containing a *cholinergic antagonist* blocks the parasympathetic cholinergic innervation of the pupillary constrictors, leaving the pupillary dilators (sympathetic) unopposed. The pupil then dilates.

A generalized stimulation of the sympathetic division elicits the "*fight or flight response.*" Believed to function as a defense mechanism in animals, this generalized response includes components such as an increase in heart rate and heart contractility, an increase in blood flow to somatic muscles, pupillary dilation, a sticky, mucoid salivary secretion, and cold sweaty palms. A generalized parasympathetic response, in contrast, is more *vegetative* or *anabolic*—slower heart rate, increase in blood flow to the gastrointestinal tract, and pupillary constriction. Table 18–1 summarizes some of the responses of target organs to sympathetic and parasympathetic stimulation.

CARDIOVASCULAR SYSTEM

The *heart* is a good example of dual, antagonistic autonomic innervations. The *parasympathetic innervation* is from branches of the vagus nerves via the *cardiac plexus*. Fibers from the plexus reach the atrium and the sinoatrial and atrioventricular nodes. Stimulation of this parasympathetic innervation leads to cardiac deceleration or *bradycardia*. Along with the slowing of the beat, a *reduction in the force of contraction* and a *reduction in the ventricular output* (blood volume per beat) occur. In comparison, stimulation of the *sympathetic innervation* (cardiac nerves from the cervical ganglia) leads to cardiac acceleration or *tachycardia*. Accompanying this is an *increase in contractile force* and an *increase in the volume of blood* pumped per beat.

Automomic innervation affects the *coronary arteries* both directly and indirectly. Under normal conditions, the *indirect effect* is more important. During the *sympathetic stimulation* of the heart, an increase occurs in the rate of metabo-

TABLE 18-1

Responses of Selected Effector Organs to Autonomic Innervation

EFFECTOR ORGAN	SYMPATHETIC STIMULATION	PARASYMPATHETIC STIMULATION
Heart	Increased heart rate (β_1)*	Decreased heart rate
	More contractile force (β_1)	Reduced contractile force
	More output volumee (β_1)	Reduced output volume
Coronary Arteries		
Direct effect (innervation)	Superficial constriction (α)	Slight dilation
	Deep vessel dilation (β_2)	
Indirect effect (metabolic)	Generalized vasodilation	Generalized constriction
Systemic Blood Vessels		
Skeletal muscle	Mostly vasodilation (β_2)	No detectable response
Integument	Vasoconstriction (α)	Dilation (face,blushing)
Visceral organs	Vasoconstriction (α)	Vasodilation
Nasal mucosa	Vasoconstriction (α)	Vasodilation
Eye		
Iris	Dilation (mydriasis) (α_1)	Constriction (miosis)
Ciliary muscle	Relaxation (far vision) (β)	Contraction (near vision)
Tarsal muscles	Contraction (α)	
Lacrimal gland	Vasoconstriction (α)	Secretion of tears and vasodilation
Integument		
Erector pili mm.	Contraction (α)	—
Apocrine glands	Secretion (α)	—
Sweat glands	Palms of hands (α), rest of body (M_2-AChR)†	—
Respiratory System		
Bronchioles	Dilation (β_2)	Constriction
Bronchial glands	Decreased secretion (β_1)	Increased secretion
	Increased secretion (β_2)	
Salivary Glands	Mucus secretion (α)	Serous secretion
	Vasoconstriction (α)	Vasodilation
Gastrointestinal Tract		
Peristalsis	Inhibition (α_1)	Stimulation
Sphincters	Contraction (α)	Relaxation
Blood flow	Vasoconstriction (α)	Vasodilation
Intrinsic glands	—	Increased secretion
Liver	Glycogenolysis and gluconeogenesis	Glycogenesis
Pancreas		
Acinar cells	Decreased secretion (α)	Increased secretion
Islet (β) cells	Decreased secretion (α_2)	—
	Increased secretion (β_2)	—
Urinary Bladder		
Detrusor muscle	—	Contraction
Sphinctor muscle	Contraction (α)	Relaxation
Reproductive Organs		
Male	Smooth muscle component of ejaculation (α)	Erection of penis
		Accessory gland secretion
Female	Smooth muscle component of orgasm; cervical dilation	Engorgement of clitoris and bulbs of vestibule
		Glandular secretion

* Adrenergic receptor type is indicated in ( ).
† Most sweat gland innervation is cholinergic sympathetic with muscarinic receptors (see text).

lism, which in turn modulates local blood flow by *dilating the coronary vessels*. This effect increases the blood flow to the more active heart muscles. In contrast, with *parasympathetic stimulation*, a corresponding decrease in metabolism occurs, which *constricts the coronary vessels* and decreases the blood flow to the less active muscle.

The *direct effects* of the autonomic innervation are less significant and often are confusing, because they differ from the indirect effects. The limited effect of *direct parasympathetic stimulation* of the coronary arteries is one of *slight vasodilation*. The effect of *direct sympathetic stimulation* on coronary vessels varies, and much depends on the balance between α- and β-adrenergic receptors in the coronary vessel wall. Stimulation of the α-receptors leads to *vasoconstriction*, whereas stimulation of the β-receptors leads to *vasodilation*. Normally, a preponderance of β-receptors is noted in the deep muscle tissue. More α-receptors are found in the superficial layers. Thus, the direct effects of sympathetic stimulation are a dilation of the deep muscle arteries and a constriction of the superficial vessels. *In both the parasympathetic and the sympathetic innervations, the direct effects are of less significance and usually are masked by the stronger indirect effects* (see Table 18–1).

SYSTEMIC BLOOD VESSELS

The autonomic innervation of systemic blood vessels also demonstrates the contrasting effects of the sympathetic and parasympathetic divisions. In keeping with the "fight-or-flight" appellation given the sympathetic division, *sympathetic stimulation* leads to *vasodilation* of vessels in the *somatic muscles*, but it also leads to a *vasoconstriction* of the *cutaneous blood vessels* as well as the vessels of the *digestive system* and the *lungs*. In contrast, the *parasympathetic innervation* of blood vessels produces only *vasodilation*: dilation of vessels to the *digestive system*, to the *glands* in the head, to the *face* (*blushing*), to the *kidneys*, to the *nasal mucosa*, and to other *erectile tissue*. Little or no parasympathetic innervation of the blood vessels to somatic muscle exists (see Table 18–1).

EYE

The *eye* also receives both sympathetic and parasympathetic innervation. *Parasympathetic preganglionic fibers* reach the eye as the GVE component of the *oculomotor nerve* and synapse on postganglionic neurons in the *ciliary ganglion*. The postganglionic fibers form the *short ciliary nerves* that enter the eyeball and innervate the *pupillary constrictors* (*miosis*) and the *circumferential muscles of the ciliary body*. When stimulated, this innervation relaxes the tension on the suspensory ligaments of the lens, allowing the lens to become more convex and more suitable for near vision.

The parasympathetic innervation of the muscles of the ciliary body and the pupillary constrictors are part of the *accommodation reflex*. This reflex has three components: a somatomotor response, the convergence of the eyes, and two visceromotor responses, pupillary constriction and making the lens more convex.

Postganglionic *sympathetic fibers* reach the orbit via the sympathetic plexus surrounding the ophthalmic artery. These fibers innervate the *radial muscles of the iris* and the *superior* and *inferior tarsal muscles* (smooth muscles in the upper and lower eyelids). Upon stimulation, the radial muscles of the iris *dilate the pupils* (*mydriasis*). The tarsal muscles *widen the palpebral fissure*. Most of the eyelid musculature, the orbicularis oris and levator palpebrae superioris, are striated muscle (see Fig. 18–6).

The *lacrimal gland* receives both sympathetic and parasympathetic innervation. These autonomic postganglionic fibers reach the orbit indirectly by way of the lacrimal nerve and innervate the *lacrimal gland* (see Fig. 18–6). Contrasting effects exist between the two innervations. *Sympathetic* stimulation *constricts* the blood vessels of the glandular tissue, whereas *parasympathetic* stimulation both *dilates* the blood vessels and stimulates the *secretion of tears* (see Table 18–1).

INTEGUMENT

The autonomic innervation to the *integument* or skin is *anatomically sympathetic*. Preganglionic fibers arise from the neurons of the *intermediolateral cell column* of the *thoracolumbar spinal cord*, and the postganglionic neurons are in the *paravertebral sympathetic chain*. Pharmacologically, however, many of these postganglionic fibers meet the criteria for parasympathetic neurons.

The *noradrenergic sympathetic innervation* of the skin produces *vasoconstriction* of the *superficial* and *deep vessels*; stimulates *secretion of apocrine glands*; *contraction of erector pili muscles*, producing "goose bumps"; and stimulates *secretion* of *palmar sweat glands*, especially during emotional stress. However, the remaining postganglionic sympathetic fibers are *cholinergic* and innervate *sweat glands*. These postganglionic neurons meet all the pharmacological criteria for parasympathetic postganglionic neurons, although anatomically they are sympathetic. We recognize the dichotomy and refer to these as *cholinergic sympathetic postganglionic neurons.*

Throughout the body, *postganglionic sympathetic fibers* reach the integument by way of the gray communicating rami of the sympathetic chain and distribute with the *segmental spinal nerves.* In the head region, the sympathetic innervation arises from the carotid plexuses, and these postganglionic fibers follow the terminal branches of these arteries. Many subsequently join the *branches of cranial nerves*, principally the trigeminal, and distribute to the skin (see Table 18–1).

RESPIRATORY SYSTEM

Autonomic innervation of the *lungs* and *pulmonary vessels* is similar to the heart. Extensive *pulmonary plexuses* are continuous with the cardiac plexuses and represent a mixture of sympathetic postganglionic fibers, vagal parasympathetic preganglionic fibers, and general visceral afferent fibers.

Stimulation of *sympathetic* fibers *dilates* the *pulmonary bronchioles*, whereas stimulation of *parasympathetic* fibers *constricts* the *bronchioles* and *increases* the rate of *secretion* of the numerous glandular cells along the pulmonary tree. The actual process of respiration, the inhalation and exhalation of air, is a somatic motor response; however, the *autonomic innervation modulates the efficiency of the respiratory process.* Little evidence exists of the autonomic nervous system having a significant role in the regulation of pulmonary blood flow.

SALIVARY GLANDS

Salivary glands have two types of secretory cells: *serous* and *mucous.* Both secretions are under autonomic regulation. Serous cells produce a thin watery fluid that contains digestive enzymes, whereas mucous cells produce a thick, mucus secretion. The major salivary glands of the head (the parotid, submandibular, and sublingual glands) contain both mucous and serous cells, although the population of mucous cells in the parotid gland is very small. Many small, unnamed glands occur in the oral, pharyngeal, and nasal cavities and contain both types of secretory cells. The *sympathetic* innervation stimulates the secretion by the *mucous cells*, and the *parasympathetic* innervation stimulates the secretion by the *serous cells.* Stress or fear will activate the sympathetics, with an increase in mucus production. Eating and even the thought of eating activate the parasympathetics, with an increase in the serous secretion or "salivation." In addition, sympathetic stimulation leads to vasoconstriction of the glandular vessels and parasympathetic stimulation leads to vasodilation and an increase in blood flow to the glandular tissue (see Table 18–1).

GASTROINTESTINAL TRACT AND INTRINSIC GLANDS

Within the wall of the *gastrointestinal tract* are two prominent plexuses: the *myenteric plexus of Auerbach* and the *submucosal plexus of Meissner.* The *myenteric plexus* is between the outer muscle layers of the gastrointestinal tract and totally surrounds the entire length of the tract, from the oral esophagus to the internal anal sphincter. The *submucosal plexus* is between the mucosal and muscular tunics of the gastrointestinal tract. This plexus totally surrounds the tract from the gastroduodenal junction to the internal anal sphincter. Together, these plexuses, their extensive interconnections and their afferent and efferent connections constitute the *enteric nervous system.*

Several reasons exist for considering these peripheral plexuses of neurons and nerve fibers as a "nervous system." This system contains more than postganglionic parasympathetic neurons, preganglionic parasympathetic fibers, and postganglionic sympathetic fibers; it also contains many interneurons and primary visceral afferent (GVA) neurons. Extensive interconnections occur between these neuronal elements. When isolated from the CNS, the *enteric nervous system* continues to function reflexly, controlling peristalsis, gastrointestinal gland secretion, and blood flow modulation. This elaborate network of ganglionic plexuses is isolated from surrounding intercellular fluids in much the same manner as the brain is isolated within the "blood-brain barrier."

Although the *enteric nervous system* can operate in isolation, normally efferent signals from both the parasympathetic and sympathetic divisions drive it. However, these efferent signals are subject to more modulation within the *enteric nervous system* than in other peripheral ganglionic plexuses of the autonomic nervous system. *Parasympathetic preganglionic fibers* synapse in the enteric nervous system, and *postganglionic fibers* innervate the muscular and glandular tissues of the gastrointestinal tract. *Parasympathetic stimulation leads to vasodilation, increased peristalsis, and increased secretion by gastrointestinal glands.* These actions all aid in the digestion of food and its passage through the gastrointestinal tract. In contrast, *sympathetic stimulation leads to vasoconstriction, inhibition of peristalsis, and contraction of the involuntary gastrointestinal sphincters* (see Table 18 – 1).

The pattern of *neurotransmitter distribution* in neurons of the enteric nervous system is complex. *Cholinergic preganglionic fibers* and *cholinergic postganglionic parasympathetic neurons* localize throughout the system. All the *noradrenergic fibers* are axons of *sympathetic postganglionic neurons* from the prevertebral ganglia. *Serotoninergic* and *dopaminergic* neurons are intrinsic to the enteric nervous system as are *GABAergic* neurons. All three localize within both plexuses. From *15 to 20 different neuropeptides,* probable neurotransmitters, co-transmitters, and neuromodulators, localize within the enteric nervous system. Some of the more abundant include *cholecystokinin (CCK), vasoactive intestinal peptide (VIP), substance P (SP), neuropeptide Y (NPY), neurotensin (NT), somatostatin (SOM), dynorphin (DYN), and enkephalin-related peptides.* Many of these co-localize with each other and with other neurotransmitters. The exceedingly complex pattern of co-localization gives a "*chemical signature*" to specific, small subpopulations of neurons and neuronal processes. At present, the functional significance of specific combinations of neurotransmitters is unknown but under intense investigation.

PANCREAS AND LIVER INNERVATION

Stimulation of the *parasympathetic innervation* to the *pancreas* increases the secretion of digestive juices, whereas stimulation of the *sympathetic innervation* inhibits secretion. In the *liver*, stimulation of the *sympathetic innervation* promotes *glycogenolysis* and *gluconeogenesis*, whereas stimulation of the *parasympathetic innervation* promotes *glycogenesis* (see Table 18 – 1).

URINARY BLADDER

The bladder receives both *somatomotor and visceromotor innervation.* The somatomotor innervation is to the external sphincter and the perineal muscles via the internal pudendal nerve from the sacral spinal cord. This innervation provides a voluntary control mechanism to override the bladder-emptying reflex that stretch receptors evoke when the bladder becomes full. *Parasympathetic neurons* provide the motor component for the *bladder-emptying reflex,* through the innervation of smooth (detrusor) muscles in the bladder wall. The *sympathetic innervation* is principally vascular and has little to do with normal bladder function (see Table 18 – 1).

REPRODUCTIVE ORGANS

Normal functioning of the male genital system requires intact innervation by both the parasympathetic and sympathetic components of the autonomic nervous system. Stimulation of the *parasympathetic component* leads to *erection* of the penis and active *secretion* by the accessory glands, the prostate gland, and the seminal vesicles. The *sympathetic innervation* is responsible for a motor component of *ejaculation,* the expulsion of semen through the contraction of smooth muscles in the accessory glands and their ducts. Ejaculation also is accompanied by clonic spasm of the striated bulbospongiosus and ischiocavernous muscles in the body of the penis, a reflex triggered by the pressure of semen entering the urethra. Thus, the reflexive responses associated with ejaculation are a combination of somatomotor and visceromotor reflexes, with the visceromotor components being *sympathetic.*

Normal functioning of the female genital system also requires intact innervation by both divisions of the autonomic nervous system. Stimulation of the *parasympathetic component* is responsible for *engorgement of the clitoris* (the homologue of the penis); the *bulbs of the vestibule*; and, to a lesser extent, the vascular tissue within the inferior wall of the *vagina.* In addition, *parasympathetic stimulation* results in *secretion* by the labial, vestibular, vaginal, and cervical glands. During female *orgasm,* clonic spasm occurs in the bulbospongiosus and ischiocavernous muscles and in the muscles within the inferior vaginal wall, along with a dilation of the cervical canal that can last for up to several hours. These responses in the female, as in the male, are a combination of somatomotor and visceromotor (*sympathetic*) reflexes. Other complex and less understood responses, by both the parasympathetic and sympathetic divisions, exist.

The only response of the testes, the ovaries, and the body of the uterus to either sympathetic or parasympathetic stimulation is vasomotor (see Table 18–1).

ADRENAL MEDULLA

The *adrenal medulla* differentiates from primitive neuroblasts that migrate from the developing celiac ganglion. Instead of differentiating into neurons, these cells become the chromaffin cells of the adrenal medulla, an endocrine gland. These chromaffin cells receive sympathetic preganglionic innervation, and upon stimulation they release epinephrine (80%) and norepinephrine (20%) by exocytosis. The catechol amines then diffuse into the capillary beds and sinusoids of the gland and enter the general circulation. The effect of the release is similar to that of a generalized sympathetic stimulation. Destruction of the adrenal medulla is not life threatening because other sympathetic mechanisms are able to compensate for the loss.

Anatomy of the Hypothalamus

GENERAL FEATURES

The *hypothalamus*, although a small subdivision of the diencephalon, is a multifunctional center for control of visceromotor and endocrine activity. First, the hypothalamus is an important *integrator* and *modulator* of *autonomic activity*, including the integration of visceromotor responses during the expression of emotions. Second, it is a very sensitive *sensory transducer*, containing neurons with specialized receptors that respond to changes in temperature or osmolality or in the level of specific hormones in the general circulation. Third, the hypothalamus, through a vascular portal system, *regulates endocrine functions* of the *adenohypophysis*. Fourth, the hypothalamus through specific neurosecretory cells *functions as an endocrine organ*, producing and releasing oxytocin and vasopressin (antidiuretic hormone, ADH), from the posterior lobe of the pituitary, the neurohypophysis.

Chemical communication is an essential ingredient of nervous system function. Throughout most of the nervous system, this communication is "short ranged," with the chemical messengers (neurotransmitters) traversing the very narrow synaptic cleft before interacting with the postsynaptic receptor. Hypothalamic neurons, in comparison, use a variety of chemical messengers: short-ranged neurotransmitters at synaptic junctions, "medium-ranged" hypothalamic hypophysiotropic hormones (HHHs); and "long-ranged" neurohormones (oxytocin and vasopressin). Although the neurotransmitters act over very short distances, HHHs act over distances measured in millimeters. After release in the hypothalamus, the hypophyseal portal system transports them to the adenohypophysis. The neurohormones, in contrast, enter the general circulation and travel throughout the body.

ANATOMY

The slit-like third ventricle divides the hypothalamus in the sagittal plane. On the medial or ventricular surface of the diencephalon, the *hypothalamic sulcus* marks the boundary between the dorsal thalamus above and hypothalamus below (Fig. 18–7). Although the third ventricle sharply defines the medial surface of the hypothalamus and the ventral surface of the brain defines the inferior margin, the other boundaries are less distinct.

Lateral Boundaries. Basal forebrain structures, such as the substantia innominata and the nuclei of the anterior perforated substance, form the lateral boundaries of the anterior part of the hypothalamus. Portions of the subthalamus form the lateral boundaries of the posterior part of the hypothalamus (see Figs. 7–20 and 7–21).

Anterior Boundaries. The hypothalamus extends to the lamina terminalis in the midline and into basal portions of the forebrain on either side of the lamina terminalis, becoming continuous with the septal nuclei and the bed nuclei of both the stria terminalis and the anterior commissure (see Fig. 7–22). Although the anterior most portions of the hypothalamus are actually in the forebrain (telencephalon), the entire hypothalamus is considered to be diencephalic.

Posterior Boundaries. The midbrain and portions of the subthalamus form the posterior boundaries of the hypothalamus (see Fig. 18–7).

In Weigert-stained preparations, the hypothalamus appears homogenous. Most of the fiber con-

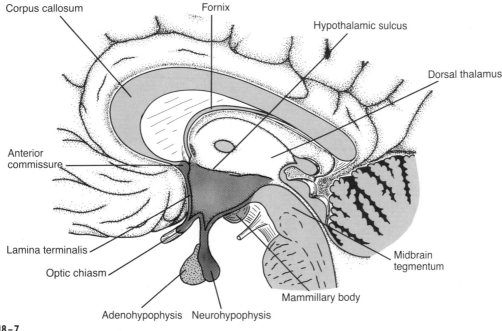

Corpus callosum

Fornix

Hypothalamic sulcus

Dorsal thalamus

Anterior commissure

Lamina terminalis

Optic chiasm

Adenohypophysis   Neurohypophysis

Mammillary body

Midbrain tegmentum

FIGURE 18-7

A midsagittal section through the brain at the level of the diencephalon illustrating the midline boundaries of the hypothalamus. Hypothalamus and neurohypophysis are shaded red. See text for details.

nections between the hypothalamic nuclei and between the hypothalamus and other parts of the brain are thin, poorly myelinated fibers and are not visible with myelin stains. Two prominent exceptions exist, the *fornix* and the *mammillothalamic tract*. Both of these pathways are very heavily myelinated and are visible with Weigert stains (see Figs. 7–20, 7–21, and 7–22).

DIVISIONS

The hypothalamus has *three zones* from the medial ventricular surface to the lateral margin: the *periventricular zone*, the *medial zone*, and the *lateral zone* (Fig. 18–8A). The *periventricular zone* is very thin and consists of many small, poorly defined nuclear groups that line the ventricular surface of the hypothalamus. The passage of the fornix through the hypothalamus, extending from the anterior commissure to the mammillary bodies, is an approximate landmark for the boundary between the *medial zone* and *lateral zone*. Hence, the medial zone extends from the periventricular zone to the more laterally situated fornix. The portion of the hypothalamus lateral to the fornix is the lateral zone.

Based on the presence of identifiable anatomical structures visible on the ventral and medial surfaces, the hypothalamus has *three regions* along the anterior-posterior axis, the *chiasmatic region*, the *tuberal region*, and the *mammillary region* (Fig. 18–8B and Table 18–2). The *chiasmatic region* (*pars chiasmatica*) is the most anterior region of the hypothalamus, bounded ventrally by the *optic chiasm*. The *mammillary region* (*pars mammillaris*) is the most posterior region, bounded ventrally by the *mammillary bodies*. The middle region, between the mammillary bodies and the optic chiasm, contains the *tuber cinereum* and is the *tuberal region* (*pars tuberalis*). The *median eminence* is the central part of the tuber cinereum and the origin of the *infundibular process* and the *neurohypophysis* (*posterior pituitary*, *pars nervosa* of the *pituitary*).

Thus, the hypothalamus has three segments in the anteroposterior direction; and three more in the mediolateral direction; the *chiasmatic, tuberal*, and *mammillary regions* and the *periventricular, medial*, and *lateral zones*. Combinations of these terms are helpful to define, anatomically, nine small "blocks" of the hypothalamus, in a part of the brain that lacks more striking ana-

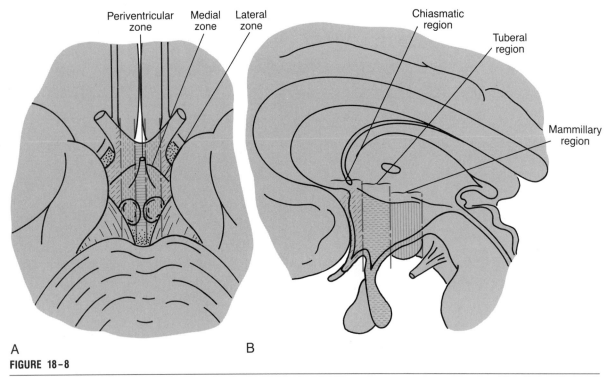

Periventricular zone · Medial zone · Lateral zone · Chiasmatic region · Tuberal region · Mammillary region

A   B

FIGURE 18–8

Division of the hypothalamus into zones and regions. *A*, Periventricular, medial, and lateral zones as viewed from the ventral surface of the brain. *B*, Chiasmatic, tuberal, and mammillary regions as viewed in the midsagittal plane. See text for details.

tomical landmarks (e.g., lateral-tuberal, medial-chiasmatic, and so forth).

NUCLEAR ORGANIZATION

Many nuclear groups are visible using Nissl stains within the otherwise homogenous-appearing hypothalamus. Most of the differentiated nuclear groups are in the medial zone. The organization of the lateral and periventricular zones is not as well defined (see Table 18–2).

Within the *chiasmatic region* are two very prominent nuclei, with large neurons that contain prominent, dense Nissl bodies, the *paraventricular nucleus* and the *supraoptic nucleus* (see Fig. 18–9). Both of these nuclei contain neurons with neurosecretory functions. These neurons send axonal processes down the infundibular stalk and into the neurohypophysis. On stimulation, these endings release neurohormones into the circulation (see the following discussion). The *paraventricular nucleus* is a broad, flat nuclear group, oriented parallel to the third ventricle in the superior portion of the hypothalamus close to the hypothalamic sulcus. Although principally in the

medial zone, portions of the paraventricular nucleus extend into the periventricular zone. The *supraoptic nucleus*, in comparison, is smaller and caps the optic chiasm on either side of the midline. Portions of this nucleus extend into the lateral zone. A less well-defined nuclear group, the *anterior nucleus*, occupies much of the space between the paraventricular and supraoptic nuclei. Immediately rostral to the anterior nucleus and extending into portions of both medial and lateral zones anterior to the optic chiasm is the *preoptic area*. It is difficult to define specific nuclear groups within the preoptic area (see Fig. 18–9).

The smaller neurons of the medial zone in the *tuberal region* form two major nuclei: the *dorsomedial nucleus* and the *ventromedial nucleus*. Besides these large nuclei, several smaller nuclei extend into the more ventral regions of the tuber cinereum, including the dopaminergic *arcuate nuclei* of the hypothalamus (see Fig. 18–9).

The medial zone of the *mammillary region* contains two major nuclear groups, the *posterior nucleus* with its large neurons and a very prominent nuclear complex, the *mammillary nuclei* or

TABLE 18-2

Principal Nuclei of the Hypothalamus

NUCLEUS OR AREA	LOCATION AND PRESUMED FUNCTION
Chiasmatic Region	
Preoptic area	Contains many small nuclear groups; located in rostral portion of the chiasmatic region.
Paraventricular nucleus	Prominent nucleus in the chiasmatic region has neurosecretory functions and produces the neurohormones oxytocin and vasopressin.
Supraoptic nucleus	Prominent nucleus located immediately above the lateral margin of the optic chiasm has neurosecretory functions and produces oxytocin and vasopressin
Suprachiasmatic nucleus	Small midline nucleus above the optic chiasm implicated in patterns of circadian rhythms.
Anterior nucleus	Ill-defined group of nuclei occupying the area between the paraventricular and supraoptic nuclei.
Tuberal Region	
Dorsomedial nucleus	Large group of small neurons in the dorsal part of the medial zone.
Ventromedial nucleus	Large group of small neurons in the ventral part of the medial zone.
Arcuate nucleus	A small group of dopaminergic neurons located in the basal portion of the tuber cinereum.
Mammillary Region	
Posterior nucleus	Prominent nucleus of large neurons occupying most of the medial zone dorsal to the mammillary complex.
Mammillary nuclei	A complex of three to four nuclei that forms the mammillary body elevations on the ventral surface of the hypothalamus. They receive extensive projections from the hippocampus via the fornix and have an extensive projection to the anterior nuclei of the dorsal thalamus via the mammillothalamic tract.

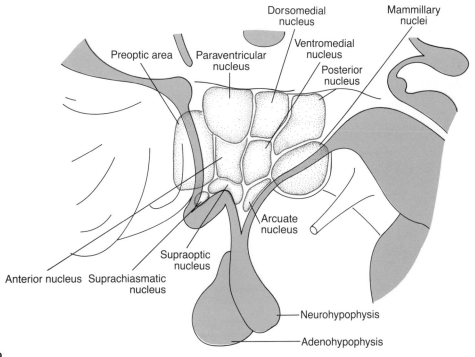

FIGURE 18-9

The principal nuclear groups of the medial zone. The nuclei of the periventricular zone and the lateral hypothalamus are not illustrated. See text for details.

nucleus, this often is subdivided into three or four nuclei (see Fig. 18–9).

FIBER PATHWAYS

Most of the fibers entering and leaving the hypothalamus are small, unmyelinated or very lightly myelinated axons. These are difficult to stain and are equally difficult to trace. Two exceptions are the very heavily myelinated *fornix* and *mammillothalamic tract*, and both appear as prominent tracts in Weigert-stained preparations of the brain stem (see Figs. 7–20 and 7–21). Although most of the pathways can be classified as either afferent or efferent (input or output) to the hypothalamus, *all* contain reciprocal connections, some more than others. Two pathways, the *medial forebrain bundle* and the *stria medullaris thalami*, are difficult to classify as either afferent or efferent with respect to the hypothalamus, because they make comparable connections in each direction (Table 18–3).

The *medial forebrain bundle* is a loosely organized and diffuse group of small, unmyelinated to lightly myelinated fibers that run in an anteroposterior direction through the *lateral hypothalamus*, interconnecting the *basal forebrain, hypothalamus*, and lower centers in the *brain stem*. Fibers in the medial forebrain bundle both arise from and terminate on neurons in all three areas,

TABLE 18–3

Principal Efferent and Afferent Pathways* of the Hypothalamus

		EFFERENT PATHWAYS
Hypothalamocerebellar path	*From*	Dorsomedial nucleus, dorsal and lateral areas
	To	Cerebellar nuclei and cortex
Hypothalamospinal tract	*From*	Paraventricular nucleus, also dorsomedial, ventromedial, and posterior nuclei
	To	Preganglionic neurons of brain stem and spinal cord
Mammillointerpeduncular tract	*From*	Mammillary nuclei
	To	Ipsilateral interpeduncular nucleus
Mammillotegmental tract	*From*	Mammillary nuclei and surrounding nuclei
	To	Midbrain tegmentum
Mammillothalamic tract	*From*	Mammillary nuclei
	To	Anterior nuclei of dorsal thalamus
Periventricular bundle	*From*	Periventricular nuclei
	To	Frontal cortex and lower brain stem
Tuberoinfundibular tract	*From*	Arcuate nuclei, other nuclei of tuberal region
	To	Infundibular stalk of neurohypophysis
		AFFERENT PATHWAYS
Cerebellohypothalamic path	*From*	Cerebellar nuclei
	To	Dorsal, lateral, and posterior areas and dorsomedial nucleus
Fornix†	*From*	Hippocampus
	To	Anterior hypothalamus and septal area to mammillary nuclei
Mammillary peduncle	*From*	Converging, ascending sensory pathways
	To	Mammillary nuclei
Retinosuprachiasmatic tract	*From*	Retina
	To	Suprachiasmatic nucleus
Stria terminalis	*From*	Amygdaloid nuclei
	To	Medial preoptic area
Thalamohypothalamic tract	*From*	Dorsomedial and midline nuclei of thalamus
	To	Lateral preoptic area, other hypothalamic nuclei
Ventral amygdalohypothalamic tract	*From*	Amygdaloid nuclei
	To	Numerous hypothalamic nuclei
		RECIPROCAL PATHWAYS
Medial forebrain bundle	*Interconnects*	Frontal lobes, basal forebrain, hypothalamus, and midbrain
Stria medullaris thalami	*Interconnects*	Supraoptic nucleus, preoptic area, and septal area with the habenular nucleus

* Although most are reciprocal to some degree, pathways are grouped by the primary direction of information flow, see text for details.
† The fornix also contains the prominent cholinergic septohippocampal pathway.

with the most extensive contributions made by neurons of the hypothalamus and septal area.

The *stria medullaris thalami* is a fiber tract running along the superomedial margin of the dorsal thalamus and interconnecting the habenula with the anterior hypothalamic and septal areas. Extensive reciprocal connections occur between neurons of the *habenula* and those of the *supraoptic nucleus*, the *preoptic area*, and the *septal area* (Fig. 18–10).

Connections between the *hypothalamus* and the *cerebellum* are both afferent and efferent. Some represent reciprocal connections but others do not. Neurons in the *dorsomedial nucleus and dorsal and lateral areas of the hypothalamus* project to the *cortex and nuclei of the cerebellum*, the *hypothalamocerebellar pathway*. These *histaminergic fibers* end in all three layers of the cerebellar cortex and have collaterals that project to the cerebellar nuclei. The pattern of termination in the cerebellar cortex is similar to that of the serotoninergic and adrenergic projections

from the brain stem raphe nuclei and the locus ceruleus (see Chapter 17). In addition, significant projections arise from the *cerebellar nuclei* to the *posterior, dorsal, and lateral areas and the dorsomedial nucleus of the hypothalamus*, the *cerebellohypothalamic pathway* (see Table 18–3).

Efferent Pathways

The hypothalamus is the origin of descending nerve fibers that synapse directly on sympathetic and parasympathetic preganglionic neurons in the brain stem and spinal cord. This pathway, the *hypothalamospinal tract*, arises principally from the *paraventricular nucleus*. Contributions also arise from neurons in the *dorsomedial, ventromedial, and posterior nuclei* and from numerous, scattered nuclei as well. Most of these descending fibers synapse with *preganglionic neurons* in ipsilateral *GVE nuclei or columns of the brain stem and spinal cord*. Although this pathway represents a direct connection between hypothalamic neu-

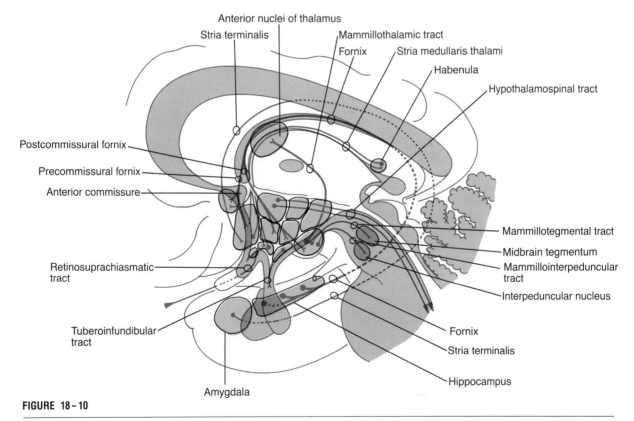

FIGURE 18–10

Some of the major afferent and efferent pathways of the hypothalamus. Not illustrated are the medial forebrain bundle, periventricular bundle, mammillary peduncle, and ventral amygdalohypothalamic tract, and the reciprocal connections with the cerebellum. See text for details.

rons and the preganglionic neurons, it represents only a small part of the descending influences of the hypothalamus on the preganglionic neurons. Most of the descending signals from the hypothalamus travel in poorly defined, multisynaptic pathways that are difficult to trace anatomically. All these descending hypothalamic pathways, both the direct and the indirect, contain small diameter, poorly myelinated axons.

The mammillary nuclei are the origin of three efferent pathways, the most prominent of which is the *mammillothalamic tract* (*mammillary fasciculus*). The mammillothalamic tract is a dense bundle of large, well-myelinated nerve axons projecting *from the mammillary nuclei to the anterior nuclei of the dorsal thalamus* (see Fig. 18–10). These thalamic nuclei, in turn, project to cingulate, subcallosal, and parolfactory gyri of the limbic forebrain and to portions of the hippocampal formation. The two other efferent pathways arising from the mammillary nuclei descend into the brain stem. The *mammillointerpeduncular tract* contains axons arising from neurons of the *mammillary nuclei and descending to the interpeduncular nucleus*, situated in the ventral midbrain, immediately lateral to the interpeduncular fossa. The *mammillotegmental tract* courses dorsal to the mammillointerpeduncular tract and *ends in nuclei of the midbrain reticular formation, the tegmentum*. Although all three pathways are basically efferent, extensive reciprocal connections occur (see Table 18–3).

The *periventricular bundle*, by many criteria, is a reciprocal rather than an efferent pathway. However, descending fibers extend into the lower levels of the medulla and into the spinal cord. Therefore, we will consider it as efferent. This is a loose network of fibers at the level of the hypothalamus, situated immediately lateral to the third ventricle, within the substance of the periventricular zone. Fibers in this network *interconnect* the various *nuclei of the periventricular zone* with each other and with the *frontal cortex* and *lower brain stem*. The descending fibers enter the periaqueductal gray of the midbrain and continue into lower levels of the brain stem as the *dorsal longitudinal fasciculus of Schütz* (see Figs. 7–9, 7–10, 7–11, 7–12, and 7–13 and see Table 18–3).

The *tuberoinfundibular tract* arises from the *arcuate nuclei* and other small nuclei of the tuberal region. Axons from these neurons extend into the *infundibular stalk* of the neurohypophysis where they end. Stimulation of these neurons leads to the release of one or more of the HHHs

in at the nerve terminal. The vessels in the hypophyseal portal system pick up the HHH and transport it to the *adenohypophysis* (*anterior pituitary*), where it modulates the release of a trophic hormones (see subsequent discussion of the parvocellular neurosecretory system) (see Table 18–3).

Afferent Pathways

The *fornix* is a major source of afferent projections to the hypothalamus. Axons of *pyramidal cells*, deep in the temporal lobe, leave the hippocampal formation to form the *fimbria of the fornix* and then the *fornix* proper. As the fornix leaves the surface of the hippocampus, it curves dorsomedially to meet the fornix from the opposite side immediately below the corpus callosum. At this point, a few of the fibers cross to the opposite side in the *hippocampal commissure*, but most continue uncrossed to the ipsilateral hypothalamus. Beyond the hippocampal commissure, the fornix continues in a forward direction but curves ventrad toward the anterior commissure and the lamina terminalis. At the anterior commissure, the fornix splits. Some of the fibers pass in front of the anterior commissure, the *precommissural fornix*; however, most of the fibers pass behind the anterior commissure as the *postcommissural fornix*. Fibers of the *precommissural fornix* end in the *preoptic and anterior hypothalamic areas* as well as the *septal nuclei* of the basal forebrain. Most of the fibers of the *postcommissural fornix* curve in a posterior and ventral direction and run through the hypothalamus along the approximate boundary between medial and lateral zones to end in the *ipsilateral mammillary nuclei*. During its course through the substance of the hypothalamus, the postcommissural fornix gives off many fibers to other nuclei between the anterior commissure and the mammillary nuclei (see Fig. 18–10 and Table 18–3). Most of the fibers in the fornix run from the hippocampal formation to the hypothalamus and basal forebrain, however, some run toward the hippocampus. The most significant of these is a bundle of cholinergic fibers, the *septohippocampal tract*, that runs within the fornix from the *septal nuclei to the hippocampus* (see Chapter 22).

The *mammillary peduncle* represents a convergence of fibers from *ascending sensory systems* in the tegmentum of the midbrain. These fibers, representing many sensory systems, project from the *midbrain to the mammillary nuclei* as the mammillary peduncle. This pathway is the principal source of sensory information for the hypothalamus (see Table 18–3).

The very small *retinosuprachiasmatic tract* projects from the *retina* to the *suprachiasmatic nucleus*. This retinal projection travels in the optic nerve and enters the hypothalamus at the optic chiasm. The direct visual information from this pathway has a role in the modulation and regulation of circadian rhythms and estrous cycle patterns (see Table 18–3).

The *stria terminalis* is a long arcing pathway extending from the *amygdaloid nuclei*, near the anterior pole of the temporal lobe, to the hypothalamic nuclei in the *medial preoptic area*. These fibers run along the medial margin of the caudate nucleus at its boundary with the dorsal thalamus and follow the same course as the vena terminalis (see Fig. 18–10). Along the base of the stria terminalis, adjacent to the stria and the underlying hypothalamus, is the *bed nucleus of the stria terminalis*. This nucleus is part of the basal forebrain, but it sends fibers to both the hypothalamus and the amygdaloid complex in the temporal lobe (see Table 18–3).

The *ventral amygdalohypothalamic tract* is another tract between the amygdaloid nuclei and the hypothalamus. These afferents from the amygdaloid complex pass directly through the *sublenticular portion* of the *internal capsule* and into the hypothalamus, a much more direct route than that taken by the stria terminalis (see Table 18–3).

Projections from the dorsal thalamus to the hypothalamus are generally diffuse; however, those from the *dorsomedial nucleus* and the *midline nuclei* of the thalamus compose the *thalamohypothalamic tract*. These fibers project principally to the *lateral preoptic area* of the hypothalamus, although they make more diffuse connections with many other hypothalamic nuclei (see Table 18–3).

Functions of the Hypothalamus

LOCALIZATION OF FUNCTION

The precise localization of many functions within the hypothalamus is difficult because of the very small size of the hypothalamus and because of the complex pattern of pathways entering, exiting, and passing through the structure. Clinical cases of lesions that involve the hypothalamus often involve adjacent and functionally related structures (basal forebrain, amygdala, ventral

striatum, limbic system, and midbrain), which further complicate the correlation between the structural damage and the functional deficit. The correlation between structure and function is the result of laboratory experiments and extrapolation of results to the human nervous system, when consistent with the anatomy and the clinical data.

Several generalities often are made about the localization of function within the hypothalamus. The *anterior hypothalamus* regulates primarily *parasympathetic functions*, and the *posterior hypothalamus* regulates primarily *sympathetic functions*. Although an oversimplification, stimulating anterior portions of the hypothalamus elicits, *preferentially, parasympathetic responses*; stimulating posterior portions of the hypothalamus elicits *both sympathetic and parasympathetic responses*. The descending parasympathetic fibers pass through the posterior regions of the hypothalamus, and the stimulation of "sympathetic centers," therefore, affects these descending parasympathetic fibers. In addition, many projections go to the parasympathetic preganglionic neurons in the brain stem nuclei that originate from neurons in the frontal lobe, basal forebrain, ventral striatum, and septal area. Many of these fibers also pass through the substance of the hypothalamus, as they descend to the brain stem. Stimulation of these hypothalamic areas also affects these fibers.

Neurons in the *parvocellular* part of the *paraventricular nucleus* form the single largest concentration of "autonomic upper motor neurons." Other neurons, scattered in many other hypothalamic nuclei, also project to brain stem and spinal cord levels, but those of the paraventricular nucleus are the best documented. These efferent neurons are a mixture of both *sympathetic* and *parasympathetic upper motor neurons*.

Parasympathetic and sympathetic innervations have nearly opposite effects on effector organs, yet these upper motor neurons intermix within the same nuclei. As many as 15% of these paraventricular neurons project to *both sympathetic and parasympathetic nuclei*, through collateral branches. For example, some descending axons have collaterals to the dorsal motor nucleus of the vagus (parasympathetic) en route to the thoracic intermediolateral cell column (sympathetic). This arrangement insures the simultaneous inhibition of one and excitation of the other. *The same neuron and its transmitter can have opposite effects on different postsynaptic neurons.* The receptor and not the transmitter determines the nature of the postsynaptic response—receptors coupled to different second messenger systems or to different ion channels. In addition, inhibitory interneurons may be involved in the circuitry of one of the nuclei. The importance resides in the simultaneous excitation of one and inhibition of the other. For example, the simultaneous excitation of neurons associated with cardiac acceleration (sympathetic) and inhibition of those associated with cardiac deceleration (parasympathetic).

MAGNOCELLULAR NEUROSECRETORY SYSTEM

Neurons in both the *supraoptic nucleus* and the *paraventricular nucleus* are the principal producers of two important circulating neurohormones, *oxytocin* and *vasopressin* (*antidiuretic hormone, ADH*). *Oxytocin* stimulates the *contraction of myometrial and myoepithelial cells* of the mammary glands (the milk-ejection reflex) and the uterus (contractions at parturition). *Vasopressin*, in contrast, is a potent *vasoconstrictor and antidiuretic*. Separate clusters of specialized neurons, the *magnocellular neurosecretory cells* (*MNCs*) synthesize each of these peptides. A different neural and humoral mechanism regulates the production and release of each hormone (Fig. 18–11).

Following synthesis in the cell body, the MNC stores the neurohormone in colloid-filled vesicles and transports these vesicles down axons to the nerve terminal. The axons form the *hypothalamoneurohypophysial tract*; these axons pass down the infundibular stalk and end as enlarged terminals adjacent to the capillaries in the *neurohypophysis* (*posterior pituitary*). Upon stimulation of the neuronal cell body in the hypothalamus, the terminals in the neurohypophysis release the hormone into the general circulation. The *MNCs*, the *hypothalamoneurohypophysial tract*, and the *neurohypophysis* together constitute the *magnocellular neurosecretory system*.

The sites of hormone production are not limited to MNCs of the paraventricular and supraoptic nuclei but also include scattered MNCs in small adjacent nuclei that produce one or the other of the hormones. Both the oxytocin MNCs and the vasopressin MNCs contain other peptides that are co-released with the neurohormones. The physiological significance of these other peptides is not known.

Although *vasopressin MNCs* are sensitive to changes in circulating plasma osmolality, they are not nearly as sensitive as neurons in the *organum vasculosum* (a small cluster of highly vascularized neurons in the lamina terminalis), the *subfornical organ* (a small cluster of neurons covered by a columnar ependymal layer and situated in the anterior wall of the third ventricle between the columns of the fornix), and the *periventricular neurons* (in the anteroventral part of the lateral wall of the third ventricle). These neurons are examples of *neurons within the CNS* that are capable also of *functioning as primary afferent receptors*. The *osmosensitive neurons* in all three of these structures respond to very small changes in the osmolality of the blood. These neurons, in turn, project to the MNCs that produce vasopressin.

The vasopressin MNCs receive adrenergic projections from the ventrolateral portion of the caudal medulla, the *A1 group of adrenergic neurons*. These neurons receive information from the *carotid chemoreceptors* and *baroreceptors* (glossopharyngeal and vagus nerves) that has been relayed in the *nucleus of the solitary tract*. Another afferent source triggering the release of vasopressin is the elevation in level of *circulating angiotensin II* that follows a vascular hemorrhage. Angiotensin II acts directly on neurons in the *subfornical organ* that excite vasopressin MNCs, thus increasing the release of vasopressin in the neurohypophysis.

The *oxytocin MNCs* receive afferent projections from *serotoninergic neurons* of the *midbrain raphe*. Additional afferents to the oxytocin MNCs arise from neurons of the hypothalamic *arcuate nuclei* and a few from the *subfornical organ*. All three nuclear groups respond to the stimulus of suckling, but the pathways for this afferent information and that related to parturition are unknown.

PARVOCELLULAR NEUROSECRETORY SYSTEM

The *adenohypophysis* (*anterior pituitary*) produces six hormones—four of which are tropic hormones, hormones that stimulate or regulate the function of other endocrine glands (see Table 18–4). The production and release and the inhibition of release of these hormones by the adenohypophysis are under the *humoral control* of the hypothalamus. Small groups of neurons in the hypothalamus, many in the region of the tuber cinereum, synthesize one of seven *HHHs*. Of the seven, five are well-characterized peptides and one is the catechol amine, dopamine. The neu-

FIGURE 18-11

The magnocellular neurosecretory cells (MNCs), parvocellular neurosecretory cells (PNCs), and hypophyseal vasculature.

Large MNCs from the paraventricular and supraoptic nuclei send varicosed axons into the neurohypophysis. These varicosities contain neurosecretory material en route to the nerve terminal. When stimulated, the MNCs release oxytocin or vasopressin into the capillary beds of the neurohypophysis and into the general circulation.

In contrast, small PNCs of the tuberal region send axons into the neurohemal zone of the median eminence. When stimulated, the PNCs release hypothalamic hypophysiotropic hormones (HHHs) into the capillary bed formed from the superior hypophyseal arteries in the neurohemal zone. Instead of entering the general circulation, these hormones are transported by a series of portal veins to the venous sinusoids of the adenohypophysis. Once in the adenohypophysis, the HHHs stimulate or inhibit the release of adenohypophysial trophic hormones. This unique vascular system is the hypothalamohypophysial portal system. See text for details.

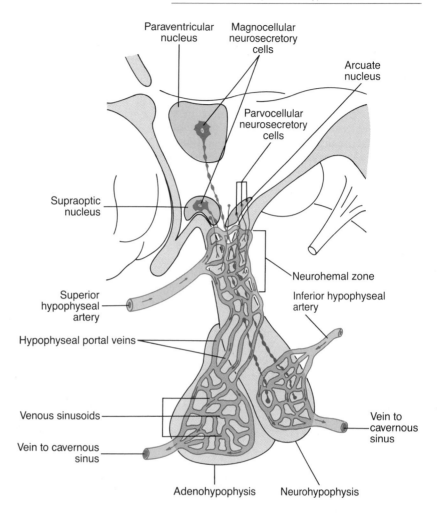

TABLE 18-4

Humoral Regulation of the Adenohypophysis

ADENOHYPOPHYSEAL HORMONE	HYPOTHALAMIC HYPOPHYSIOTROPIC HORMONES
Adrenocorticotropic hormone (ACTH)	Corticotropin-releasing hormone (CRH)
Growth hormone (GH) (somatotropin)	Growth hormone-release-inhibiting hormone (GHRIH, somatostatin)
	Growth hormone–releasing hormone (GHRH)
Thyrotropic hormone (TSH)*	Thyrotropin-releasing hormone (TRH)
Prolactin	Prolactin-inhibiting hormone (PIH) (dopamine)
	Prolactin-releasing hormone (PRH)
Follicle-stimulating hormone (FSH)	Gonadotropin-releasing hormone (GnRH) is identical with follicle-stimulating hormone releasing–hormone (FSHRH). GnRH stimulates the release of both FSH and LH.
Luteinizing hormone (LH)†	Gonadotropin-releasing hormone (GnRH), identical with luteinizing hormone–releasing hormone (LHRH). GnRH stimulates the release of both FSH and LH.

*The older abbreviation for thyrotropic hormone (formerly thyroid stimulating hormone) is retained to avoid confusion with the abbreviation for thyroid hormone.

†Previously known as interstitial cell-stimulating hormone (ICSH) in the male. Nomenclature now uses only GnRH, because the molecule is the same, male or female.

rons that produce the HHHs are small, lack the large colloid-filled vesicles of the MNCs, and are known as *parvocellular neurosecretory cells (PNCs)* (see Fig. 18 – 11).

The *parvocellular neurosecretory system* consists of the *PNCs* and the unique *hypophyseal portal system*, the vascular channels that carry the HHHs to the adenohypophysis following their release in the hypothalamus by the PNCs. The *superior hypophyseal arteries*, branches of the internal carotid, enter the basal portion of the median eminence and form into a dense *plexus of capillary loops* in the *neurohemal zone* of the *median eminence*. The blood in this capillary bed picks up the released HHHs and carries them through a network of small venous channels linking the hypothalamus with the venous sinusoids of the adenohypophysis. This network, the capillary bed of the neurohemal zone, the venous channels, and the venous sinusoids of the adenohypophysis constitute the *hypophyseal portal system* (see Fig. 18 – 11). Because this vascular portal system is very small in volume, the release of small amounts of the HHH by the hypothalamus produces a high concentration in the adenohypophysis — many orders of magnitude higher than the release of the same amount of hormone into the general circulation.

THERMOREGULATION

Thermoregulation, the control of body temperature, is an example of integrated *autonomic, neuroendocrine, somatomotor,* and *behavioral responses*. The hypothalamus is a central control center for these mechanisms and an important sensory transducer. Among other things, *destruction of the hypothalamus leads to the inability to regulate properly body temperature.*

Many neurons throughout the brain and spinal cord are temperature sensitive. Their firing rates change in response to very small changes in the temperature of the circulating blood. In addition, peripheral temperature sensors exist throughout the body that transmit information on both body temperature and environmental temperature via the somatosensory system. However, the *temperature-sensitive neurons* in the CNS, and those in the hypothalamus in particular, are sensitive to very small changes in temperature ($<0.1°$ C). These sensory neurons of the hypothalamus are in close contact with fine capillary beds within the neural tissue.

A hierarchy of control of body responses to temperature changes exists, with each level subject to modulation by higher centers and with the hypothalamus as the CNS control center. Body responses to changes in temperature fall into two categories: *heat dissipation responses* that tend to lower the body temperature and *heat conservation responses* that tend to increase the body temperature.

Heat dissipation responses include such mechanisms as *peripheral vasodilation*, the *sweating response*, the somatovisceral response of *accelerated respiration,* and the general behavior response of *decreased somatomotor activity*. Stimulation of areas in the anterior hypothalamus elicits most of these responses.

Heat conservation responses are mechanisms such as *peripheral vasoconstriction, increased heart rate, increased body metabolism,* and the general behavioral response of *increased somatomotor activity*. One additional heat conservation response involves somatic muscle tissue, *shivering*. This mechanism is not understood; however, the response requires the hypothalamus, because damage to the hypothalamus abolishes the shivering response. Stimulation of areas in the posterior half of the hypothalamus elicits most of these responses. The *increased body metabolism is a neuroendocrine mechanism*. The hypothalamus releases more TRH into the portal system, triggering an adenohypophyseal release of thyrotropic hormone that in turn stimulates the thyroid gland to release additional thyroxin and triiodotyrosine.

Although some division of labor exists between areas, e.g., anterior for heat dissipation and posterior for conservation, the *medial preoptic area* is critical for the visceral responses to temperature challenges. The medial preoptic area, however, does not affect the behavioral mechanisms. These mechanisms are abolished or impaired with damage to the lateral hypothalamic area.

Even with hypothalamic damage, local reflexes are still responsive to some of the larger changes in temperature, i.e., the somatovisceral reflex of vasoconstriction observed when placing one's hand in cold water. These local responses are not an effective homeostatic mechanism for the maintenance of a constant body temperature. For this, the hypothalamus is essential.

BODY FLUID REGULATION AND THIRST

The regulation of body fluid includes a broad range of biological responses from osmoregulation at the cellular and tissue level to initiating a behavioral drive to seek and consume water at the organismic level. In a broad sense, all these responses are to thirst, although we normally think of thirst as the behavioral drive elicited by the sensory stimulus of a dry mouth.

Four categories of stimuli elicit the thirst responses. The first is *an increase in plasma osmolality*, a condition that stimulates CNS osmoreceptors. The second is *a decrease in plasma volume*, or *hypovolemia*, as might occur from a vascular hemorrhage, a condition that stimulates both the baroreceptors and the production and release of angiotensin II by the kidneys. The third is *primary afferent sensory information* (GVA fibers of the glossopharyngeal nerve) to the nucleus of the solitary tract. The fourth category is *behavioral or cognitive factors*, such as the sight of a drink, factors involving limbic and neocortical mechanisms associated with conditioning and learning.

Sensory signals, from *carotid baroreceptors* (sensing a blood pressure drop as occurs in hypovolemia) and from *GVA receptors* in the oral and pharyngeal mucosa (sensing "dryness"), reach the *paraventricular nucleus*, the *supraoptic nucleus*, and the *lateral area of the hypothalamus* after relay in the *nucleus of the solitary tract*. This arrangement provides a direct route for the sensory information to reach the hypothalamus. Our conscious appreciation of the dry-mouth sensation, however, involves the relay of this information to the primary sensory cortex.

Osmoreceptors are CNS neurons that are able to detect very small changes in the plasma osmolality. These neurons, found in the *hypothalamus* and the *subfornical organ*, are an important class of receptors for the regulation of body fluid. The subfornical organ has major projections to the paraventricular and supraoptic nuclei and to the lateral area of the hypothalamus as well as many limbic and basal forebrain structures.

Angiotensin II levels in the circulating plasma are another important sensory signal in the regulation of body fluids. Following hemorrhage and reduction in plasma volume, circulating levels of angiotensin II rise. Neurons in both the *subfornical organ* and in the *medial preoptic area* of the hypothalamus have *angiotensin II receptors* and respond to changes in circulating levels of this hormone. Although angiotensin II has direct vascular pressor effects (increasing blood pressure principally through vasoconstriction), the vasopressor effects from stimulating angiotensin-sensitive neurons in the medial preoptic area and the subfornical organ are much greater.

The *behavioral or cognitive stimuli* for thirst

originate in the *cerebral cortex* and the *limbic system*. These probably influence the hypothalamus through projections to both the *lateral* and *medial areas*, areas containing reciprocal connections with limbic, basal forebrain, and frontal cortical areas. Direct connections also exist between the subfornical organ and these areas, providing a potential pathway for angiotensin II–stimulated, hypovolemic thirst to reach behavioral and somatomotor areas. Sensory information reaching the primary sensory cortex also provides associational input to those cortical and limbic areas responsible for the behavioral aspects of thirst drives.

Only a few of the connections between the afferent stimuli discussed previously and the efferent responses by the body to thirst are known. The hypothalamus, however, coordinates these responses. The *efferent responses to thirst fall into four categories*: (1) *autonomic* or *visceromotor (GVE)*, (2) *magnocellular neurosecretory cells (MNC)*, (3) *parvocellular neurosecretory cells (PNC)*, and (4) *behavioral*. The initial response varies with the initial stimulus, however, if the stimulus persists or is intense, the hypothalamus recruits other responses as well.

Baroreceptor reflexes are typical of autonomic or visceromotor responses. Stimulation of baroreceptors elicits vasopressor responses through the descending *hypothalamospinal tract* and other multisynaptic descending pathways to the sympathetic preganglionic fibers in the *intermediolateral cell column* of the spinal cord. The visceromotor responses are principally vasopressor and include *vasoconstriction, increased heart rate*, and *increased force in the contraction of the heart*. Additional visceromotor activities in response to thirst stimuli include the *release of catechol amines from the adrenal medulla* and other fluid conservation responses, such as an *inhibition of body sweating*, although adrenergic palmar sweating may occur.

The *MNC* response is one of the most important responses to thirst stimuli. The stimulation of *vasopressin-producing MNCs* in both the *supraoptic* and *paraventricular nuclei* increases the levels of circulating vasopressin. These higher levels have strong *vasopressor effects*, principally vasoconstriction and lead to higher blood pressure. Vasopressin also has strong *antidiuretic effects*. These hypothalamic nuclei receive strong projections from the subfornical organ and the medial preoptic area, thus an elevation in vasopressin levels is one of the initial responses to both hyperosmolality and hypovolemia. The nucleus of the solitary tract, a GVA processing station, also has strong projections to both the supraoptic and paraventricular nuclei, thus providing a direct route for sensory-stimulated increases in vasopressin.

The *PNC* response leads to an increase in circulating adrenal corticosteroids. The largest concentration of PNCs associated with the production of *corticotropin-releasing hormone (CRH)* is in the *paraventricular nucleus*. The release of CRH into the hypophyseal portal system leads to an increase in the release of *ACTH* by the *adenohypophysis*. ACTH, in turn, stimulates the release of *corticosteroids* from the cortex of the *adrenal gland*. Among other properties, the corticosteroids have vasopressor effects. One of the corticosteroids, cortisol, also raises blood glucose levels. Information about hyperosmolality, hypovolemia, and GVA thirst sensations all project to the paraventricular nucleus.

The *behavioral responses* to thirst are complex. Cognitive mechanisms or conditioned responses eliciting the thirst drive involve the *limbic system* and the *neocortex*. The initiation of somatomotor responses directed at the seeking and consumption of water involves the cerebral cortex, basal ganglia, and cerebellum, as do all somatomotor responses. However, the hypothalamus becomes a modulator and coordinator of those responses to the thirst drive. These mechanisms may involve some of the reciprocal connections between the hypothalamus and cerebellum. These connections appear to have vasopressor effects and other vasoregulatory functions.

REGULATION OF FOOD INTAKE

The hypothalamus plays an important role in eating behavior; however, the mechanism of this control is unknown. For many years, the ventromedial nucleus was considered a "satiety center" and the lateral area of the hypothalamus a "feeding center." Further data, however, raise questions about the validity of these roles. One fact remains firm—the *paraventricular nucleus* regulates food intake but through a mechanism yet to be defined. The involvement of the paraventricular nucleus is not surprising because it is a principal efferent nucleus of the hypothalamus. Pancreatic insulin release stimulates feeding behavior, and vagal efferents to the pancreas stimulate insulin release. Projections from the paraventricular nucleus and from other hypothalamic nuclei modulate these vagal efferents through projections to preganglionic neurons in the dorsal

motor nucleus of the vagus. In addition, the release of norepinephrine in medial regions of the hypothalamus also stimulates insulin release and initiates feeding behavior. These norepinephrine projections (some to the parvocellular portion of the paraventricular nucleus) originate principally in the locus ceruleus of the brain stem.

The presence of insulin receptors in neurons of the hypothalamus makes it likely that these neurons monitor circulating levels of insulin and respond accordingly. To date, however, the mechanism whereby the hypothalamus regulates eating behavior in response to the body's needs is not known. The hypothalamus is important in feeding. Pathology of the hypothalamus can lead to many eating disorders as can pathology of the closely interconnected structures of the limbic system.

CIRCADIAN RHYTHM AND THE BIOLOGICAL CLOCK

The *suprachiasmatic nucleus* is the circadian rhythm generator. Although it receives direct retinal input via the retinosuprachiasmatic projections and indirect input via the lateral geniculate nucleus, these projections only "lock" the rhythm into a precise 24-hour cycle. The loss of visual input does not abolish the circadian rhythm; however, the rhythm no longer remains "locked" to a day-night period but is "free running," with a regular cyclic pattern that is close to but not equal to 24 hours. Other afferents to the suprachiasmatic nucleus include serotoninergic projections from the midbrain raphe nuclei; however, the function of these projections is unknown. The mechanism of the generation of the circadian rhythm by this biological clock is not understood; however, projections from this nucleus regulate those mechanisms, principally neuroendocrine, that follow a circadian pattern.

SEXUAL BEHAVIOR AND REPRODUCTION

Centers within the hypothalamus control many patterns of sexual differentiation, both endocrinological and behavioral. In the adult, the hypothalamus, principally through the *PNC system* and the *hypothalamic-hypophyseal-gonadal axis*, modulates *humoral, behavioral, and physiological patterns related to sexual behavior and reproduction*.

In early development, the hypothalamus is "female." In the normal, genetic *female* this leads to the differentiation of a system that *produces and releases gonadotropin-releasing hormone (GnRH) in a cyclical pattern.* This activity, in turn, stimulates the *release of follicle-stimulating hormone (FSH) and luteinizing hormone (LH) by the adenohypophysis.* This cyclic pattern, beginning at the onset of puberty, regulates the menstrual cycle, the production of estrogen and progesterone, and ovulation.

The exposure of the hypothalamus to circulating androgens during early postnatal life in the normal genetic *male* alters the development, and the hypothalamus takes on "male" characteristics. Beginning at puberty in the normal male there is a *continuous, low-level release of GnRH* from PNCs in the hypothalamus. GnRH, in turn, leads to the production and release of FSH and LH by the adenohypophysis. In the male, these gonadotropins stimulate spermatogenesis, testosterone production, and the development of secondary sexual characteristics.

Exposure of a genetic female to androgens during this critical period of perinatal development results in the hypothalamus differentiating into a "male" structure. Morphological changes occur in several nuclei of the medial preoptic and suprachiasmatic areas, changes that are characteristic of the normal male hypothalamus. At puberty, the "androgenized" female will be sterile and acyclic and will release GnRH in a tonic pattern characteristic of the male.

The *medial preoptic* and *suprachiasmatic areas* generate the characteristic cyclic pattern of gonadotropic hormone release in the female. These nuclei receive many inputs from higher cortical and limbic centers as well exteroceptive stimuli, including direct retinal projections to the suprachiasmatic nucleus. The day-night (light-dark) patterns generated by this input may be responsible for the observation that Eskimo women often become acyclic. They frequently do not ovulate during the period of extended darkness characteristic of the Arctic winter. In addition, the strong limbic system and neocortical projections can alter the normal female cyclic pattern, which often is apparent during periods of physical or emotional stress.

EMOTIONAL EXPRESSION AND THE LIMBIC SYSTEM

Emotions trigger a complex of mental and physiological responses, and many of the physiological responses require the autonomic nervous system for their expression. Strong projections are sent from the limbic system to the hypothalamus. These limbic-hypothalamic projections provide the afferent signals for the visceromotor responses, be they tears of joy or the sweaty palms and sticky mouth of fear. The magnitude of the autonomic response to emotions, such as love, hate, anger, rage, fear, grief, sadness, and joy, varies from individual to individual and so does the degree to which an individual is able to override the autonomic responses at the neocortical level, i.e., "control one's emotions" (see Chapter 22).

Brain Stem, Cerebellar, and Cortical Influences

BRAIN STEM AND PRESSORECEPTOR REFLEX

Within the brain stem a central pattern generator (CPG), or a central oscillator circuit, generates a pattern of rhythmic discharges in autonomic cardiovascular neurons. Superimposed on this basic pattern is the pulse-synchronized baroreceptor afferent activity. Thus, the intrinsic brain stem circuitry generates a basic pattern. The baroreceptor reflex modulates or "locks in" the pattern to the appropriate rate and degree of heart muscle contraction. As with other motor systems, this reflex modulation of a basic pattern also is subject to further modulation from higher centers, i.e., the hypothalamus and the cerebral cortex.

Two important brain stem centers for the regulation of cardiovascular function are the *pressor center* and the *depressor center*. These centers act in concert to maintain an adequate systemic blood pressure. The *pressor center*, in the lower pontine reticular formation and extending into the lateral medullary reticular formation, generates a constant rhythmic pattern of excitation to *preganglionic sympathetic vasoconstrictor* and *cardiac accelerator neurons.* Another name for the pressor center is the *rostral ventrolateral medullary reticular formation*, although it includes a part of the caudal pontine tegmentum. Descending reticulospinal neurons from the pressor center, projecting to the intermediolateral cell column of the thoracic spinal cord, have pacemaker qualities, i.e., a rhythmic pattern of discharge.

The *depressor center* is in the medial and more caudal portion of the medulla, the *caudal ventromedial medullary reticular formation*, and extends from the level of the facial colliculus to the obex of the medulla. The depressor center also is tonically active, exciting *vagal preganglionic cardiac decelerator neurons* in the dorsal motor nucleus of X. Considerable overlap occurs between the two areas, creating an intermediate zone that elicits either pressor or depressor responses on stimulation. The opposite but complementary actions of the two centers provide a mechanism for increasing or decreasing heart rate and blood pressure to meet the body's demands.

The *arterial baroreceptor reflex* integrates the activities of the pressor and depressor centers for the maintenance of an appropriate blood pressure and heart rate. The *glossopharyngeal* and *vagus nerves* transmit baroreceptor information from pressor receptors in the *carotid sinus, vena cava, aortic arch*, and *auricle of the heart* to the *solitary nucleus* in the medulla. This information reflexly modulates the activity of both the pressor and depressor centers. These centers, in turn, modulate the level of excitement of the preganglionic neurons that drive the cardiovascular responses. In addition, the baroreceptor locks in the rhythmic pattern of pressor and depressor centers to the physiological needs of the system. Without this reflex, the rhythmic pattern would be free running.

With a *decrease* in *blood pressure*, there is a corresponding *decrease in baroreceptor discharge* that leads to a synchronous *increase in the sympathetic firing rate* and a *decrease in the parasympathetic firing rate*. The increase in sympathetic activity, driven by the pressor center, leads to increases in heart rate, heart stroke volume, and peripheral vascular tone. Simultaneously, the depressor center becomes less active and there is a corresponding decrease in vagal activity.

The reverse is true when there is an *increase* in *blood pressure*. An *increase in baroreceptor discharge* leads to a synchronous *decrease in sympathetic firing rate* and an *increase in parasympathetic firing rate*. The decrease in sympathetic firing reduces peripheral vascular tone, and the increase in parasympathetic firing slows the heart rate and reduces the stroke volume. Both the sympathetic and parasympathetic systems act in concert to provide the fine balance between pressor and depressor responses. This fine balance between agonist and antagonistic effects is just as important for the smooth functioning of the cardiovascular system as it is for the smooth execution of motor acts by the somatomotor system.

Without input from higher brain centers, above the pons, the cardiovascular system functions and maintains a regular pulse rate and a constant blood pressure. Damage to either of the medullary centers or to the solitary nucleus leads to a drop in blood pressure and a loss of vital reflex control.

CEREBELLAR INFLUENCE ON AUTONOMIC ACTIVITY

The *hypothalamocerebellar* and *cerebellohypothalamic pathways* provide direct connections between the integrative centers for visceromotor and somatomotor activity. The cerebellum is active in the planning, coordination, and execution of somatomotor activity. Through these direct connections, the visceromotor system can *anticipate the visceromotor needs of somatic tissue and continuously monitor the demands of new steady states*, i.e., metabolic and vasoregulatory requirements of specific muscle groups during a somatomotor activity, in progress or anticipated. These direct connections probably represent only a fraction of the interaction between these two centers, because both have extensive connections with the brain stem reticular formation. The general pattern of cerebellar projections to the hypothalamus suggests that these interactions involve the planning and coordination of a broad spectrum of visceromotor responses besides those involving the cardiovascular system.

CORTICAL MODULATION OF AUTONOMIC FUNCTION

The human brain has the capacity to override many, if not all, visceromotor activities that normally are considered reflexive or involuntary. For example, many Hindu yogis are able to exert "voluntary" control over such functions as heart rate, blood pressure, respiration, gastrointestinal motility, and sphincter control. They achieve this state, however, only through intense concentration and practice. Normal function does not require this type of "mind-over-body" control. However, these abilities do illustrate that the neural connections and pathways for that potential control exist. This control also implies that we may be unaware of existing, but subtle, neocortical modulations of autonomic function.

Disorders of Autonomic Function

HYPOTHALAMUS AND BRAIN STEM DISORDERS

Because the hypothalamus is small, lesions of this regulatory station of autonomic function usually involve several nuclei and pathways. Therefore, even small lesions can produce a variety of symptoms, depending on the specific area or areas damaged. Thus, the following disorders may occur in various combinations following damage to the hypothalamus.

Homeothermy, the maintenance of a constant body temperature, is often impaired following damage to the hypothalamus. *Hyperthermia*, from the *inability to dissipate body heat*, is the most common. If the involvement is hypothalamic, local spinal reflexes remain intact, e.g., vasodilation of the hand after exposure to warm water. These reflexes, however, are not sufficient for the homeostatic regulation of body temperature.

Diabetes insipidus often is a consequence of hypothalamic damage. This disorder is characterized by the production of copious amounts of dilute urine (*hyposthenuria*) and an insatiable thirst and the incessant drinking of large amounts of water (*polydipsia*). Most often, diabetes insipidus involves either insufficient production or release of *vasopressin*. This may result from the loss of the specific MNCs that produce vasopressin or from damage to the paraventricular and supraoptic nuclei or to the tuberoinfundibular tract. Damage to the nuclei or the tract produces a concomitant loss of *oxytocin*, clinically apparent only during parturition and lactation.

A number of sleep disorders, *narcolepsy, insomnia, hypersomnia*, and other changes in the normal sleep rhythm, may accompany damage to the hypothalamus. These disorders are also symptomatic of damage to lower brain stem centers. When they are caused by hypothalamic damage, other symptoms of hypothalamic malfunction accompany the sleep disorders.

A full range of eating disorders often accompany hypothalamic damage. These range from *bulimia*, a ravenous, insatiable appetite for food, to *anorexia nervosa*, a lack appetite for food and an intense fear of becoming fat. Both disorders may be accompanied by periods of binge eating followed by induced vomiting to rid the body of the food. The latter often leads to *cachexia* or a general wasting due to malnutrition, with an accompanying *amenorrhea* in the female patient. The last may be secondary to the cachexia or may be caused by an alteration in the parvocellular neurosecretory cell system and gonadotropin release from the anterior pituitary. The eating disorders, in the absence of other evidence of hypothalamic dysfunction, may be psychogenic.

Hypothalamic malfunction during normal *growth* and *development* can lead to a number of disorders associated with hypofunction of the anterior pituitary. These result from alterations in the PNC system and the production of HHHs, e.g., *dwarfism* due to insufficient growth hormone and *delayed puberty* due to insufficient gonadotropin. *Adiposogenital dystrophy* (*Fröhlich's syndrome*) is a genetic disorder of hypothalamic function, present from birth and characterized by an obesity, especially around the shoulders and hips, and a generalized genital hypoplasia and immaturity.

The midbrain region, the *pretectal area* in particular, is essential for the parasympathetic pupillary light reflex. Damage to the pretectal area will abolish this reflex, producing the *Argyll Robertson pupil*, an effect that is almost always bilateral. The retina is sensitive to light (the patient can see); however, the pupils do not constrict in response to light stimuli. Usually, however, the pupillary constriction associated with the accommodation reflex is intact. Because the constrictor mechanism can be activated by accommodation, both the preganglionic and postganglionic fibers must be intact. The accommodation reflex, however, does not utilize the pretectal area. This pathway involves the visual stimulation of cortical areas and an undefined pathway from the cortex to the Edinger-Westphal nucleus of the oculomotor complex. The retina remains sensitive to light and vision is intact; however, the pupils do not contract in response to light but do contract in response to accommodation.

Lower brain stem damage, especially to the *vasopressor* and *vasodepressor* centers, may include episodes of *paroxysmal hypertension* or *orthostatic hypotension*. Both are often associated with space-occupying lesions of the posterior cranial fossa.

Familial dysautonomia (*Riley-Day syndrome*) is a rare autosomal recessive disorder. Although the effects of the disease include more than just the autonomic nervous system, the principal clinical signs are those of autonomic dysfunction. Some of the altered functions include an inability to regulate blood pressure, with the patient having alternating periods of *episodic hypertension* and *hypotension. Hyperthermia, hyperhidrosis,* and *reduced lacrimation* are present to varying degrees. A number of additional CNS problems may occur, such as epileptic seizures, dysarthria, incoordination, and insensitivity to pain. The molecular nature of the single-gene deficit remains unknown.

PERIPHERAL DISORDERS OF AUTONOMIC FUNCTION

Aganglionic megacolon (*Hirschsprung's disease*) is one of the most common anorectal congenital malformations. This results from a failure of neural crest cells to migrate to the distal part of the developing colon and rectum, leading to the *absence of Meissner's and Auerbach's plexuses from the distal bowel.* The extent of the deficiency is variable; it may involve the entire colon and rectum or only the distal most portion, including the internal anal sphincters. Normally, smooth muscle cells of the internal anal sphincter act as signal oscillators, generating their own sinusoidal waves of contraction that keep the internal sphincter closed. The sphincter relaxes reflexly, following distension of the lower bowel, a signal that is transmitter through Auerbach's plexus and is independent of spinal cord innervation. This reflex is absent in Hirschsprung's disease. In addition, the absence of enteric neurons in the lower bowel results both in a lack of muscle tone and peristalsis. These factors combine to produce a distended colon (megacolon), lacking in motility and prone to impaction.

Horner's syndrome results from an interruption of the *sympathetic innervation to the head and neck.* The interruption of the sympathetic innervation can be due to damage to the postganglionic sympathetics from the cervical ganglia (primarily the superior cervical ganglion), to the ganglion itself, to the preganglionic fibers, or to the descending central pathways en route to the intermediolateral cell column of the thoracic cord. The basic symptoms are as follows:

1. *Miosis* or pupillary constriction is due to the unopposed parasympathetic innervation of pupillary constrictors.
2. *Ptosis* of the upper eye lid is due to a loss of sympathetic innervation to the superior tarsal muscle.
3. *Anhidrosis,* or a lack of sweating, is due to a loss of innervation to the sweat glands.

4. *Facial flushing* is due to a loss of tone in the peripheral blood vessels of the face, leading to passive vasodilation.

If the loss of sympathetic innervation is unilateral, these symptoms are all ipsilateral. Because cocaine blocks the re-uptake of NE, eye drops containing cocaine are useful in testing for Horner's syndrome. When the drops are applied, the denervated or affected eye will not dilate but will remain constricted. The parasympathetic constrictors are acting unopposed. With the loss of sympathetic innervation, no release of NE occurs; hence, blocking the re-uptake of a neurotransmitter that is not being released has no effect.

If the postganglionic neurons are intact and if the lesion involves either the descending central pathways to the intermediolateral cell column or the preganglionic sympathetic fibers, drops containing hydroxyamphetamine, which promotes the release of NE, will dilate both eyes, assuming the postganglionic neurons are intact. If the lesion is postganglionic, the affected pupil will fail to dilate with the hydroxyamphetamine.

When the lesion involves either the postganglionic fibers or the ganglion, the target muscles (pupil dilators) become more sensitive, a phenomenon known as *denervation supersensitivity.* This phenomenon is demonstrable in a patient with Horner's syndrome, which is the result of a postganglionic lesion. With phenylephrine drops, an NE agonist, central or preganglionic lesions show equal dilation of both eyes. The postganglionic innervation is intact, and the target has not developed the supersensitivity due to denervation. However, when these drops are applied to a patient's eye with postganglionic involvement, the affected eye will dilate more than the normal eye because it is now more sensitive to the neurotransmitter agonist.

If there is a *loss of parasympathetic innervation to the eye* with the sympathetic innervation intact, the pupillary dilators will be unopposed in their action. Under these conditions, the pupil dilates (*mydriasis*) more than normal and the pupillary light reflex is absent. The pupillary constriction that normally accompanies the accommodation reflex is also absent, with the affected eye remaining dilated while the pupil of the unaffected eye constricts. If the oculomotor nerve, carrying the parasympathetic preganglionic fibers, is involved, problems occur with the extraocular musculature and the movement of the affected eye (see Chapter 19). Involvement of the ciliary ganglion and the postganglionic parasympathetic fibers affects only the pupil.

SUGGESTED READING

Furness, J. B., I. J. Llewellyn-Smith, J. C. Bornstein, and M. Costa (1988). Chemical neuroanatomy and the analysis of neuronal circuitry in the enteric nervous system. In *Handbook of Chemical Neuroanatomy*, Volume 6. *The Peripheral Nervous System*, A. Björklund, T. Hökfelt, and C. Owman (Editors). Elsevier Biomedical Publishers, New York, pp. 161–218.

An excellent review of the enteric nervous system. This chapter with many references integrates the neurochemical and morphological features of this complex "peripheral nervous system" and sets the stage for future studies addressing the relation of function to the chemical anatomy.

Haines, D. E., P. J. May, and E. Dietrichs (1990). Neuronal connections between the cerebellar nuclei and hypothalamus in *Macaca fascicularis*: Cerebello-visceral circuits. J. Comp. Neurol., 299: 1065–122.

In this article, the authors discuss the functional implications of the direct interconnections between the cerebellum and the hypothalamus for the regulation of visceromotor responses and their coordination with somatomotor activity. This article contains numerous references.

Renaud, L. P. (1987). Magnocellular neuroendocrine neurons: update on intrinsic properties, synaptic inputs and neuropharmacology. Trends Neurosci. 10: 498–502.

A mini-review of the advances in our understanding of the mechanisms regulating the activity of the magnocellular neurosecretory cells. Special emphasis is on the intrinsic and synaptic mechanisms that regulate their firing patterns and rate.

Swanson, L. W. (1987). The hypothalamus. In *Handbook of Chemical Neuroanatomy*, Volume 5. *Integrated Systems of the CNS*, Part I, A. Björklund, T. Hökfelt, and L. W. Swanson (Editors). Elsevier Biomedical Publishers, New York, pp. 1–124.

A review with many references of the advances in our understanding of the circuitry of the hypothalamus. Special emphasis is on the relation of this circuitry to the various endocrine, autonomic, and behavioral functions integrated by the hypothalamus.

CRANIAL NERVES

19

Synopsis of the Cranial Nerves

OCULOMOTOR, TROCHLEAR, AND ABDUCENS NERVES (III, IV, AND VI)

TRIGEMINAL NERVE (V)

FACIAL NERVE (VII)

GLOSSOPHARYNGEAL NERVE (IX)

VAGUS NERVE (X)

SPINAL ACCESSORY NERVE (XI)

HYPOGLOSSAL NERVE (XII)

This chapter contains a review of the cranial nerves, excluding those of special sense: the optic nerve (Chapter 11), the vestibulocochlear nerve (Chapter 12) and the olfactory nerve (Chapter 13). Many of the cranial nerves are "mixed," i.e., they contain more than one functional component. Other chapters present some of the same material as in this chapter, but from the perspective of the functional system and not the perspective of the cranial nerve as an entity. This chapter integrates the previous material for each cranial nerve and considers the peripheral course of each nerve. The clinical consequences of damage to either peripheral or central components of the nerve are discussed.

Oculomotor, Trochlear, and Abducens Nerves (III, IV, and VI)

Three cranial nerves, the *oculomotor, trochlear,* and *abducens* (*cranial nerves III, IV,* and *VI*),

provide *somatic motor innervation* to the *extraocular musculature*, the striated muscles that move the eyeball and raise the eyelid, and *parasympathetic visceral motor innervation* to the eye (Table 19–1). Of the seven muscles, the oculomotor nerve innervates five, and the trochlear and abducens nerves innervate one each. Because these striated muscles are not of pharyngeal arch origin, the functional motor component is *general somatic efferent* (*GSE*).

The oculomotor nerve exits the brain stem ventrally, into the interpeduncular fossa; the trochlear nerve exits from the dorsal surface of the brain stem, below the inferior colliculus; and the abducens nerve, from the ventral surface, at the medullopontine junction (Fig. 19–1).

In addition to the GSE component, the *oculomotor nerve* contains the *general visceral efferent* (*GVE*) preganglionic axons that synapse in the *ciliary ganglion* before innervating the *pupillary constrictors*, producing miosis, and the *muscles of the ciliary body*, producing accommodation (see Table 19–1).

TABLE 19–1

Functional Components of the Cranial Nerves*

CRANIAL NERVE	COMPONENTS	CNS NUCLEUS AND PERIPHERAL TARGET
Oculomotor nerve (cranial nerve III)	GSE	*Oculomotor nucleus.* Motor innervation to all extraocular muscles except the superior oblique and lateral rectus.
	GVE	*Edinger-Westphal nucleus.* Parasympathetic innervation of the eye. Preganglionic fibers synapse in the ciliary ganglion.
Trochlear nerve (cranial nerve IV)	GSE	*Trochlear nucleus.* Motor innervation to the superior oblique muscle.
Abducens nerve (cranial nerve VI)	GSE	*Abducens nucleus.* Motor innervation to the lateral rectus muscle.
Trigeminal nerve (cranial nerve V)	SVE	*Motor nucleus of cranial nerve V.* Branchiomotor innervation of the muscles of mastication, tensor tympani muscle, and tensor veli palatini muscle.
	GSA	*Spinal nucleus of cranial nerve V.* Somatic afferent innervation of the face, buccal mucosa, and anterior two thirds of the tongue.
		Main sensory nucleus of cranial nerve V and mesencephalic nucleus of V. Proprioceptive innervation of muscles of mastication.
Facial nerve (cranial nerve VII)	SVE	*Facial nucleus.* Branchiomotor innervation of the muscles of facial expression.
	GVE	*Superior salivatory nucleus.* Preganglionic fibers to the sphenopalatine ganglion; parasympathetic innervation of lacrimal, nasal, and palatine glands.
		Preganglionic fibers to the submandibular ganglion; parasympathetic innervation of sublingual and submandibular glands.
	GVA	*Nucleus of solitary tract.* Afferent innervation of the soft palate and nasal cavity.
	SVA	*Nucleus of solitary tract.* Taste to the anterior two thirds of the tongue.
	GSA	*Spinal nucleus of cranial nerve V.* Somatic afferent innervation of the external auditory meatus and external ear.
Glossopharyngeal nerve (cranial nerve IX)	SVE	*Nucleus ambiguus.* Branchiomotor innervation of the stylopharyngeus muscle.
	GVE	*Inferior salivatory nucleus.* Preganglionic fibers to the otic ganglion; parasympathetic innervation of parotid gland.
	GVA	*Nucleus of solitary tract.* Afferent innervation of the pharyngeal mucosa and the posterior third of tongue.
	SVA	*Nucleus of solitary tract.* Taste to the posterior third of tongue.
	GSA	*Spinal nucleus of cranial nerve V.* Somatic afferent innervation of external auditory meatus and external ear.
Vagus nerve (cranial nerve X)	SVE	*Nucleus ambiguus.* Branchiomotor innervation of laryngeal musculature.
	GVE	*Motor nucleus of cranial nerve X.* Preganglionic fibers for the parasympathetic innervation of thoracic and abdominal viscera.
	GVA	*Nucleus of solitary tract and the dorsal sensory nucleus of cranial nerve X.* Afferent innervation of the laryngeal mucosa and of the thoracic and abdominal viscera.
	SVA	*Nucleus of solitary tract.* Taste to the epiglottis (fetus and newborn).
	GSA	*Spinal nucleus of cranial nerve V.* Somatic afferent innervation of the external auditory meatus, external ear, and meninges.
Spinal accessory nerve (cranial nerve XI)	SVE	*Spinal accessory nucleus.* Branchiomotor innervation of portions of the trapezius and sternomastoid muscles.
Hypoglossal nerve (cranial nerve XII)	GSE	*Hypoglossal nucleus.* Somatic motor innervation of tongue musculature.

* The cranial nerves of special sense, optic (II), vestibulocochlear (VIII), and olfactory (I), are reviewed in Chapters 11, 12, and 13, respectively.

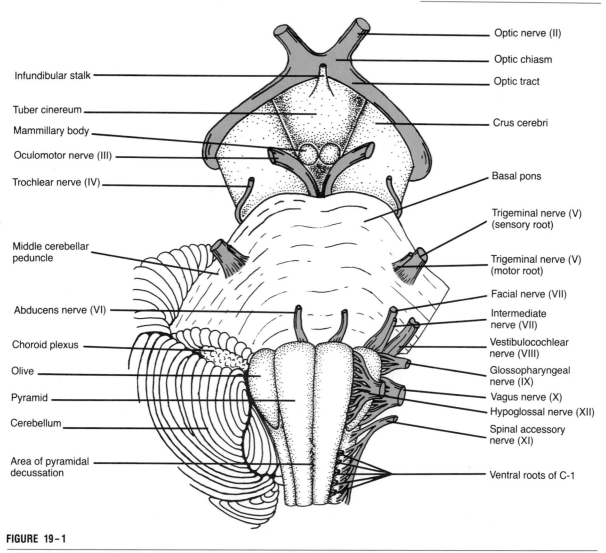

Infundibular stalk

Tuber cinereum

Mammillary body

Oculomotor nerve (III)

Trochlear nerve (IV)

Middle cerebellar peduncle

Abducens nerve (VI)

Choroid plexus

Olive

Pyramid

Cerebellum

Area of pyramidal decussation

Optic nerve (II)

Optic chiasm

Optic tract

Crus cerebri

Basal pons

Trigeminal nerve (V) (sensory root)

Trigeminal nerve (V) (motor root)

Facial nerve (VII)

Intermediate nerve (VII)

Vestibulocochlear nerve (VIII)

Glossopharyngeal nerve (IX)

Vagus nerve (X)

Hypoglossal nerve (XII)

Spinal accessory nerve (XI)

Ventral roots of C-1

FIGURE 19–1

Ventral view of the brain stem illustrating the cranial nerves. The "bulbar" component of the spinal accessory nerve (aberrant vagal fibers) is shown merging with the main trunk of the spinal accessory nerve. This bundle of fibers joins the vagus nerve as the two nerves pass through the jugular foramen. See text for details.

ANATOMY OF THE GENERAL SOMATIC EFFERENT COMPONENT

The *GSE* fibers of the oculomotor nerve arise from the *oculomotor nucleus* situated near the midline of the midbrain at the level of the superior colliculus. This nuclear complex is bounded ventrally and laterally by the medial longitudinal fasciculus (MLF) and dorsally by the periaqueductal gray (Fig. 19–2). The GSE component of

this nucleus contains individual subnuclei for each of the extraocular muscles. The *superior rectus muscle* receives innervation from neurons in a contralateral subnucleus; the *levator palpebrae superioris muscle*, from a medial subnucleus; and the *inferior rectus, medial rectus,* and *inferior oblique muscles* receive innervation from neurons in ipsilateral subnuclei (Fig. 19–3). The axons from these lower motor neurons arch in a ventral direction, through the substance of the

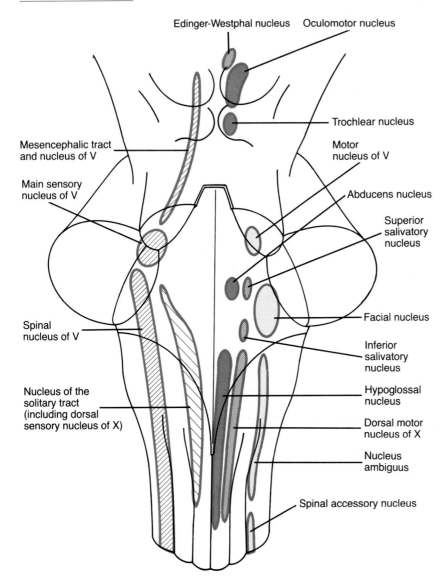

Edinger-Westphal nucleus   Oculomotor nucleus

Mesencephalic tract
and nucleus of V

Main sensory
nucleus of V

Spinal
nucleus of V

Nucleus of the
solitary tract
(including dorsal
sensory nucleus of X)

Trochlear nucleus

Motor
nucleus of V

Abducens nucleus

Superior
salivatory
nucleus

Facial nucleus

Inferior
salivatory
nucleus

Hypoglossal
nucleus

Dorsal motor
nucleus of X

Nucleus
ambiguus

Spinal accessory nucleus

FIGURE 19-2

Schematic of the main nuclei of the cranial nerves. The sensory nuclei are on the left, motor nuclei on the right. The nucleus of the solitary tract contains what some investigators consider a separate nucleus, the dorsal sensory nucleus of X. This distinction is not made in this text.

The mesencephalic tract and the nucleus of V along with the main sensory and spinal nuclei of V are general somatic afferent (GSA). The nucleus of the solitary tract is general visceral afferent (GVA) and special visceral afferent (SVA). The oculomotor, trochlear, abducens, and hypoglossal nuclei are general somatic efferent (GSE). The Edinger-Westphal nucleus, the superior and inferior salivatory nuclei, and the dorsal motor nucleus of X are general visceral efferent (GVE). The motor nucleus of V, the facial nucleus, the nucleus ambiguus, and the spinal accessory nucleus are special visceral efferent (SVE). See text for details.

midbrain and red nucleus, and exit the central nervous system (CNS) in the *interpeduncular fossa* (see Fig. 19–1).

The *oculomotor nerve* courses anteriorly from the interpeduncular fossa, pierces the dura mater, and courses in the lateral wall of the *cavernous sinus*. The nerve continues along the lateral and superior margin of the cavernous sinus and enters the orbit through the *superior orbital fissure*. Once in the orbit, the oculomotor nerve passes through the *common tendinous ring* and splits into *superior* and *inferior divisions* (Fig. 19–4). The common tendinous ring is a circumferential band of tendinous tissue that loosely surrounds the optic nerve. The four rectus muscles arise

from this ring, and the ring is anchored to the posterior wall of the orbit. The superior oblique and levator palpebrae superioris muscles arise separately from the posterior wall of the orbit, and the inferior oblique muscle arises from the floor of the orbit. The *inferior division* of the oculomotor nerve innervates the *inferior rectus*, *inferior oblique*, and *medial rectus muscles*; the *superior division* innervates the *superior rectus* and *levator palpebrae superioris* muscles (see Fig. 19–4).

The *GSE* fibers of the trochlear nerve arise from the *trochlear nucleus*. This nucleus lies near the midline of the midbrain at the level of the inferior colliculus and is bounded ventrally by the

FIGURE 19-3

The oculomotor nucleus illustrating the subnuclei innervating specific extraocular muscles of the right eye. *A*, Lateral view from the right side.

B, Dorsal view. Note that the superior rectus muscle receives innervation from neurons in a contralateral subnucleus and the levator palpebrae superior muscle from a medial subnucleus. Axons from these neurons form the superior division of the oculomotor nerve. The inferior rectus, medial rectus, and inferior oblique muscles receive innervation from neurons in ipsilateral subnuclei. Their axons form the inferior division of the oculomotor nerve. (Adapted with permission from R. Warwick, J. Com. Neurol., 98: 449–503, 1953.)

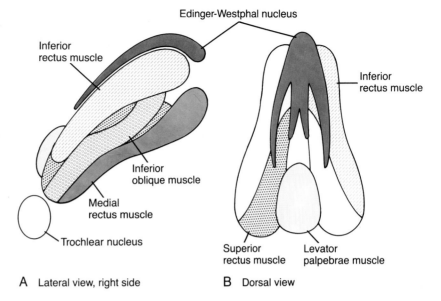

A   Lateral view, right side   B   Dorsal view

MLF and dorsally by the periaqueductal gray (see Fig. 19–2). Unlike other cranial nerves, the fibers of the trochlear nerve curve laterally and dorsally to *exit from the dorsal surface of the brain stem*, in the anterior medullary velum immediately below the inferior colliculus. In following this course, the nerve fibers curve around the cerebral aqueduct and decussate as they exit the brain stem (see Figs. 7–3 and 7–4). The *trochlear nerve* swings ventrally around the cerebral peduncle; courses anteriorly to pierce the dura mater; and courses in the lateral wall of the cavernous sinus, immediately below the oculomotor nerve. The trochlear nerve enters the orbit through the superior orbital fissure but above the common tendinous ring. Within the orbit, the trochlear nerve crosses over the levator palpebrae superioris and superior rectus muscles to innervate the *superior oblique muscle* (Fig. 19–5).

The *GSE* fibers of the abducens nerve arise from the *abducens nucleus*. This nucleus, like the two preceding nuclei, lies near the midline of the brain stem but at the level of the pontine tegmentum (see Fig. 19–2). The nucleus lies immediately under the *facial colliculus*, looping fibers of the facial nerve (see Fig. 1–25). The efferent fibers from the abducens nucleus arch ventrally and somewhat caudally to exit near the ventral midline at the medullopontine junction (see Fig. 19–1). From there, the *abducens nerve* courses anteriorly; pierces the dura mater; and enters the cavernous sinus, medial and inferior to the troch-

lear nerve and immediately below the internal carotid artery. Unlike the oculomotor and trochlear nerves that run in the lateral wall of the sinus, the abducens nerve courses within the cavernous sinus and is more vulnerable to injury following thrombosis of the cavernous sinus. The abducens nerve also enters the orbit through the superior orbital fissure, passes through the common tendinous ring lateral to the optic nerve, and innervates the *lateral rectus muscle* (see Fig. 19–5).

ANATOMY OF THE GENERAL VISCERAL EFFERENT COMPONENT

The *GVE* component of the *oculomotor nerve* arises from the *Edinger-Westphal nucleus*, situated dorsal and medial to the rostral portion of the main body (GSE) of the oculomotor complex (see Figs. 19–2 and 19–3). Axons from these *preganglionic parasympathetic neurons* enter the orbit with the main body of the oculomotor nerve, follow the inferior division of the nerve, and enter the *ciliary ganglion* (see Fig. 19–4). *Postganglionic parasympathetic* fibers from the ciliary ganglion form a number of *short ciliary nerves*, enter the eyeball, and innervate the pupillary constrictor muscle (*miosis*) and the circumferential muscle of the ciliary body (*accommodation*).

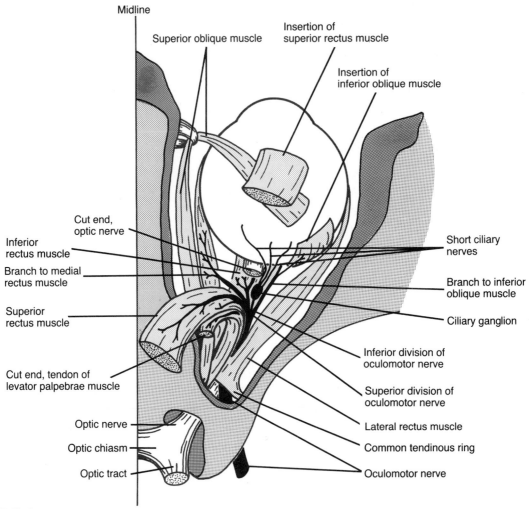

FIGURE 19-4

The orbit showing the oculomotor nerve entering through the tendon ring, lateral to the optic nerve, and splitting into two divisions. The superior division is to the superior rectus and levator palpebrae superior; the inferior is to the medial rectus, inferior rectus, and inferior oblique. The general visceral efferent (GVE) component and the ciliary ganglion (lateral to optic nerve) with short ciliary nerves are included.

Other nerve fibers pass through the ciliary ganglion en route to and from the eyeball. *Somatosensory fibers* leave the eyeball, pass through the ganglion, and join the nearby nasociliary branch of the ophthalmic division of the trigeminal nerve. *Sympathetic postganglionic fibers* reach the orbit as part of a nerve plexus surrounding the ophthalmic artery. These fibers pass through the ciliary ganglion, join both the long and short ciliary nerves, and provide the sympathetic innervation to the eyeball.

PROPRIOCEPTIVE INNERVATION OF EXTRAOCULAR MUSCLES

The smooth movement of the eye requires extensive proprioceptive information. The extraocular muscles are rich in muscle spindles. Some primary afferent fibers course with the oculomotor, trochlear, and abducens nerves; however, these are a very small percentage of the spindle afferents. Most of the spindle afferents travel with orbital branches of the ophthalmic division of the

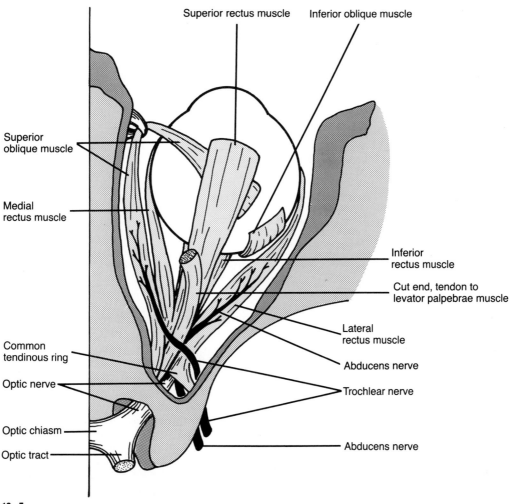

Superior rectus muscle

Inferior oblique muscle

Superior oblique muscle

Medial rectus muscle

Inferior rectus muscle

Cut end, tendon to levator palpebrae muscle

Lateral rectus muscle

Abducens nerve

Trochlear nerve

Common tendinous ring

Optic nerve

Optic chiasm

Optic tract

Abducens nerve

FIGURE 19-5

The orbit showing the *trochlear nerve* entering above the tendon ring and crossing over the superior rectus muscle and levator palpebrae superior muscle to innervate the superior oblique muscle. The *abducens nerve* enters through the ring to innervate the lateral rectus muscle.

trigeminal nerve (cranial nerve V) and reach the CNS as a GSA component of the trigeminal nerve. The cell bodies of these primary afferent neurons reside not in a ganglion but in the *mesencephalic nucleus of V* (see subsequent discussion).

CONTROL OF EYE MOVEMENT

Eye movements are very delicate and under fine control, a fact supported by the very small size of the motor units in the extraocular muscles and the large number of muscle spindles. Many eye movements are reflexive in nature, but volitional

commands readily override them. Because of the complex nature of the eye movements, the volitional movements incorporate many of the reflex mechanisms. Any single eye movement involves a complex symphony of synchronized excitations and inhibitions of the lower motor neurons that drive the extraocular muscles.

Each of the extraocular muscles, the four rectus muscles, and the two oblique muscles moves the eye in one of six directions (Table 19–2). Hence, the movement of the eye in any single direction is a vectorial summation of excitations (agonists) and inhibitions (antagonists). In addition, the vector of movement of the eye by any single

TABLE 19-2

Principal Eye Movements by the Extraocular Muscles

EYE MUSCLE	UNOPPOSED MOVEMENTS WITH EYE CENTERED	CRANIAL NERVE
Lateral rectus	Abducts the eye (moves *out*).	VI
Medial rectus	Adducts the eye (moves *in*).	III
Inferior rectus	Moves the eye down and adducts the eye. Rotates superior pole toward the temporal area.* (Moves *down* and *in*.)	III
Superior rectus	Moves the eye up and adducts the eye. Rotates superior pole toward the nose.* (Moves *up* and *in*.)	III
Superior oblique	Moves the eye down and abducts the eye. Rotates superior pole toward the nose.* (Moves *down* and *out*.)	IV
Inferior oblique	Moves the eye up and abducts the eye. Rotates superior pole toward the temporal area.* (Moves *up* and *out*.)	III

* These muscles also impart a rotational component, about the visual axis, to the overall movement of the eyeball.

muscle differs with the position of the eye. For example, with the eye centered, the superior rectus muscle both adducts the eye and moves the eye upward; however, with the eye abducted 23 degrees, the muscle moves the eye only upward.

The controlled relaxation of the antagonistic muscles is as important to smooth movement of the eye as is the smooth contraction of the agonist muscles. Although the circuitry is complex and much is unknown, several important components of eye movement can be described.

GAZE CENTERS

Within the brain stem are two areas known as *gaze centers*. these centers coordinate the *conjugate movement* of the two eyes in either the horizontal plane (*lateral gaze center*) or the vertical plane (*vertical gaze center*). In a sense, these are comparable to central pattern generators (CPGs) found at spinal and brain stem levels for patterned movements of the trunk and extremities.

The *lateral gaze center* resides in the pontine tegmentum, specifically the *paramedian pontine reticular formation*, *PPRF*, which is a part of the *nucleus reticularis pontis caudalis*. The *PPRF* is immediately rostral to the abducens nucleus and adjacent to the MLF. When stimulated, the PPRF excites motor neurons in the ipsilateral abducens nucleus, innervating the lateral rectus muscle, and excites motor neurons in the contralateral subnucleus of the oculomotor complex,

innervating the medial rectus muscle. These signals travel from the PPRF to the nuclei in the MLF, resulting a *conjugate movement of the two eyes* in the horizontal plane, an *abduction (lateral movement) of the ipsilateral eye and a synchronized adduction (medial movement) of the contralateral eye*. The actual mechanism is more complex, but these two muscles are the principal components. Besides excitation, there is also synchronous inhibition of the antagonistic muscles.

The *vertical gaze center* coordinates the conjugate movement of the two eyes in the vertical plane (upward and downward). Vertical gaze is more complex. The movement requires the synchronous excitation or inhibition of four muscles: the *superior* and *inferior rectus muscles* and the *superior* and *inferior oblique muscles* (see Table 19-2). Although not as well defined as the lateral gaze center, the vertical gaze center resides in the *periaqueductal gray* at the level of the superior colliculus, near the oculomotor complex. Projections from the vertical gaze center terminate in the trochlear nucleus (superior oblique muscle) and in the subnuclei of the oculomotor complex that innervate the inferior oblique muscle and the superior and inferior rectus muscles.

SACCADES, SMOOTH PURSUIT, AND VISUAL FIXATION

Saccades are very rapid (30 to 50 msec duration), voluntary eye movements. These occur when we read a printed page, scan a map, or look at the world around us. The eyes move in a very quick, darting fashion. The slower, *smooth pursuit movement* is possible only when the eye becomes *fixed* on an object and the eyes are *tracking* the object across the visual field. Without visual fixation, eye movements are saccadic in nature. Smooth pursuit movement requires visual fixation and is a reflex involving visual association areas.

VESTIBULAR-MEDIATED OCULOMOTOR REFLEXES

The vestibular system plays an important role in eye movement. Whenever the head moves in space, the vestibular nuclei signal the abducens, trochlear, and oculomotor nuclei via the MLF and *provide corrective eye movements that keep the eyes oriented in a horizontal plane and fixed on an object* (see Fig. 12–27). For example, as the head turns, the eyes tend to turn in the opposite direction, remaining fixed on an object. When the head turns to the point where the object is out of the field of vision, the eyes, in a rapid or saccadic movement, fix on a new object in visual space. If the head and body rotate, this reflex becomes more dramatic, with slow pursuit movement in the direction opposite the rotation, keeping the eyes fixed on an object, followed by a rapid snap of the eyes in the direction of rotation to fix on a new object. *The rapid or saccadic movement is always in the direction of the movement.* If the rotation continues, the process is repeated, always with the slow tracking movement keeping the eye fixed on an object and with the rapid saccade in the direction of the movement to fix on a new object. This sequence of slow and fast movements that continues for the duration of the rotation is the *vestibulo-oculomotor reflex (VOR)* or *nystagmus.*

Nystagmus is named for the direction of the fast component. For example, left nystagmus has the fast component of the movement to the patient's left. The vestibular nuclei drive the slow pursuit component. The PPRF drives the saccade. Visual association areas of the cerebral cortex, including the frontal eye fields, drive the PPRF. When the rotation stops, there is a brief period of *postrotatory nystagmus*, a nystagmus in the opposite direction because of the momentum of the endolymph in the semicircular canals. This causes a stimulation that mimics movement in the opposite direction, as the endolymph "catches up" with the semicircular canals.

VOLUNTARY EYE MOVEMENTS AND FRONTAL EYE FIELDS

The *frontal eye fields (FEFs)* are integral to visual tracking and to the initiation and coordination of voluntary eye movements. The generation of voluntary eye movements by the FEFs provides a mechanism for a cortical override of the more rigidly controlled saccadic movements generated at the level of the brain stem. This mechanism, however, can not override the saccadic movements of nystagmus. Because the *FEFs* are the cortical targets for the *oculomotor circuits* associated with the basal ganglia, these circuits of the basal ganglia probably function in the planning and execution of oculomotor activity. Both through these loops and direct intercortical pathways, the FEFs have extensive connections with the premotor area, the middle temporal visual area, and the dorsolateral prefrontal cortex.

If there is unilateral damage to one FEF, both eyes will deviate toward the side of the lesion. The eyes can't be turned in the opposite direction. Because these losses are transitory, it appears that the contralateral FEF can take over the function of both FEFs.

ACCOMMODATION REFLEX

The *accommodation reflex* occurs when the focus of the eyes moves from a distant object to a near object or when an object on which the eyes are fixed moves from a distant location to a near location. During the shift in focus from the distant to the near, *three motor events occur.* First is *ocular convergence.* This is a somatic motor response by the extraocular muscles, principally a contraction of both medial rectus muscles. A pathway from visual cortical areas to the oculomotor nuclei, by way of the superior colliculus, drives this motor response. Second, the *lens becomes more convex.* This event is due to the parasympathetic contraction of the circumferential muscles of the ciliary body, relaxing the tension on the suspensory ligaments and permitting the lens to round up. Third is *pupillary constriction.* This, too, is a parasympathetic response, a contraction of the pupillary constrictor muscles. Both parasympathetic responses involve the pretectal area. The entire course of the reflex loop is not understood. However, visual stimuli must reach the visual cortex, and cortical signals must reach the superior colliculus (somatic motor response) and the pretectal area (visceral motor response).

412 Cranial Nerves

EXTERNAL OPHTHALMOPLEGIAS

Oculomotor paralysis or *paresis* occurs following damage to the oculomotor nerve. *External strabismus* occurs, and the affected eye is turned down and out, owing to the unopposed action of the lateral rectus and superior oblique muscles (see Table 19–2). In addition, drooping of the eyelid, *ptosis*, occurs because of paralysis of the levator palpebrae superioris muscle. An interruption of the parasympathetic innervation of the pupillary constrictors and the ciliary muscles in the affected eye accompanies these somatic motor losses. This results in a *loss of the pupillary light reflex*, leading to a *dilated pupil* due to the unopposed action of the sympathetic innervation of the pupillary dilators. All three components of the accommodation reflex are lost, owing to an interruption of all the necessary efferent nerves.

Trochlear nerve paralysis or *paresis* occurs following damage to the trochlear nerve. Because only the superior oblique muscle is affected, *external strabismus* is produced, with the eye rotating up and out, owing to the unopposed action of the inferior oblique muscle. Usually, the patient compensates by tilting the head (the chin points away from the side of the affected eye) to avoid the *diplopia* or "double vision." On examination, the patient is unable to move the affected eye downward and outward (see Table 19–2).

Abducens nerve paralysis or *paresis* occurs following damage to the abducens nerve and affects only the lateral rectus muscle. This deficit produces an *internal strabismus*, with the eye tending to deviate toward the nose because of the unopposed action of the medial rectus. The patient is unable to fully abduct the affected eye and may tend to rotate the head toward the affected side to avoid diplopia. Some limited lateral movement of the eye is noted, because both the superior and inferior oblique muscles have a minor abductive component (see Table 19–2). The long intracranial course of the abducens nerve makes it susceptible to damage in cases of increased intracranial pressure. Its location within the cavernous sinus makes it vulnerable to damage following a cavernous sinus thrombosis.

CENTRAL OPHTHALMOPLEGIAS

Damage to some of the brain stem areas, nuclei, gaze centers, and superior colliculus often affects both eyes, because the structures are close to the midline. Damage to the superior colliculus, among other symptoms, interferes with the verti-cal gaze center. A loss of conjugate upward movement of the eyes takes place. Damage to the PPRF may produce an associated loss of lateral conjugate gaze movements. Similarly, damage to the MLF between the abducens nuclei in the pons and the trochlear and oculomotor nuclei in the midbrain alters the lateral gaze response and lead to a complex nystagmus due to the interruption of many of the vestibulo-oculomotor fibers.

Trigeminal Nerve (V)

The *trigeminal nerve* (*cranial nerve V*) is the largest of the cranial nerves and is the nerve that developmentally supplies the first branchial or pharyngeal arch. Two functional components are in the trigeminal nerve, a *branchiomotor* (*special visceral efferent, SVE*) component, innervating the muscles of mastication, and a *somatosensory* (*general somatic afferent GSA*), component. The GSA fibers innervate the entire face, from the lower margin of the mandible to the top of the scalp and laterally to the anterior portion of the pinna of the ear, including the anterior wall of the external auditory meatus. The trigeminal innervates most of the dura mater (Fig. 19–6).

ANATOMY

The *trigeminal nerve* leaves the brain stem through the middle of the brachium pontis in a ventrolateral location (see Fig. 19–1). The fibers of the trigeminal form two distinct and separate bundles at this level, the *portio major*, carrying the primary afferent fibers, and the smaller *portio minor*, carrying the branchiomotor fibers to the muscles of mastication.

Within 1 to 2 cm of the brain stem, the trigeminal nerve swells to form the very large *trigeminal ganglion* (*gasserian ganglion* or *semilunar ganglion*), which contains the cell bodies of the pseudounipolar primary sensory neurons. The trigeminal ganglion, lying in a depression in the floor of the middle cranial fossa, is functionally the "dorsal root ganglion" of the face.

As the fibers exit the trigeminal ganglion, they form three primary divisions: the *ophthalmic division* (V_1) innervating the upper portion of the face; the *maxillary division* (V_2) innervating the mid-face region; and the *mandibular division* (V_3) innervating the lower facial region (see Fig. 10–17). The motor fibers travel with the mandibular division. The ophthalmic and maxillary divisions carry only sensory fibers (see Fig. 19–6).

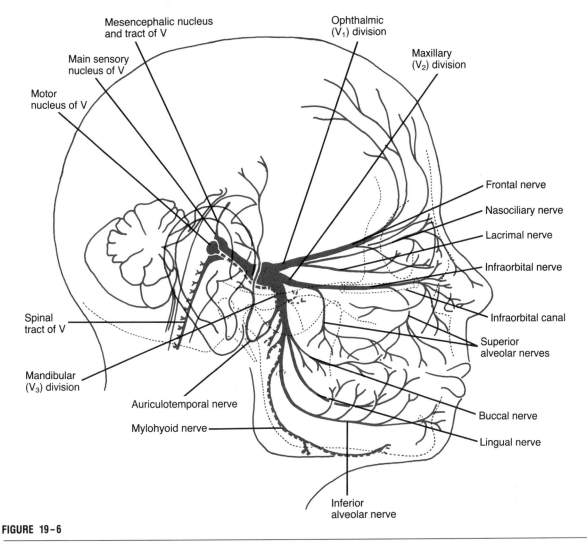

FIGURE 19-6

The course and distribution of the principal divisions and branches of the trigeminal nerve. GSA, solid red line; SVE, dotted red line.

PERIPHERAL COURSE

The *ophthalmic division,* V_1 leaves the trigeminal ganglion, passes through the dura, and enters the lateral wall of the cavernous sinus. The ophthalmic division runs forward in the lateral wall of the cavernous sinus below the trochlear and oculomotor nerves. Continuing forward, V_1 enters the orbit through the superior orbital fissure and divides into three terminal branches: the *nasociliary, lacrimal,* and *frontal nerves* (see Fig. 19-6). The *nasociliary nerve* supplies the external surface of the nose, anterior nasal cavity, ethmoid sinuses, and medial eyelids along with branches that pass through the ciliary ganglion to provide GSA innervation to the eyeball. This GSA innervation to the eyeball includes the cornea, an innervation that is important to the blink reflex. The *lacrimal nerve* carries information from the lateral part of the upper eyelids, the conjunctiva and the lacrimal gland. The *frontal nerve* provides GSA innervation to the frontal sinuses, the upper eyelid, the bridge of the nose, and the forehead.

The *maxillary division,* V_2, after leaving the trigeminal ganglion and entering the cavernous sinus, runs forward and slightly down to enter the foramen rotundum, in the pterygoid bone, and the pterygopalatine fossa. The main portion of the division continues forward as the *infraorbital nerve,* enters the infraorbital canal, and emerges from the skull through the infraorbital foramen (see Fig. 19–6). Within the pterygopalatine fossa, the maxillary division gives rise to other smaller terminal branches, the *zygomatic, pterygopalatine*, and *posterior superior alveolar nerves*. The *infraorbital nerve* provides cutaneous GSA innervation to the upper lip and to the medial cheek and lateral nose areas. This nerve also gives rise to the *middle* and *anterior superior alveolar nerves* that provide GSA innervation to the teeth in the maxilla. The *zygomatic nerve* provides GSA innervation to the area over the zygomatic arch and the lateral forehead and anterior temporal area. The *pterygopalatine nerve* provides GSA innervation to the posterior nasal cavity, the nasal septum, and the hard and soft palates.

The *mandibular division*, V_3, is the largest of the three divisions and contains all the motor (SVE) fibers besides the GSA fibers. The mandibular division leaves the cranial vault through the foramen ovale. Immediately after leaving the skull, this division gives off a recurrent branch to the dura that re-enters the skull through the foramen spinosum. At its point of exit from the skull, the mandibular division lies anteromedial to the temporomandibular articulation and close to the origin of the pterygoid muscles as well as the tensor and levator veli palatini muscles. Several small branches, the *nerves to the muscles of mastication*, containing both SVE and GSA fibers, run to the four muscles of mastication (the temporal, masseter, lateral pterygoid, and medial pterygoid) and to the tensor veli palatini and tensor tympani muscles.

The main terminal branches of the mandibular division include the sensory (GSA) *auriculotemporal, buccal, lingual*, and *inferior alveolar nerves* and the mixed (SVE and GSA) *mylohyoid nerve*. The mylohyoid nerve innervates the mylohyoid muscle and the anterior belly of the digastric muscle. This nerve arises from the inferior alveolar nerve (see Fig. 19–6). The *nerves to the muscles of mastication* also carry GSA information, principally proprioceptive, from the muscles of mastication. The *auriculotemporal nerve* carries GSA information from the side of the head and scalp, the anterior wall of the external auditory meatus, and the external surface of the tympanic membrane. The *buccal nerve* carries GSA information from the mucosa of the mouth and gums. The *lingual nerve* carries GSA information from the anterior two thirds of the tongue, and the *inferior alveolar nerve* carries information from the teeth of the lower jaw. The *mylohyoid nerve* carries proprioceptive informa-

tion (GSA) from and supplies motor innervation (SVE) to the mylohyoid muscle and the anterior belly of the digastric muscle.

The trigeminal nerve gives rise to several small *meningeal nerves*. Often, one or two arise from the proximal portion of the mandibular division, although one or two may arise from the proximal portion of the maxillary division. The meningeal nerves re-enter the cranial vault through the foramen spinosum and provide GSA innervation to the dura mater of the anterior and middle cranial fossae.

AUTONOMIC "HITCHHIKERS"

Many branches of the trigeminal nerve pick up "hitchhikers," bundles of nerve fibers, principally autonomic, as they course to their target areas. Sympathetic postganglionic fibers from the plexus on the internal carotid artery and parasympathetic preganglionic fibers from the greater petrosal branch of the facial nerve form the *nerve of the pterygoid canal* and enter the *pterygopalatine ganglion*. The parasympathetic preganglionic fibers synapse in this ganglion.

Postganglionic parasympathetic and sympathetic fibers join the adjacent *maxillary division* of the trigeminal nerve. Parasympathetic fibers to the glands of the nasal cavity, palate, and pharynx are distributed with branches of the maxillary division of the trigeminal nerve. Others, after a brief ride with the maxillary division, "change nerves" and join the *lacrimal nerve* of the *ophthalmic division* and provide autonomic innervation to the lacrimal gland (see Fig. 18–6).

The parasympathetic preganglionic fibers of the *chorda tympani nerve* join the *lingual nerve* of the *mandibular division* and hitch a ride to the *submandibular ganglion*, where they synapse. The postganglionic fibers innervate the sublingual and submandibular salivary glands.

Preganglionic parasympathetic fibers in the lesser petrosal nerve, which is glossopharyngeal in origin, enter the *otic ganglion* and synapse. Postganglionic fibers hitch a ride on the *auriculotemporal nerve*, as it passes the otic ganglion, and travel to the parotid gland. Sympathetic postganglionic fibers also join the auriculotemporal nerve, as it bifurcates to surround the middle meningeal artery (see Fig. 18–6). Although the trigeminal nerve does not have an autonomic, GVE, component as it leaves the brain stem, damage to some of the peripheral branches can produce autonomic deficits because of the hitchhikers.

BRAIN STEM NUCLEI

The trigeminal nerve has three sensory nuclei: the *spinal nucleus of cranial nerve V*, the *main sensory nucleus of cranial nerve V* (*chief* or *principal nucleus of cranial nerve V*), and the *mesencephalic nucleus of cranial nerve V*, in addition to the motor nucleus of cranial nerve V (Figs. 19–2 and 19–7).

Nearly half the afferent fibers from the trigeminal ganglion enter the brain stem, descend in the *spinal tract of cranial nerve V*, and terminate in the *spinal nucleus of cranial nerve V*. The spinal tract of cranial nerve V is a descending bundle of primary afferent fibers that merges imperceptibly with the dorsolateral fasciculus in the upper cervical segments of the spinal cord. In general, these are small fibers, comparable to type-Aδ and type-C fibers that make up the lateral division of the dorsal root in the spinal cord. Most carry information from pain and temperature receptors. Within the brain stem, the spinal tract of cranial nerve V courses near the dorsolateral

surface and extends caudad from the point of entry of the trigeminal nerve to the upper cervical segments of the spinal cord (see Fig. 19–7).

Of the remaining afferent fibers (large, myelinated type-Aβ fibers), most bifurcate with an ascending branch ending in the *main sensory nucleus of cranial nerve V* and a descending branch ending in the more rostral levels of the *spinal nucleus of cranial nerve V*, principally the *pars oralis*. These fibers are comparable to the medial division of the dorsal root and transmit various mechanoreceptive-mediated sensations, principally discriminative touch (see Fig. 19–7).

The *spinal nucleus of cranial nerve V* is a long column of neurons extending from the point of entry of the trigeminal nerve to the upper cervical spinal cord. This nucleus lies immediately deep to the spinal tract of cranial nerve V, and in the cervical spinal cord it merges with and becomes indistinguishable from the substantia gelatinosa (laminae I through IV) of the dorsal horn. The spinal nucleus of cranial nerve V contains three subdivisions: the *pars oralis* composes the

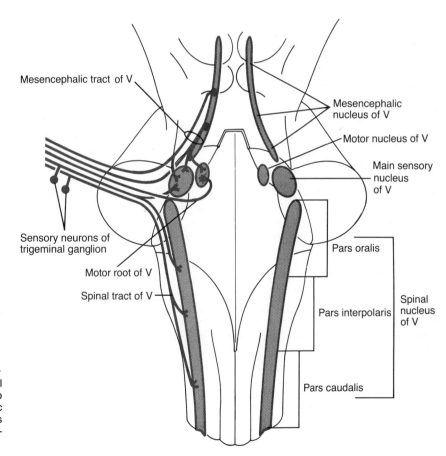

FIGURE 19–7

The nuclei of the trigeminal nerve. Note that there are no synapses in the mesencephalic nucleus of V, and the neurons are pseudounipolar primary sensory neurons.

rostral third of the nucleus; the *pars interpolaris* the middle third; and the *pars caudalis*, the caudal third (see Fig. 19–7). Pain and thermal sensations localize in the caudal portion of the spinal nucleus of cranial nerve V, whereas tactile sensations localize in the more rostral portions of the nucleus. A dorsal-ventral somatotopic organization to the spinal nucleus is evident, with fibers from the ophthalmic division ending throughout the ventral portion of the nucleus, the mandibular division in the dorsal portion, and the maxillary division in the middle.

The *main sensory nucleus of cranial nerve V* lies immediately rostral to its spinal nucleus in the mid-pons (see Fig. 19–7). Anatomically and functionally, the main sensory nucleus is the homologue of the dorsal column nuclei. The main sensory nucleus of cranial nerve V also is somatotopically organized in a manner similar to its of the spinal nucleus.

The *mesencephalic nucleus of cranial nerve V* is not a true nucleus; it lacks synapses and contains the cell bodies of displaced primary, pseudounipolar sensory neurons. These cell bodies, together with their central and peripheral processes, form the *mesencephalic tract* and *nucleus of V*, a thin column of pseudounipolar neurons adjacent to a small bundle of myelinated nerve fibers. These extend rostrally from the point of entry of the trigeminal nerve to the level of the oculomotor nuclei and superior colliculi in the midbrain. This nucleus and associated fiber tract lies along the lateral margin of the periaqueductal gray (see Figs. 19–2 and 19–7).

Most of the peripheral processes of the neurons of the mesencephalic nucleus of V exit with the motor root of the trigeminal nerve and accompany the motor branches to the muscles of mastication, where they end in muscle spindles and other proprioceptive receptors. The central processes of these neurons project to the *main sensory nucleus of cranial nerve V* and to the *motor nucleus of cranial nerve V*, the latter for reflex connections with the motor neurons (see Fig. 19–7).

The *motor nucleus of cranial nerve V* contains SVE branchiomotor neurons that innervate the muscles of mastication via the *portio minor* and the *mandibular division* (see Fig. 19–6). As with other motor nuclei, it contains both α- and γ-motor neurons.

CLINICAL DISORDERS

Paralysis or *paresis* of the muscles of mastication is readily detectable by palpation after the patient clenches the jaw. If the involvement is peripheral, the jaw will deviate toward the side of the lesion, the loss in bite strength will be unilateral, the muscles will be flaccid, and the muscle mass will atrophy with time. If it is an upper motor neuron lesion, the jaw reflex will be hyperactive. Other than this sign, the lesion may be undetectable. Alternatively, a bilateral weakness may be apparent, because the corticobulbar projections are a combination of crossed and uncrossed fibers (see Fig. 15–7). With a peripheral lesion, there also will be a loss of sensation to the area of the face supplied by the mandibular division (see Fig. 10–17).

Sensory deficits (loss of pain, temperature, and touch to the face) are useful in localizing damage to the trigeminal and its major divisions, because there is little overlap in the peripheral distribution of the fibers. One of the most common clinical problems is *trigeminal neuralgia*. With trigeminal neuralgia periods of severe, shooting pain are experienced. The pain localizes to one side of the face and involves the area of innervation of one or more of the divisions of the trigeminal nerve, usually the maxillary or mandibular divisions. The origin of the pain is not known. However, in severe cases, severing of the spinal tract of cranial nerve V in the lower medulla below the level of the inferior olive offers relief. The pars caudalis of the spinal nucleus of cranial nerve V receives principally pain fibers. Interruption of the spinal tract fibers at this level eliminates pain and some temperature sensation, while leaving the tactile sensations intact.

In localizing injury to branches of the trigeminal nerve, the integrity, or the lack thereof, of the autonomic innervation to salivary glands and lacrimal glands is valuable information. If damage occurs peripheral to the hitchhikers joining the nerve, an autonomic loss accompanies the sensory loss (see Fig. 18–6).

As with other sensory ganglia, the trigeminal ganglion is vulnerable to the infection of *herpes zoster*. This virus infection results in considerable pain and ulceration of the skin and mucous membranes supplied by the affected fibers. The ophthalmic division is most frequently affected.

Facial Nerve (VII)

The *facial nerve (cranial nerve VII)* has two parts, a facial nerve proper and an adjacent nerve root (the intermediate nerve, or the intermediate root of the facial nerve). The *facial nerve* and the *intermediate nerve* exit together from the ventrolateral surface of the brain stem at the medullo-pontine junction (see Fig. 19–1).

The *facial nerve* is the motor nerve to the muscles of facial expression. These muscles develop from the second branchial (pharyngeal) arch, and their innervation is therefore branchio-motor, or *special visceral efferent* (*SVE*). The *intermediate nerve* contains three sensory components: *general visceral afferent* (*GVA*), *special visceral afferent* (*SVA*, taste), and *general somatic afferent* (*GSA*), and a parasympathetic preganglionic visceromotor component, *general visceral efferent* (*GVE*). The intermediate nerve is sometimes called the sensory root of the facial nerve. This is a misleading term, because the nerve contains GVE fibers (Fig. 19–8).

PERIPHERAL COURSE

The *facial* and *intermediate nerves* exit the brain stem together and pass through the internal auditory meatus to enter the *facial canal* within the petrous portion of the temporal bone. The *geniculate ganglion*, containing cell bodies of the primary GSA, GVA, and SVA neurons, is in the facial canal. The central processes of these neurons enter the CNS as part of the intermediate nerve.

In the facial canal, the facial nerve gives rise to three branches: the *greater petrosal nerve*, the *nerve to the stapedius muscle*, and the *chorda tympani nerve*. At the level of the geniculate ganglion, GVE and GVA fibers from the intermediate nerve form the *greater petrosal nerve* and leave the facial canal. The greater petrosal nerve joins the deep petrosal nerve (sympathetic postganglionic fibers from the carotid plexus), forming the *nerve of the pterygoid canal* (*vidian nerve*). This nerve enters the pterygoid canal en route to the pterygopalatine ganglion (see Fig. 19–8 and Fig. 18–6). As the facial nerve traverses the facial canal it gives off the small *nerve to the stapedius muscle*, providing branchiomotor, SVE, innervation to the stapedius muscle. The third branch of the facial nerve contains GVE and SVA fibers and forms the *chorda tympani nerve*. After leaving the middle ear cavity, the chorda tympani nerve joins the lingual nerve to carry SVA taste sensation from the anterior two thirds of the tongue and GVE parasympathetic preganglionic fibers to the submandibular ganglion.

As the *facial nerve* exits the skull through the stylomastoid foramen, it runs through the body of the parotid gland and forms into many terminal branches that provide the branchiomotor, SVE, innervation to the muscles of facial expres-sion (see Fig. 19–8). At the point of exit, the facial nerve consists only of SVE fibers plus the very small GSA component destined for the pinna of the ear and external auditory meatus. *The facial nerve does not provide the parasympathetic innervation of the parotid gland. Instead this innervation reaches the parotid gland by way of the glossopharyngeal nerve, the otic ganglion, and the auriculotemporal branch of the trigeminal nerve* (see Fig. 18–6). Within the parotid gland, terminal branches of the facial nerve travel together with terminal branches of the auriculotemporal nerve, providing mixed motor and sensory innervation to the face and the muscles of facial expression.

SPECIAL VISCERAL EFFERENT (BRANCHIOMOTOR) COMPONENT

The large *facial nucleus* contains motor neurons that innervate muscles derived from the embryonic mesenchyme of the second branchial (pharyngeal) arch. These branchiomotor, SVE, neurons are the major component of the facial nerve. Muscles innervated include the facial expression muscles (the mimetic musculature), the stylohyoid muscle, the posterior belly of the digastric muscle, and the stapedius muscle of the middle ear.

Within the substance of the parotid gland, the *facial nerve* divides into six primary branches. Although some variation exists, usually these six branches are identifiable. The *temporal nerve* innervates the muscles in the upper face, including the frontalis and orbicularis oris muscles, the *zygomatic nerve* innervates the muscles in the middle portion of the face; and the *buccal nerve* innervates the cheek muscles, including the buccinator muscle. The *mandibular nerve* innervates the muscles of the lower face; and the *cervical nerve*, the muscles below the chin, including the platysma muscle. The relatively small *nerve to the digastric muscle* innervates the posterior belly of the digastric muscle and the stylohyoid muscle. The *posterior auricular nerve* innervates the occipitalis and posterior auricular muscles (see Fig. 19–8).

GENERAL VISCERAL EFFERENT COMPONENT

The facial nerve is one of four cranial nerves with a *GVE*, parasympathetic preganglionic motor component. The preganglionic neurons of the *facial nerve* are in the *superior salivatory nucleus*,

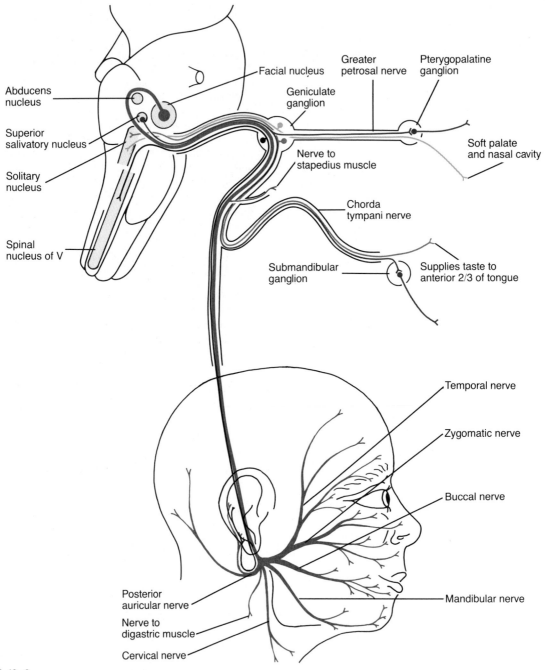

FIGURE 19-8

The course and distribution of the facial nerve and its primary branches. See text for details. SVE, dark red line; GVE, dark gray line; GVA, light red line; GSA, black line; and SVA, medium red line.

just rostral to the medullopontine junction (see Fig. 19–2). These preganglionic fibers exit the brain stem as a component of the *intermediate nerve* and subsequently leave the facial nerve as one of two branches, the *greater petrosal nerve* or the *chorda tympani nerve*.

Near the geniculate ganglion, the *greater petrosal nerve* leaves the facial nerve and the facial canal, enters the cranial cavity through the hiatus of the facial canal, and runs toward the internal carotid artery. There, it joins the deep petrosal nerve (sympathetic fibers from the internal carotid plexus) to form the *nerve of the pterygoid canal* (*vidian nerve*). After passing through the pterygoid canal, this nerve enters the palatine fossa, where the preganglionic parasympathetic fibers synapse in the *pterygopalatine ganglion*. From there, postganglionic fibers provide parasympathetic innervation to many *nasal, oral*, and *palatine glands* besides the *lacrimal gland*. Postganglionic fibers reach the lacrimal gland by first hitching a ride with the maxillary division of the trigeminal nerve and then with the lacrimal nerve, a terminal branch of the ophthalmic division of the trigeminal nerve (see Fig. 19–8 and Fig. 18–6). Traveling with the GVE fibers are GVA fibers (see the following discussion).

The *chorda tympani nerve* leaves the facial nerve and the facial canal and enters the *tympanic cavity*. It then crosses the lateral wall of the middle ear and runs under the mucous membrane on the inner surface of the tympanic membrane and over the manubrium of the malleus. Anteriorly, it exits the middle ear cavity, passes through the petrotympanic fissure, leaves the skull, and passes along the medial surface of the spine of the sphenoid bone. From there, the fibers of the chorda tympani nerve join the *lingual nerve*, a terminal branch of the *trigeminal nerve* (see Fig. 19–8). These preganglionic fibers synapse in the *submandibular ganglion*. From that ganglion, postganglionic fibers provide parasympathetic innervation to the *submandibular* and *sublingual glands* and other neighboring, smaller salivary glands in the oral cavity (see Fig. 19–8 and Fig. 18–6). The chorda tympani nerve also contains SVA fibers that innervate the anterior two thirds of the tongue (see subsequent discussion).

SPECIAL VISCERAL AFFERENT COMPONENT

The *facial nerve* contains an *SVA* component that carries taste information from the anterior two thirds of the tongue. The cell bodies of these primary sensory neurons are in the *geniculate ganglion*, at the genu of the facial nerve and within the petrous portion of the temporal bone. The distal processes of these sensory neurons reach the tongue by traveling with the chorda tympani and lingual nerves. Once there, they distribute to the taste buds along the anterior two thirds of the tongue (see Fig. 19–8). The chorda tympani nerve also contains the preganglionic parasympathetic fibers (GVE) from the superior salivatory nucleus (see previous discussion).

The central processes of the SVA neurons enter the brain stem as part of the *intermediate nerve*, immediately lateral to the motor root of the facial nerve at the medullopontine junction, just rostral to the inferior olive. These central afferent processes enter the ipsilateral *solitary tract* and terminate in the rostral portion of the *nucleus of the solitary tract* (see Fig. 19–8). The *gustatory nucleus* is another name for this region of the solitary nucleus.

GENERAL VISCERAL AFFERENT COMPONENT

The *GVA* component of the *facial nerve* is very small. The *primary sensory neurons* are in the *geniculate ganglion*, and their central processes enter the brain stem with the *intermediate nerve*. The peripheral processes course with the *greater petrosal nerve* and innervate the nasal cavity, the sinus cavities, and part of the soft palate. On entering the brain stem, the central processes of these GVA neurons join the *solitary tract* and synapse in the *nucleus of the solitary tract* (see Fig. 19–8).

GENERAL SOMATIC AFFERENT COMPONENT

The *facial nerve* has a GSA component, albeit small. Within the mastoid bone, peripheral GSA fibers join with a comparable component of the vagus nerve to form the auricular nerve and to innervate a very small area on the pinna of the ear and in the external auditory meatus. The primary sensory neurons are in the *geniculate ganglion*. The central processes of these neurons enter the CNS with the *intermediate nerve* and join the descending *spinal tract of cranial nerve V* to end in the *spinal nucleus of cranial nerve V* (see Fig. 19–8). When these fibers join the spinal tract of cranial nerve V, they course in the dorsal most portion, immediately adjacent to the fibers of the mandibular division of cranial nerve V. These fibers carry sensory information for pain, temperature, and touch.

CLINICAL DISORDERS

Motor innervation of the muscles of facial expression is the principal function of the facial nerve. Accordingly, the most common symptom from damage to the nerve, nucleus, or corticobulbar projections is a paralysis or paresis of these muscles. Involvement of the components of the intermediate nerve serves to localize the point of damage to the facial nerve.

Facial palsy is an *impairment (paresis)* or *a total paralysis of some or all of the muscles of facial expression.* With damage to the facial nerve or the facial nucleus, the paralysis is ipsilateral to the insult and flaccid, i.e., lower motor neuron damage. With time, there is an accompanying muscle atrophy. Normal facial wrinkles and creases due to the insertion of the muscles into the skin disappear, giving the affected side a smooth and expressionless appearance.

The patient is unable to close the affected eye. If there is a lack of tearing (see subsequent discussion), the cornea tends to dry out. The corner of the mouth tends to droop, and there is a tendency for the patient to drool out of that corner of the mouth. Damage to only certain of the terminal branches of the facial nerve leads to a loss of only those muscles innervated. Similarly, nuclear lesions, if partial, may involve selected muscle groups because specific subnuclei of the facial nucleus innervate specific target muscles or muscle groups. The term *Bell's palsy* describes a facial palsy resulting from damage to the facial nerve at some point at or beyond the nerve's exit from the skull through the stylomastoid foramen. Typically, Bell's palsy does not involve the components of the intermediate nerve (see the following discussion).

Supranuclear facial palsy has a very characteristic feature, *a sparing of the upper muscles of facial expression* (above the level of the palpebral fissure). Corticobulbar projections to facial neurons innervating the upper muscles of facial expression are both crossed and uncrossed, whereas those to neurons innervating the lower muscles of facial expression are all crossed. Hence, lesions affecting the corticobulbar projections produce a *contralateral* paralysis of the lower muscles of facial expression and spare the upper muscles. Patients are able to close both eyes and wrinkle both brows. In addition, because it is an upper motor neuron lesion, there is no accompanying atrophy of the muscles and there is a retention of facial reflexes, i.e., the patient's ability to smile reflexly or show other emotional expressions.

Loss of taste in the anterior two thirds of the tongue in combination with a facial palsy indicates damage to the facial nerve central to the exit of the chorda tympani nerve. Also, the loss of the preganglionic parasympathetic fibers to the submandibular ganglion causes *diminished salivation.* However, this sign may be difficult to detect, because the parotid gland is functional. The loss of taste and diminished salivation without motor palsy suggest involvement only of the chorda tympani nerve. When *anesthesia of the tongue* accompanies the loss of taste and diminished salivation, an involvement of the lingual nerve (a terminal branch of the trigeminal nerve) is likely. An accompanied *loss of tearing* (lacrimal gland innervation) occurs only if the facial nerve lesion is central to the geniculate ganglion. Lacrimal gland innervation is via the greater petrosal nerve. *Hyperacusis*, an increase in auditory sensitivity on the affected side, often occurs if there is a paralysis of the stapedial muscle. This indicates involvement of the facial nerve central to the stapedial nerve (see Fig. 19–8).

Glossopharyngeal Nerve (IX)

The *glossopharyngeal nerve (cranial nerve IX)*, as the name implies, innervates portions of the tongue (*glossus*) and the pharynx. Although one of the smallest cranial nerves, the glossopharyngeal nerve contains five functional components. The glossopharyngeal nerve carries *special visceral afferent (SVA*, taste) information from the tongue, *general visceral afferent (GVA)* information from the tongue and pharyngeal wall, and *general somatic afferent (GSA)* information from the external ear. In addition, the glossopharyngeal nerve contains a small *special visceral efferent (SVE*, branchiomotor) component and a larger *general visceral efferent (GVE)* parasympathetic preganglionic component that innervates the parotid gland (see Fig. 19–9).

PERIPHERAL COURSE

The *glossopharyngeal nerve* emerges from the brain stem as a series of five or six small nerve rootlets, immediately dorsal to the inferior olive

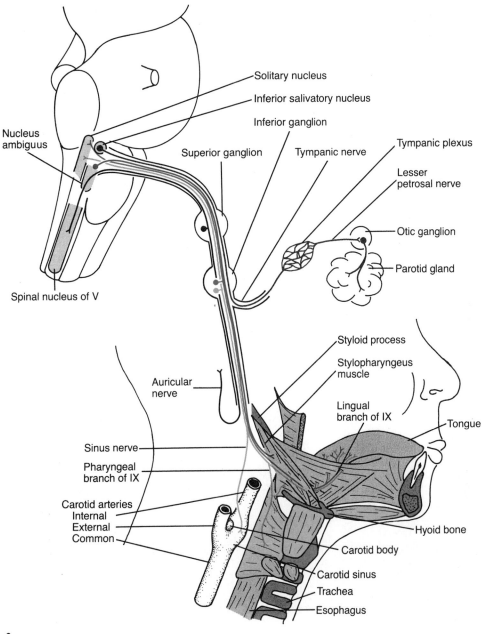

FIGURE 19-9

The course and distribution of the glossopharyngeal nerve and its primary branches. See text for details. Components same colors as in Fig. 19-8.

(see Fig. 19-1). These rootlets are immediately rostral to the rootlets that form the much larger vagus nerve. The glossopharyngeal nerve exits the cranial vault through the jugular foramen and emerges immediately posterior to the styloid pro-cess. Within the jugular foramen, two small swellings representing sensory ganglia are visible in the nerve, the very small *superior ganglion*, containing GSA neurons, and the somewhat larger *inferior ganglion* (*petrosal ganglion*), containing both GVA and SVA neurons (see Fig. 19–9).

Immediately below the inferior ganglion, as the glossopharyngeal nerve exits from the skull, it gives off its first branch, the *tympanic nerve*. This is a small nerve that immediately enters the tympanic cavity and crosses the medial wall of the middle ear as the *tympanic plexus*. These fibers then re-enter the cranial vault as the *lesser petrosal nerve* only to exit the skull again and terminate in the *otic ganglion*, immediately medial to the mandibular division of the trigeminal nerve near the foramen ovale. Postganglionic parasympathetic fibers from the otic ganglion hitch a ride with the auriculotemporal branch of the trigeminal nerve to supply the *parotid gland*. The tympanic nerve also contains a few GVA fibers that innervate the mucous membranes of the tympanic cavity and eustachian tube. These GVA fibers are not illustrated in Figure 19–9. The glossopharyngeal gives off another small branch that joins with the auricular branch of the vagus to provide GSA innervation to a small area on the pinna of the ear and in the external auditory meatus (see Fig. 19–9).

The main trunk of the glossopharyngeal nerve descends along the lateral wall of the pharynx. As the nerve swings anteriorly and medially toward the base of the tongue, it gives off many branches containing GVA fibers that enter the *pharyngeal plexus*. The terminal branch of the glossopharyngeal nerve enters the posterior third of the tongue, providing both SVA (taste) and GVA innervation. Before entering the tongue, the glossopharyngeal nerve also supplies a motor branch (SVE) to the adjacent *stylopharyngeus muscle* and a sensory branch (GVA) to the *carotid sinus* (see Fig. 19–9). The glossopharyngeal nerve may also make a small contribution to the nerve to the carotid body, the last being principally vagal.

SPECIAL VISCERAL EFFERENT COMPONENT

The branchiomotor neurons, composing the *special visceral efferent* (*SVE*) component of the glossopharyngeal nerve, reside in the *nucleus ambiguous* (see Fig. 19–2). Axons from these neurons exit with the glossopharyngeal nerve rootlets, travel with the main body of the nerve, and form the very small *nerve to the stylopharyngeus muscle*, the one muscle innervated by the glossopharyngeal nerve (see Fig. 19–9).

GENERAL VISCERAL EFFERENT COMPONENT

The *preganglionic parasympathetic neurons* of the glossopharyngeal nerve are in the *inferior salivatory nucleus* of the medulla, immediately rostral to the large dorsal motor nucleus of the vagus nerve (see Fig. 19–2). Preganglionic fibers leave the glossopharyngeal nerve below the inferior ganglion as the *tympanic nerve* en route to the tympanic plexus and proceed to the *otic ganglion*, which is situated immediately inferior to the foramen ovale. Postganglionic fibers from the otic ganglion hitch a ride with the *auriculotemporal nerve* to provide parasympathetic innervation to the *parotid gland* (see Fig. 19–9).

SPECIAL VISCERAL AFFERENT COMPONENT

The *glossopharyngeal nerve* innervates the taste buds on the posterior third of the tongue. The *inferior ganglion* contains the visceral afferent neurons, both general (GVA) and special (SVA). The peripheral processes of the SVA fibers follow the main route of the glossopharyngeal nerve to the base of the tongue and innervate taste buds in the posterior third of the tongue and a few rudimentary taste buds in the adjacent pharyngeal wall (see Fig. 19–9). The central processes of these SVA neurons enter the brain stem with the other components of the glossopharyngeal nerve and terminate in the rostral portion of the ipsilateral *solitary nucleus* (*gustatory nucleus*) (see Fig. 19–9).

GENERAL VISCERAL AFFERENT COMPONENT

The *glossopharyngeal nerve* innervates much of the pharyngeal mucosa and the posterior third of the tongue. The anterior two thirds is somatic and, therefore, innervated by the GSA component of the trigeminal nerve. A small sensory branch from the glossopharyngeal nerve innervates the pressure receptors of the *carotid sinus*. These sensory nerves form the afferent arms of reflex loops that modulate blood pressure.

The primary sensory neurons (GVA) of the glossopharyngeal nerve reside in the *inferior* (*petrosal*) *ganglion* (see Fig. 19–9). The central processes of the GVA neurons enter the brain stem and join the *solitary tract* (*fasciculus*), and they synapse in the *solitary nucleus*.

GENERAL SOMATIC AFFERENT COMPONENT

The *GSA* component of the glossopharyngeal nerve is very small, joins the auricular branch of the vagus nerve, and innervates a very small area on the pinna of the ear and in the external auditory meatus. The primary sensory neurons are in the *superior ganglion* of the glossopharyngeal nerve. The central processes of these neurons enter the CNS, join the descending *spinal tract of cranial nerve V* and synapse in the *spinal nucleus of cranial nerve V* (see Fig. 19–9). When these fibers join the spinal tract of cranial nerve V, they course in the dorsal most portion, immediately adjacent to the fibers of the mandibular division of cranial nerve V. These fibers carry sensory information for pain, temperature, and touch.

CLINICAL DISORDERS

A lesion affecting only the glossopharyngeal nerve is rare but would result in both a *loss of taste* sensation on the ipsilateral *posterior third of the tongue* and a marked reduction in the serous secretion of the *ipsilateral parotid gland*. Some reduction of sensibility in the pharynx occurs. The vagus nerve may contribute some sensory fibers to the pharyngeal plexus; however, most of the vagal fibers are motor (see subsequent discussion). The *loss of* (or reduction in) *the gag reflex* usually is a cardinal sign of glossopharyngeal damage. Stroking the lateral wall of the pharynx near the tonsilar fossa normally elicits the gag reflex. Damage to the glossopharyngeal nerve eliminates part of the sensory arm of the reflex.

Vagus Nerve (X)

The *vagus nerve (cranial nerve X)* is one of the largest of the cranial nerves. Although it is primarily a visceromotor nerve, providing *general visceral efferent (GVE)* innervation to the thorax and most of the abdomen, it also is the branchiomotor nerve for the fourth, fifth, and sixth branchial or pharyngeal arches during embryonic development, providing *special visceral efferent (SVE)* innervation to the muscles of the pharynx and larynx in the adult. Accompanying both the GVE and SVE fibers are an abundance of *general visceral afferent (GVA)* fibers. They carry sensory information principally from the pharynx and

larynx as well as some of the GVA innervation to the thoracic and abdominal viscera (Fig. 19–10).

Most of the sensory innervation of the thoracic and abdominal viscera is conducted to the dorsal root ganglia in association with the sympathetic innervation. This factor provides the anatomical basis for referral of pain to somatic dermatomes (see Chapter 10). Two additional very small sensory components exist, a *general somatic afferent (GSA)* component, innervating the external ear, and a vestigial *special visceral afferent (SVA)* component, innervating taste buds on the epiglottis, most of which disappear soon after birth (see Fig. 19–10). This combination of five functional components, *SVE, GVE, GVA, SVA,* and *GSA* is the same combination in the facial and glossopharyngeal nerves (see Table 19–1).

PERIPHERAL COURSE

The *vagus nerve* emerges from the brain stem as a series of nerve rootlets just dorsal to the inferior olive and immediately caudal to the glossopharyngeal nerve and rostral to the spinal accessory nerve (see Fig. 19–1). These rootlets collate to form the large vagus nerve, and the nerve exits from the cranial vault through the *jugular foramen*. The caudal most bundle of rootlets initially courses with the spinal accessory nerve, and they were inappropriately considered as the bulbar root of the spinal accessory nerve (see Fig. 19–1). These fibers, however, leave the spinal accessory nerve and join the vagus, as the two nerves come into proximity passing through the jugular foramen.

The vagus nerve has two sensory ganglia, situated immediately below the jugular foramen. The more superior and smaller ganglion, the *superior (jugular) ganglion*, contains primary afferent neurons that are *GSA*; the inferior and larger ganglion, the *inferior (nodose) ganglion*, contains primary visceral afferent neurons, both the *GVA* and the vestigial *SVA* components (see Fig. 19–10).

The *main trunk of the vagus nerve* descends in the neck, within the carotid sheath, lateral to the internal carotid and common carotid arteries, and medial to the jugular vein. The vagus nerve remains in the carotid sheath until it enters the thoracic cavity. The major target of innervation is the viscera of the thorax and abdomen. The details of the course of the vagus nerve in the thorax and abdomen are presented in Chapter 18.

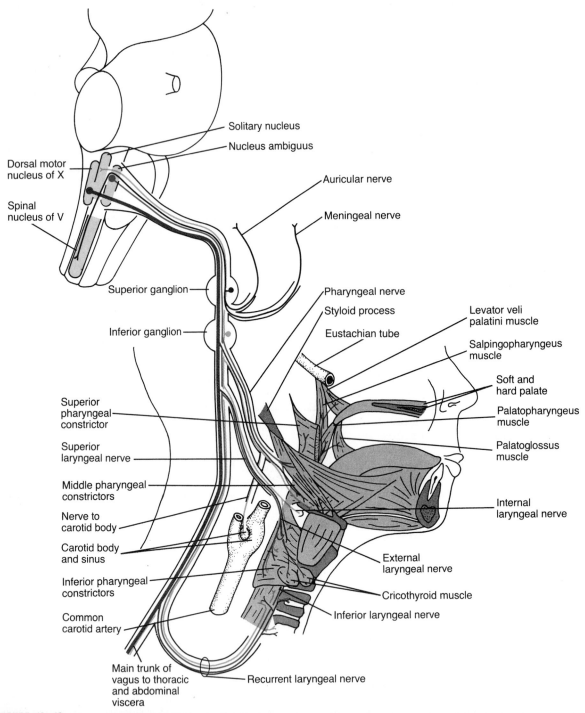

FIGURE 19–10

The course and distribution of the vagus nerve and its primary branches. The vestigial special visceral afferent (SVA) component is omitted from this illustration. Chapter 18 reviews the course and distribution of parasympathetic fibers to the viscera. See text for details. Components same colors as in Fig. 19–8.

CERVICAL BRANCHES

Immediately below the superior ganglion, the *auricular nerve* leaves the vagus, turning posterosuperiorly toward the external ear. This branch anastomoses with similar branches from the facial and glossopharyngeal nerves to provide the small *GSA* innervation to a part of the pinna of the ear and the external auditory meatus. The *meningeal nerve* is another small, recurrent branch that also leaves the vagus immediately below the superior ganglion, turns, and re-enters the cranial vault through the jugular foramen to innervate the dura of the posterior cranial fossa (see Fig. 19–10).

The *pharyngeal nerves* leave the vagus below the inferior ganglion and swing toward the anterior surface of the pharynx, as they continue to descend in the neck while giving off small terminal branches that form the *pharyngeal plexus*. The vagal contributions to the pharyngeal plexus are principally the *SVE* branchiomotor fibers to all the muscles of the pharynx and soft palate except the stylopharyngeus muscle (glossopharyngeal nerve) and tensor veli palatini muscle (trigeminal nerve). Some *GVA* fibers supply to the pharynx and soft palate; however, most of the sensory innervation is supplied by the glossopharyngeal nerve. The vagus also contributes *GVE* preganglionic parasympathetic innervation to glands in the pharyngeal mucosa (see Fig. 19–10).

The *superior laryngeal nerve* descends along the lateral wall of the pharynx before dividing into two terminal branches, the *internal laryngeal nerve* and the *external laryngeal nerve*. The internal laryngeal nerve enters the larynx through the thyrohyoid membrane and provides sensory innervation (*GVA*) to the mucosa of the larynx, down to the level of the vocal cords. The external laryngeal nerve provides branchiomotor (*SVE*) innervation to the inferior pharyngeal constrictor muscle and the cricothyroid muscle of the larynx (see Fig. 19–10).

The *recurrent laryngeal nerves*, the principal motor nerves to the larynx (*SVE*), descend to the thoracic cavity where the right nerve loops around the subclavian artery and the left nerve loops around the aortic arch. After making these loops, both recurrent laryngeal nerves ascend toward the larynx in the groove between the trachea and the esophagus. The terminal branch, the *inferior laryngeal nerve*, enters the larynx and innervates all the intrinsic musculature of the larynx (*SVE*), except the cricothyroideus muscle. Several smaller branches (*GVA* and *GVE*) go to

the trachea and esophagus. One or more small inferior cardiac rami may arise from the recurrent laryngeal nerve; on the right side, the inferior cardiac rami may arise from the main trunk of the vagus.

SPECIAL VISCERAL EFFERENT COMPONENT

The *nucleus ambiguus* contains the motor neurons that innervate all the *muscles of the pharynx* and of *the larynx*. The vagus nerve innervates all this musculature except the stylopharyngeus (glossopharyngeal) and tensor veli palatini (trigeminal) muscles.

GENERAL VISCERAL EFFERENT COMPONENT

The vagus nerve provides the parasympathetic *general visceral efferent* (*GVE*) innervation to the mucous glands of the larynx and the visceral contents of the entire thoracic cavity as well as most of the abdominal cavity. The preganglionic neurons of the vagus nerve are in the large *dorsal motor nucleus of the vagus nerve* (*dorsal motor nucleus of cranial nerve X*). These preganglionic fibers exit the brain stem with the other rootlets of the vagus and leave the cranium with the main trunk of the vagus nerve to descend into the thoracic cavity within the *carotid sheath*. As the vagus enters the thoracic cavity, it gives off many branches to the various plexuses associated with the visceral organs of the thorax and abdomen. These preganglionic fibers synapse with *postganglionic neurons* in small ganglionic patches, situated largely within the walls or supporting connective tissues of the target organs. The vagus supplies the parasympathetic innervation to all the *thoracic* and *abdominal viscera*, except the descending and sigmoid colon, rectum, and anus (see Fig. 18–4).

SPECIAL VISCERAL AFFERENT COMPONENT

The facial and glossopharyngeal nerves provide most of the taste bud innervation. However, during development, a small number of taste buds form on the epiglottis and receive vagal innervation. This *SVA* component of the *vagus nerve* is very small in humans and probably absent in most adults. The primary afferent neurons are in the *inferior ganglion* of the vagus, just below the jugular foramen where the vagus exits the cranial cavity. Distal processes of the SVA neurons descend with the main trunk of the vagus nerve, leave with the pharyngeal branch of the vagus, enter the posteroinferior portion of the pharyngeal plexus, and terminate in the taste buds of the epiglottis. Central processes enter the brain stem with the main portion of the vagus nerve and terminate in the rostral portion of the ipsilateral *solitary nucleus* (*gustatory nucleus*) (see Figs. 19–2 and 13–6).

GENERAL VISCERAL AFFERENT COMPONENT

The primary sensory *GVA* neurons of the vagus nerve are in the *inferior ganglion*. The peripheral processes provide sensory innervation to the mucosal linings of the pharynx, larynx, and soft palate. In addition, the vagus may gives rise to a small *nerve to the carotid body*. The glossopharyngeal nerve may also innervate the carotid body in addition to the carotid sinus. The central processes of these neurons enter the brain stem with the rootlets of the vagus, join the *solitary tract*, and synapse in the *nucleus of the solitary tract* (see Fig. 19–10). A dorsomedial extension of the solitary nucleus is often separately identified as the dorsal sensory nucleus of the vagus because of some histological differences. In addition, the latter receives principally vagal afferent fibers. We will consider it as one nucleus, the nucleus of the solitary tract. Many of the vagal connections in the nucleus of the solitary tract are associated with autonomic reflexes. Other visceral afferent fibers, especially those associated with a high degree of sensory discrimination from the pharynx and larynx, appear to synapse in the spinal nucleus of cranial nerve V.

GENERAL SOMATIC AFFERENT COMPONENT

The *vagus nerve* has a small *GSA* component. These fibers join similar branches from the facial and glossopharyngeal nerves to form the *auricular nerve* (*Arnold's nerve*) and innervate a very small area on the pinna of the ear and in the external auditory canal. The primary sensory neurons are in the *superior ganglion*, and the central processes of these neurons enter the CNS with the vagus nerve and descend in the *spinal tract of cranial nerve V* to synapse in the *spinal nucleus of cranial nerve V* (see Fig. 19–10).

When these fibers join the spinal tract of cranial nerve V, they course in the dorsal most portion, immediately adjacent to the fibers of the mandibular division of cranial nerve V. These fibers carry sensory information for pain, temperature, and touch.

CLINICAL DISORDERS

Damage to the vagus nerve, causes *loss of parasympathetic and some visceral afferent innervation to the thoracic viscera and most of the abdominal viscera.* The loss, although major, is not life threatening, and the patient survives. Spinal nerves carry the signals for visceral pain. The sensations carried by the vagus nerve are more concerned with visceromotor reflexes. *Hyperactivity of the vagus nerve* leads to *hyperacidity* and *gastric ulceration.* One treatment is a highly selective vagotomy, severing of the gastric branches of both vagus nerves.

Following damage to the vagus nerve, the most obvious symptoms are branchiomotor, SVE, deficits with the resultant paralysis or paresis of the pharyngeal and laryngeal musculature. An early sign of *unilateral damage to the vagus nerve* is a *persistent hoarseness in the voice* due to a *unilateral paralysis of intrinsic laryngeal musculature.* On examination, a patient with unilateral vagal damage also shows pharyngeal and soft palate involvement. The loss of muscle tone in the paralyzed levator palati muscle leads to a *drooping of the soft palate on the affected side and a deviation of the uvula away from the side of the injury due to the unopposed action of intact motor units.* The patient may have problems swallowing, *dysphagia,* with food passing into the nasal pharynx and into the trachea due to soft palate and pharyngeal muscle paralyses. However, this is often not a problem, because of other muscle actions. Damage only to the *recurrent laryngeal nerve* leads to the *hoarseness without the pharyngeal involvement.* The recurrent laryngeal nerve is vulnerable during surgical procedures in the neck region, such as a thyroidectomy.

Because the corticobulbar projections from the motor cortex to the nucleus ambiguous are bilateral, unilateral upper motor neuron damage is not apparent. Central unilateral lesions of the nucleus ambiguous usually affect other adjacent structures as well. An example is the *lateral medullary syndrome* (*Wallenberg's syndrome*), resulting from an infarct of the posterior inferior cerebellar artery. When this occurs, a number of other symptoms accompany the *hoarseness* and *dysphagia*, including *loss of pain and temperature sensation to the contralateral body (spinothalamic tract) and ipsilateral face (spinal tract and nucleus of cranial nerve V), ipsilateral hearing deficits (cochlear nuclei), nystagmus, ataxia, and nausea (vestibular nuclei).* Bilateral involvement of the nucleus ambiguus, as in amyotrophic lateral sclerosis, poliomyelitis, or brain stem tumor, produces a profound loss of swallowing ability and a loss of the gag reflex. These are life-threatening symptoms, because the patient is susceptible to asphyxia and aspiration pneumonia.

The *GSA* neurons in the vagus nerve form the auricular nerve to the external auditory meatus, which makes reflex connections with the dorsal motor nucleus of the vagus. Thus, *stimulation of the external ear can cause coughing, nausea, and even fainting.*

Spinal Accessory Nerve (XI)

The *spinal accessory nerve (cranial nerve XI)* is a motor nerve with its neurons of origin in the upper cervical segments of the spinal cord. Hence, the spinal accessory nerve is actually a special type of spinal nerve rather than a "true" cranial nerve. In the early neuroanatomical descriptions, the spinal accessory nerve had two components, *bulbar and spinal*. However, the bulbar component is an aberrant group of fibers belonging to the vagus nerve (see previous discussion). Another controversy that surrounds the spinal accessory nerve is its classification as either branchiomotor (SVE) or somatomotor (GSE). Some embryologists question the branchial arch origin of the portions of the sternomastoid and trapezius muscles innervated by the spinal accessory nerve. However, the development of the neurons in the spinal accessory nucleus follows a pattern identical to other SVE neurons and not GSE neurons (see Chapter 1). In addition, the location of the spinal accessory nucleus and the point of exit of the nerve fibers are consistent with the SVE classification.

ANATOMY

The *spinal accessory nerve* contains one functional component, the *SVE* or branchiomotor component. The *spinal accessory nucleus* is in the dorsolateral portion of the ventral horn (lamina VII), in a direct line with the nucleus ambiguus of the medulla (see Fig. 19–2). The *spinal accessory nucleus extends from the lower medulla*

through the first five or six cervical segments. Axons leaving the nucleus course briefly in a dorsomedial direction before making a 180 degree bend to exit the spinal cord laterally, immediately dorsal to the denticulate ligaments, midway between the dorsal and ventral roots (Fig. 19–11).

The emerging fibers collate, as they ascend parallel to the spinal cord and enter the cranial vault through the *foramen magnum*. Once in the cranial vault, the fibers of the *spinal accessory nerve* curve downward to exit the skull through the *jugular foramen*. At the curvature, a group of SVE fibers of the vagus nerve, and arising from the nucleus ambiguus, join the spinal accessory nerve and enter the jugular foramen. *Where the spinal accessory nerve exits from the jugular foramen, it consists only of fibers from the spinal accessory nucleus.* The aberrant vagal fibers have joined the vagus nerve.

The spinal accessory nerve descends in the neck in the company of the jugular vein and enters the medial surface of the sternomastoid muscle. Before entering the muscle, fibers that are principally sensory from the upper cervical nerves join the spinal accessory nerve. Some neuroanatomists maintain that the spinal accessory nerve also receives somatomotor (GSE) fibers from these cervical nerves. For our purposes, we consider the motor component to be SVE from the spinal accessory nucleus and the sensory component to be GSA from the upper cervical nerves. After giving off branches to the sternomastoid muscle, the nerve leaves the muscle and traverses the posterior cervical triangle before entering the lower portion of the trapezius muscle.

CLINICAL DISORDERS

Clinical involvement of only the spinal accessory nerve is uncommon. However, damage to the spinal accessory nerve produces symptoms typical of lower motor neuron damage. A *flaccid paralysis or paresis* of the muscles innervated and a *subsequent atrophy* of the muscles occur with time. When the damage is unilateral, the patient displays a weakness in rotating the head down and away from the side of injury, i.e., sternomastoid muscle weakness. Damage to the entire nerve or the branch innervating the trapezius produces a paresis of the trapezius muscle, resulting in a slight droop of the affected shoulder and an inability to shrug that shoulder. The patient has reduced force when elevating the arm and shoulder against pressure and is unable to elevate

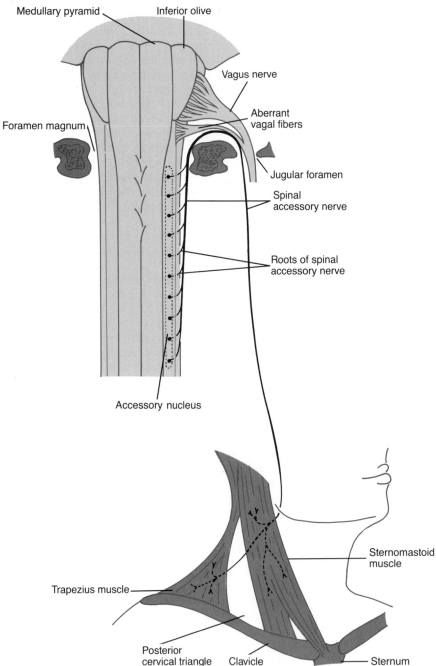

Medullary pyramid

Inferior olive

Vagus nerve

Aberrant vagal fibers

Foramen magnum

Jugular foramen

Spinal accessory nerve

Roots of spinal accessory nerve

Accessory nucleus

Sternomastoid muscle

Trapezius muscle

Posterior cervical triangle   Clavicle   Sternum

FIGURE 19-11

The course and distribution of the spinal accessory nerve and its branches. Note the aberrant vagal fibers ("bulbar root of the spinal accessory nerve") traveling with the spinal accessory nerve only to join the vagus, as the two nerves pass through the jugular foramen. See text for details.

it above the horizontal plane. At the point where the spinal accessory nerve crosses the posterior triangle of the neck it is a small, thin nerve, rendering it vulnerable to damage during extensive neck surgery, such as radical neck dissection for removal of a tumor and removal of cervical lymph nodes. No paresis of the sternomastoid muscle occurs when the injury is only to the branch innervating the trapezius muscle.

Upper motor neuron lesions produce a contralateral paresis of the muscles, because the descending corticospinal fibers cross in the pyramidal decussation of the lower medulla before reaching the spinal accessory nucleus. Addition-

FIGURE 19-12

The course and distribution of the hypoglossal nerve and its branches. The hypoglossal nerve innervates the intrinsic musculature of the tongue and the extrinsic muscles (genioglossus, hyoglossus, and styloglossus).

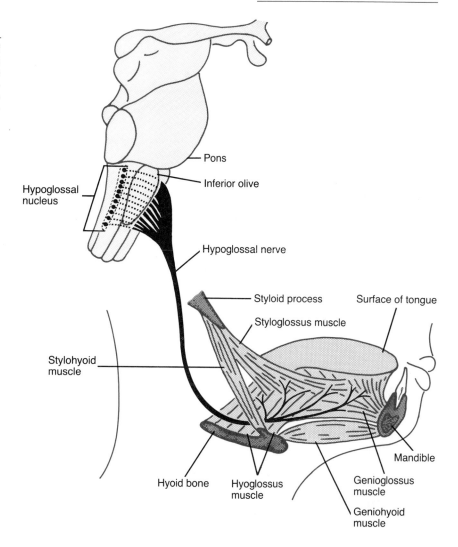

Pons

Inferior olive

Hypoglossal nucleus

Hypoglossal nerve

Styloid process

Surface of tongue

Styloglossus muscle

Stylohyoid muscle

Hyoid bone

Hyoglossus muscle

Mandible

Genioglossus muscle

Geniohyoid muscle

ally, no muscle atrophy occurs, because the lower motor neurons in the spinal accessory nucleus are intact. An upper motor neuron lesion affecting only the spinal accessory nerve is very rare.

Hypoglossal Nerve (XII)

ANATOMY

The *hypoglossal nerve (cranial nerve XII)* is principally a motor nerve with only one functional component (*GSE*), and it innervates the musculature of the tongue (Fig. 19–12). The lower motor neurons of the hypoglossal nerve are in the *hypoglossal nucleus*, a GSE motor nucleus found in the medulla, close to the midline and immediately beneath the floor of the fourth ventricle (see Fig. 19–2). The presence of the nucleus is visible on the ventricular surface of the medulla as an elevation, the *hypoglossal trigone* (see Fig. 7–4).

Axons of the motor neurons leave the nucleus in a ventral and slightly lateral direction, exiting the brain stem between the inferior olive and the medullary pyramids as a row of small fascicles of fibers (see Fig. 19–1). These fascicles collate, forming the *hypoglossal nerve* and exit the cranial vault through the hypoglossal canal. The hypoglossal nerve descends in the neck to about the level of the hyoid bone, where it curves forward and enters the body of the tongue to innervate the muscles, specifically the hyoglossus, genioglossus, and styloglossus, along with the intrinsic musculature of the tongue (see Fig. 19–12).

A number of nerve fibers from the first and second cervical nerves join the hypoglossal nerve for a short distance, as it descends in the neck. Before the nerve turns forward to enter the tongue, these fibers leave the hypoglossal nerve, forming two branches, a nerve to the geniohyoid and thyrohyoid muscles and the superior root of the ansa cervicalis, which innervates other infrahyoid muscles. Besides these somatic motor fibers, some *sympathetic postganglionic fibers* from the cervical ganglia of the sympathetic chain join the hypoglossal nerve and distribute to the vasculature of the tongue and to some of the small glands within the oral mucosa. Clinically, these are insignificant.

Some question about the motor "purity" of the hypoglossal nerve has been raised. A few sensory neurons, innervating muscle spindles of the tongue, reside within the substance of the hypoglossal nerve. These are of little clinical significance, because most of the proprioceptive innervation of the tongue is by way of the lingual nerve, a branch of the mandibular division of the trigeminal nerve.

CLINICAL DISORDERS

Damage to the hypoglossal nerve or nucleus produces symptoms typical of lower motor neuron damage—*flaccid paralysis* of the muscles normally innervated and *subsequent atrophy* of the muscles. If the damage is unilateral, the *tongue always deviates toward the side of the lesion*, when protruded. Because the intact genioglossus muscle of the opposite side thrusts the tongue forward, it deviates toward the impaired side, because of a lack of opposition from the affected muscle.

Upper cervical motor fibers travel with the hypoglossal nerve and innervate the geniohyoid muscle and the infrahyoid muscles. Damage to the hypoglossal nerve in the neck, before the point where the cervical root fibers split off, results in a loss of innervation to these muscles in addition to the muscles of the tongue.

Upper motor neuron lesions produce a contralateral paralysis of the tongue musculature, because the descending corticobulbar fibers cross en route to the hypoglossal nucleus. No muscle atrophy occurs, because the lower motor neurons remain intact.

SUGGESTED READING

Brodal, A. (1957). *The Cranial Nerves: Anatomy and Anatomicoclinical Correlations.* Blackwell Scientific Publications, Oxford.

This brief monograph is an excellent review of the neuroanatomical and gross anatomical features of all the cranial nerves. Both the anatomy and clinical correlations are dealt with clearly and concisely. The neurological deficits are related to the anatomy.

Wilson-Pauwels, L., E. J. Akesson, and P. A. Stewart (1988). *Cranial Nerves: Anatomy and Clinical Comments.* B. C. Decker, Inc. Toronto.

This textbook provides an excellent bridge between the gross anatomy and neuroanatomy of the cranial nerves. The many excellent illustrations provide a clear picture of the peripheral course of each cranial nerve. It is especially suited for those students who have not yet studied gross anatomy.

Part

VII

HIGHER INTEGRATIVE
CENTERS

Chapter

20

The Thalamus and Thalamocortical Projections

ANATOMY OF THE THALAMUS
MORPHOLOGICAL DIVISIONS OF THE THALAMUS
GENERAL PRINCIPLES OF THALAMIC ORGANIZATION
FUNCTIONAL CONNECTIONS OF THE THALAMIC NUCLEI

The *dorsal thalamus*, or simply the *thalamus*, is one of four anatomical subdivisions of the diencephalon. Situated at the rostral end of the brain stem, the thalamus functions as a principal relay station for information destined for the ipsilateral telencephalon, composed of the cerebral cortex and the basal ganglia. In lower vertebrates, with a minimum of cortical development, the thalamus is a center of higher nervous activity and assumes some limited integrative and perceptual functions. Higher vertebrates have a marked increase in cortical development and a corresponding increase in the size and degree of differentiation of the thalamus. These changes are direct reflections of increases in ascending sensory pathways and in reciprocal thalamocortical and corticothalamic connections. Although some integrative and perceptual functions may be retained by the thalamus, in humans and other higher vertebrates they are minimal in comparison with those carried out at the cortical level.

Anatomy of the Thalamus

The *thalamus* is one of a symmetrical pair of ovoid structures located in the diencephalon,

dorsal to the hypothalamus and ventral to the transverse cerebral fissure. The hypothalamic sulcus, in the lateral wall of the third ventricle, marks the medial boundary between the hypothalamus below and the thalamus above (Fig. 20-1). The left and right thalami are separated medially by the third ventricle and bounded laterally by the posterior limb of the internal capsule (Fig. 20-2). The two thalami usually join medially at the interthalamic adhesion. Although this represents a continuity of tissue mass, no direct fiber connections are made between the two. The thalamus is bounded anteriorly by the head of the caudate nucleus and the genu of the internal capsule and posteriorly by the midbrain. Immediately ventral to the thalamus and sandwiched between the thalamus, hypothalamus, and pretectal area is the ventral thalamus or subthalamus.

In its role as a relay station, the thalamus makes connections with many diverse functional systems—a heterogeneity that is reflected in the large number of specialized nuclei. This chapter focuses on those principles of organization and connections that are common to most, if not all, thalamic nuclei. Although the anatomical location and primary connections of the thalamic

433

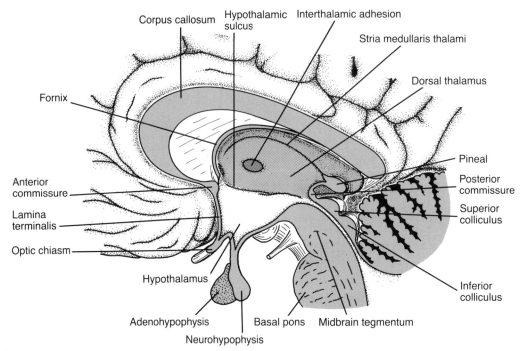

FIGURE 20-1

A midsagittal section through the brain stem and the corpus callosum. The right dorsal thalamus (red) is illustrated in relation to other diencephalic structures, the right cerebral hemisphere, and the rostral portion of the midbrain. Cut surfaces are gray.

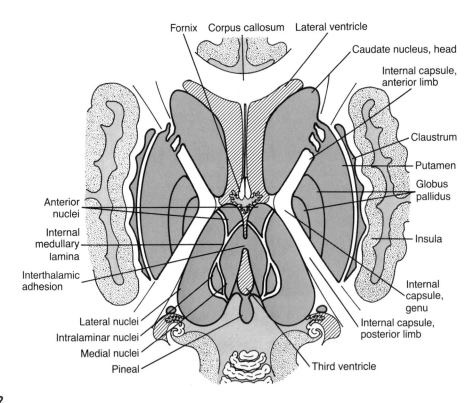

FIGURE 20-2

A horizontal section through the brain at the level of the dorsal thalamus, pineal, and basal ganglia. Note the relation of the thalamus (red) to the internal capsule, basal ganglia, and third ventricle.

434

nuclei are dealt with in this chapter, chapters reviewing the specific functional systems consider in greater detail the organization and projections of specific nuclei or groups of nuclei (see Chapters 10 to 18).

Morphological Divisions of the Thalamus

A thin sheet of myelinated nerve fibers, the *internal medullary lamina*, runs through the center of the thalamus, roughly dividing the component nuclei into groups of *medial nuclei* and *lateral nuclei* (Figs. 20–2 and 20–3). At the rostral end of the thalamus, the internal medullary lamina splits into two rostral wings, partially encapsulating the *anterior nuclei*. A group of *posterior nuclei*, the *midline nuclei* lining the ventricular surface, and the *intralaminar nuclei* embedded within the internal medullary lamina complete the division of the thalamus into six primary groups of nuclei (Table 20–1).

INTRALAMINAR NUCLEI

The internal medullary lamina is much thinner than that depicted in the illustration and is visible as a dark line in Weigert-stained sections (Fig. 20–4). Embedded within the lamina is a group of nuclei, collectively called the *intralaminar nuclei*, the most prominent of which is the *centromedian nucleus* (*CM*). Other intralaminar nuclei include the *parafascicular nucleus* (*PF*), the *paracentral nucleus*, the *centrolateral nucleus*, (*CL*) and the *central medial nuclei*. The parafascicular nucleus surrounds the habenulointerpeduncular tract (fasciculus retroflexus of Meynert) and is adjacent to the more laterally placed centromedian nucleus.

ANTERIOR NUCLEI

The *anterior group* is the most rostral of the thalamic nuclei. This group is subdivided into *anterior ventral* (*AV*), *anterior medial* (*AM*), and *anterior dorsal* (*AD*) *nuclei*. However, the connections and functions of these nuclei are similar enough to consider them collectively as the *anterior nuclei* (see Fig. 20–3).

LATERAL GROUP OF NUCLEI

The *lateral group*, the largest of the nuclear groups, is further subdivided into *lateral* and *ventral divisions* (see Fig. 20–3 and Table 20–1). The *ventral division* of the lateral group contains

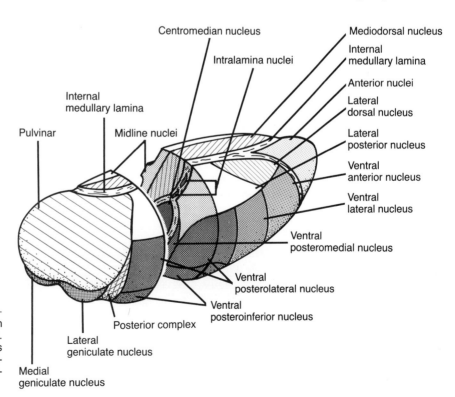

FIGURE 20–3

Three-dimensional representation of the right dorsal thalamus. Most of the major nuclear groups are represented. The ventral posterosuperior nucleus is not illustrated.

Centromedian nucleus
Intralamina nuclei
Mediodorsal nucleus
Internal medullary lamina
Anterior nuclei
Lateral dorsal nucleus
Lateral posterior nucleus
Ventral anterior nucleus
Ventral lateral nucleus
Ventral posteromedial nucleus
Ventral posterolateral nucleus
Ventral posteroinferior nucleus
Posterior complex
Lateral geniculate nucleus
Medial geniculate nucleus
Midline nuclei
Internal medullary lamina
Pulvinar

TABLE 20–1

Principal Nuclei of the Dorsal Thalamus

LATIN NOMENCLATURE	ABBREVIATION	COMMON NOMENCLATURE
Anterior Group		
n. anterior ventralis	AV	anterior ventral n.
n. anterior medialis	AM	anterior medial n.
n. anterior dorsalis	AD	anterior dorsal n.
Medial Group		
n. medialis dorsalis	MD	mediodorsal n.
Lateral Group — Lateral Division		
n. lateralis dorsalis	LD	lateral dorsal n.
n. lateralis posterior	LP	lateral posterior n.
Lateral Group — Ventral Division		
n. ventralis anterior	VA	ventral anterior n.
n. ventralis lateralis	VL	ventral lateral n.
n. ventralis posterior	VP	ventral posterior n.
n. ventralis posterolateralis	VPL	ventral posterolateral n.
n. ventralis posteromedialis	VPM	ventral posteromedial n.
n. ventralis posteroinferiores	VPI	ventral posteroinferior n.
n. ventralis posterosuperioris	VPS	ventral posterosuperior n.
Posterior Group		
pulvinar	—	pulvinar
n. corpus geniculati medialis	MGN	medial geniculate n.
n. corpus geniculati lateralis	LGN	lateral geniculate n.
n. posterior thalami	PO	posterior complex (zone)
Intralaminar Nuclei		
n. centrum medianum	CM	centromedian n.
n. parafascicularis	PF	parafascicular n.
n. paracentralis	—	paracentral n.
n. centralis lateralis	CL	centrolateral n.
n. centralis medialis	—	central medial n.
Midline Nuclei		
n. paraventricularis	—	paraventricular n.
n. reuniens	—	reuniens n.
n. parataenialis	—	parataenial n.
n. centralis medialis	—	central medial n.

n., nucleus.

those nuclei in the ventral portion of the lateral thalamus, whereas the *lateral division* of the lateral group contains those nuclei immediately dorsal to the ventral division, even though their name is "lateral." The original names were based on the relative positions of these nuclei in lower animal forms. The relative positions of some of the groups have shifted in humans—owing in large part to a relative increase in the ventral nuclei and their associated sensory and motor systems. Because the functional connections are similar, the original names are retained.

Lateral Division of the Lateral Group

The *lateral division* of the *lateral group* contains two nuclei of interest. The *lateral dorsal nucleus* (*LD*), the most rostral of the group, is functionally related to the anterior nuclei and lies immediately posterior to that group. The larger and more posterior *lateral posterior nucleus* (*LP*) makes up the remainder of the lateral group (see Fig. 20–3).

Ventral Division of the Lateral Group

The *ventral division* of the *lateral group* contains three major nuclei. The *ventral anterior nucleus* (*VA*), the most rostral of the ventral nuclei, lies immediately behind the anterior nuclei, separated from them by the internal medullary lamina. The *ventral lateral nucleus* (*VL*), often called the ventral intermediate nucleus, is immediately posterior to the ventral anterior nucleus. VL is subdi-

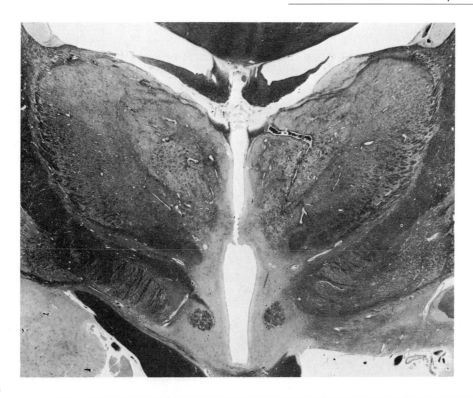

FIGURE 20–4

Transverse section through a human brain stem at the level of the interthalamic adhesion and the optic chiasm. Weigert stain. Compare with Figure 7–21.

vided into *anterior* and *posterior divisions*, *VLa* and *VLp*, respectively. Both VA and VL are part of the somatic motor system.

The *ventral posterior nucleus* (*VP*) relays somatosensory information to the cerebral cortex and contains medial, lateral, superior, and inferior subdivisions of nuclei. These sensory relay nuclei are the *ventral posterolateral nucleus* (*VPL*), the *ventral posteromedial nucleus* (*VPM*), the *ventral posterosuperior nucleus* (*VPS*), and the *ventral posteroinferior nucleus* (*VPI*). Collectively, VPL, VPM, VPS, and VPI compose the *ventrobasal complex* (see Fig. 20–3).

POSTERIOR GROUP OF NUCLEI

The *posterior group* contains four nuclei. The largest and most dorsal is the *pulvinar*. Immediately below the posterior margin of the pulvinar are two small but very important sensory relay nuclei, the *medial geniculate nucleus* (*MGN*) (*medial geniculate body*) and the *lateral geniculate nucleus* (*LGN*) (*lateral geniculate body*). Just rostral to the geniculate nuclei, but deep to the pulvinar and immediately behind the ventral

basal complex, is the *posterior complex* or *posterior zone* (*PO*) (see Fig. 20–3).

MEDIAL AND MIDLINE NUCLEI

Medial to the internal medullary lamina are two groups of nuclei, the *medial group* and the *midline nuclei*. The midline nuclei line the ventricular surface of the thalamus and include the *paraventricular nuclei*, the caudal portions of which belong to the epithalamus and are continuous with the periaqueductal gray of the midbrain; the *parataenial nucleus*; the *medial central nucleus*, forming the interthalamic adhesion; and the more ventrally placed *reuniens nucleus*. In humans, only one nucleus of the medial group is of major significance, the *mediodorsal nucleus* (*MD*). This very large nucleus occupies most of the space between the midline nuclei and the internal medullary lamina (see Fig. 20–3).

RETICULAR NUCLEI

Covering the lateral, anterolateral, and ventrolateral surfaces of the thalamus, between the thalamus and the internal capsule, is another sheet of myelinated fibers, the *external medullary lamina.* Embedded within this lamina is a group of small nuclei, collectively called the *reticular nuclei of the thalamus,* or simply, the *reticular nucleus* (see Fig. 20–4). *This inconspicuous, but important, nuclear complex is neither anatomically nor functionally related to the brain stem reticular formation.* Neurons of the *reticular nucleus* make extensive *reciprocal connections with all the nuclei of the dorsal thalamus,* however, they do not project to the cerebral cortex. The functional organization and connections of the reticular nucleus differ from other nuclei of the dorsal thalamus. The reticular nucleus makes extensive connections with other nuclei of the dorsal thalamus, and it receives collateral input from the thalamocortical, corticothalamic, thalamostriate, and pallidothalamic fibers.

General Principles of Thalamic Organization

Although many diverse functional systems have fibers that synapse in the dorsal thalamus en route to the cerebral cortex, three general statements can be made about thalamic organization and function.

1. *All nuclei of the dorsal thalamus receive afferent fibers from at least one extrathalamic source, and all nuclei have efferent projections to the cerebral cortex.* To this extent, all can be considered relay nuclei. The older concept of two classes of thalamic nuclei, association and relay, is no longer applicable.

2. *Thalamic nuclei relay all information destined for the cerebral cortex,* except for the olfactory pathway, the ascending extrathalamic cortical modulatory systems (see Chapter 21).

3. *Few, if any, connections exist between the major nuclei of the thalamus,* except for the extensive interconnections between the intralaminar nuclei.

SPECIFIC AND NONSPECIFIC THALAMIC AFFERENTS

The subcortical input to the thalamic nuclei can be divided into two categories, *specific* and *nonspecific.* The principal afferent pathways of the major sensory systems are examples of the *specific afferents* (e.g., medial lemniscus, optic tract, and brachium of the inferior colliculus). In the case of each of these systems, ascending fibers carrying the sensory information synapse in a precise topographic fashion within a specific relay nucleus of the thalamus. Thalamic relay neurons, in turn, project to the cortex in a highly ordered fashion, resulting in a very precise cortical representation of the sensory field (e.g., visual, somatosensory, and auditory).

The *nonspecific afferents* lack the order and precision of the specific pathways. These afferent projections are not confined to a specific relay nucleus. The fiber terminals of nonspecific pathways tend to concentrate in one or more thalamic nuclei but usually synapse in many other nuclei as well, including the principal sensory nuclei. Examples of the nonspecific afferents include ascending noradrenergic and serotoninergic projections from the brain stem locus ceruleus and the raphe nuclei, respectively. The noradrenergic terminals from the neurons of the locus ceruleus are heaviest in the AV nucleus, although significant terminals occur in other nuclei as well, including the ventrobasal complex and the intralaminar nuclei. Similarly, serotoninergic fibers, principally from neurons of the dorsal raphe nucleus, have terminals in the LGN and in many other nuclei of the dorsal thalamus.

SPECIFIC AND NONSPECIFIC THALAMIC EFFERENTS

Thalamocortical efferent projections also can be subdivided into specific and nonspecific categories. *Specific efferent projections* arise from a single thalamic nucleus. They project, in an ordered and defined pattern, to a restricted area of the cerebral cortex. This category includes thalamocortical projections from specific sensory relay nuclei, such as MGN, LGN, and VPL. *Nonspecific efferent* projections are more diffuse and not limited to a single cortical area. Although they may have a higher concentration of terminals in one region, the distribution of the fibers is widespread.

As a general rule, *each cortical area receives both specific and nonspecific thalamocortical efferent* projections—a well-defined, specific projection from a principal thalamic nucleus and a more diffuse, nonspecific projection from another thalamic source. No general pattern is observed. Nonspecific projections can originate from several sources, including principal relay nuclei.

RECIPROCAL THALAMOCORTICAL-CORTICOTHALAMIC CONNECTIONS

A precise system of reciprocal thalamocortical-corticothalamic projections exists. When a thalamic relay neuron projects to a cortical area, a cortical pyramidal cell from that area of the cortex sends a corticothalamic fiber to the same thalamic nucleus. These precise, *point-to-point reciprocal connections are present for both specific and nonspecific thalamocortical projections.*

LAMINAR TERMINATIONS OF THALAMOCORTICAL PROJECTIONS

The laminar pattern of thalamocortical terminations is different for the specific and nonspecific projections. *Specific thalamic efferent projections* to the *highly granular cortical areas* (primary sensory areas) end in *layer IV.* Specific thalamic efferent projections to *agranular cortical areas* (motor cortex) avoid layer IV and end in *layer III.* Those thalamic efferents to *other cortical areas* end in *both layers III and IV. Nonspecific thalamic efferent projections,* from the more diffusely projecting thalamic nuclei, end principally in *layer I.* Both the specific and nonspecific thalamic efferent projections to the cerebral cortex send collateral terminals to the deeper layers, *layers V and VI* (see Chapter 21).

The results of electrophysiological studies have led to several hypotheses about the functional significance of laminar segregation. The diffuse projections to layer I are probably associated with cortical excitability. Those terminals in layers V and VI make monosynaptic connections with pyramidal cells that give rise to the reciprocal corticothalamic projections. This corticothalamic feedback system may, in turn, regulate the subsequent flow of information to that particular cortical area. Because the intracortical processing of afferent information begins in Layers III and IV, the specific thalamic projections to these layers probably represent the first step in information processing at the cortical level. The excitatory neurotransmitters, glutamate and aspartate, are the principal transmitters in the corticothalamic leg of this loop. The thalamocortical transmitter is unknown.

RETICULAR NUCLEUS AND MODULATION OF THALAMIC ACTIVITY

Anatomically, the reticular nucleus covers the lateral, anterolateral, and ventrolateral surfaces of the thalamus as a sheet of neurons, two or three cells thick, embedded in the external medullary lamina (see Fig. 20–4). From this unique neuroanatomical location, the reticular nucleus monitors the activity of the dorsal thalamus. Thalamocortical projections and reciprocal corti-

cothalamic connections for all thalamic nuclei pass through the reticular nucleus, and most give off collateral terminals en route. In addition, the thalamostriatal projections of the intralaminar nuclei and their reciprocal pallidothalamic fibers also have collaterals, which terminate in the reticular nucleus. Other afferent projections to the reticular nucleus include projections from the deep nuclei of the pretectal area.

The topography of connections in the reticular nucleus is not as precise as that observed in thalamic relay nuclei. However, collaterals of thalamocortical fibers, and their reciprocal corticothalamic fibers, from a particular thalamic nucleus all end in the same area of the reticular nucleus. Reticular neurons from this area project back to that same thalamic nucleus. Although some overlap occurs, specific areas of the reticular nucleus are "dominated" by connections with particular thalamic relay nuclei.

Thus, the neurons of the reticular nucleus monitor the level of activity in both the thalamus and the cerebral cortex. These inhibitory, GABAergic neurons, through inhibition of thalamic relay neurons, can modulate the flow of information from the thalamus to the cortex. This activity probably is more important in the regulation of both thalamic arousal level and information flow from thalamus to cortex than in the processing of sensorimotor information. The reticular nucleus has a high concentration of nicotinic cholinergic receptors. The reticular neurons are sensitive to acetylcholine, however, the source of the cholinergic input has not been identified.

THALAMIC NEURONS

Large relay neurons and smaller interneurons are the principal neuronal cell types of the major thalamic nuclei. The relay neurons, or projection cells, are relatively large (20 to 50 μm), with numerous large, symmetrically radiating dendrites (Fig. 20–5A). The dendrites have characteristic stump-like protrusions, the sites of synaptic contact with the primary afferent fibers. These protrusions are longer, thicker and less common than the dendritic spines of striatal "spiny cells" or cortical pyramidal cells. Relay neurons have a large, well-developed axon that projects to the cerebral cortex. A few collaterals from axons of thalamic relay neurons terminate in the nucleus of origin. Collaterals to the reticular nucleus are more common.

Relay neurons from different nuclei are subtle variations of the same general theme. In some of

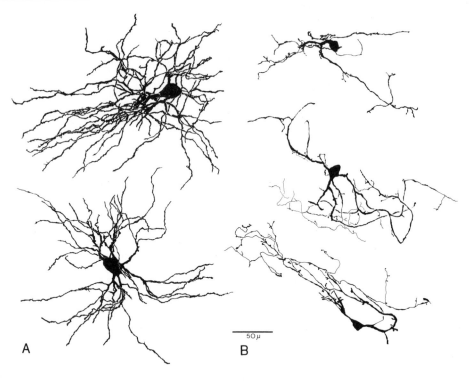

FIGURE 20-5

Golgi preparations of the primate lateral geniculate nucleus. Relay neurons (A) and interneurons (B) illustrate morphological features common to neurons of many thalamic nuclei (see text). (Courtesy of Drs. Michael Conley and Vivien Casagrande, Vanderbilt University, Nashville, Tennessee.)

the major nuclei, relay neurons have been classified as large and small, with the larger neurons projecting to cortical layer IV and the smaller ones to layer I. These would be specific and nonspecific thalamic efferents, respectively. In the LGN, for example, some relay neurons have dendritic trees confined to a single lamina of the nucleus, whereas others radiate across laminar boundaries. In the same nucleus, subtle variations in the morphology of relay neurons correlate with the receipt of fibers from different types of retinal ganglion cells. Individual thalamic nuclei have different information-processing needs. These differences may be reflected in variations in this basic design.

Small interneurons (10 to 20 μm), with thin, locally ramifying axons, account for about 25% of the neurons in the thalamus (Fig. 20-5B). Similar to relay neurons, these cells have specializations that are specific to individual nuclei, specializations that reflect particular information-processing needs. The neuronal population also contains numerous cells with size and dendritic properties intermediate to those described as relay

cells or interneurons. Their numbers and characteristics also vary from nucleus to nucleus.

THALAMIC CIRCUITRY

The ascending afferent fibers branch within the target nucleus, ending in large, prominent synaptic bulbs on dendritic protrusions of relay neurons and on the dendrites of interneurons. These asymmetrical synapses, with presynaptic terminals that contain small clear vesicles, are excitatory. The reciprocal corticothalamic fibers have numerous synaptic terminals on both the primary dendrites of the relay neurons and on the dendritic branches of the interneurons. These excitatory synapses, with asymmetrical membrane thickenings and clear spherical synaptic vesicles, use either glutamate or aspartate as the neurotransmitter. Axon terminals from neurons in the reticular nucleus of the thalamus form inhibitory, GABAergic synapses on the soma or proximal dendritic segments of the relay neurons.

A characteristic feature of the thalamic circuitry is the *glomerulus,* or *synaptic island,* that surrounds the primary synapse between the ascending afferent fiber to the thalamus and the thalamic relay neuron. Contained within this cluster, in addition to the afferent terminal and dendritic protrusion of the relay cell, are many small dendritic processes of interneurons and axon terminals of interneurons. Many of the dendritic processes contain synaptic vesicles.

Most of these small dendritic processes of the interneurons in the glomerulus are postsynaptic to the primary afferent fiber. Some, however, are presynaptic to the relay neuron, forming dendrodendritic synapses; some are presynaptic to dendritic terminals of interneurons, also forming dendrodendritic synapses; and others are postsynaptic to axon terminals from other interneurons. The entire synaptic complex is surrounded by an astrocytic capsule. The unusual grape-like appendages, characteristic of the Golgi preparations of thalamic interneurons (see Fig. 20–5), are clusters of these small dendritic processes.

These synaptic relationships are summarized in Figure 20–6. The thalamic afferent fiber (*A*) has its terminal (*T1*) on the dendritic process (*D*) of the relay neuron (*R*). This complex is surrounded by the many small dendritic processes (*T2*) of the interneuron (*I*) and the axon terminal (*F*) of the interneuron. The entire complex is enveloped by an astrocytic capsule (*G*). Axon terminals from cortical neurons (*C*) and reticular neurons (*Rt*) are shown in a typical synaptic relation to the relay neuron.

Functional Connections of the Thalamic Nuclei

NONSPECIFIC NUCLEI

Intralaminar Nuclei

The intralaminar nuclei have many features in common. All are heavily interconnected. The

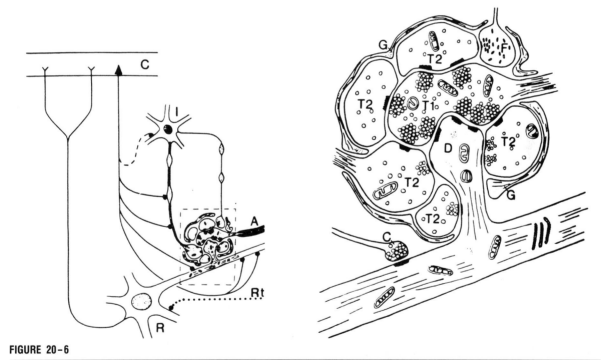

FIGURE 20–6

Synaptic relationships typical of the majority of thalamic nuclei. Dendritic protrusions (*D*) of thalamocortical relay cells (*R*) receive the terminals (*T1*) of ascending afferent fibers (*A*) and the presynaptic dendrites (*T2*) of interneurons (*I*). Presynaptic dendrites and probably conventional dendrites of interneurons are also postsynaptic to the afferent fiber terminal and sometimes to one another (not shown).

Axons of interneurons also terminate (*F*) mainly on presynaptic dendrites. The complex synaptic aggregation tends to be ensheathed in astrocytic processes (*G*). Outside this synaptic complex, corticothalamic terminals (*C*) end on relay cell dendrites and on presynaptic dendrites of interneurons. On the relay cell, most cortical terminals are distally situated. Terminals of reticular axons (*Rt*) also terminate on or close to the somata of relay neurons. (Reproduced with permission from E. G. Jones, *Handbook of Physiology*, Section 1, Volume III, p. 173, 1984.)

connections include only other intralaminar nuclei of the dorsal thalamus. The intralaminar nuclei are the only group of thalamic nuclei to have significant intrathalamic connections.

All have well-organized, heavy projections to the striatum: the caudate and the putamen. These projections connect areas of the intralaminar and striatal nuclei—areas that receive corticothalamic and corticostriatal projections from a common cortical area. In other words, corticothalamic and corticostriatal fibers, arising from a particular cortical area, project to regions of the intralaminar nuclei and striatum that are interconnected by intralaminar-striatal projections.

All of the intralaminar nuclei have reciprocal thalamocortical projections. These are diffuse and not confined to restricted regions of the cortex, although each nucleus has a dominant cortical area. The *central medial* and *paracentral nuclei* project to the medial and rostral portions of the frontal lobe, including the anterior limbic areas and the cingulate gyrus. The *parafascicular nucleus* projects to the rostral and lateral areas of the frontal lobe; the *centromedian nucleus*, to the motor and premotor areas; and the *centrolateral nucleus*, to the somatosensory and other parietal areas, with some projections as far posterior as the occipital visual cortex. The heaviest projections are to motor-related areas and the lightest, to sensory areas.

A number of the subcortical afferents to the intralaminar nuclei are well defined. Afferents go to all intralaminar nuclei from the deep nuclei of the cerebellum, except for the parafascicular nucleus and that portion of the centrolateral nucleus that receives somatosensory fibers. The centromedian and parafascicular nuclei, however, are the only ones to receive afferents from the globus pallidus. Additional afferents arise in the brain stem reticular formation, the pontine parabrachial nucleus, the substantia nigra, the deep layers of the superior colliculus, and the deep nuclei of the pretectum and the ascending spinothalamic tract.

Pain pathways end in a number of the intralaminar nuclei. However, a precise somatotopic localization is not seen. These pain afferents are from both the direct *spinothalamic tract* and the diffuse multisynaptic ascending pathways within the *brain stem reticular formation*. Functionally and anatomically, the intralaminar nuclei are diencephalic extensions of the brain stem reticular formation. Intralaminar neurons project both to the striatum and to widespread areas of the cortex, including the somatosensory areas. *These connections suggest a role in sensorimotor inte-* *gration.* In addition, many of the widespread cortical projections of intralaminar relay neurons are part of a general *cortical arousal* mechanism.

Midline Nuclei

The connections of the midline nuclei are the least well documented of the thalamic nuclei. As a group, they project to both the striatum and the cerebral cortex. The cortical projections are diffuse and nonspecific, although individual nuclei have a cortical region of preference. As with all thalamocortical projections, these are reciprocal. The parataenial nucleus, situated beneath the more rostral portion of the stria medullaris thalami, projects to the hippocampus, the hippocampal rudiments, and the nucleus accumbens of the basal forebrain. The other midline nuclei project to anterior, middle, and posterior areas of the medial surface of the cerebral cortex. Afferents to the midline nuclei are poorly defined. In addition to ascending adrenergic and serotoninergic fibers from the brain stem, there are diffuse projections from the pretectal area and reciprocal connections with the hypothalamus and epithalamus. Functionally, a role in the integration of visceral activities has been proposed.

SPECIFIC NUCLEI

Somatosensory Relay

The *ventral posterolateral, posteromedial, posterosuperior*, and *posteroinferior nuclei* (*VPL, VPM, VPS*, and *VPI*), collectively known as the *ventrobasal complex*, are the principal somatosensory relay nuclei. This nuclear complex is highly ordered, with a precise topographic representation of the contralateral half of the body and a separation of the sensory modalities. Sensations of light touch, pressure, and joint movement, carried by the medial lemniscus, spinothalamic tract, and spinocervicothalamic tract, terminate in VPL and VPI. Those carried by the trigeminal lemniscus end in VPM. VPS receives sensory input exclusively from proprioceptors. Topographically, VPM represents the head; VPL, the remainder of the body, with the more medial portion of VPL containing the upper extremity arm representation and the lateral portion, the lower extremity. The entire body is represented in both VPS and VPI. Both levels of thalamic organization, topography, and sensory modality are preserved in the thalamocortical projections. These projections terminate in the primary somatosensory cortex, S-I (Brodmann's areas 3, 1, and 2), and in the secondary somatosensory cortex, S-II (Fig. 20–7).

The *posterior complex* or zone, *PO*, is involved in the perception of painful or noxious stimuli. PO is included with the somatosensory relay nuclei even though it may receive afferents from other sensory systems as well. The thalamocortical projections from PO end in the retroinsular area, a secondary somatosensory area. Additional afferents include projections from the inferior colliculus, medial lemniscus, and MGN. Physiologically, neurons in this complex respond to high threshold somatosensory and auditory stimuli and have properties consistent with an involvement in central nervous system (CNS) pain mechanisms. The ventrobasal complex and PO are reviewed in detail in Chapter 11.

Gustatory Relay

Taste sensation signals, originating in the solitary nucleus and relayed in the parabrachial nucleus of the dorsal pons, terminate in the *parvocellular division* of the *ventral posteromedial nucleus* (*VPMpc*), an area unresponsive to somatic stimuli and often referred to as the *basal ventromedial nucleus for taste*. Thalamocortical projections end in the tongue region of S-I and S-II as well as in the retroinsular area of the cortex. See Chapter 13 for detailed review.

Vestibular Relay

Two nuclei of the *ventrobasal complex* receive vestibular afferents. The *pars oralis* of the *ventral posterolateral nucleus* (*VPLo*) and the *ventral posteroinferior nucleus* (*VPI*) receive significant projections from the vestibular nuclei and relay the information principally to Brodmann's area 3a in the postcentral gyrus, immediately adjacent to the primary motor cortex. Although VL receives a major contribution from ascending vestibular afferents, these are motor in function and probably do not contribute to a conscious appre-

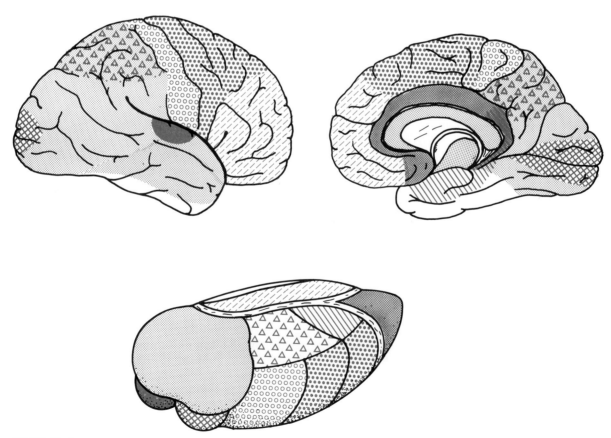

FIGURE 20–7

Summary of the thalamocortical projections from some of the principal thalamic relay nuclei. Cortical shading (red) represents the projection area of the corresponding thalamic nuclear group.

ciation of vestibular sensory information (see Chapter 12).

Auditory Relay

The *medial geniculate nucleus* (*MGN*) receives afferent fibers from the inferior colliculus. These auditory projections end in the appropriate iso-frequency lamina of the MGN, producing a highly ordered, bilateral, tonotopic representation of the cochlea within the nucleus. Thalamocortical projections from MGN terminate in the primary auditory cortex (A-I), the transverse temporal gyri (Brodmann's areas 41 and 42) (see Fig. 20–7). The tonotopic organization of the MGN is preserved in the cortical representation of audition in A-I. Additional auditory thalamocortical projections end in the surrounding secondary auditory area (A-II), in an area of the insular cortex, and in a third auditory area (A-III) found in the head region of S-II. A-II and A-III are not represented in Figure 20–7.

The *MGN* contains three subdivisions: *ventral* (*MGNv*), *medial* (*MGNm*), and *dorsal* (*MGNd*). *MGNv* is the principal cortical relay nucleus and contains the precise tonotopic representation. MGNv accurately relays information on sound intensity and sound frequency and on the binaural properties of the sound stimulus. *MGNd* is less well defined, and the tonotopic organization is not as precise as that of MGNv. The response properties of these neurons are complex. The tonotopic organization of *MGNm* also is not precise, and the nucleus receives projections from both the auditory and the nonauditory neurons of the brain stem, with a major contribution from the superior olivary complex (see Chapter 12).

Visual Relay

The *lateral geniculate nucleus* (*LGN*) is the principal thalamic relay nucleus for the visual system, receiving projections from retinal ganglion cells. The projections to this six-layered nucleus form a specific *visuotopic map* of the contralateral visual hemifield (see Chapter 11). Neurons from all six layers of the LGN then relay this visual information to the *primary visual cortex* (*V-1*) (Brodmann's area 17).

Although the primary function of the LGN is the accurate transmission of visual information from the retina to the primary visual cortex, a second and equally important function is the regulation of the flow of visual information to

V-1. A combination of feed-forward and feedback inhibitory circuits, along with extensive cortico-geniculate (corticothalamic) projections, regulate this flow of information.

The largest single source of afferents to the LGN is the corticothalamic projections from the visual cortex, exceeding the number reaching the LGN from the retina. These cortical projections may have an important role in arousal, in regulating the level of visual attention, and in modulating the flow of information from the LGN to V-1.

Motor Relay

In the dorsal thalamus, the three nuclear groups are associated with the somatic motor system: the *ventral anterior nucleus* (*VA*) and both the *anterior* and *posterior divisions* of the *ventral lateral nucleus* (*VLa* and *VLp*). The *VLp* receives well-defined afferents from the cerebellum, specifically from the globose, emboliform, and dentate nuclei. This thalamic nucleus then projects selectively to the *premotor cortex* (*PMC*) and to the *primary motor cortex* (*M-I*) (Brodmann's area 4 and part of 6) (see Fig. 20–7 and Fig. 15–1). Both *VA* and *VLa* receive afferents from the globus pallidus (GPi) and the substantia nigra. Neurons in these thalamic nuclei, in turn, project selectively to the *supplementary motor area* (*SMA*) (part of Brodmann's area 6) (see Fig. 20–7 and Fig. 15–1). In addition, both VLa and VLp receive less specific afferents from the medial lemniscus, spinothalamic tract, and vestibular nuclei. Nonspecific thalamocortical projections from VLa and VLp go to the primary somatosensory cortex and frontal lobe areas rostral to the motor areas (Brodmann's areas 8 and 9). The projections of VA are not as well defined.

Limbic Relay

The three nuclei of the *anterior nuclear group* and the *lateral dorsal nucleus* (*LD*) are relay nuclei for limbic system circuits. The *anterior group* receives afferents from the mammillary nuclei of the hypothalamus via the very prominent mamillothalamic tract. Thalamocortical projections from the *anterior nuclei* terminate in the cingulate gyrus, the subcallosal gyrus and parolfactory gyri of the limbic forebrain, the retrosplenial portion of the cingulate gyrus, and the hippocampus on the medial surface of the temporal lobe (see Fig. 20–7). *LD* receives afferents from the limbic forebrain and septal areas via the stria medullaris thalami, and thalamocortical projections from LD end in the posterior and retrosplenial portions of the cingulate gyrus and in the parahippocampal gyrus of the temporal lobe (see Fig. 20–7). Some of these projections overlap with those from the anterior nuclei.

As with most of the nuclei of the dorsal thalamus, we know little about the specific neurotransmitters involved. The *anterior nuclei* contain the highest concentration of muscarinic cholinergic receptors in the thalamus, but the source of these cholinergic afferents has not been identified.

Mediodorsal Nucleus

The *mediodorsal nucleus* (*MD*) is the largest and most prominent of the medial nuclei in humans. The relative size and importance of this nucleus parallels frontal lobe development. Principal afferents are from the anterior hypothalamus and the amygdaloid complex. Additional afferents arise in the septal nuclei, the nucleus of the diagonal band, and the pretectal area of the midbrain. Thalamocortical projections terminate throughout most of the frontal lobe, from the supraorbital cortex to the area just rostral to the motor areas (see Fig. 20–7). The amygdala projects to the same area of the frontal cortex. A point-to-point relation exists between areas in the amygdala, MD, and frontal cortex (see Chapter 22).

Influence of Brain Stem Reticular Formation

Stimulation of the brain stem reticular formation facilitates transmission at many thalamic relay nuclei. However, few demonstrable afferents go directly to these nuclei from the brain stem reticular formation. The facilitation may be due to a reduction in the level of inhibition of thalamic relay neurons. One hypothesis involves a reticular formation inhibition of the inhibitory reticular nucleus of the thalamus. However, no direct connections between the brain stem reticular formation and the reticular nucleus of the thalamus are demonstrable. The only demonstrable afferents from the brain stem reticular formation are the diffuse serotoninergic and adrenergic projections from the dorsal raphe and locus ceruleus, principally to the intralaminar nuclei. The influence of the reticular formation may be indirect. By acting on the intralaminar nuclei, the brain stem reticular formation could indirectly influence thalamic activity by way of intralaminar projections to the cerebral cortex, the striatum, or the reticular nucleus of the thalamus. Such a pathway would account for the long latency between the stimulation of the brain stem reticular formation and the disinhibition of thalamic relay neurons.

SUGGESTED READING

Jones, E. G. (1984). Organization of the thalamocortical complex and its relation to sensory processes. In *Handbook of Physiology*. Section I. *The Nervous System*. Volume III. *Sensory Processes*, Part 1, I. Darian-Smith (Editor), American Physiological Society, Bethesda, pp. 149–212.

This review develops the concept that the dorsal thalamus is a heterogeneous structure associated with many diverse functional systems. The general principles of organization, applicable to many of the thalamic nuclei, are developed.

Jones, E. G. (1983). The thalamus. In *Chemical Neuroanatomy*. P. C. Emson (Editor), Raven Press, New York, pp. 257–293.

Changing concepts of thalamic organization are presented. The differences between specific and nonspecific nuclei are clarified. This review includes a discussion of the role of the reticular nucleus of the thalamus in the modulation of thalamic activity.

Chapter

21

Cerebral Cortex

The cerebral cortex, the center of higher neural function, is most highly developed in humans. The cortex is the most complex region of the brain. Until relatively recently, this complexity discouraged many researchers, and few studies addressed the functional organization of the cerebral cortex. However, the results of an increasing amount of new research on the cerebral cortex have begun to shed some light on this organization.

Estimates of the number of neurons in the adult human cerebral cortex range from 14 to 16 billion, with about two thirds of these neurons being small pyramidal cells. Unlike the cerebellar cortex, where many of the interconnections between the different neurons and fibers are well documented, much of the very complex "wiring" of the cerebral cortex remains a mystery. Even after further research, there is still no single,

unifying theory of functional organization that "fits" all of the cortical areas.

This chapter reviews the largest and the phylogenetically most recent portion of the cerebral cortex, the *neocortex* or the *neopallium*. The older cortical areas, the *archicortex* (*archipallium*) and the *paleocortex* (*paleopallium*) that make up less than 10% of the human cerebral cortex, are discussed as part of the *limbic system* (see Chapter 22).

Development

In the 5th week of fetal development, the *telencephalic vesicles*, the forerunners of the cerebral hemispheres, grow out from the dorsolateral margin of the forebrain like a pair of balloons. During the following 2 to 3 months of fetal life, these vesicles grow more rapidly than the rest of the brain—a growth that is primarily planar and one that dramatically increases the surface area of the vesicle.

In the early stages of cortical development, the walls of the telencephalic vesicles, although very thin, contain the same three primary layers as other regions of the developing neural tube: (1) an inner *germinal layer*, (2) a middle *mantle layer*, and (3) an outer *marginal layer*. However, the fate of the three layers is quite different from that of the brain stem or spinal cord. The *germinal layer* produces the early neuroblasts that migrate into the *mantle layer*. However, at 8 to 10 weeks of development, the neuroblasts of the mantle layer migrate into the outer *marginal layer* and differentiate at the surface of the vesicle as a sheet of telencephalic gray matter, the *cerebral cortex*. The *mantle layer*, now devoid of neuroblasts, becomes the *white matter* of the cerebral hemisphere and is deep to the superficial gray matter. The white matter contains cortical associational and commissural fibers as well as cortical afferent and efferent fibers. The *germinal layer* ultimately differentiates into the *ependymal layer*, as it does in the brain stem.

As differentiation proceeds, the neurons of the cerebral cortex form up to six histologically distinct layers by the 6th to 8th month of fetal development. All of the *neocortex* has six layers, whereas the *archicortex* and *paleocortex* have from three to five layers (see Chapter 22).

As the balloon-like cerebral hemispheres enlarge in surface area, owing to the overall planar growth pattern of the walls, they soon are thrown into a series of folds, with the surfaces of the folds forming the *gyri* and the depths of the folds the *sulci*. The early signs of gyri and sulci are apparent as early as 6 months of fetal life (see Fig. 1–20). In the adult, the cerebral cortex has a surface area of 2000 to 2500 cm², of which only about a third is visible from the surface, the remainder being buried in the depths of the sulci and fissures. In the adult, the sheet of gray matter or cortex is thickest on the crests of the gyri (4.5 to 5.0 mm) and thinnest in the depths of the sulci (1.2 to 1.6 mm).

In early growth and development, the phylogenetically older cortical areas, the archicortex and paleocortex, develop first and are disproportionately large. However, as development proceeds, the neocortex grows more rapidly and displaces the older cortical areas to the more medial portions of the hemisphere.

Subdivisions

ANATOMICAL AND PHYLOGENETIC SUBDIVISIONS

Based on *histological and phylogenetic criteria*, the three principal regions or subdivisions of the cerebral cortex are the *archicortex (archipallium)*, *paleocortex (paleopallium)*, and *neocortex (neopallium)*. The archicortex's hippocampal formation contains three distinct histological layers and is the oldest region phylogenetically. The *paleocortex*, principally olfactory in nature, has from three to five cortical layers, including the *piriform area* (the *lateral olfactory gyrus*, the *uncus*, and the *anterior portion* of the *parahippocampal gyrus*). The *neocortex* is the newest cortical area, phylogenetically, and contains six distinct histological layers. In humans, the neocortex constitutes over 90% of the cerebral cortex. The *archicortex* and *paleocortex* often are referred to as *allocortex*, and the *neocortex* is referred to as *isocortex*.

GEOGRAPHICAL SUBDIVISIONS

Each cerebral hemisphere is divided, *geographically*, into lobes: *frontal lobe, parietal lobe, occipital lobe, temporal lobe*, and *insula*. These divisions are based on geography and do not represent functional or cytoarchitectural divisions (Figs. 21–1 and 21–2). An overlapping "lobe," and one defined as part of a functional system and not by its geography, is the *limbic lobe* (see Chapter 22).

The *frontal lobe* extends forward from the central sulcus and makes up about a third of the total cortical tissue. Included in the frontal lobe are the *primary motor area (M-I)*; the *supplementary motor area (SMA)*; the *premotor cortex (PMC)*; the *frontal eye field (FEF)*; and the most anterior portion of the frontal lobe, rostral to the motor areas, the *prefrontal area*.

The *parietal lobe* extends posteriorly from the central sulcus to the occipital lobe and inferolaterally to the temporal lobe. Included in the parietal lobe are the somatosensory cortical areas, the *primary somatosensory area (S-I)*, the *secondary somatosensory area (S-II)*, and the *retroinsular area*, along with both the *posterior parietal motor area* and the *posterior parietal visual area*.

The *occipital lobe* occupies the posterior portion of the hemisphere and extends anteriorly to the parietal and temporal lobes. Included in the

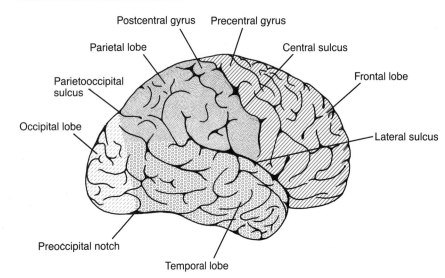

FIGURE 21-1

Lateral view of the right cerebral hemisphere illustrating the major cortical lobes. Frontal lobe, diagonal lines; parietal lobe, stipple; occipital lobe, dashed lines; temporal lobe, open circles.

occipital lobe are the *primary visual area* (*V-1, calcarine cortex*) and the *prestriate visual areas* (*V-2, V-3,* and *V-4*).

The *temporal lobe* is bounded superiorly by the lateral sulcus and the parietal lobe and posteriorly by the occipital lobe. Included in the temporal lobe are the *primary auditory area* (*A-1*), the *secondary auditory areas*, and the *middle temporal visual area* (*MT*). Geographically involved with the temporal lobe are a number of components of the limbic lobe.

The *insula* is a cortical area buried in the depths of the lateral sulcus and is immediately superficial (lateral) to the basal ganglia. The insula is visible only when the overlying *frontal, parietal,* and *temporal opercula* are spread apart or cut away (see Fig. 8–2).

The *limbic lobe,* although defined in relation to the *limbic system,* forms an inner ring of cortical tissue on the medial surface of each hemisphere with components that *geographically* belong to the frontal, parietal, and temporal lobes. In the

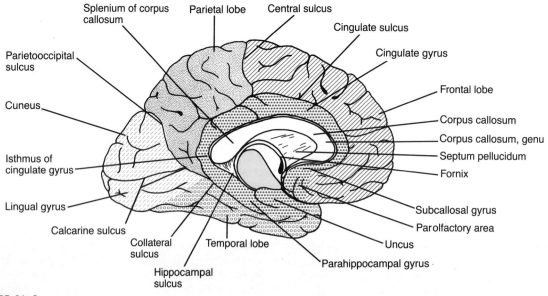

FIGURE 21-2

Midsagittal view of the left cerebral hemisphere illustrating the major cortical lobes. Frontal lobe, diagonal lines; parietal lobe, stipple; occipital lobe, dashed lines; temporal lobe, open circles; limbic lobe, filled circles.

limbic lobe are the *parolfactory area*, the *subcallosal area*, the *cingulate gyrus*, the *parahippocampal gyrus*, the *uncus*, and the *hippocampal formation* (see Fig. 21–2).

CYTOARCHITECTURAL SUBDIVISIONS

Certain primary sulci appear early in development and are consistent from brain to brain. A number of these form the boundaries for dividing the brain into lobes—central sulcus, lateral sulcus, and parieto-occipital sulcus. However, the overall pattern of gyri and sulci is quite variable.

Much less variable, however, is the cytoarchitectural organization of the cortex.

Although the entire neocortex contains six basic layers, a number of differences occur in the cytoarchitecture. Based on these differences, the human cerebral cortex has been divided into as many as 200 histologically distinct areas. Subtle differences are observed in regional cytoarchitecture, but these differences are constant from brain to brain. This pattern of *areal differences* forms the basis of many cytoarchitectural maps of the human cerebral cortex (Fig. 21–3). These areas are subsequently discussed in greater detail.

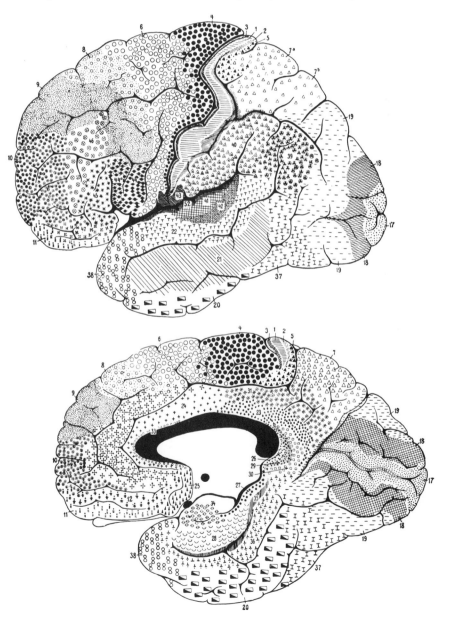

FIGURE 21-3

Brodmann's cytoarchitectural map of the human cerebral cortex as first presented in 1909. Upper figure is the lateral view of the cerebral hemisphere; lower figure is the medial view. (Reproduced with permission from K. Brodmann, *Vergleichende Lokalisationslehre der Grosshirnrinde in ihern Prinzipien dargestellt auf Grund des Zellenbaues*, J. A. Barth, Leipzig, 1925.)

Histological Organization of the Neocortex

CORTICAL NEURONS

Although over 14 billion neurons are found in the human cerebral cortex, most cortical neurons are one of four cell types: *pyramidal cells* (Fig. 21–4), *granule cells* (Fig. 21–5), *fusiform cells*,

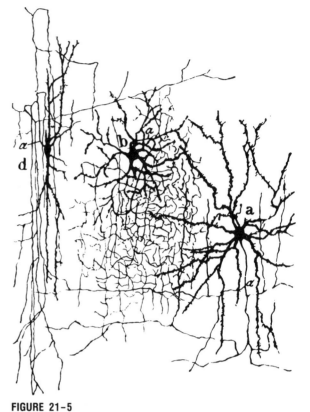

FIGURE 21–5

Several varieties of cortical interneurons or granule cells drawn by Ramon y Cajal from a Golgi-stained preparation. (Reproduced with permission from S. Ramon y Cajal, *Histologie du Système Nerveux*, Tome II. Translated by L. Azoulay. Instituto Ramon y Cajal, Madrid, 1955.)

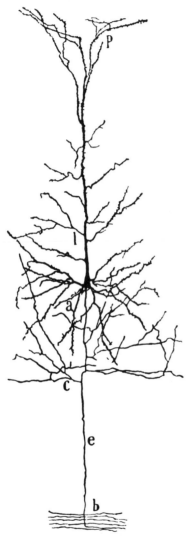

FIGURE 21–4

A typical cortical pyramidal cell drawn by Ramon y Cajal from a Golgi-stained preparation. a, basal dendrites; b, white matter; c, axon collaterals; e, axon leaving cortex; l, apical dendrite with branches; p, terminal branches of apical dendrite. (Reproduced with permission from S. Ramon y Cajal, *Histologie du Système Nerveux*, Tome II. Translated by L. Azoulay. Instituto Ramon y Cajal, Madrid, 1955.)

and *horizontal cells*. Some classifications describe many more cells, but most are variations of one of these basic types. The greatest variation in cell type is found in the granule cell classification. Granule cells, as used here, refer to all nonpyramidal cells, except the very characteristic fusiform cell of layer VI and the horizontal cell of layer I. Many terms, e.g., stellate, multipolar, chandelier, bitufted, double bouquet, bipolar, and basket, often further modified with the descriptive terms spinous or aspinous, are chosen to describe the nonpyramidal cells of the neocortex. No two cortical neurons are the same; hence, many varieties of shape and size exist within each of these categories. For most purposes, especially in an introductory text, a simplified classification with four basic cells types is sufficient.

The *pyramidal cell* is by far the most abundant of the cortical neuron types and the most characteristic neuron of the cerebral cortex (see Fig.

21–4 and Figs. 2–2*A*, 2–3, and 2–4*A*). The most prominent features of pyramidal cells include their *conical-shaped soma* (triangular in section), with the apex of the cone always pointing toward the surface of the cortex, and a very prominent *apical dendrite* arising from the tip of the cone. The apical dendrites of pyramidal cells are variable in length, with many extending to the more superficial layers of the cortex.

In addition to the apical dendrite, pyramidal cells also have many *basal dendrites* that radiate from the base of the cone-shaped soma. The pyramidal cell *axon* arises from the base of the soma or often from the proximal portion of a basal dendrite. Pyramidal cells are the principal efferent neurons of the cerebral cortex. Because of this factor, most pyramidal cell axons descend into the *white matter* of the cortex. From the white matter, axons of these neurons may project to other cortical areas of the same hemisphere (*intrahemispheric associational fibers*); to the opposite cortical hemisphere (*commissural association fibers*); or, via the internal capsule, to the lower levels of the central nervous system (CNS) (*cortical efferent fibers*).

Pyramidal cells have one or more collateral axonal branches that terminate near the cell soma or ascend for variable distances in the cortex before terminating. The size of the soma of most pyramidal cells ranges from 10 to 50 μm high, the notable exception being the giant *pyramidal cells of Betz*. These huge *Betz cells* have soma heights of 80 to 150 μm and are found only in layer V of the primary motor cortex.

The second most abundant cell type of the cerebral cortex is the *granule cell* or *stellate cell* (see Fig. 21–5 and Fig. 2–4*C*). These neurons are multipolar, polygonal cells of relatively small size. Somas range from 4 to 10 μm in diameter. The dendrites radiate from the soma in all directions, giving many of them a star-shaped or stellate appearance. Within this classification are two subcategories, the *Golgi type I* and *Type II granule cells*. *Golgi type I neurons* are simply granule cells with *long axons* that extend beyond the dendritic tree, and *Golgi type II neurons* are granule cells with *short axons* that usually do not extend beyond the dendritic tree (see Figs. 2–2*B* and 2–2*C*). The axonal processes of many of the *Golgi type I granule cells* display specialized patterns that often are the bases of further subclassification. For example, some with cell bodies in the deeper layers of the cortex have axons that ascend toward the surface of the cortex and terminate in the outer three layers of the cortex.

These are often called the *Martinotti cells*. Other Golgi type I granule cells have axons that give off long, horizontally running collaterals. Axon terminals from these collaterals envelop the somata of nearby pyramidal and granule cells, with a characteristic basket-like terminal arbor (similar to cerebellar basket cells). These are often called *basket cells of the cerebral cortex*.

Fusiform cells (*spindle cells*) are found principally in the deepest layer (VI) of the cortex and are small, cigar-shaped cells with their long axes at right angles to the surface of the cortex. These neurons also have a long *apical dendrite*, with some extending to the cortical surface. Axons of fusiform cells arise from the lower part of the cell soma and descend into the white matter. In addition to the apical dendrite, fusiform cells have variable numbers of dendrites radiating from the cell soma. Often, fusiform cells are classified as "modified pyramidal cells."

The fourth neuronal cell type found in the cerebral cortex is the *horizontal cell of Cajal*, or simply the *horizontal cell*. These neurons, limited to layer I (the outer or molecular layer) of the cortex, have relatively long axons that run parallel to the surface of the cortex. These axons also branch and terminate in the outer cortical layer. The dendritic tree of the horizontal cell is small, and it also resides in the outer layer of the cortex.

LAMINAR ORGANIZATION

An uneven distribution of types and sizes of neurons combined with horizontal patterns of incoming afferent fibers and axons of local neurons gives the cortex a laminar pattern of organization. In the *neocortex*, six well-defined cortical layers are found, numbered I through VI, from the pial surface to the deepest layer, adjacent to the white matter (Figs. 21–6, 21–7, and 21–8). *Layer I*, the *molecular layer*, is the most superficial; immediately deep to layer I is *layer II*, the *external granular layer*; then, *layer III*, the *external pyramidal layer*; followed by *layer IV*, the *internal granular layer*; then, *layer V*, the *internal pyramidal layer*; and *layer VI*, the *multiform* or *fusiform layer*. Immediately deep to layer VI is the *cortical white matter*, composed of nerve fibers entering and exiting the overlying cortex. As the names of the layers imply, they are characterized by an abundance of one or more of the cortical neuron cell types.

Layer I, the *molecular layer*, contains an abundance of nerve processes, both dendritic and axonal, and a relative paucity of neuronal cell

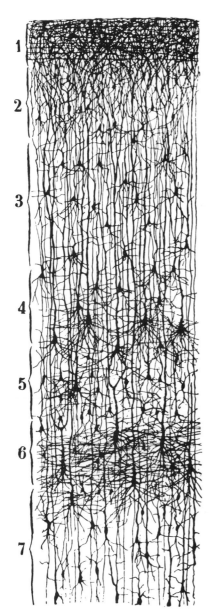

FIGURE 21-6

The appearance of layers in the parietal cortex of a 1-month-old infant as drawn by Ramon y Cajal. Laminar designations of Ramon y Cajal differ slightly from those of Brodmann and those of this text. Layers 3 and 4 of Ramon y Cajal are approximately equivalent to layer III. Thus, layer 1 is the molecular layer (layer I); layer 2, the outer granular layer (layer II); layers 3 and 4, the outer pyramidal layer (layer III); layer 5, the inner granular layer (layer IV); layer 6, the inner pyramidal layer (layer V); and layer 7, the fusiform layer (layer VI). (Reproduced with permission from S. Ramon y Cajal, *Histologie du Système Nerveux*, Tome II. Translated by L. Azoulay. Instituto Ramon y Cajal, Madrid, 1955.)

bodies, with those that are present being small. The most characteristic neuronal cell type is the *horizontal cell*. Horizontal cells have a small, fusiform body and a sparse dendritic tree that remains within layer I. These neurons have a long axon, up to several millimeters, with numerous long collateral branches. Both the axon and its branches spread over the cortical surface. Many small *Golgi type II granule cells* are scattered among the neuronal cell processes of layer I. Their axons terminate within the immediate vicinity of the neuron, rarely leaving layer I, the molecular layer.

Layer I contains a dense, horizontal plexus of axonal and dendritic nerve endings. In addition to the dendritic trees of the horizontal and granule cells intrinsic to the layer, the terminal branches of the apical dendrites from many pyramidal and fusiform cells of the deeper cortical layers spread out parallel to the surface in layer I. Terminal axonal processes from cortical association fibers, terminal branches of ascending granule cell axons, and ascending monoaminergic axons from neurons in the brain stem provide most of the remaining neuronal processes that contribute to the plexus of layer I, the molecular layer (see Figs. 21-6 and 21-7).

Layer II, the *external granular layer*, has two characteristic features: (1) an abundance of small, densely packed neurons and (2) a paucity of myelinated fibers. Of the neurons, most are very small *granule cells* (both *Golgi type I* and *type II*). The remainder are very small pyramidal cells, with apical dendrites extending into layer I and axons terminating in the deeper layers of the cortex. Axons of some granule cells descend to deeper layers of the cortex; however, a few have axons that ascend and ramify within the plexus of layer I, the molecular layer (see Fig. 21-7).

Layer III, the *external pyramidal layer*, contains numerous medium to medium-large *pyramidal cells* and a small number of *granule cells*. The pyramidal cells tend to be arranged according to size, with the medium cells most superficial and the larger cells deeper. The apical dendrites of these pyramidal cells ascend to layer I. Axons of most of the layer III pyramidal cells descend through the cortex, forming cortical association fibers, both callosal and intrahemispherical. Before leaving the cortex, most pyramidal cell axons have many collaterals: recurrent collaterals terminating near the cell of origin and collaterals branching profusely within deeper cortical layers (see Figs. 21-4, 21-7, and Fig. 15-3).

Layer IV, the *internal granular layer*, is the

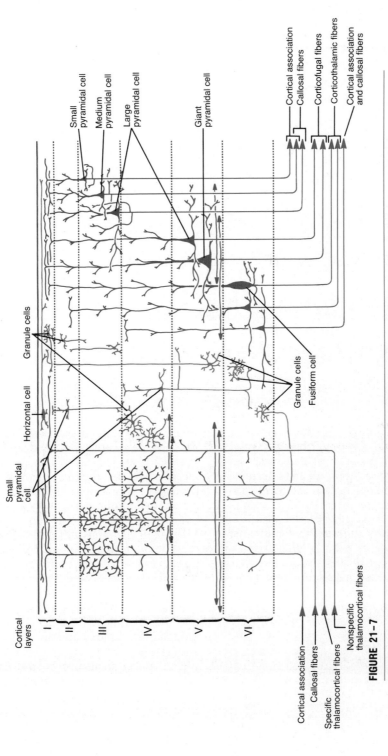

FIGURE 21–7

Some of the principal components of the neocortical circuitry. Cortical afferents are illustrated on the left; cortical efferents, on the right. In the center are a few of the component neurons of the local cortical circuitry. See text for details.

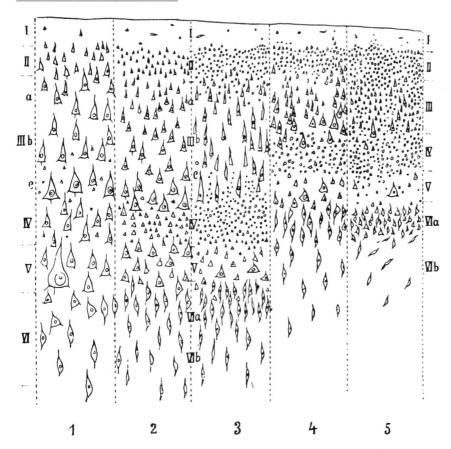

FIGURE 21-8

Five basic types of cortex are illustrated: (1) agranular-pyramidal, (2) granular-pyramidal, (3) granular-parietal, (4) polar, and (5) granular. See text for details. (Reproduced with permission from C. F. von Economo, *The Cytoarchitectonics of the Human Cerebral Cortex*, Oxford Medical Publications, London, 1929.)

principal "receiving station" of the cortex, i.e., the site of termination of specific thalamocortical projections. Although thalamic afferents also terminate in other layers as well, all have terminal branches in layer IV. The single most characteristic histological feature of layer IV in a myelinstained section is a dense, horizontal plexus of myelinated nerve fibers (mostly thalamic afferents) that form the *outer band of Baillarger*. In the primary visual cortex (area 17), the *outer band of Baillarger* is especially prominent and is known as the *stripe of Gennari*. The prominence of this band or "stripe" is the reason why area 17 is frequently called the *striate cortex* (see Chapter 11).

Additionally, layer IV has an abundance of *granule cells*, both the *Golgi type I* and *Golgi type II*. The abundance of granule cells and the relative thickness of layer IV vary from one cortical area to the next. A thick layer IV and an abundance of granule cells are characteristic of primary sensory areas. Most of the granule cell axons terminate within layer IV, although some project to deeper layers. A few *pyramidal cells*,

small to medium in size, also reside in layer IV. Most of these project to the deeper cortical layers, V and VI (see Figs. 21-7 and 21-8).

Layer V, the *internal pyramidal layer*, is the principal efferent layer of the cortex and is thickest in the motor cortical areas. This layer contains mostly medium-to-large *pyramidal cells*. Most of their axons descend through the cortical white matter to the internal capsule en route to lower centers of the brain, the brain stem, and the spinal cord. These corticofugal fibers arising from layer V include corticostriate, corticobulbar, and corticospinal fibers as well as most of those to other brain stem centers, such as the pons, reticular formation, and tectum (see Figs. 21-6 and 21-7).

The apical dendrites of the larger pyramidal cells extend to layer I, where they contribute to the dense horizontal plexus. In the primary motor cortex, area 4, some pyramidal cells are huge. Many of these have cell bodies that exceed 100 μm in height. These are the *giant pyramidal cells of Betz*, numbering about 34,000 in the human. These neurons originally were thought to be the major contributor to the corticospinal tract; however, their axons account for only about 2% of the 1.7 million efferent fibers in the corticospinal tract (see Chapter 15).

Scattered among the pyramidal cells of layer V are a number of *granule cells*, some with axons that ascend to the more superficial layers. Within layer V and near the border between layers V and VI is a dense band of myelinated fibers that form a horizontal plexus, the *inner band of Baillarger*. This band contains collaterals from the axons of cortical association and callosal fibers, en route to their principal site of termination, layers II and III, and horizontal axon collaterals from layer V pyramidal cells (see Fig. 21–7).

Layer VI, the *multiform* or *fusiform layer*, contains a large number of *fusiform cells*. Each of these spindle-shaped cells have the long axis of the cell body at a right angle to the surface of the cortex. The fusiform cells, ranging from very small to large, all have an apical dendrite that arises from the end of the cell pointed toward the cortical surface. The apical dendrites of fusiform cells extend toward the surface of the cortex, with those from larger cells reaching the dense horizontal plexus of layer I. Those from the smallest fusiform cells remain within layer VI. In addition to the fusiform cells, layer VI contains a mixture of medium-sized *pyramidal cells* and a large variety of *granule cells*. The axons of some *Golgi type I granule cells* enter the cortical white matter, forming short cortical association fibers, usually terminating in cortical areas within a few centimeters of their origin. The *fusiform cells* and *pyramidal cells* of layer VI are the principal sources of *corticothalamic fibers* and contribute to the intrahemispheric *cortical association fibers* (see Fig. 21–7).

Immediately deep to layer VI is the *cortical white matter*. This central core of white matter contains the axons of all cortical afferent and cortical efferent fibers, including the cortical association fibers, both callosal and intrahemispheric.

FIBER PATTERNS AND CORTICAL AFFERENTS AND EFFERENTS

Within the gray matter of the cerebral cortex, nerve fibers form two distinct patterns. The first is a pattern of delicate *radial bundles*, small clusters of nerve fibers at right angles to the cortical surface. These small radial bundles, largest in diameter in the deepest layers and tapering toward the surface, represent small clusters of

axons entering and leaving the cortex, the cortical afferents and efferents. The other pattern is one of *horizontal bands*, bundles of nerve fibers parallel to the cortical surface, containing terminal branches of cortical afferent axons; axon collaterals; and, in some cases, horizontally spreading dendritic trees. Although horizontally running fibers are in nearly every layer, the three most prominent horizontal bands are the *horizontal plexus* of layer I, the *outer band of Baillarger* in layer IV, and the *inner band of Baillarger* in layer V (see Fig. 21–7).

The *thalamocortical projections* from *specific thalamic nuclei* terminate principally in layer IV of the primary sensory cortical areas. In the motor cortex ,where layer IV is poorly developed, these projections terminate principally in layer III. In other areas, these projections terminate in both layers III and IV, with most terminating in IV. The *thalamocortical projections* from the *nonspecific, intralaminar, and midline thalamic nuclei*, however, terminate principally in layer I. All thalamocortical projections have collaterals to layers V and VI. Medium-size pyramidal and fusiform cells in layer VI give rise to most of the reciprocal *corticothalamic projections* (see Fig. 21–7).

With the exception of the corticothalamic fibers, most *corticofugal fibers* arise from layer V. These corticofugal fibers include *corticospinal, corticobulbar, corticopontine, corticotectal, corticorubral, corticoreticular, corticohypothalamic,* and *corticostriate* projections (see Fig. 21–7).

The two varieties of *cortical association fiber* are *callosal* and *intrahemispheric*. The *callosal association fibers* arise principally from the larger pyramidal cells deep in layer III, with some contributions from neurons in layer VI, and project to the corresponding point in the opposite hemisphere via the corpus callosum. These association fibers end in all layers of the cortex, with the axonal branches forming a columnar-shaped terminal arbor 200 to 300 μm in diameter. The greatest accumulation of these callosal association terminals is in layers III and IV and the least in layers V and VI. *Intrahemispheric association fibers*, in comparison, arise from the smaller pyramidal cells of the more superficial part of layer III, with some contributions from layers II, IV, and VI. These association fibers terminate principally in layer III, with most contributing collateral terminals to layers IV and VI (see Fig. 21–7).

A final category of cortical afferents is the *extrathalamic cortical modulatory systems*. Fibers forming these systems arise from small groups of neurons situated in the brain stem or basal forebrain. Their axons project directly to the cerebral cortex. Most of these ascending fibers arch over the surface of the cortex, branching profusely and terminating in nearly all of the layers of the cortex. There are, however, differences in the specific termination patterns between these six modulatory systems (see subsequent discussion).

The *horizontal plexus* is a network of terminal dendritic trees and axons in layer I, and it contains few myelinated fibers. Contributing to the horizontal plexus are the dendritic trees of the horizontal and granule cells, intrinsic to the layer, and the terminal branches of the apical dendrites of pyramidal and fusiform cells, located in the deeper layers. Axonal contributions include branches from nonspecific thalamocortical fibers and projections from extrathalamic cortical modulatory systems (see Fig. 21–7).

The *outer band of Baillarger* is a horizontal plexus of myelinated nerve fibers, most prominent in layer IV of primary sensory cortical areas. Most of these fibers represent specific thalamocortical projections. The *inner band of Baillarger* is a dense horizontal band of myelinated nerve fibers in layer V, near the border between layers V and VI. This band, less prominent than the outer band of Baillarger, contains axon collaterals from cortical association fibers as well as horizontal collaterals of the axons of layer V pyramidal cells (see Fig. 21–7).

The Cortex as a Mosaic

BASIC TYPES OF CORTEX

The six layers are present in all areas of the neocortex. However, marked variations occur in the cellular composition, the total cortical thickness, and the relative thickness of the different layers. Variations in these features are the bases for defining five basic types of cortex: *agranular-pyramidal, granular-pyramidal, granular-parietal, polar,* and *granular* (see Fig. 21–8).

In the *agranular-pyramidal type*, or simply the *agranular cortex*, a predominance of *pyramidal cells* occurs in nearly every layer with a corresponding paucity of granule cells. Both outer and inner pyramidal cell layers (layers III and V) are well developed and thick. The inner granule cell layer, layer IV, is nearly absent. These cortical areas are among the thickest in the cerebral hemisphere and are typified by the *primary motor area*, Brodmann's area 4 (see Fig. 21–8).

The *granular-pyramidal type* (*frontal type*) of cortex has six well-differentiated layers, has many large pyramidal cells in layers III and V, and has a very prominent inner granular layer, layer IV. The *frontal lobe* (rostral to area 4) and portions of the *superior parietal area* (posterior to the somatosensory area) are examples of the granular-pyramidal type (see Fig. 21–8).

The *granular-parietal type* of cortex also has six well-differentiated layers. The pyramidal cells, however, are small to medium in size. An abundance of granule cells occurs in all layers. The *inferior parietal lobe* and the *superior temporal gyrus* are typical examples of granular-parietal cortex (see Fig. 21–8).

The *polar type* of cortex, although having six distinct layers, is one of the thinnest. This cortical type is rich in granule cells but poor in pyramidal cells. Much of the cortex making up the *prefrontal* and *occipital poles*, excluding area 17, is polar-type cortex. This includes the basal and medial frontal gyri and many areas of the occipital lobe, including secondary visual areas (areas 18 and 19) but excluding area 17 (see Fig. 21–8).

In the *granular type* of cortex, *granule cells* predominate to the near exclusion of the pyramidal cells. Both the outer and inner granule cell layers (layers II and IV) are thick, with layer IV highly differentiated. In some areas, such as the primary visual cortex, as many as four sublaminae are identifiable (see Chapter 11). The inner and outer pyramidal cell layers (layers III and V) are nearly absent from these very thin cortical areas. The *primary sensory areas* (V-1, S-I, and A-1, visual, somatosensory, and auditory, respectively) are examples of the granular type of cortex (see Fig. 21–8).

The *granular* and *agranular cortical areas* represent two extremes of neocortical differentiation. Both are highly specialized for their particular function. *Motor cortical areas* typify the *agranular cortex* or are variations of the same basic pattern. These areas are a major source of descending corticobulbar and corticospinal systems and have important connections with the basal ganglia and the cerebellum via corticostriate and corticopontine projections. Accordingly, these areas have well-developed efferent layers, the inner and outer pyramidal layers (layers III and V). *Primary sensory areas* typify the *granular cortex*. These areas receive primary sensory information relayed from the specific sensory relay nuclei of the dorsal thalamus. Thus, the inner granular layer, the cortical "receiving station," is the most highly differentiated and the most prominent of the cortical layers. The specializations of granular and agranular cortex are such that often it is difficult to differentiate all six layers; hence, these cortical areas, representing two extremes, are known as *heterotypic cortex*. All six layers are more clearly demarcated in the remainder of the neocortex, and these cortical areas are known as *homotypic cortex*.

CYTOARCHITECTURAL MOSAIC

Within the five general types of neocortex, many smaller subtypes exist with very characteristic anatomical, physiological, and functional properties. Within these subtypes or areas, similarities exist both in the cytoarchitecture and in the physiological response properties of the neurons. In addition, similarities are found in the extrinsic and intrinsic neuronal connections. As we learn more about the relationships between the structure and the physiology of specific areas, we can assign unique functions to each area and specific roles for many of these areas in information processing and in overall behavior patterns.

The cytoarchitectural differences between areas of the cerebral cortex have been the bases for many cortical "maps." By utilizing subtle differences in the relative size and neuronal composition of the layers of the cortex, *the human cerebral cortex can be defined as a mosaic of cytoarchitecturally distinct areas.* The definitions and criteria for differentiating areas have varied with the investigator. Some of the maps divide the cerebral hemisphere into as many as 200 definable regions or areas. The most widely used map when referring to specific areas of the cortex, however, is the map of Brodmann (see Fig. 21–3), devised in 1909.

Although Brodmann's map is over 80 years old, it is still quite useful in defining specific areas. These areas can be related to specific functions. Brodmann, employing only cytoarchitectural criteria, divided the cortex into over 50 areas. These areas, referred to by number, are consistent in their relative location from brain to brain. In addition, since their initial description, many of these areas correlate well with specific cortical functions, e.g., area 4 (primary motor); areas 3, 1, and 2 (primary somatosensory); area 17 (primary visual); and area 6 (supplementary motor area and premotor cortex). Many areas remain a mystery with regard to specific functions; however, it is likely that investigators have not yet asked the appropriate questions. Brod-

mann's map may not be the ideal map of the cortex, but it is still the most widely used when referring to specific areas of the cortex.

FETAL DEVELOPMENT AND ESTABLISHMENT OF MOSAIC PATTERN

The initial establishment of the mosaic pattern of cortical areas takes place in early development. The germinal layer, immediately bordering on the ventricle, establishes very early in development, a two-dimensional blueprint for the mosaic of cortical areas in the adult. The early neuroblasts are the precursor cells for a series of radially oriented ontogenetic columns of differentiating neuroblasts that eventually form the neurons of layers I through VI of that column. The columnar arrangement of the neurons, combined with a radial orientation of the afferent and efferent bundles of fibers, gives the cortex a columnar pattern of organization, a pattern that is more apparent in some cortical areas than in others. The ultimate size of a particular cytoarchitecturally distinct area depends on the number of proliferative units and, hence, on the number of ontogenetic columns contributing to the area.

Although the genetic blueprint for the mosaic is established early, the numbers of neurons and the final patterns of cells in any particular area are determined by extrinsic factors, such as the afferent input and the establishment of viable efferent projections. The patterns of both neuronal excitation and inhibition during development play important roles in this differentiation process. In addition, increasing evidence exists that these patterns of excitation and inhibition are essential for the maintenance of the differentiated state. If these patterns vary—even in the adult—certain "plastic" changes in the organization occur. The functional properties of neurons and the characteristics of small cortical areas are in a dynamic state and may change with alterations in the input-output systems.

Cortical Information Processing

CORTICAL CIRCUITRY

Although tremendous advances have been made in our understanding of cortical interconnections, it is premature to make generalizations about the common features of cortical columnar organization. Whether the more general features are common to all cortical areas also is unknown. It is, however, clear that the cerebral cortex is a mosaic of columnar units, each with a unique combination of afferent and efferent connections. The manner in which individual columns process information and interact with adjacent columns or other cortical areas is not clear.

The many cytoarchitecturally different areas also vary in neuronal composition; hence, the circuitry within columns from one area must be different from that in another area. The degree of similarity in the detailed circuitry among columns in the same area, the primary motor cortex for example, is largely unknown. There probably are features in common in the processing of information from one area to the next. However, because of the anatomical differences between areas, each column is a unique "piece" in the cortical mosaic.

Certain features of the afferent and efferent connections are common to nearly all of the cortical columns. All maintain reciprocal connections with the dorsal thalamus, and the cortical association fibers for all areas originate and terminate in similar cortical laminae. The specific bits of information entering a column, however, are unique to that column.

The circuitry and functional properties of the neurons in columns, or cortical modular units, are not static. The afferent input, both cortical and subcortical, and the establishment of functional efferent connections are the factors that initially determine the characteristics of these areal units. These functional connections are also essential for the maintenance of the unit's physiological characteristics. If the properties of these connections change, even in the adult, so will the physiological characteristics of the unit. Thus, small cortical areas or modules are in a dynamic state and retain their ability to change as the nature of their connections change.

For some systems, e.g., vision, a considerable amount of data is available about information processing at the cortical level. The general applicability of these features to other systems, however, remains uncertain. The known general features of cortical information processing are discussed in the appropriate chapter for that system (see Chapters, 10, 11, 12, 13, and 15).

CORTICAL NEUROCHEMISTRY

Of the cortical neurons, the majority are either *glutaminergic* or *GABAergic*. All of the efferent neurons, both those projecting to other cortical areas and those projecting to subcortical parts of the CNS, are excitatory and utilize glutamate as the neurotransmitter. Inhibitory cortical neurons are an important part of the circuitry in all areas of the cortex. Just as inhibitory signals are essential for the transmission of crisp signals in ascending afferent pathways, inhibitory signals are essential for the processing of information at the level of the cortex. These cortical inhibitory signals are generated by *GABAergic interneurons*. Nearly 30% of all cortical interneurons use gamma-aminobutyric acid (GABA) as the primary neurotransmitter.

This population of inhibitory interneurons or granule cells represents a very heterogenous population of morphological cell types. About 20% of these GABAergic interneurons have a peptide co-transmitter, adding a further dimension of chemical heterogeneity to the complexity of the cortical circuitry.

Neuropeptides are an abundant class of neurotransmitters in the cerebral cortex. Most of the *interneurons* in the cortex are *peptidergic*. The GABAergic interneurons contain some of these neuropeptides as co-transmitters. In other interneurons, the peptides appear to be the only chemical neurotransmitters. Other peptides found in the cortex are co-transmitters at the nerve terminals of monoaminergic neurons that project directly from the brain stem to the cortex. In all, over 60 different peptides reside in the interneurons and nerve terminals of the cerebral cortex. Often, several neuroactive peptides localize within the same cortical interneuron and are co-transmitters. The most common peptides with a neurotransmitter role in the cortex include *vasoactive intestinal peptide* (*VIP*), *cholecystokinin* (*CCK*), *corticotropin-releasing hormone* (*CRH*), *substance P* (*SubP*), and *somatostatin* (*SOM*), along with many opioid peptides (*dynorphins* and *enkephalins*).

Many neurotransmitters act at the level of the cerebral cortex but are within the nerve terminals of the neurons that project to the cortex from the brain stem and basal forebrain. Many of these are neurons belonging to the extrathalamic cortical modulatory systems (see subsequent discussion). These include the neurotransmitters *acetylcholine*, *norepinephrine*, *serotonin*, *dopamine*, and *histamine*. No neurons intrinsic to the cerebral cortex appear to use these neurochemical transmitters.

RAPID SIGNALING

Glutamate and GABA are the primary neurotransmitters for most of the neurons intrinsic to the cerebral cortex. Both transmitters have cortical receptors that respond rapidly. All three glutamate receptors (NMDA, QA, and KA) and the $GABA_A$ receptor are ligand-gated ion channels (see Chapter 5). These receptors have response latencies measured in microseconds. Their durations of response range from 1 to 2 msec. These are the only ligand-gated ion channel receptors in the cerebral cortex, limiting all of the rapid cortical signaling to glutamate and GABA. The other neurotransmitters found in the cerebral cortex utilize second-messenger coupled receptors.

SLOW RESPONSES AND MODULATORS

Except for the "fast" synapses containing the glutamate and $GABA_A$ receptors, the remaining neurotransmitter receptors in the cerebral cortex are coupled to second-messenger systems. Some of these systems activate or inhibit adenyl cyclase, others activate phospholipase C with the stimulation of the phosphatidylinositol cascade (see Chapter 5).

Response latencies for the second-messenger coupled systems range from 100 to 250 msec. The duration of the response can range from a few milliseconds to minutes to hours or even days. Those receptors with the shortest latency and with the shortest duration of response usually are coupled to the activation of an ion channel by a protein kinase–catalyzed phosphorylation reaction. The activation of the ion channel leads to the generation of either an excitatory postsynaptic potential (EPSP) or an inhibitory postsynaptic potential (IPSP). The duration of the channel's activation is dependent on the intracellular activity of protein phosphatases, enzymes that reverse the phosphorylation reaction.

Other postsynaptic responses coupled to second-messenger systems may be of much longer duration. These can range from a local alteration of membrane properties to the activation of gene transcription. These types of responses are more prolonged and may be sustained for hours or even days by the postsynaptic neuron. Such changes may not alter the membrane potential— there is no demonstrable EPSP or IPSP—but they may alter the physiological properties of the postsynaptic neuron. Thus, the membrane potential of the postsynaptic neuron may not be changed, but its sensitivity to another neurotransmitter may have increased or decreased.

At the molecular level, the physiological properties of neurons are very plastic. Stimulated by synaptic activity, second-messenger systems in the postsynaptic neuron are continually "fine tuning" or *modulating* the response properties of the cell, adapting the cortical neuron to the conditions of the moment. Ion channels and chemical receptors undergo frequent modification, rendering them either more or less sensitive in accord with the physiological state of the neuron.

These same second-messenger systems also play an active role in the regulation of gene expression. Neurotransmitter-activated second-messenger systems can initiate or enhance the transcription of mRNAs for the synthesis of specific receptors, enzymes, and ion channels and other molecules involved in neuronal communication. This role is the most complex dimension of neuronal communication, but one that may be of importance in the regulation of complex cortical processes, such as learning and memory.

Modulation of Cortical Activity by Extrathalamic Neurons

Stimulation of the brain stem's reticular formation changes the slow wave, cortical EEG pattern to one of low-voltage, fast waves. In early studies, these changes were believed to reflect a cortical *arousal* or *activating function*. Little, however, was known about the neurons or circuits involved.

Later, neurons from the brain stem reticular formation were observed projecting directly to the cerebral cortex without first synapsing in the dorsal thalamus. Also, as noted in Chapter 20, "nonspecific" thalamic nuclei receive extensive input from the brain stem reticular formation. The relay neurons in these nuclei project to both the cerebral cortex and to the striatum. Collectively, the two reticular formation projection systems, reticulothalamocortical and reticulocortical, became known as the *reticular activating system*.

At least six neurochemically distinct, extrathalamic projection systems reach the cerebral cortex monosynaptically, *without* a relay in the dorsal thalamus. Of these, three arise from the brain stem reticular formation, two from the hypothalamus, and one from the basal forebrain. In addition, the pattern of cortical projections and terminations for all six of these systems is tangential and highly divergent, with axons of individual neurons terminating in broad cortical areas. This pattern contrasts with the precise topography maintained by the radial/columnar pattern of the specific thalamocortical projections. All six of these extrathalamic projection systems appear to modulate cortical activity. Accordingly, the phrase *extrathalamic cortical modulatory systems* is a better and more accurate description of these systems than the more restrictive phrase "reticular activating system."

GENERAL FEATURES OF EXTRATHALAMIC CORTICAL MODULATORY SYSTEMS

Each of the six systems arises from a small nucleus or region of the brain stem or forebrain, and the neurons of each system project directly to the cerebral cortex. The neurons within each system employ the same principal neurochemical transmitter. As the systems project directly to the cerebral cortex, the axons branch profusely and the systems become highly divergent. The terminal boutons of these ascending axons appear to form traditional synaptic-like contacts with the dendrites of target neurons in the cortex. This finding is best documented for the noradrenergic, serotoninergic, and cholinergic systems.

These nuclei or clusters of chemically defined neurons do not always correspond to the more traditional, neuroanatomically defined, brain stem nuclei (see Chapter 7). As a result, there is an alternative nomenclature for these chemically defined groups of neurons: A1, A2, . . . A15 refer to specific clusters of noradrenergic or dopaminergic neurons; B1, B2, . . . B8, to serotoninergic groups; and Ch1, Ch2, . . . Ch6, to cholinergic groups. Where possible, this text utilizes both the traditional neuroanatomical nomenclature and the alternative neurochemical designation.

One system, arising principally from the *nucleus basalis* of the basal forebrain, uses *acetylcholine (ACh)*; a second, from the *locus ceruleus* of the pontine reticular formation, uses *norepinephrine (NE)*; a third, from the *midbrain raphe nuclei*, uses *serotonin (5-HT)*; a fourth, from the *ventral midbrain*, uses *dopamine (DA)*; and the two arising from *hypothalamic nuclei* use *histamine* and *GABA*, respectively as a primary neurotransmitter. Some evidence exists that several of these cortical projections have one or more peptides as co-transmitters. This information, although not unexpected, is not fully documented (Figs. 21–9 and 21–10). The presence of one or more co-transmitters in projection neurons from a particular nucleus could add a dimension of chemical selectivity to an otherwise diffuse-appearing system.

Certain *similarities* exist in the cortical projections: all six are highly divergent with a single neuron projecting to large, functionally unrelated, areas of the cortex; branches of these projection neurons terminate in nearly all of the cortical laminae; and all appear to have modulatory influences on the activity of neurons in the cerebral cortex.

Noradrenergic System

The noradrenergic system is the best defined of the six modulatory systems. In the medulla and pons of the human brain stem, six nuclear groups

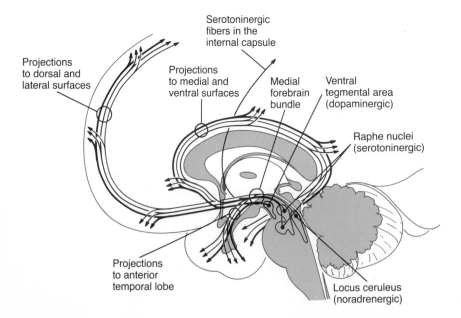

FIGURE 21–9

Three extrathalamic cortical modulatory systems are illustrated: the noradrenergic projections from the locus ceruleus, the serotoninergic projections from the raphe nuclei, and the dopaminergic projections from the ventral tegmental area. See text for details.

FIGURE 21-10

Three extrathalamic cortical modulatory systems are illustrated: the cholinergic projections from the nucleus basalis and both the histaminergic and GABAergic projections from the posterior hypothalamus. See text for details.

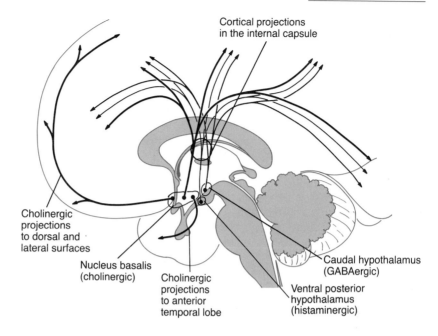

Cortical projections in the internal capsule

Cholinergic projections to dorsal and lateral surfaces

Nucleus basalis (cholinergic)

Cholinergic projections to anterior temporal lobe

Caudal hypothalamus (GABAergic)

Ventral posterior hypothalamus (histaminergic)

contain noradrenergic neurons. Of these, the largest complex is the *noradrenergic locus ceruleus complex*, containing noradrenergic cell groups *A4* and *A6*. Although all of the direct noradrenergic projections to the neocortex arise from the locus ceruleus, this nucleus also projects to nearly every level of the neuraxis, from the olfactory bulb to the spinal cord.

In the human brain stem, approximately 13,000 noradrenergic neurons of the locus ceruleus send axons to each cerebral hemisphere. Most arise from the ipsilateral nuclear complex with a small contribution from the contralateral nucleus. These projections ascend through the central portion of the *midbrain tegmentum* and, at the level of the diencephalon, join other fibers in the *medial forebrain bundle*. Besides innervating the entire cortex (neocortex, paleocortex, and archicortex), these noradrenergic fibers innervate nearly every nuclear group of the basal forebrain area, including all of the olfactory structures.

After reaching the diencephalon, the cortical projections from the locus ceruleus follow one of three pathways (see Fig. 21-9). One population of fibers continues rostrally with the medial forebrain bundle into the frontal pole of the hemisphere. These fibers spread out, arching in a rostrocaudal direction to cover the entire frontal, dorsal, and lateral aspects of the neocortex. A second group of fibers also arches in a caudal direction but above the corpus callosum. These fibers spread out to innervate the more medial and ventral surfaces of the hemisphere, including the hippocampal formation. A third group of

noradrenergic fibers reaches the temporal lobe, including the entorhinal cortex, in the accompaniment of fibers destined for the amygdaloid complex (see Fig. 21-9).

Serotoninergic System

Of the six cortical modulatory systems, the *serotoninergic system* contains the most fibers and provides the densest innervation to the cortex. Most of the serotoninergic neurons of the human brain are in an extensive complex of brain stem nuclei situated near the midline of the medulla, pons and midbrain, the *raphe nuclei*. Of these, only the *dorsal raphe nucleus, B7*, of the midbrain and pons and the *median raphe nucleus, B6* and *B8*, of the pons contribute to the cortical projection system (see Fig. 21-9). Like the noradrenergic system, many serotoninergic neurons in these nuclei project to nearly every level of the CNS. In addition, many serotoninergic neurons contain one or more peptide co-transmitters. These have been best defined for the serotoninergic projections to the spinal cord (see Chapter 5). However, it is likely that neurons in the cortical projection system also contain one or more different peptide co-transmitters.

The serotoninergic projections ascend through the central portion of the midbrain tegmentum and, at the level of the diencephalon, join noradrenergic and other fibers in the *medial forebrain bundle*. Besides innervating the entire cortex (neocortex, paleocortex, and archicortex), this *ventral ascending serotoninergic pathway* innervates nuclear groups in the thalamus, hypothalamus, basal ganglia, and basal forebrain area, including olfactory structures. A smaller group of serotoninergic fibers, principally from neurons in the dorsal raphe nucleus, forms the *dorsal ascending serotoninergic pathway*. These fibers ascend immediately ventral to the cerebral aqueduct, beneath the periaqueductal gray, in the *dorsal longitudinal fasciculus of Schütz*. After ascending to the level of the hypothalamus, the fibers join those of the dorsal pathway in the medial forebrain bundle.

At the level of the diencephalon, the cortical projections of the serotoninergic system follow a path similar to that of the noradrenergic system (see Fig. 21–9). One population of fibers ascends rostrally into the frontal pole of the hemisphere where they arch in a rostrocaudal direction to cover the entire frontal, dorsal, and lateral aspects of the neocortex. Other fibers reach cortical areas via the internal capsule; still others arch over the corpus callosum to innervate the medial and ventral surfaces of the hemisphere, including the hippocampal formation. Additional projections reach the temporal lobe, including the entorhinal cortex, in the accompaniment of fibers destined for the amygdaloid complex (see Fig. 21–9).

The pattern of cortical termination of the serotoninergic projections is one of greater total density than that of the noradrenergic system. Although all areas and laminae of the cortex receive serotonergic projections, the pattern, like that of the noradrenergic system, is not uniform throughout the primate cortex. In general, the pattern of serotonergic terminals complements that of the noradrenergic system. Areas and laminae with the greatest density of noradrenergic terminals receive few serotonergic terminals. Conversely, the areas and laminae with the highest concentrations of serotoninergic terminals contain few noradrenergic terminals.

Dopaminergic System

The principal *dopaminergic neurons* associated with cortical modulation reside in the midbrain. The largest of these dopaminergic nuclei is the *pars compacta* of the *substantia nigra* (*SNc*) or *A9*. The other two mesencephalic nuclei containing dopaminergic nuclei are the more caudolateral *retrorubral nucleus* (*A8*) and the more rostromedial *ventral tegmental area* (*A10*) (see Fig. 21–9). Although identifiable as three separate nuclei, many investigators consider all three nuclei to be part of a single complex. These mid-

brain dopaminergic nuclei contain neurons that project to the telencephalon. Collectively, they form the *mesotelencephalic dopaminergic system*. Within this large projection system are three components: *mesostriatal*, *mesolimbic*, and *mesocortical*.

The *mesostriatal component*, better known as the *dopaminergic nigrostriatal system*, functions to reinforce cortically initiated motor activity (see Chapter 16). The *mesolimbic component* ascends in the medial forebrain bundle and distributes to many structures in the limbic system, principally in the telencephalon (see Chapter 22). The *mesocortical component* was the last of the three components described and includes projections to all areas of the *neocortex*.

Some parts of the neocortex belong to the "functionally defined" limbic system. Therefore, the terms mesolimbic and mesocortical often describe the same projections—the dopaminergic, limbic system projections to the cingulate gyrus or the areas of the prefrontal cortex. In this text, when the main subject is the neocortex, these projections are called *mesocortical*. When the limbic system is discussed, these same projections are termed *mesolimbic*. All these fibers reach the target cortical areas by way of the *medial forebrain bundle* and travel to their final cortical destinations in the company of the noradrenergic and serotoninergic fibers (see Fig. 21–9).

Dopaminergic projections to the neocortex are not uniform. The primary visual, auditory, and somatosensory cortical areas receive the fewest mesencephalic dopaminergic projections. Most of their terminals concentrate in the outer layers, principally layer I. Secondary and tertiary sensory areas, in comparison, receive dense projections with terminals in all layers, except layer IV. Projections to prefrontal cortical areas as well as temporal and parietal association areas are dense as well. The heaviest projections, however, are to the motor cortical areas. In these areas, the distribution of terminals is uniform, including dense projections to layer IV.

Cholinergic System

The basal forebrain contains four populations of cholinergic neurons with projections to the cerebral cortex (see Fig. 21–10). The principal source of cholinergic fibers to the neocortex is the large *nucleus basalis of Meynert* (*Ch4*). More than 90% of the neurons in this nucleus are cholinergic. These neurons project to all areas of the *cerebral cortex*, principally through the internal capsule.

Some also reach the temporal lobe, including the entorhinal cortex, in the accompaniment of noradrenergic and other fibers destined for the amygdaloid complex (see Fig. 21–10). The nucleus basalis in the human brain occupies most of the substantia innominata and lies immediately ventral to the lentiform nuclei.

About 10% of the neurons of the *medial septal nucleus* are cholinergic (*Ch1*). These send axons to the *hippocampal formation* of the temporal lobe by way of the *fornix*. The vertical and horizontal limbs of the *nucleus of the diagonal band of Broca* (*Ch2* and *Ch3*) project also to the hippocampal formation and other limbic structures. Cholinergic neurons account for about 70% of the neurons in the vertical limb of this nucleus but only 1% of the neurons in the horizontal limb (see Fig. 21–10).

In Alzheimer's disease and in senile dementia of the Alzheimer's type, a dramatic and selective loss of the cholinergic neurons in the nucleus basalis of Meynert occurs. A similar loss occurs in some forms of Parkinson's disease that are accompanied by dementia. However, in Huntington's chorea, another degenerative disorder accompanied by dementia, no significant loss of neurons in the nucleus basalis of Meynert is noted. Thus, in Alzheimer's disease, the loss of cholinergic neurons may be a secondary change and not the primary cause of dementia. An alternative explanation is that dementia can result from the selective loss of more than one population of neurons projecting to or residing in the cerebral cortex. In Alzheimer's disease and in Huntington's chorea, different populations of neurons with different neurochemical properties are lost, but the result is the same.

Histaminergic and GABAergic Systems

Of the six extrathalamic cortical modulatory systems, the *histaminergic* and *GABAergic* systems are the least well documented. Preliminary studies show that both systems arise from neurons in the posterior hypothalamus and both have diffuse projections to the cerebral cortex (see Fig. 21–10). Both systems also appear to have a modulatory influence on cortical activity.

The principal population of *histaminergic neurons* lies in the *ventral posterior hypothalamus*, encompassing portions of the arcuate, dorsomedial, ventromedial, and posterior nuclei. This small group of neurons sends fibers to nearly every region of the CNS, including extensive projections to the cerebral cortex. The cortical projections appear to contain one or more cotransmitters, including such neurotransmitters as 5-HT, GABA, adenosine, and several neuropeptides.

A small population of large *GABAergic neurons* in the *caudal hypothalamus* is located immediately rostral to the mammillary nuclei. These GABAergic neurons project diffusely to the entire cerebral cortex. Details regarding these projections are not yet clear, hampered in part by the large number of intrinsic cortical neurons that are GABAergic. The postsynaptic receptors at most of these GABAergic synapses are the second-messenger coupled $GABA_B$ receptor (see Chapter 5).

MODULATORY ACTIVITY

These extrathalamic cortical modulatory systems do not appear to send specific signals to the cerebral cortex. Instead, their role is that of a *modulator of cortical activity*. The physiological properties of these ascending signals are best understood for the noradrenergic and serotoninergic systems. Firing of *noradrenergic neurons* in the locus ceruleus, for example, *enhances the selectivity and magnitude of the response of cortical neurons to primary afferent information*. Instead of producing a postsynaptic potential, these synapses alter the membrane properties of the postsynaptic cortical neuron. The cortical neuron becomes more responsive to the incoming primary afferent signals. This response occurs in two ways: first, there is an increase in the sensitivity of the cortical neuron to the afferent signal, and second, there is a decrease in the rate of spontaneous firing of the cortical neuron. Not only does the noradrenergic signal render the cortical neuron more receptive or sensitive, but it reduces the background, thus increasing the "signal-to-noise" ratio. Because this system enhances the response of target cells, these noradrenergic projection neurons are called *enablers*. The firing pattern of the locus ceruleus neurons becomes higher during alerting and arousing situations, rendering the cortex more responsive to afferent information under those circumstances.

The projections of all six of the extrathalamic cortical modulating systems are divergent, with individual neurons projecting to a broad, seemingly unspecific area of the cortex. Within the cortex, small, radially orientated, peptidergic cortical interneurons interact synergistically with this global monoaminergic innervation and receive afferent signals. Thus, the subthreshold noradrenergic stimulation of the cortical target neurons in combination with stimulation of peptidergic interneurons that also receive primary afferent signals may provide a mechanism for a localized intensification of the primary afferent signals.

Noradrenergic projections appear to interact selectively with cortical interneurons containing *vasoactive intestinal peptide* (*VIP*), whereas cortical interneurons with *somatostatin* appear to have a similar synergistic role in the *cholinergic innervation* of the cortex. Currently, specific interneurons have not been identified for the other four systems. The combination of (1) the global subthreshold modulation of target pyramidal cells by the extrathalamic projection neurons and (2) the synergistic innervation of local radially oriented peptidergic interneurons may add the requisite dimension of specificity to an otherwise diffuse system.

The *serotoninergic innervation* of the cortex is complementary to the noradrenergic system in many ways. Although the two systems appear complementary in fiber distribution and density of terminals, no direct evidence exists that their effects are opposite. *Raphe neurons exhibit a pattern of activity that more directly correlates with the general behavioral state, relating more to the sleep-wake cycle. The noradrenergic system correlates more strongly with the phasic activity associated with alerting and attentiveness.*

Much less is known about the functional correlates of the other extrathalamic cortical modulatory systems. Some evidence exists that the *dopaminergic system* functions in response to behavior involving the orientation and the initiation of movement; the *cholinergic system* functions in response to behavior involving motivation and, perhaps, emotions. How this evidence is related to the strong clinical correlation between the loss of cholinergic neurons from the nucleus basalis and senile dementia is unknown.

None of these projection systems are part of the mainstream in either the sensory or motor pathways. Their nuclei do, however, receive collateral input from both major ascending and descending pathways. Exactly how the collateral input affects the level of cortical excitation is unknown.

Specialized Cortical Areas

Much of what is known about the localization of function in the cerebral cortex comes from clinical studies of patients with focal damage to spe-

cific cortical areas. Other information comes from the direct stimulation of and recording from specific cortical areas of the human brain. These electrophysiological studies are often a necessary component of corrective neurosurgical procedures.

Newer, noninvasive procedures, such as positron emission tomography (PET) scanning, are beginning to provide more insight into regional cortical activity under a variety of pharmacological and behavioral situations. Our ability to localize specific functions and specific steps in the processing of information will increase as these techniques improve. These procedures offer the potential of localizing the sequential activation of specific loci within the CNS during the processes of learning and storing information.

Memory is a very complex process and involves many areas in both the limbic lobe and the neocortex. Because of the extensive involvement of the limbic lobe, memory is discussed in Chapter 22.

PRIMARY SENSORY AREAS

The *primary sensory areas* of the cortex are those highly granular cortical areas that receive afferent projections from specific thalamic sensory relay nuclei. These areas are receiving stations for primary information. Here, it is sorted and relayed to the appropriate secondary sensory areas for processing. The best documentation of the sorting of primary sensory information and its subsequent processing through secondary sensory areas is for the visual system. These basic principles of sensory information sorting and processing are probably similar for other sensory systems. Chapter 11 contains a detailed account of visual information processing at the cortical level.

The primary sensory area for the somatosensory system is *S-I*, the postcentral gyrus, or Brodmann's *areas 3, 1*, and *2*. The primary receiving station for visual information is *V-1*, the striate cortex, or Brodmann's *area 17*. The auditory system uses *A-1*, Brodmann's *areas 41* and *42*, as its primary area. The one for taste is found in Brodmann's *area 43* (see Fig. 21–3). These primary sensory areas are reviewed in detail in Chapters 10, 11, 12, and 13. In general, primary sensory areas contain precise maps of the sensory information. In S-I, this is a somatotopic map of the contralateral body; in V-1, it is a visuotopic map of the contralateral visual hemifield; and in A-1, it is a tonotopic map.

SECONDARY SENSORY AREAS

Secondary sensory areas of the cortex usually surround or are adjacent to the primary sensory area. Most secondary areas do not receive primary sensory projections from the thalamus but receive presorted sensory information via dense reciprocal connections with the appropriate primary area. Many secondary areas retain some of the "map-like" properties of the primary sensory areas. Additionally, they process specific dimensions or qualities of the information and often integrate this information with that from other modalities or systems.

With the visual system as an example, immediately adjacent to the primary visual cortex (*area 17*) are the secondary visual areas, the prestriate visual areas, *V-2, V-3,* and *V-4* (Brodmann's *areas 18* and *19*). Completing the secondary visual areas is the *middle temporal visual area (MT)*. MT is anterior to area 19 on the lateral surface of the hemisphere, along the boundary between occipital and temporal lobes and includes part of *area 39* (see Fig. 21–3).

The visual system is a good example of combined hierarchical and parallel information processing. Parallel streams of different bits of visual information project from the retina, to the lateral geniculate nucleus of the thalamus, and then to the primary visual cortex. At the level of area 17, further segregation and sorting of this information occurs before it projects to the secondary cortical areas and, finally, to the tertiary visual areas in the parietal and temporal lobes. Three of these parallel streams of information have been studied in detail and are good examples of the combination of parallel and hierarchical types of information processing. The first stream answers the question of *where it is* and the second stream, *what it is*. The third carries information about color. For details, see Chapter 11.

MOTOR AREAS

At least five cortical areas have a major role in motor function: the primary motor cortex, *M-I* (the precentral gyrus, Brodmann's *area 4*); and four secondary motor areas. The secondary motor areas include (1) the premotor cortex, *PMC* (most of *area 6* on the lateral surface of the hemisphere); (2) the supplementary motor area, *SMA* (the medial and superolateral portion of *area 6*); (3) the frontal eye fields, *FEF* (an area in the posteroinferior region of *area 8*); and (4) the posterior parietal motor area, *PMA* (*areas 5* and

7) (see Fig. 21–3, also see Chapter 15 and Fig. 15–1).

A principal function of *M-I* is the execution of *specific, well-defined motor responses*. Neurons in the *secondary motor areas (SMA)* elicit more *complex motor responses*. Secondary motor areas *program* the more complicated movements and send this information to the primary motor area *and* directly to the brain stem and spinal cord.

Each secondary area is involved in a different dimension of the planning and initiation of motor activity. The major afferents to *SMA* include a substantial input from the basal ganglia. These projections, from the *globus pallidus* and the pars reticulata of the *substantia nigra,* are by way of the anterior division of the *ventral lateral nucleus (VLa)* of the thalamus. In contrast, the major afferents to *PMC* are from cortical association areas and the *cerebellum,* the latter being relayed by the posterior division of the *ventral lateral nucleus (VLp)* of the thalamus. For details about the organization and function of the motor cortical areas, see Chapter 15.

INTERPRETATIVE OR ASSOCIATION AREAS

In the cerebral cortex, those areas that are not strictly motor or sensory (as previously defined) are *cortical association areas*. The human cerebral cortex contains a vast amount of association cortex, much more than that of any other animal. The principal distinguishing feature between the human brain and that of the higher primates is the large quantity of association cortex.

The association cortex, or association areas, provides humans with our *intellectual capacity,* our *ability to reason and plan ahead,* and our *language and communication skills*. Our greater *ingenuity and resourcefulness,* our *individual personalities,* and our *ability to make decisions based on past experiences* are also functions of these association areas.

The measurement and assessment of many of these functions is not as subject to analysis as the measurement of sensory information processing. In addition, a broad spectrum of individual differences exists in the human capacity for many of these functions. Thus, the ability to localize these functions and to understand the information processing associated with these functions is much less precise.

The two cerebral hemispheres are not identical, either anatomically or functionally. The left hemisphere is generally the *dominant hemisphere*.

Certain cortical functions tend to reside in either the dominant or nondominant hemisphere. Language and mathematical skills, for example, are principally a dominant hemisphere function, whereas musical skills are a nondominant hemisphere function. This finding is the basis for the colloquial reference to the analytical person as "left-brained" and the creative person as "right-brained." These functions are *lateralized*, that is, they are principally in one hemisphere or the other. Emphasis in this section is on functions generally shared by both hemispheres. The lateralized cortical functions are discussed in the following section.

Our understanding of most of the following localizations is based on *loss* of function resulting from injury, neurosurgical procedures, or disease. With a deficit in function following damage to a focal area, we *presume* that the area lost is essential for the function lost. Most of these clinical findings are supported by experimental data from studies on primates.

POSTERIOR PARIETAL ASSOCIATION CORTEX

The *posterior parietal association cortex* is that part of the parietal lobe posterior to the somatosensory cortex and immediately rostral to the prestriate visual areas of the occipital cortex and consists of Brodmann's *areas 5, 7, 39,* and *40* (see Fig. 21–3). With damage to this area, the principal deficit is one of *neglect, neglect of the contralateral body and contralateral extrapersonal space.* Motor and most sensory pathways are crossed. The left motor areas in the cortex control movement of the right half of the body. Similarly, left somatosensory cortex receives information from the right half of the body, and the left visual cortex receives information about the right visual hemifield.

This neglect has several dimensions: *sensory, motor, cognitive,* and *attentional.* The degree to which these components are expressed varies from patient to patient and depends on subtle differences in both the amount and specific area of the posterior parietal cortex involved and the duration of recovery time since the initial insult.

Patients with posterior parietal lobe lesions typically ignore or neglect contralateral parts of the body. They groom and dress only the ipsilateral side. In the extreme, a patient in bed may even perceive the opposite half of his or her body as that of another person. The patient also has problems forming mental images of objects palpated with the contralateral hand, *astereognosis.*

Little loss occurs in the capacity to discriminate, tactually or visually. The major deficit is an inability to match the object palpated with the contralateral hand with an identical object noted visually. This is a deficit in the ability to *associate* the tactile image with the visual image rather than a perceptual deficit.

Visual reconstructions from memory show a similar neglect of contralateral extrapersonal space. When the patient is asked to imagine himself or herself in front of his or her home and to describe the scene looking down the street to the left, the patient will describe only the ipsilateral side of the street (ipsilateral relative to the side of the brain lesion). When asked to turn around, mentally, and look in the other direction, the description still will contain only the ipsilateral side of the street; only now, it is the other side of the street. The complete visual memory is intact, but the *ability to assemble the pieces* for the contralateral half of extrapersonal space is lacking. When asked to draw an object, usually only the ipsilateral half of the object is drawn. If the object is a clock, for example, often only the ipsilateral half of a clock face is drawn, often with all 12 numbers on one half of the face.

Ataxia often accompanies posterior parietal lesions, usually with a general absence of volitional movement of the contralateral limbs, except movements such as bipedal locomotion that have a large reflexive component. When patients become aware of an object in the contralateral hemifield of extrapersonal space—after turning the head—they invariably reach for the object with the ipsilateral hand, rather than the contralateral hand, even though the contralateral hand is much closer. Most of the contralateral motor function is intact, although often ataxic. The deficit is principally in the *neglect to use* or *to initiate movement* in the contralateral limbs.

Many accompanying sensory deficits diminish with time, but the sensory neglect remains. The patients have trouble paying *attention* to the contralateral world around them or to the contralateral half of their bodies. This effect is one of being unable to disengage one's attention from the ipsilateral surround or unable to turn one's attention to the contralateral surround. This *attentional neglect is the single most characteristic feature of posterior parietal lobe damage.*

TEMPORAL ASSOCIATION CORTEX

The *temporal association cortical areas* include all of the temporal lobe except the primary auditory area, Brodmann's areas 41 and 42. Based on function, it is convenient to divide the temporal associational cortex into three areas: the *superior*, the *inferior*, and the *anteromedial temporal association areas*. The *superior temporal association area* is essentially Brodmann's *area 22*. The *inferior temporal association area* includes Brodmann's *areas 20, 21*, and *37*. The *anteromedial temporal association area* contains Brodmann's *areas 27, 28, 34, 35, 36*, and *38* (see Fig. 21–3). The anteromedial area contains principally the temporal lobe components of the limbic system (see Chapter 22).

The *superior temporal association area* is crucial in the *understanding of speech and the perception of written language*. These are a function of the dominant hemisphere and detailed in the following discussion of lateralization. In addition to language comprehension, the superior temporal association area has a role in auditory discrimination. Because of the bilateral nature of the auditory representation in the adjacent primary auditory cortex, these deficits are extremely difficult to assess.

Temporal lobe damage also leads to difficulty in the performance of visually cued tasks requiring a high degree of *visual discrimination*. Most of this impairment is due to damage in the *inferior temporal association area*, an area with strong reciprocal connections to the prestriate visual areas, the pulvinar and the posterior parietal lobe. In order for the deficit to be apparent, the task must require a very high level of visual perception. Usually, the patient is unaware of the deficit until specifically tested. More prominent deficits are the *short-term memory losses* following lesions to the inferior temporal area. Although both left and right temporal lobe lesions produce these deficits, the nature of the loss is markedly different. Damage to the *right temporal lobe* produces severe deficits in *short-term visual memory*. If the lesion is in the *left temporal lobe*, the visual loss is not as severe, but a pronounced deficit occurs in *short-term verbal memory*. The partitioning of these deficits reflects the lateralization of the language skills to the left hemisphere. The long-term memory losses that often accompany temporal lobe removal appear to involve the loss of both the inferior and anteromedial temporal association areas (see Chapter 22).

An unusual, but striking deficiency from temporal lobe lesions is a condition known as *prosopagnosia*, or the inability to recognize familiar faces, including one's own reflection in a mirror. The disorder is not due to a loss of visual perception, and the patient still can recognize family and friends from the sounds of their voices.

Prosopagnosia most frequently accompanies *bilateral* lesions of the *inferior temporal lobe*, near the temporal-occipital junction, including Brodmann's *area 37* (see Fig. 21–3).

PREFRONTAL ASSOCIATION CORTEX

The *prefrontal association cortex* contains all of the frontal lobe rostral to the motor areas—in front of Brodmann's area 6. This includes Brodmann's *areas 8, 9, 10, 11, 12, 24, 25, 32, 33, 44, 45, 46*, and *47*. The deficits arising from prefrontal lobe lesions fall into two general categories: (1) *problem-solving deficits* and (2) *emotional deficits*.

The *problem-solving deficits* often are quite subtle. Patients may show no deficits on standard intelligence tests, but deficits are demonstrable when the patients attempt complicated tasks, especially those that require a change in approach or strategy during the task. If only one frontal lobe is involved, the patient may seem to ignore or neglect the contralateral hemifield of extrapersonal space, a deficit that resembles lesions to the posterior parietal lobe. Another factor contributing to the patient's problem-solving deficit is the inability to deal with distractions and to concentrate on a single task. Related to the problem solving deficits is the patient's *inability to make an informed decision*. These patients simply are unable to assemble facts and data about a particular subject and to come to a conclusion based on the facts and data.

The *emotional deficits* are probably the most characteristic of the frontal lobe deficits. Often, the patients display bizarre, socially unacceptable behavior. Their emotional state is very labile and unpredictable. Family and friends often find these emotional and personality changes to be the most upsetting.

Attempts to localize these deficits to specific areas of the prefrontal area suggest that the problem-solving deficits involve the dorsolateral prefrontal area, including Brodmann's area 9. The orbitofrontal region is more directly associated with emotional disturbances. The latter area, when stimulated in the human, leads to strong emotional reactions and to autonomic nervous system responses. Both the orbitofrontal and dorsolateral areas of the prefrontal area have strong efferent projections to areas of the basal forebrain and basal ganglia that are associated with the limbic system and emotions. In addition, the prefrontal area is the only neocortical area known to have direct projections to the hypothalamus. Both areas have strong reciprocal connections with the mediodorsal nucleus of the dorsal thalamus and with other areas of the neocortex. These reciprocal cortical connections for the dorsolateral area are widespread and include many neocortical areas, whereas those for the orbitofrontal area are principally with components of the limbic system.

Lateralization of Cortical Functions

The two hemispheres have specializations in function that distinguish one from the other and are sometimes reflected in an anatomical asymmetry. *Lateralization* refers to this functional dominance of one hemisphere over the other.

Much of what we know about lateralization in the human brain comes from the study of patients under one of four conditions. These conditions are *loss of cortical tissue, commissurotomy, hemispheric anesthesia,* or *electrical stimulation.* The *tissue losses* usually result from neurosurgical removal, trauma, or infarct. A *commissurotomy* is the surgical transection of the cortical commissures, a procedure performed in the treatment of some forms of epilepsy. In this procedure, all three commissures (corpus callosum, anterior commissure, and hippocampal commissure) are cut. Following a commissurotomy, the two hemispheres remain intact but the avenues of interhemispheric communication no longer exist. The *anesthesia of one cortical hemisphere,* following injection of amobarbital (Amytal) into an internal carotid artery, produces contralateral hemiparesis, hemianesthesia, and hemianopsia for about 10 minutes. The other hemisphere, however, remains conscious and in control of its half of the body. This procedure allows the neurosurgeon to identify the dominant hemisphere and thereby avoid procedures that alter language capacity. Neurosurgeons also use *electrical stimulation* of the cortex to confirm essential surgical landmarks. The results of these stimulations continue to contribute to our understanding of the localization of cortical function in the human brain.

Results from these procedures, however, limit our efforts to understand the function of the normal, intact brain. Although these studies indicate many lateralized functions, the intact brain may not be as lateralized as these studies suggest. The corpus callosum is the largest single bundle of nerve fibers in the CNS, and interhemispheric communication is the largest input-output system

in the cerebral cortex. Tissue removal, commissurotomy, and hemispheric anesthesia create situations in which the strong reciprocal, intrahemispheric connections are absent or depressed. In the normal, intact brain, one cortical area does not operate in isolation from its contralateral counterpart. Although one hemisphere may be dominant for a particular function, both contribute to information processing through these reciprocal connections.

Considerable variation exists both between the degree of lateralization of different functions and the degree to which a given function is lateralized in particular individuals. Some lateralizations are so strong that an individual is unable to initiate specific processes without the dominant hemispheric area. Written and spoken language skills are good examples.

HEMISPHERIC DOMINANCE

The localization of *speech centers* is the traditional criterion for defining the *dominant cerebral hemisphere.* Most individuals have highly lateralized areas for language skills. Even for language skills, however, a wide range of variation exists from individual to individual in the *degree* of lateralization. For most, language skills are so lateralized that loss of the dominant hemispheric area leads to a total loss of function. At the other extreme are those few individuals who have no hemispheric dominance and either hemisphere can initiate language skills. Currently, we do not know why one hemisphere becomes dominant for a particular function. Whether the anatomical differences that exist are the result of or the cause of the lateralization is not known.

In 96% of normal, right-handed individuals and in 70% of normal, left-handed individuals, the *left hemisphere* contains the *language centers.* These individuals are "left hemisphere dominant." Damage to the language centers of the left hemisphere produces marked deficits in language skills, whereas damage to the contralateral area does not. Of the 30% of left-handed individuals who are not left hemisphere dominant, one half are right hemisphere dominant and the other half are bilateral dominant—neither hemisphere is speech dominant. An anatomical asymmetry, an enlargement of a cortical area containing one of the language centers, often accompanies functional lateralization. On the superior surface of the temporal lobe, in the depths of the lateral fissure, the area immediately posterior to the primary auditory cortex forms the *planum tem-*

porale. The planum temporale contains a major portion of Wernicke's area, one of the important language centers. In 65% of normal human brains, the left planum temporale is larger than the right; in 24%, they are the same size; and in 11%, the left planum temporale is smaller than the right.

LANGUAGE LATERALIZATION AND APHASIA

Damage to the dominant hemisphere from trauma, infarct of the middle cerebral artery, or tumor usually produces some form of *aphasia.* The aphasic changes accompany many motor and sensory deficits that reflect the areas and extent of the damage. *Aphasia* is a general term for a *loss of or impairment in the ability to use or understand language,* either written or spoken. The specific aphasic changes observed reflect the area of the dominant hemisphere damaged. Rarely does a patient "fit" the description of any one of the classic types of aphasia. Patients usually have deficits that include components from several classic descriptions.

Many additional factors make the classification of an individual case difficult. These include cognitive differences (e.g., intellect, basic knowledge, original language skills), differences in degree of language lateralization, and differences in both the size and location of the actual lesion. The following descriptions of *motor, sensory,* and *conduction aphasia* illustrate some basic features in the cortical organization of language mechanisms.

Motor aphasia (*expressive aphasia, Broca's aphasia*) is the loss of the ability to express one's thoughts in spoken words. Motor aphasia involves damage to *Broca's area,* an area of the frontal lobe at the posterior end of the inferior frontal gyrus, immediately above the lateral fissure (Brodmann's area 44 and part of 45) (Figs. 21–3 and 21–11). If the damage is severe, the patient is mute. In less severe cases, the patient is able to speak, but haltingly and with very few words, often repeating isolated words or parts of words. *If damage is limited to the frontal lobe area, an understanding of both spoken or written language remains intact.* Here, the deficit is in the mechanics of speaking.

Agraphia, the inability to express one's thoughts in writing, often accompanies motor aphasia. The patient may be able to form single letters but cannot combine them into meaningful words. Frequently, a contralateral hemiparesis of the face and hand, due to the involvement of the adjacent motor cortical area, accompanies motor aphasia.

Sensory aphasia (*receptive aphasia, Wernicke's aphasia*) is *the loss of the ability to understand language, spoken or written,* including gestures and musical sounds. *Sensory aphasia* involves a lesion of *Wernicke's area.* Two definitions of Wernicke's area are in general use. One definition includes only the posterior portions of the superior and middle temporal gyri (portions of Brodmann's areas 21 and 22); a broader definition also includes the angular and part of the supramarginal gyri (Brodmann's area 39 and portions of 40) (see Figs. 21–3 and 21–11). We prefer the broader definition in this textbook.

With *sensory aphasia,* the spontaneous speech of the patient is fluent, with good articulation.

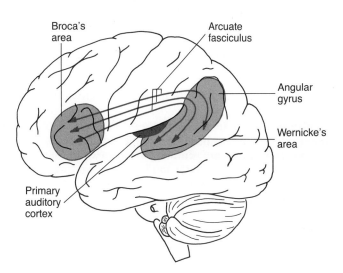

FIGURE 21-11

The left cerebral hemisphere illustrating the relative locations of Broca's area and Wernicke's area and the angular gyrus. The arcuate fasciculus is also shown. See text for details.

The patient, however, uses inappropriate words or uses them in the wrong sequence. If one is not attentive to what the patient is actually saying, the speech pattern seems normal. The mechanical aspects are normal—the rate, rhythm, and intonation—but the content is jargon. It contains inappropriate words, often in meaningless sequences. Usually the patient is unaware of this problem because of *an impairment in language comprehension.*

Patients with sensory aphasia have difficulty comprehending speech sounds or combinations of speech sounds. In addition, there may be semantic problems of associating the correct meaning with a word or sound. *The ability to associate a meaning with a perceived sound requires an intact Wernicke's area.*

Alexia is a form of sensory aphasia. A loss of the ability to understand written language has occurred because of a lesion in the angular gyrus of the dominant hemisphere. *Dyslexia* is an incomplete alexia, with a loss of reading ability to levels below that expected, based on the individual's overall intelligence and abilities. *Dyslexia* also refers to a congenital reading deficiency or a deficiency observed during the initial learning of reading skills, in contrast to the loss of acquired reading skills. Because the angular gyrus is critical for the integration of visual, auditory, and tactile information, lesions in the area produce deficits in reading, writing, and speaking. The patients are unable to convert visual symbols into either spoken or written language, although the motor mechanisms for speaking and writing are intact. In addition, most patients with lesions in the angular gyrus cannot employ their tactile sense to recognize block letters or combinations of block letters (words) after touching them with their fingers. They lack the ability to convert these tactile "images" into language symbols with an associated meaning.

Conduction aphasia is characterized by fluency in spontaneous speech and normal comprehension of spoken and written language. However, the patients are *paraphasic* (use incorrect words) and much of what is said is jargon. Patients often have difficulty in naming people and objects. Many symptoms are similar to sensory aphasia, except the patients understand written and spoken language and know what they want to say. These patients are often frustrated because they are very much aware that what they are trying to say is coming out as jargon. This, in turn, leads to a reluctance on the patient's part to respond to the examiner's questions.

Conduction aphasia is due to a lesion in the pathway that connects Broca's and Wernicke's areas, usually in the suprasylvian region, immediately above the lateral or sylvian fissure. This pathway, the *arcuate fasciculus*, is actually the inferior fibers of a larger cortical bundle, the superior longitudinal fasciculus (see Fig. 21–11 and Fig. 8–8). Because of its location, facial and limb movement apraxia (inability to carry out purposeful movements without muscle paralysis) often accompanies damage to the arcuate fasciculus.

In considering the various language centers and forms of aphasia, a simple metaphor may be helpful. Imagine a business executive (Wernicke's area) dictating a memo to a secretary (Broca's area). If Wernicke's area dictates garbage, Broca's area will have nothing but garbage to type (sensory aphasia). If Broca's area can't hear what Wernicke's area is dictating, the memo will not say what Wernicke's area wanted it to say (conduction aphasia). If the word processor in Broca's area breaks down, the message from Wernicke's area can't be typed (motor aphasia).

OTHER DOMINANT HEMISPHERE FUNCTIONS

Mathematical and computational skills also lateralize to the dominant hemisphere. Patients with severe damage to the left hemisphere, especially in the parietal associational areas, suffer from *acalculia*, an inability to perform simple arithmetical calculations. Intellectual functions involving decisions and problem solving based on analytical data and rational, symbolic thought processes tend to lateralize to the dominant hemisphere as well. These functions are not as strongly lateralized as are the language skills (Fig. 21–12).

NONDOMINANT HEMISPHERE FUNCTIONS

The nondominant hemisphere has some capacity for independent language comprehension and has a latent potential for developing language skill centers similar to those of the dominant hemisphere. In the intact normal brain, both hemispheres function in concert during the processing of language-related information. Immediately following surgical removal of the dominant hemisphere, patients become aphasic. With time and training, they are able to recover many lost language skills, indicating a latent capacity for lan-

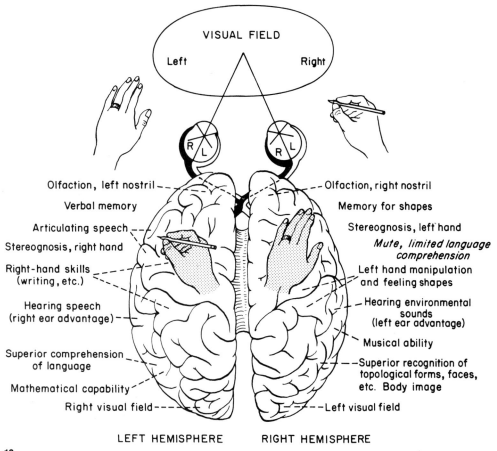

VISUAL FIELD

Left   Right

Olfaction, left nostril
Verbal memory
Articulating speech
Stereognosis, right hand
Right-hand skills (writing, etc.)
Hearing speech (right ear advantage)
Superior comprehension of language
Mathematical capability
Right visual field

Olfaction, right nostril
Memory for shapes
Stereognosis, left hand
Mute, limited language comprehension
Left hand manipulation and feeling shapes
Hearing environmental sounds (left ear advantage)
Musical ability
Superior recognition of topological forms, faces, etc. Body image
Left visual field

LEFT HEMISPHERE   RIGHT HEMISPHERE

FIGURE 21-12

Schematic summary of lateralized functions revealed by psychological tests of patients with commissurotomies and other patients. See text for details. (Reproduced with permission from A. F. Fuchs, and J. O. Phillips, Association cortex. In H. D. Patton, A. F. Fuchs, B. Hille, A. M. Scher, and R. Steiner (Editors), *Textbook of Physiology*, Volume 1, 21st Edition, W. B. Saunders Co., Philadelphia, 1989.)

guage in the remaining hemisphere. This type of recovery is much more rapid and complete in children, suggesting that a loss of functional plasticity occurs with maturation and aging.

The nondominant hemisphere is much more adept at the recognition of complex, three-dimensional structures and patterns. This recognition can be visual or tactile or a combination of the two (left visual field and left hand, if the right hemisphere is nondominant). In addition, the recognition of faces or images lateralizes more to the nondominant hemisphere.

Although the intellectual functions of the dominant hemisphere utilize rational and symbolic thought processes, those of the nondominant hemisphere involve more nonverbal, intuitive thought processes. In essence, the left hemisphere is more analytical, whereas the right hemisphere

is more intuitive. Related to the intuitive processes are the lateralization of creative and artistic abilities, including musical ability, to the nondominant hemisphere (see Fig. 21-12).

SPLIT BRAIN

The term *split brain* describes the outcome of a commissurotomy. Following the surgical transection of the cortical commissures, the patients appear to lead normal, functional lives with no detectable alterations in personality, intellect, or behavior. This surgical procedure has been relatively successful in providing the patient with relief from severe epileptic seizures. More subtle testing, however, will demonstrate distinct impairments related to the interhemispheric transfer of information. A total separation of function of the two hemispheres occurs in nearly every cognitive or psychic activity. The processes of learning and memory proceed separately in the two hemispheres. Each hemisphere maintains its own consciousness with its own independent methods of processing information, "thinking," and responding to the external world.

For example, both hemispheres recognize visual stimuli in the contralateral visual fields; however, the processing and utilization of that information is different in the two hemispheres. Assume the visual stimulus is a composite picture of a face, the left half being that of an old man and the right half that of a young woman. When the stimulus is presented so that each half of the composite face is in a different visual field, the right visual cortex will "see" only the image of the old man (left visual field), whereas the left visual cortex will "see" only the young woman's image (right visual field).

The image perceived by the patient depends on what the patient intends to do with the visual information. If asked to describe the image, using speech centers, the description is invariably that of the young woman. If the patient is asked to identify the image by pointing to the correct picture in a group of pictures, the one selected is usually that of the old man. In essence, the half of the brain that is best suited for the task at hand takes over. Because the left half saw only the young woman and speech centers are in the left hemisphere, the description could only be that of the woman. Because the nondominant, right hemisphere saw only the old man, any use of the image by a function lateralized to the right hemisphere would use only the image of the old man. Pointing to the correct image from a group of images (facial recognition) lateralizes more to the nondominant hemisphere.

Each hemisphere functions independent of the other. Information is not exchanged and memory recall is limited to events recorded only in that hemisphere. Thus, when the recall mechanism employs a function lateralized to the left, only the memory stored in the left hemisphere can be accessed. The same is true for recall from the right hemisphere.

Brain Waves and the Electroencephalogram

CORTICAL NEURONAL ACTIVITY

Neurons are excitable cells, cells that maintain a membrane potential and generate action poten-

tials. The action potentials produce postsynaptic potentials, which in turn lead to postsynaptic membrane currents. Most neurons maintain a spontaneous rate of firing and express their level of excitation or inhibition with an increase or decrease in this rate (see Chapters 3 and 4). These activities are readily measured in *individual cortical neurons* by impaling them with *microelectrodes*.

Macroelectrodes, when placed on the surface of the cortex, *measure summated electrical changes from the population of neurons* in the underlying area. These measured changes are principally summations of ionic currents generated by postsynaptic potentials on the thousands of neurons within the immediate vicinity of the recording electrode. The action potential appears to contribute little to the cortical potential. Most investigators believe that the long, vertically orientated dendrites of the pyramidal cells are the largest contributors to the postsynaptic currents as measured from the surface of the cortex. Because the cerebral cortex contains 12 to 14 billion neurons, there is a significant amount of cortical electrical activity, even during states of "rest." These recordings of electrical responses from surface cortical macroelectrodes are *electrocorticograms* (*ECoGs*).

These summated changes in cortical electrical potential are measurable with macroelectrodes placed on the surface of the scalp as well. After the electrical signals pass through the meninges, cerebrospinal fluid, skull, and scalp, they are markedly attenuated. Recorded tracings of these diminished electrical potentials (now in microvolts) produce rhythmic, wave-like patterns known as *brain waves*. The simultaneous tracing of these brain waves from many electrodes placed over the surface of the scalp is an *electroencephalogram* or, simply, an *EEG* (Fig. 21–13).

For the normal human, EEG frequencies range from 0.5 to 30 Hz with changes in potential difference of from 10 to 200 μV. As a rule, the lower the frequency, the larger the change in voltage; the higher the frequency, the smaller the change in voltage. *Beta waves*, for example, are a high-frequency, low amplitude wave, whereas *delta waves* are a low-frequency, high amplitude wave.

TYPES AND PROPERTIES

Although the frequencies and amplitudes of the brain waves in the EEG form a complex pattern, several major wave patterns occur with regularity. These patterns correlate with specific states of

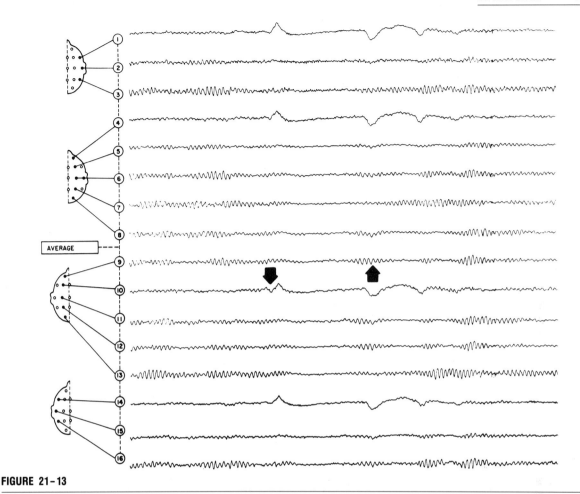

FIGURE 21-13

An electroencephalogram (EEG) from a normal individual. Left side of the figure illustrates the electrode position for each tracing. Note the prominent alpha spindles principally in the tracings from occipital and parietal leads. When the eyes are opened (downward arrow) the alpha activity diminishes, only to reappear when the eyes are closed (upward arrow). (Reproduced with permission from W. E. Crill, The cerebral cortex, consciousness, and sleep. In H. D. Patton, J. W. Sundsten, W. E. Crill, and P. D. Swanson (Editors), *Introduction to Basic Neurology*, W. B. Saunders Co., Philadelphia, 1976.)

cortical activity. The *alpha waves* have a frequency of 8 to 13 Hz. They often wax and wane in amplitude, forming symmetrical, spindle-shaped patterns. Alpha spindles are typical of the EEG from normal and awake, but very relaxed, individuals. These waves are recorded most frequently from the occipital and parietal regions of the cortex (see Fig. 21-13). *Beta waves* are the fastest of the brain waves with frequencies of 18 to 30 Hz. These high-frequency, low amplitude waves are characteristic of an intense mental activity or a high level of afferent stimulation to the cortex (see Fig. 21-13). Beta waves are recorded most frequently from the frontal and parietal regions of the cortex. *Delta waves* have the lowest frequency and are defined as any brain wave slower than 3.5 Hz. These low-frequency,

high amplitude waves are typical for an adult during deep sleep, an infant, or an individual with a serious brain disorder. *Theta waves* also have a relatively low frequency, 4 to 7 Hz. The theta wave pattern is frequently found in normal children and in adults, during sleep or emotional stress.

PATTERNS DURING NORMAL LEVELS OF CORTICAL ACTIVITY

The pattern of the EEG is a reflection of the level of cortical activity. During periods of intense mental activity, the characteristic pattern of the EEG is one of high-frequency, low amplitude *beta waves*. When individuals are relaxed and at rest with their eyes closed, *alpha waves* or *alpha spindles* are a characteristic feature (see Fig. 21–13). During periods with high levels of afferent stimulation, beta waves are a characteristic feature. Figure 21–13 demonstrates the shift from alpha spindles to beta waves when the relaxed patient opens his or her eyes (afferent stimulation). Different stages of sleep have very characteristic EEG patterns with many *delta* and *theta waves*. These are discussed in the following section.

CLINICAL USE

The EEG provides a useful, noninvasive clinical tool for the evaluation of cortical function. Abnormalities in the overall pattern of brain waves help to localize brain tumors, evaluate areas of brain damage following an infarct, and analyze sleep patterns. Most recently, abnormal brain waves, or an absence of brain waves, have become one of the criteria for brain death. Areas of

brain wave instability or abnormal patterns often reflect trigger points for epileptic seizures. During an actual seizure, the brain wave pattern changes dramatically. These patterns often include high voltage polyspikes and spikes superimposed on low-frequency, high amplitude synchronous wave patterns (Fig. 21–14).

Sleep

We normally spend from one fourth to one third of our lives sleeping. Today, as throughout history, many people are intrigued by the study of sleep. Over the centuries, many theories have been put forth to explain sleep. These theories have ranged from ones that considered sleep a state resembling death to ones that considered sleep a state of active mentation in which behavioral patterns are rehearsed. Scientists have a massive amount of data about the sleeping state,

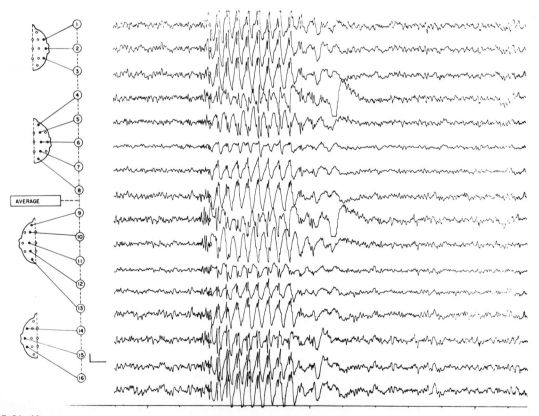

FIGURE 21–14

An electroencephalogram (EEG) showing bilaterally synchronous onset of polyspike, spike, and wave activity in a 38 year-old man during a generalized seizure. Calibration units are 50 μV and 500 msec. Left side illustrates the electrode position for each tracing. (Reproduced with permission from W. E. Crill, Epilepsy and seizure states. In H. D. Patton, J. W. Sundsten, W. E. Crill, and P. D. Swanson (Editors), *Introduction to Basic Neurology*, W. B. Saunders Co., Philadelphia, 1976.)

with much of this data obtained during the last 30 to 40 years. Agreement on the basic mechanisms of sleep, however, is still lacking. We lack a clear definition of the neurobiological mechanisms of sleep, and we do not understand the physiological purposes for some sleep stages.

AN ACTIVE AND CIRCADIAN BRAIN FUNCTION

Normal adults sleep from 6 to 8 hours per night, in a rather predictable circadian pattern. Superimposed on the sleep pattern are other circadian rhythms, such as body temperature and hormone production levels. These rhythms normally maintain a constant temporal relation to the sleep-wake cycle. When individuals are placed in a constant environment, one that excludes environmental cues, such as light-dark cycles and temperature changes and other cues that might suggest the time of day, their biological clocks become free running. Most individuals drift into a sleep-wake cycle of about 25 hours duration. Under these conditions, other circadian rhythms, such as body temperature, maintain the same temporal relationship to the sleep-wake cycle. A few individuals, however, settle into longer sleep-wake patterns, some lasting up to 32 to 34 hours. In these individuals, the other biorhythms, such as body temperature, become uncoupled from the sleep-wake cycle and maintain a 25- to 26-hour cyclic pattern of their own. This temporal de-synchronization indicates that these biorhythms are driven by different biological clocks.

Despite the duration of the sleep-wake cycle, the overall pattern of a night's sleep is the same. During the sleeping period, an individual passes through four to six alternating periods of *slow wave sleep* followed by *rapid eye movement (REM) sleep*. Slow wave sleep lacks visual dreams and is the deepest. REM sleep is a period of visual dreams and is the lightest. Individuals waking up spontaneously are most likely to do so during REM sleep.

STAGES

The first period of sleep is *slow wave sleep*, (*non-REM sleep* or *dreamless sleep*). Slow wave sleep consists of four stages (I, II, III, and IV) of increasingly deep sleep, each with a characteristic EEG pattern. The overall progression is from fast, low amplitude, asynchronous brain waves to slow, large amplitude, synchronous brain waves (Fig. 21–15). One characteristic of stage II sleep is the appearance of *sleep spindles* (see Fig. 21–

15). Another feature of the changing EEG pattern is a progressive increase in proportion of theta waves followed by an increase in delta waves. The term *delta wave sleep* often is employed for stages III and IV.

As the brain waves become slower, the depth of sleep becomes greater, as defined by the intensity of the stimulus necessary to wake an individual. Simultaneously, heart rate and blood pressure drop to low, stable values and respiration becomes slow and deep. A typical individual spends 40 to 50 minutes passing from stage I to stage IV of slow wave sleep. After reaching stage IV, there is a reversal in the pattern and the individual passes sequentially back through stages III and II. After reaching stage II, the EEG of the individual approaches the asynchronous pattern of stage I. Associated with the onset of the asynchronous EEG pattern is a dramatic change in the individual's physiological state. This new stage of sleep is *REM sleep*.

REM sleep, also known as *rapid eye movement sleep*, *paradoxical sleep*, or *dream sleep*, is a stage in which the EEG pattern returns to a high-frequency, low amplitude wave, more characteristic of the awake state or stage I. Associated with REM sleep is a general loss of somatic muscle tone, except the middle ear muscles and the extraocular muscles. During this period, there are movements of the eyes: occasional rapid, saccadic-like movements superimposed on a basic pattern of slow-rolling, undulating movements. The eye movements are the basis for the name, rapid eye movement or REM sleep.

Each period of REM sleep is a period of visual dreaming, but the content of the dream is not stored in memory. Therefore, effective recall of the dream is limited to those times when the individual is awakened during or immediately after REM sleep. During REM sleep, respiration becomes irregular, shallow, and more rapid. In addition, several autonomic nervous system responses, both parasympathetic and sympathetic, develop. These include a general increase in both heart rate and blood pressure. A decrease occurs in blood flow to the gastrointestinal tract, but an increase occurs in blood flow to both the brain and the external genitalia. The latter leads to penile erection; however, this is not related to the content of REM sleep dreams. Sex therapists often utilize this physiological correlate of REM sleep to differentiate between physical and psychological causes of impotence.

During the first cycle of sleep stages, the period of REM sleep is brief, lasting from 5 to 15 minutes. The total time elapsed for one cycle,

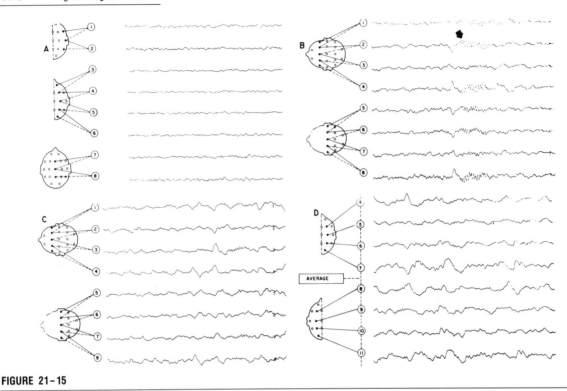

FIGURE 21-15

Sequential electroencephalogram (EEG) records show the change in brain wave pattern with the stages of sleep. *A*, Stage I; *B*, stage II; *C*, stage III; and *D*, stage IV. Note the appearance of sleep spindles in *B* (arrow). (Reproduced with permission from W. E. Crill. The cerebral cortex, consciousness, and sleep. In H. D. Patton, J. W. Sundsten, W. E. Crill, and P. D. Swanson (Editors), *Introduction to Basic Neurology*, W. B. Saunders Co., Philadelphia, 1976.)

from the beginning of slow wave sleep through the first period of REM sleep, is 90 to 110 minutes. Following REM sleep, the individual again passes through the successive stages of slow wave sleep, stages II through IV; then passes back to stage II in reverse sequence; and then enters another period of REM sleep. This sequential pattern continues throughout the night. However, with each 90- to 110-minute cycle, the duration of the REM sleep component becomes longer. Later periods of REM sleep may last 40 to 60 minutes. Concurrent with the rise in duration of REM sleep is a decline in duration of the deeper stages of slow wave sleep. Often, stages III and IV are absent during the last cycle of sleep.

If subjects are awakened at the onset of REM sleep and allowed to return to sleep, they return to the first stages of slow wave sleep. This feature has been employed experimentally to deprive subjects of REM sleep. After deprivation of REM sleep for up to 16 days, subjects appear perfectly normal and perform well on a battery of physical and psychological tests. When they return to a normal, uninterrupted sleep pattern, however, these individuals show *REM rebound*. It is as if their systems attempt to make up for the loss in REM sleep. Their sleep patterns contain very long periods of REM sleep interposed between periods of normal slow wave sleep. The *longer the deprivation*, the *stronger the rebound* phenomenon. These studies suggest that REM sleep is important, but we do not know why.

Many theories have been put forth to explain the purpose of REM sleep. Freud believed that dreams accompanying REM sleep were a way of working through upsetting stimuli from the previous day and were a harmless way of releasing repressed impulses. Other scholars suggest that dreams occurring in REM sleep serve to reinforce weak neuronal circuits and to strengthen important memories and experiences from the previous day. A later theory suggests that during sleep the brain is systematically erasing informational errors that have inadvertently accumulated and that the dreams of REM sleep are only a reflection of this data purging process.

NEUROBIOLOGICAL BASIS

Many pathways and nuclei in the CNS are important for sleep. The actual circuitry, however, is not clear and some evidence is contradictory. Neither the receptors nor the afferent signals that trigger the response of sleep are known. Many factors or events can leave us feeling "sleepy" or "tired." We often feel tired after a hard day's work (physical or mental) and after dealing with a stressful situation, or when we are simply bored. Drowsiness often follows a large meal or descends like clockwork as bedtime approaches. We understand a few of the physiological changes that accompany these varied states—changes in blood flow and biological rhythms. It remains unclear (1) how these physiological states and bodily changes signal the CNS, (2) how the nervous system processes this information, and (3) what the actual triggers might be for the sleeping state.

Cortical brain wave patterns define the various stages of sleep. One characteristic of slow wave sleep is the appearance of sleep spindles (see Fig. 21–15). We do know that *spindle activity* in the cortex is due to the *synchronous bursting activity of thalamocortical neurons*. As long as the thalamocortical neurons are in a bursting pattern, afferent signals cannot pass through the thalamus to reach the cortex. *GABAergic neurons* of the *reticular nucleus of the thalamus*, through the cyclic generation of long duration IPSPs on thalamocortical neurons, are the *pacemakers for thalamocortical bursting activity*. Any modulation of these GABAergic oscillators should, therefore, effectively modulate sleep.

At least four of the *extrathalamic cortical modulatory systems* are important in the regulation of sleep: the *serotoninergic, noradrenergic, cholinergic*, and *histaminergic* systems (see Figs. 21–9 and 21–10). In addition, other neurons of the *brain stem reticular formation* that project to the thalamus, hypothalamus, basal forebrain, and spinal cord have important roles in the sleep process. All ascending afferent and descending efferent systems send axon collaterals to the brain stem reticular formation. The reticular formation is therefore constantly "aware" of external and internal environments and motor actions both planned and in progress. How the reticular formation integrates this information and uses it to modulate sleep patterns is unknown.

At least four "sleep centers" have been described in the brain stem. Most have been defined through either laboratory experiments or clinical observations. Two of these reside in the hypothalamus and two in the brain stem reticular formation.

Damage to the *preoptic nucleus of the hypothalamus* produces *insomnia*, whereas *stimulation* of the nucleus with serotonin induces *slow wave sleep*. Damage to neurons in the *ventrolateral posterior hypothalamus*, in comparison, produces transient sleep. The latter area includes the *histaminergic projections to the cerebral cortex* (see Fig. 21–10). The neurons from this posterior hypothalamic area have arousal properties through both (1) the direct excitatory, histaminergic projections to the cerebral cortex and (2) indirect excitatory, projections to the brain stem reticular formation. Some evidence exists that the preoptic nucleus induces sleep indirectly through inhibition of the excitatory neurons of the posterior hypothalamus.

The *serotoninergic* projections from neurons in the *raphe nuclei* of the brain stem reticular formation are important for sleep. If either the neurons or the projection fibers are destroyed, animals are unable to sleep. Although there is some recovery, it's only a fraction of the initial level. These serotoninergic neurons project both to the *cerebral cortex* (see Fig. 21–9) and to the *preoptic nucleus* of the hypothalamus. If the synthesis of serotonin is blocked (with parachlorophenylalanine) animals will deplete reserve stores of serotonin within a few days and are then unable to sleep. If the blocking of serotonin synthesis continues, however, there is an almost complete recovery after 8 to 9 days, *even though the brain levels of serotonin remain depleted*. Obviously, the serotoninergic pathways are important for sleep, but it appears that alternative pathways are able to compensate for their loss.

The *cholinergic neurons* of both the *nucleus basalis* in the basal forebrain and the *dorsolateral tegmental area* (near the junction of the pons and midbrain) have a role in the sleep process. Both areas project to the reticular nucleus of the thalamus, inhibiting the spindle-generating GABAergic neurons. Stimulation of either cholinergic pathway blocks thalamocortical bursting activity, effectively disinhibiting the thalamus. In addition, the cholinergic neurons from the *nucleus basalis* project both directly to the *cerebral cortex* and descend to the *midbrain reticular formation*, many terminating in the dorsolateral tegmental area.

The *noradrenergic projections* from the *locus ceruleus* have been implicated in arousal. Stimulation of these neurons produces an asynchronous EEG pattern, characteristic of the waking state. These neurons appear to act both directly on the cerebral cortex (see Fig. 21–9) and indirectly via a depolarization of the thalamic neurons, thereby terminating their bursting activity. Most locus ceruleus neurons, however, are not active during REM sleep. Their activity correlates more closely with states of arousal. During REM sleep, the motor cortex is active, but an inhibition of lower motor neurons occurs at the spinal cord level, producing the atonia that accompanies REM sleep. Another population of *noradrenergic neurons*, descending from the medial part of the *locus ceruleus*, inhibits lower motor neuron activity.

Just how the pieces of this puzzle fit together to regulate the sleep cycle is unknown. Because sleep and its regulating mechanisms are so important to survival, it is likely that there is some neuronal redundancy and that alternate pathways can take over. This may account for some of the apparent contradictions.

SUGGESTED READING

Foote, S. L. and J. H. Morrison (1987) Extrathalamic modulation of cortical function. Ann. Rev. Neurosci., 10: 67–95.

This succinct review includes the direct projections to the neocortex of four aminergic systems: the adrenergic, serotoninergic, dopaminergic, and cholinergic projections from the midbrain and basal forebrain areas. In the review, these authors compare and contrast these projection systems and consider the anatomy and physiology of these diverse systems, as they may relate to normal brain function.

Geschwind, N. and A. M. Galaburda (Editors) (1984). *Cerebral Dominance.* Harvard University Press, Cambridge, 232 pages.

This book is a collection of well-written articles that deal with many aspects of cortical asymmetry. The topic of brain lateralization is approached from a number of different perspectives: anatomical, histological, physiological, behavioral, and clinical. The first section deals exclusively with the human brain. Another section reviews brain asymmetry in other species.

Massimo, A., T. A. Reader, R. W. Dykes, and P. Gloor (Editors) (1988). *Neurotransmitters and Cortical Function: From Molecules to Mind.* Plenum Press, New York, 620 pages.

The 38 chapters of this book are the result of a symposium held in 1986 and provide a comprehensive picture of our knowledge of the subject at that time. Both the fast response neurotransmitters and the neuromodulators are extensively discussed. In addition, a number of hypotheses about the neurochemical aspects of cortical function are put forth. Most of the chapters are well written and contain many references.

Rakic, P. and W. Singer (Editors) (1988). *Neurobiology of Neocortex.* John Wiley & Sons, New York, 446 pages.

The chapters in this book provide the reader with a brief, timely overview of different aspects of neocortical function. Topics range from cortical organization, areal and synaptic, to general principles of cortical operation and integrative functions. Much is presented in terms of current data and concepts, but areas of ignorance are also identified. Most chapters are well written and contain many references.

Rasmussen, T. and B. Milner (1975). Clinical and surgical studies of the cerebral speech areas in man. In *Cerebral Localization; An Otfrid Foerster Symposium.* K. J. Zülch, O. Creutzfeldt, and G. C. Galbraith (Editors). Springer-Verlag, New York, pp. 238–257.

A classic review of the localization of speech mechanisms in the human cerebral cortex by pioneers in human cerebral localization. The authors review the results of three basic, but conceptually, very different approaches: cortical stimulation, cortical ablation and hemispheric anesthesia with sodium amobarbital (Amytal).

Sperry, R., M. S. Gazzaniga, and J. E. Bogen (1969). Interhemispheric relationships: the neocortical commissures; syndromes of hemisphere disconnection. In *Handbook of Clinical Neurology, Volume 4, Disorders of Speech, Perception, and Symbolic Behavior.* P. J. Vinken and G. W. Bruyn (Editors). North Holland Publishing Company, Amsterdam, pp. 273–290.

An excellent review of the now classic studies of Roger Sperry, one of the pioneers in the study of brain lateralization through the use of the "split-brain" or patients who have undergone commissurotomies.

Chapter
22

Limbic System

The term *limbic lobe* was first used in the late 1800's by Broca, a French neuroanatomist, to describe a ring of cortical tissue that surrounds the brain stem. Broca noted that this ring of cortical tissue was a constant feature of the brains of all mammals and that it contained strong olfactory connections. Many areas belonging to Broca's limbic lobe are primitive archicortex and paleocortex.

In the human brain, Broca's limbic lobe contains the *parolfactory area*; the *uncus*; and the *subcallosal, parahippocampal,* and *cingulate gyri,* along with the underlying *hippocampal formation.* Broca believed olfaction was the principal function of these structures. Even today the hippocampal formation, the parolfactory area, the parahippocampal gyrus, and the uncus form the cortical portion of the *rhinencephalon* or "smell brain" (Table 22–1 and Fig. 22–1).

The association of the limbic lobe with behavior and expression of emotions was not made until the 1930's. Papez first proposed that cognitive activity in the neocortex influenced the expression of emotions through a series of pathways linking the cortex with the hypothalamus. In this proposal, known as the *Papez circuit*, information passed from the neocortical association areas to the hippocampus via the cingulate gyrus, the cingulum, and the parahippocampal gyrus. Following information processing in the hippocampus, signals were relayed to the mammillary nuclei of the hypothalamus via the fornix. Feedback to the cingulate gyrus and completion of the loop circuit was accomplished through the mammillo-thalamic pathway, relaying information from the mammillary nuclei to the anterior nuclei of the thalamus. The anterior nuclei, in turn, project to the cingulate gyrus. In Papez's proposal, the link with the mammillary nuclei of the hypothalamus provided a means for the regulation of autonomic nervous activity during the expression of emotions (Fig. 22–2).

TABLE 22–1

Components of the Limbic System and the Rhinencephalon

	LIMBIC SYSTEM	RHINENCEPHALON
CORTICAL AREAS		
Hippocampal formation		
Hippocampus	X	X
Dentate gyrus	X	X
Hippocampal rudiments		
Medial longitudinal stria	X	X
Lateral longitudinal stria	X	X
Induseum griseum	X	X
Fasciola cinerea	X	X
Parolfactory area	X	X
Subcallosal gyrus	X	X
Parahippocampal gyrus	X	X
Cingulate gyrus	X	
Isthmus gyrus cinguli	X	
NUCLEI OF THE SEPTAL COMPLEX		
Septal nuclei	X	X
Nucleus of the diagonal band	X	X
Bed nucleus, stria terminalis	X	X
Bed nucleus, anterior commissure	X	X
OTHER BASAL FOREBRAIN NUCLEI		
Nucleus accumbens	X	
Nucleus basalis (substantia innominata)	X	
Amygdala	X	
Ventral striatum	X	
Ventral pallidum	X	
OLFACTORY STRUCTURES		
Olfactory bulb and tract		X
Anterior olfactory nucleus		X
Medial olfactory stria and gyrus		X
Lateral olfactory stria and gyrus		X
Anterior perforated substance		X
BRAIN STEM AREAS		
Hypothalamus	X	
Dorsal thalamus		
Anterior nuclei	X	
Lateral dorsal nucleus	X	
Mediodorsal nucleus	X	
Intralaminar nuclei	X	
Habenular nuclei	X	
Interpeduncular nucleus	X	
Ventral tegmental area	X	
Locus ceruleus	X	
Raphe nuclei	X	

At nearly the same time that Papez proposed a correlation between the limbic system and emotions, Klüver and Bucy described profound behavioral changes in monkeys following the bilateral removal of most of the temporal lobe (neocortical areas, hippocampal formation, parahippocampal gyrus, uncus, and amygdala). Changes in behavior included a marked increase in both the amount and diversity of sexual activity and an increase in oral activity. The monkeys examined virtually everything orally, placing all objects in their mouths—food, inedible objects, and even live snakes and rodents. The hypersexuality included heterosexual, homosexual, and autosexual behaviors. The monkeys also became very tame and lost their fear of people, other animals, and situations that normally elicited fear responses. This collection of behavioral changes is known as the *Klüver-Bucy syndrome.*

Neurosurgeons have unilaterally and bilaterally removed the amygdaloid complex and portions of the surrounding temporal lobe from epileptic in-

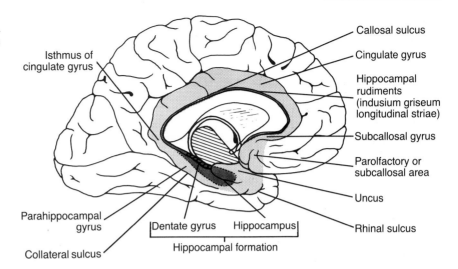

FIGURE 22-1

The cortical components of the limbic lobe.

dividuals and from those exhibiting socially unacceptable aggressive behavior. Following surgery, the behavioral changes in humans were less consistent than those in monkeys. Much more variability was noted from individual to individual. Most of the patients had one or more of the following symptoms: abnormal interest in food,

hypersexuality, and increased docility. A more normal pattern of social behavior was reported in those with a previously unacceptable pattern of social behavior. Some patients became more emotionally labile, whereas others became less labile. As discussed further in this chapter, much of the variability is probably related to the exten-

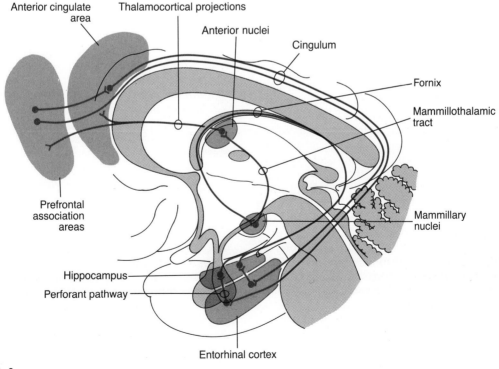

FIGURE 22-2

The principal components of the Papez circuit. See text for details.

sive and complex interconnections between the limbic areas and the multitude of very different functions associated with these areas.

Currently, we believe that the limbic system is associated with a variety of diverse functions, from behavior and emotions to memory. Because of the diverse functions of the limbic system and the complicated interconnections, it is often difficult to relate specific functions to specific components of the system. In this chapter, we first define the limbic system anatomically. This section is followed by a description of the major components of the system. Several functions of the limbic system that are difficult to localize, e.g., memory, emotion, and homeostasis, are discussed in the closing sections.

Definition

Unlike the limbic lobe, the *limbic system* contains both cortical and subcortical components. The cortical component, the *limbic lobe*, is similar to that initially described by Broca. The *subcortical components*, however, include nuclei in the basal forebrain; ventral striatum; and brain stem regions, such as the hypothalamus, epithalamus, and portions of the dorsal thalamus. Most of the *limbic system's* structures are interconnected—often by long, circuitous pathways.

A knowledge of the development of the telencephalon is helpful in the understanding of the circuitous pathways so characteristic of the limbic system (for details, see Chapter 1). In the early stages of development, the archicortical hippocampal formation lies close to target areas in the ventral forebrain and hypothalamus. It is only during the massive development of the neocortex and the corpus callosum that the archicortical hippocampal formation and the paleocortical areas of the parahippocampal gyrus are displaced to the temporal lobe. By that time, many early connections of the hippocampal and parahippocampal areas with ventral forebrain and hypothalamus areas are already established. Therefore, during displacement, these connections are drawn out, often following the course of displacement. Because of these differential growth patterns, (1) the hippocampal formation and the parahippocampal gyrus are in the medial wall of the temporal lobe and (2) the fornix and its hippocampal commissure are ventral to the corpus callosum. The displacement of the fornix and hippocampal formation is not complete, however, and some rudiments of both structures remain dorsal to the

corpus callosum (the indusium griseum and the medial and lateral longitudinal striae) (see Chapter 1).

Of the many limbic system components, only the *hippocampal formation* is unique to this system. The other structures are also components of other neuroanatomical regions or systems. The principal ones are the olfactory system (Chapter 13), the basal ganglia (Chapter 16), the autonomic nervous system and the hypothalamus (Chapter 18), the dorsal thalamus (Chapter 20), and the cerebral cortex (Chapter 21).

THE HIPPOCAMPAL FORMATION

The *hippocampal formation* contains the *hippocampus*, the *dentate gyrus*, the *subiculum*, and the *hippocampal rudiments*. In the human brain, the hippocampus and dentate gyrus are deep in the temporal lobe, parallel to but under the cover of the parahippocampal gyrus—separated from it by the *hippocampal sulcus* (Figs. 22–1 and 22–4). This relationship is more clearly visualized in a brain slice preparation (see Fig. 8–3) or in a cross section (Fig. 22–5). The *subiculum* represents a transitional strip of cortex between the hippocampus and the entorhinal area of the parahippocampal gyrus (see Fig. 22–5).

The *hippocampal rudiments* are often omitted from descriptions of the hippocampal formation. In the adult human brain, these rudiments lie dorsal to the corpus callosum and include the *indusium griseum* and the *medial* and *lateral longitudinal striae*. The *fasciola cinerea* (*gyrus fasciolaris*) represents transitional tissue connecting the dentate gyrus of the hippocampal formation with the indusium griseum (Fig. 22–3 and Table 22–1).

THE CORTICAL COMPONENTS

The *cortical components* of the limbic system, in addition to the hippocampal formation, form a ring of tissue on the medial surface of the hemisphere, surrounding the brain stem. This structure includes the *parolfactory area*, the *subcallosal gyrus*, the *cingulate gyrus*, the *isthmus gyrus cinguli* (connecting the cingulate gyrus with the parahippocampal gyrus), and the *parahippocampal gyrus*. The anterior end of the parahippocampal gyrus folds back on itself, forming the *uncus*. The uncus covers the underlying amygdala or amygdaloid nuclei (see Figs. 22–1 and 22–4).

Related to the limbic system, but usually not

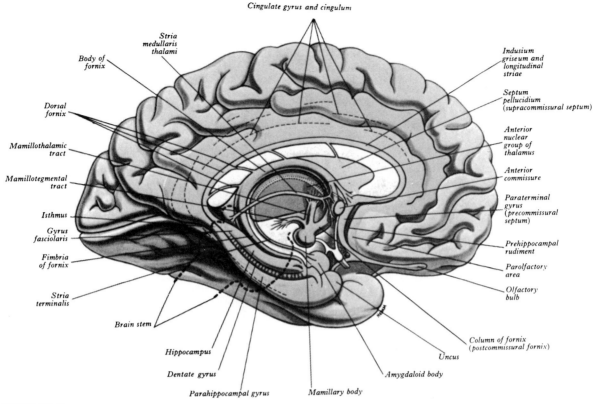

Cingulate gyrus and cingulum

Stria medullaris thalami

Body of fornix

Dorsal fornix

Mamillothalamic tract

Mamillotegmental tract

Isthmus

Gyrus fasciolaris

Fimbria of fornix

Stria terminalis

Brain stem

Hippocampus

Dentate gyrus

Parahippocampal gyrus

Mamillary body

Amygdaloid body

Uncus

Column of fornix (postcommissural fornix)

Olfactory bulb

Parolfactory area

Prehippocampal rudiment

Paraterminal gyrus (precommissural septum)

Anterior commissure

Anterior nuclear group of thalamus

Septum pellucidium (supracommissural septum)

Indusium griseum and longitudinal striae

FIGURE 22-3

A dissection of the medial surface of the cerebral hemisphere demonstrating the principal structures included in the limbic system. See text for details. (Reproduced with permission from P. L. Williams and R. Warwick, *Functional Neuroanatomy of Man*, W. B. Saunders Co., Philadelphia, 1975.)

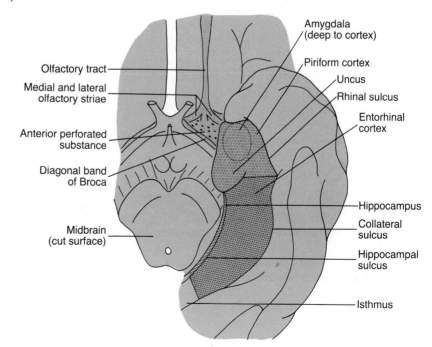

Olfactory tract

Medial and lateral olfactory striae

Anterior perforated substance

Diagonal band of Broca

Midbrain (cut surface)

Amygdala (deep to cortex)

Piriform cortex

Uncus

Rhinal sulcus

Entorhinal cortex

Hippocampus

Collateral sulcus

Hippocampal sulcus

Isthmus

FIGURE 22-4

The ventromedial surface of the temporal lobe illustrating the para-hippocampal gyrus and its subdivisions, the piriform cortex and the entorhinal cortex.

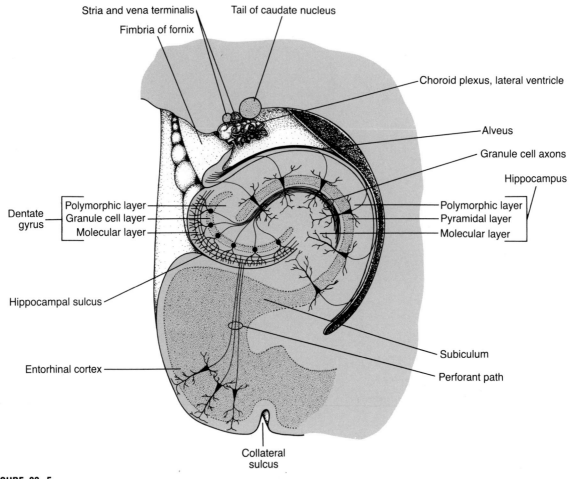

FIGURE 22–5

A transverse section through the hippocampus and dentate gyrus of the temporal lobe. A few of the principal neuronal pathways that interconnect the hippocampus, dentate gyrus, and adjacent entorhinal cortex are illustrated. The fornix is the principal efferent pathway from the hippocampal formation. See text for details.

considered a part of the limbic system, are a number of neocortical areas in the frontal and temporal lobes. These include the *orbitofrontal* and *dorsolateral prefrontal association areas*, along with the *superior, middle,* and *inferior temporal gyri*.

SEPTUM AND FOREBRAIN STRUCTURES

The *septum* has two components: the *septum pellucidum* and the *septum verum*. The *septum verum*, or true septum, extends ventrally from the septum pellucidum toward the subcallosal gyrus and contains most of the septal nuclei. Nuclei of the septal complex include the *dorsal, lateral,* and *medial septal nuclei*, the *nucleus of the diagonal band of Broca*; the *bed nucleus of the stria termi-*

nalis; and the *bed nucleus of the anterior commissure* (see Table 22–1).

Other forebrain structures that are part of the limbic system are the *ventral striatum* and the *ventral pallidum*. The *ventral striatum* contains the ventral portions of both the *caudate nucleus* and the *putamen* and all of the *nucleus accumbens* and *substantia innominata* (*nucleus basalis of Meynert*). The *ventral pallidum* contains the ventral portion of the globus pallidus (see Table 22–1).

THE AMYGDALA

The *amygdala* is a large, well defined nuclear complex in the tip of the temporal lobe deep to the uncus. During development, this nuclear complex develops as part of the basal ganglia and remains in anatomical continuity with the ventrolateral portion of the ventral striatum (see Figs. 1–19 and 8–11). Long regarded by many as a principal olfactory processing center, the amygdala now appears to be intimately involved in behavior and in regulation of autonomic and endocrine changes associated with behavior (see Table 22–1).

THE BRAIN STEM CENTERS

Many brain stem centers are involved in the functions of the limbic system, either as part of a descending efferent system or an ascending modulatory system. Most of these centers are discussed in depth in other chapters and are, therefore, mentioned only briefly.

Emotions trigger complex mental and physiological responses. Many are autonomic responses. The *hypothalamus*, as a regulator of autonomic function, coordinates and modulates many of these responses. The strong limbic system projections to the hypothalamus provide the afferent signals for the autonomic responses associated with such diverse emotional states as joy, love, hate, fear, grief, and depression.

Although all hypothalamic nuclei are part of the system, the *mammillary nuclei* and nuclei in the *preoptic area* are two of the primary targets. Limbic system efferents from the temporal lobe reach the hypothalamus via the *fornix*, the *stria terminalis*, and the *ventral amygdalohypothalamic tract*. In addition to receiving strong hippocampal projections via the fornix, the mammillary nuclei project to the anterior nuclei of the dorsal thalamus (see Fig. 22–3).

A number of nuclei in the *dorsal thalamus* are part of the limbic system. Primary among the thalamic nuclei are those in the *anterior nuclear group*, the *lateral dorsal nucleus*, and the very prominent *mediodorsal nucleus*. These nuclei process information from hypothalamic, amygdaloid, and basal forebrain nuclei that are part of the limbic system. These thalamic nuclei, in turn, project to the limbic lobe and to prefrontal and temporal association areas. Several *intralaminar thalamic nuclei* form part of the circuits that link nuclei of the ventral striatum with limbic-associated areas of the cortex.

The *habenular nuclei* (*habenula*) of the epithalamus are relay stations for information traveling from the limbic forebrain areas to the midbrain reticular formation. The principal input to the *habenula* is the *stria medullaris thalami*. This pathway carries projections mainly from the septal complex and from the preoptic and lateral areas of the hypothalamus. The major output from the habenula is the very heavily myelinated *habenulointerpeduncular tract*. These habenular efferents terminate in the *interpeduncular nucleus* and in the *raphe nuclei* of the midbrain. Some habenular neurons provide efferents to septal and hypothalamic areas as well as to the ventral tegmental area and the substantia nigra of the midbrain.

Other midbrain areas provide afferent information to the limbic system. One such example is the *mesencephalic dopaminergic system*. This system contains a *mesolimbic component* that projects principally from the *ventral tegmental area* to those cortical areas associated directly and indirectly with limbic system function. These include the limbic lobe and the prefrontal and temporal cortical association areas. Other nuclei of the *extrathalamic cortical modulatory systems* (*locus ceruleus* and *dorsal raphe*) project to the limbic lobe as well as to the septum and the amygdala.

Principal Pathways

Numerous pathways interconnect the widely separated areas of the limbic system. Many of these are reciprocal connections with the hypothalamus and provide the visceromotor component of limbic system expression. Others are cortical association pathways, both within the limbic lobe and between the limbic lobe and other cortical areas. Still other pathways interconnect the basal forebrain areas with the limbic lobe and with the hypothalamus.

Deep to the cingulate gyrus of the limbic lobe is a large cortical association bundle, the *cingulum*. The cingulum serves as a cortical association bundle for the adjacent regions of the neocortex in the frontal, parietal, and occipital lobes and in the limbic lobe. The fibers also interconnect the septal and basal forebrain areas with the parahippocampal gyrus of the temporal lobe (Figs. 22–3 and 22–6).

The *perforant pathway* is another cortical association pathway, but one not identifiable as a distinct fascicle or bundle of fibers. Fibers of the perforant pathway arise throughout Brodmann's area 28 of the *entorhinal cortex* and project through the subiculum to the adjacent *hippocampal formation*. These fibers run deep to, and at a right angle with, the hippocampal sulcus, termi-

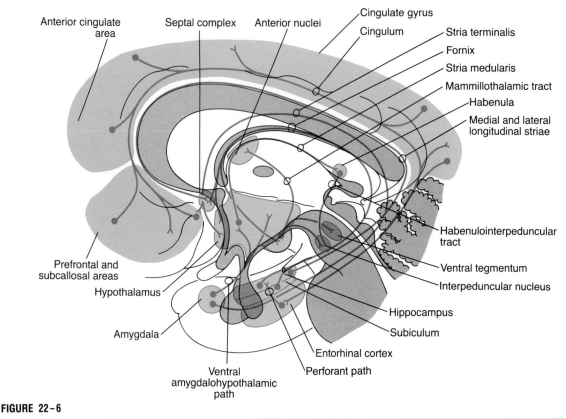

FIGURE 22-6

The principal pathways of the limbic system. See text for details.

nating in the molecular layers of both the hippocampus and the dentate gyrus (see Figs. 22–5 and 22–6).

The *anterior commissure* is a bundle of fibers that passes transversely through the lamina terminalis. Besides interconnecting the olfactory bulbs, the amygdaloid nuclei, and the anterior perforated substance, the anterior commissure contains cortical commissural fibers from parts of the parahippocampal gyri and adjacent areas of the temporal lobe.

Several other limbic pathways have prominent connections with the amygdaloid nuclei. The *stria terminalis* arises principally in the amygdaloid nuclei and follows the inner curvature of the caudate nucleus (accompanied by the vena terminalis) to the rostral forebrain area (see Figs. 22–3 and 22–6). Fibers of the stria terminalis end in the septal area, in the medial preoptic area of the hypothalamus, and in the bed nucleus of the stria terminalis.

The *ventral amygdalohypothalamic tract* is a more direct route between the amygdaloid nuclei

and the hypothalamus. These efferents leave the amygdaloid complex and pass directly through the sublenticular portion of the internal capsule and enter the hypothalamus (see Fig. 22–6).

The *diagonal band of Broca* is a band of fibers that extends caudolateral from the parolfactory area on the medial surface of the frontal lobe to the periamygdaloid area in the rostral tip of the temporal lobe. These fibers run along the lateral margin of the optic tract and form the posterior boundary of the anterior perforated substance.

The *fornix* is the principal efferent pathway from the *hippocampal formation* to the *hypothalamus* and the *septal area*. These large, heavily myelinated fibers leave the alveolar surface of the hippocampus in the temporal lobe and arch dorsomedially toward the ventral surface of the corpus callosum. Immediately ventral to the corpus callosum, the fornix from each side reaches the midline. At this point, some fibers cross to the fornix of the opposite side in the *hippocampal commissure*. Of the crossing fibers, most continue forward and terminate in the contralateral hypothalamus and septal area. A few are true commissural fibers and project to the hippocampal formation of the opposite side.

Beyond the hippocampal commissure, the fornix runs along the inferior margin of the septum pellucidum, forward and ventrad toward the anterior commissure and the lamina terminalis. At the anterior commissure, the fornix divides into two components: a *precommissural fornix* and a *postcommissural fornix*. Fibers of the precommissural fornix end in the septal area and in the more rostral nuclei of the hypothalamus. The postcommissural fibers descend through the substance of the hypothalamus, giving off branches to many hypothalamic nuclei. Most of the fibers, however, end in the mammillary nuclei (see Figs. 22–3 and 22–6). The fornix also contains fibers running toward the hippocampal formation. A major afferent pathway to the hippocampus arises from the medial septal nucleus, the *septohippocampal tract*.

During development, some fibers of the fornix remain dorsal to the corpus callosum and, along with the indusium griseum, form the *hippocampal rudiments*. These rudiments of the fornix are the *medial* and *lateral longitudinal striae*, two pairs of small bundles of myelinated fibers. These fibers run from the hippocampus over the *dorsal* surface of the corpus callosum and under cover of the indusium griseum to the septal area (see Figs. 22–3 and 22–6).

The *mammillothalamic tract* (*mammillary fasciculus*) is the most prominent of three efferent pathways arising from the mammillary nuclei of the hypothalamus. This heavily myelinated tract ends in the anterior nuclei of the thalamus. These thalamic nuclei, in turn, project to the cingulate, subcallosal, and parolfactory gyri of the limbic lobe; to the prefrontal association areas; and to portions of the hippocampal formation (see Figs. 22–3 and 22–6). The two other mammillary efferent pathways are the *mammillointerpeduncular tract* and the *mammillotegmental tract*. The mammillointerpeduncular tract projects to the interpeduncular nucleus; the mammillotegmental tract runs more dorsad, terminating in the nuclei of the midbrain tegmentum (see Figs. 22–3 and 22–6).

The *stria medullaris thalami* contains fibers that reciprocally connect nuclei of the septal and anterior hypothalamic areas with the habenular nucleus of the epithalamus. These fibers form a small, elevated ridge along the superomedial margin of the dorsal thalamus. The habenular nucleus, in turn, projects to the interpeduncular

nucleus, via the heavily myelinated *habenulointerpeduncular tract* (*fasciculus retroflexus of Meynert*). This prominent ventral projection from the epithalamus to the midbrain is the last link in a pathway from the basal forebrain and the anterior hypothalamic nuclei to the reticular formation of the midbrain (see Figs. 22–3 and 22–6).

Rounding out the limbic system pathways are two ubiquitous pathways, the *medial forebrain bundle* and the *periventricular bundle*. Both pathways are loosely organized and relatively diffuse groups of small unmyelinated to lightly myelinated fibers that interconnect the basal forebrain, septum, hypothalamus, and lower brain stem centers. Both pathways have ascending and descending fibers, and both have fibers that arise from and terminate on neurons in these areas. The most extensive contributions are made by neurons of the hypothalamus and septal area. In the diencephalon, the *medial forebrain bundle* passes through the lateral hypothalamus, whereas the *periventricular bundle* runs immediately lateral to the third ventricle, within the substance of the periventricular zone. Descending periventricular fibers enter the periaqueductal gray of the midbrain and continue into lower levels of the brain stem as the *dorsal longitudinal fasciculus of Schütz*.

Hippocampal Formation

The *hippocampus* and the *dentate gyrus* are the principal components of the *hippocampal formation*. The hippocampal formation forms a curved elevation of cortical tissue extending the entire length of the floor of the temporal horn of the lateral ventricle (see Fig. 22–1). During the development of the human brain, the rapid growth of the neocortical areas literally "rolls" the archicortical hippocampal formation into the depths of the temporal lobe (Fig. 22–7). The relative simplicity of the hippocampus has been of great interest to neuroanatomists for many years. Ramon y Cajal published one of the earlier descriptions of its histology in 1909 (Fig. 22–8).

HISTOLOGICAL ORGANIZATION OF THE DENTATE GYRUS

The *dentate gyrus* (*fascia dentata hippocampi*) differentiates from the most medial ring of cortical tissue in the developing hemisphere, immediately adjacent to the hippocampal sulcus. During development, this serrated strip of archicortex

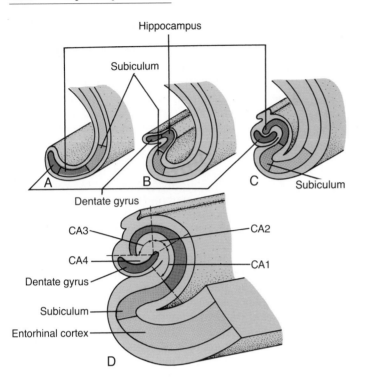

Hippocampus

Subiculum

A B C Subiculum

Dentate gyrus

CA3 CA2

CA4 CA1

Dentate gyrus

Subiculum

Entorhinal cortex

D

FIGURE 22-7

The development of the hippocampal formation and adjacent cortex of the temporal lobe. Note in (A), (B), and (C) the manner in which the archicortex forming the hippocampal formation is rolled into the depths of the temporal lobe.

With subsequent development (D), the hippocampus is divisible into four fields designated CA1, CA2, CA3, and CA4. See text for details. (Modified with permission from P. L. Williams and R. Warwick, *Functional Neuroanatomy of Man*, W. B. Saunders Co., Philadelphia, 1975.)

forms three distinct layers: an outer *molecular layer*, a middle *granular layer*, and a deep *polymorphic layer* (see Fig. 22-5). The most characteristic and abundant type of neuron in the dentate gyrus is the *granule cell*. The cell bodies of these neurons are densely packed in the granular layer. Their dendritic trees radiate into the molecular layer. These spinous dendritic processes receive synaptic input from the adjacent entorhinal cortex via the perforant path. Granule cell axons, in turn, leave the dentate gyrus and enter the molecular layer of the hippocampus as mossy fibers. Mossy fibers synapse on the proximal portion of the apical dendrite of hippocampal pyramidal cells (see Fig. 22-5). Before these axons leave the dentate gyrus, however, they give off numerous collaterals. Many of these collaterals are recurrent and ascend into the molecular layer of the dentate gyrus.

HISTOLOGICAL ORGANIZATION OF THE HIPPOCAMPUS

The *hippocampus* (*cornu ammonis* or *Ammon's horn*), also a three-layered strip of archicortex, parallels the dentate gyrus in location and development (see Figs. 22-5 and 22-7). The ventricular surface of the hippocampus, the *alveus*, is smooth and white. The alveus contains heavily myelinated axons, principally those of hippocampal pyramidal neurons, most of which enter the fimbria of the fornix. This fibrous sheet is continuous ventrally with the deep white matter of the neocortex. The three layers of the hippocampus, moving from the alveus inward, are the *polymorphic layer*, the *pyramidal cell layer*, and the *molecular layer* (see Figs. 22-5 and 22-8). The large *pyramidal cells* of the pyramidal cell layer are the most characteristic cell type in the hippocampus. These large neurons have dendritic trees that extend into the molecular layer. The basal dendrites and axons of these neurons descend into the polymorphic layer.

The *deepest layer* of the *hippocampus* is the *molecular layer*. The molecular layer contains a few neurons, relatively small and scattered, and an extensive neuropil. The neuropil contains the arborizations of the apical dendrites from the pyramidal cells in the adjacent pyramidal cell layer and a large number of axon terminals. These axon terminals include those of granule cells in the adjacent dentate gyrus, perforant path fibers from the entorhinal cortex, septohippocampal fibers, and recurrent axon collaterals from pyramidal cells (see Figs. 22-5 and 22-8). Some neuroanatomists further divide the molecular layer into three sublayers: stratum moleculare, stratum lacunosum, and stratum radiatum.

The *middle layer* of the hippocampus, the *pyramidal layer*, contains three to four rows of

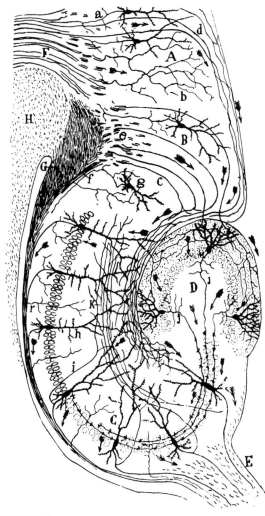

FIGURE 22-8

Some of the structure and connections of the hippocampus (Ammon's horn) as drawn by Ramon y Cajal. A, Entorhinal cortex; B, subiculum; C, hippocampus; D, dentate gyrus; E, fimbria of fornix; F, fibers of the cingulum entering the entorhinal cortex (A); K, Schaffer collaterals; a, axons entering the cingulum; b, fibers of the cingulum terminating in the entorhinal cortex; g, pyramidal cell of the subiculum; h, pyramidal cells of the hippocampus; i, ascending collaterals from the hippocampal pyramidal cells; j, granule cell axons; r, collaterals from axons in the alveus. (Reproduced with permission from S. Ramon y Cajal, *Histologie du Système Nerveux*, Tome II. Translated by L. Azoulay in 1955, Instituto Ramon y Cajal, Madrid.)

closely packed pyramidal cells. These pyramidal cells are frequently called "bitufted" neurons or "double pyramids," because of the large basal dendrites that extend deeply into the polymorphic layer (see Fig. 22-8). The axons of the pyramidal cells descend through the polymorphic

layer to reach the more superficial alveus. After running along the ventricular surface of the alveus, these fibers enter the fimbria of the fornix. These fibers terminate principally in the septal area and the anterior hypothalamus.

Another characteristic of the hippocampal pyramidal cell is the extensive collateral branching of the axon. This is particularly evident for those pyramidal cells closest to the dentate gyrus. Axons from these neurons enter the polymorphic layer and give rise to very prominent, heavily myelinated, highly branched collaterals known as *Schaffer collaterals*. Schaffer collaterals ascend through the pyramidal layer into the molecular layer. Once in the molecular layer, these collaterals spread throughout the hippocampus, synapsing with dendrites of pyramidal cells farther removed from the dentate gyrus. Many of these collaterals extend into the adjacent subiculum and the entorhinal area of the cortex (see Fig. 22-8).

The most *superficial layer*, excluding the alveus, is the *polymorphic layer*. Similar to the molecular layer, the polymorphic layer contains few neuronal cell bodies and is principally an area of extensive neuropil. Included in the neuropil are the large, bushy basal dendrites of the pyramidal cells and the highly branched collaterals of pyramidal cell axons, many of which make synaptic connections within the polymorphic layer.

Although the hippocampus is relatively uniform in structure, some subtle regional and areal differences exist in both the cytoarchitecture and the neurochemistry. Because of these differences, the transverse section of the *hippocampus* is often subdivided into regions and fields. The nomenclature was originally applied to the brains of animals in which the hippocampus lies dorsal to the corpus callosum. In the human brain, however, with the developmental displacement of the hippocampus into the temporal lobe, the hippocampus literally becomes turned over. Thus, regions that had been superior now are inferior, and regions that had been inferior are now superior. The *superior region* contains a compact pyramidal cell layer and extends about half the distance from the subiculum to the dentate gyrus. The remainder of the hippocampus is the *inferior region*. The hippocampus is divided further into four fields, designated simply by the letters CA, for cornu ammonis, and a number, 1, 2, 3, or 4. *CA1* occupies most of the superior region, *CA3* occupies most of the inferior region, and *CA2* is a small transition zone between CA1 and CA3. *CA4* is at the transition zone between the hippocampus and the dentate gyrus and is distinct from CA3 (see Fig. 22–7).

SUBICULUM

The *subiculum* is a narrow strip of cortical tissue situated between the hippocampus and the entorhinal cortex in the parahippocampal gyrus. The subiculum is a cortical transitional zone, with that part of the subiculum immediately adjacent to the hippocampus relatively simple in structure and that part immediately adjacent to the entorhinal cortex more complex. With this geographical increase in complexity, the subiculum often is subdivided into the prosubiculum (immediately adjacent to CA1 of the hippocampus), the subiculum proper, the presubiculum, and the parasubiculum (immediately adjacent to the entorhinal cortex). This text employs the term subiculum to represent the entire transitional zone between CA1 of the hippocampus and the entorhinal cortex. The subiculum, although a small area of transitional cortex, is essential for the transmission of information from the hippocampal formation to both the hypothalamus and the neocortex (see Fig. 22–6).

CORTICAL CONNECTIONS

The *hippocampal formation* has extensive connections with other regions of the cortex, both directly and indirectly via relay from adjacent areas of transitional cortex. The principal cortical afferent pathway to the hippocampal formation is the *perforant pathway*. This is a direct pathway from the *lateral entorhinal area* (Brodmann's area 28) to the hippocampal formation. Nerve fibers of the perforant pathway terminate in the *molecular layers* of both the *dentate gyrus* and the *hippocampus*. The axons of the perforant pathway synapse with the more distal portions of the dendritic trees of *both* the granule cells in the dentate gyrus and the pyramidal cells in the hippocampus.

The *cortical efferent projections* from the hippocampal formation are extensive and represent, by far, the major outflow of information from the hippocampal formation. These projections are diffuse and not identifiable as a single pathway or bundle of fibers. Many projections arise from *CA1*, *CA2*, and *CA3* of the hippocampus and terminate in areas of transitional cortex, both in the *subiculum* and the *entorhinal area*. These direct projections from pyramidal cells of the hippocampus also reach most of the cortical areas of the parahippocampal gyrus and the cingulate gyrus. Most of the hippocampal formation projections to neocortical areas, however, arise from the *subiculum*. The *subiculum* has extensive projections to *neocortical association areas* in the frontal, parietal, occipital, and temporal lobes.

SUBCORTICAL CONNECTIONS

The *fornix* is a large, heavily myelinated pathway connecting the hippocampal formation with subcortical structures, principally in the basal forebrain and hypothalamus. Most of the fibers of the fornix project from the hippocampal formation to lower centers. However, some fibers are afferents to the hippocampus and some are commissural. The latter use the fornix as a commissure to project to the hippocampal formation of the opposite side.

The heavily myelinated axons from pyramidal cells in the hippocampal formation enter the alveus en route to the fornix. These fibers, at the surface of the hippocampus, form the *fimbria of the fornix* and then the *fornix* proper. As the fornix leaves the surface of the hippocampus, it curves dorsomedially to meet the fornix from the opposite side immediately below the corpus callosum. At this point, the commissural fibers cross to the opposite side in the *hippocampal commissure* and enter the hippocampal formation of the opposite side. Most fibers of the fornix continue toward the ipsilateral basal forebrain and hypothalamic areas. A few of the fibers, however, cross in the hippocampal commissure and terminate in the contralateral forebrain and hypothalamic areas.

Rostral to the hippocampal commissure, the fornix continues in a forward direction and curves ventrad, toward the anterior commissure and the lamina terminalis. At the anterior commissure, the fornix splits. Some fibers pass in front of the anterior commissure as the *precommissural fornix*; the remainder pass behind the anterior commissure as the *postcommissural fornix*.

Fibers of the *precommissural fornix* that arise in the hippocampus proper project almost exclusively to the *lateral septal nuclei*. Other precommissural fibers of the fornix arise from areas of the subiculum and some adjacent areas of the entorhinal cortex. These project to basal forebrain areas, including the *nucleus accumbens*, the *bed nucleus of the stria terminalis*, and the *nuclei of the diagonal band of Broca*. Other subicular fibers end in *preoptic* and *anterior hypothalamic areas*.

Nearly all of the fibers in the *postcommissural*

fornix arise from the *subiculum.* At the anterior commissure, these fibers curve posterior and ventrad, running through the substance of the hypothalamus and ending in the *mammillary, arcuate,* and *ventromedial nuclei* (see Figs. 22–3 and 22–6).

The most significant of the afferent fibers in the fornix to the hippocampus are those of the *cholinergic septohippocampal tract.* These fibers are axons of neurons in the *medial septal nucleus* that terminate throughout the hippocampus and the dentate gyrus, although preferentially near the cell bodies and along the basal part of the apical dendrites. More selective in their terminations are the fibers of the *GABAergic septohippocampal tract.* These fibers also arise from the medial septal nucleus but synapse selectively with other inhibitory, GABAergic interneurons of the hippocampus. The effect of these GABAergic septohippocampal fibers, therefore, is one of disinhibition. The *chandelier cells* of the hippocampus and dentate gyrus are an example of GABAergic inhibitory interneurons. These inhibitory interneurons synapse selectively on the initial segment of axons, both from granule cells in the dentate gyrus and from pyramidal cells in the hippocampus.

The hippocampal formation also receives strong thalamic projections from the *anterior, lateral dorsal,* and *lateral posterior nuclei.* Nonspecific *intralaminar nuclei* also project to the hippocampal formation.

The hippocampal formation receives strong input from all six of the *extrathalamic cortical modulatory systems* (see Chapter 21). These include noradrenergic projections from the *locus ceruleus,* serotoninergic projections from the *raphe nuclei,* and dopaminergic projections from the *ventral tegmentum* of the midbrain (see Fig. 21–9). Cholinergic projections arise from both the *nucleus of the diagonal band of Broca* and the *nucleus basalis of Meynert.* GABAergic projections arise from the *posterior hypothalamus* and histaminergic projections from the *ventral posterior hypothalamus* (see Fig. 21–10). The dopaminergic projections are a major component of the *mesolimbic dopaminergic system.*

HIPPOCAMPAL RUDIMENTS

The *medial* and *lateral longitudinal striae* interconnect the hippocampal formation with the basal forebrain area. The projections are similar to those of the precommissural fornix but also include fibers arising from the *indusium griseum* and the *fasciola cinerea.* Neurons of the in-dusium griseum are essentially neurons of the hippocampal formation that were "left behind" during the developmental displacement of the hippocampal formation. The axons of both pairs of longitudinal striae are comparable to the precommissural fornix fibers arising from the hippocampus.

FUNCTIONS

The hippocampal formation is integral to many of the functions discussed in further sections of this chapter. A few functions, however, can be linked more with the hippocampal formation and less with the other components of the limbic system. One such function is the regulation of corticosteroid release from the adrenal gland that accompanies changes in mood and behavioral state. The normal diurnal pattern of release is controlled by autonomic mechanisms. The effectors are the parvocellular neurosecretory cells in the paraventricular nucleus of the hypothalamus (see Chapter 18). These cells release corticotropin-releasing hormone (CRH) into the hypophyseal portal system. The CRH, in turn, stimulates the systemic release of adrenocorticotropic hormone (ACTH) by cells of the adenohypophysis. The surges of adrenal corticosteroid release that occur in response to stressful situations are also due to surges of CRH release by the parvocellular neurosecretory system. *Under conditions of stress, however, the paraventricular neurosecretory cells are driven by signals from the hippocampal formation.* These signals override the normal pattern of release, providing the necessary surges of adrenal corticosteroids to meet behavioral situations. These hippocampal signals probably involve the *subiculohypothalamic fibers* in the postcommissural fornix.

Cortical Components

Collectively, the cortical components of the limbic system make up the *limbic lobe.* In addition to the archicortical *hippocampal formation* (see previous discussion), the limbic lobe contains several paleocortical and neocortical areas.

PARAHIPPOCAMPAL GYRUS—PIRIFORM AND ENTORHINAL AREAS

The terminology for the limbic system and its cortical components is often confusing. *Rhinencephalon* is frequently used incorrectly as a synonym for *limbic system.* Both are defined by function rather than by geography, and both "share" many forebrain structures.

Rhinencephalon means "smell brain," and for all species it includes those central nervous system (CNS) structures concerned with olfaction. In animals that have a keen sense of smell, such as rodents, the differences between the rhinencephalon and the limbic system are relatively clear. For the human, however, olfaction is not an essential or primary sense and the differences are not as distinct. Many homologous structures in the human brain, although retaining some olfactory connections, are involved in other functions such as emotions, homeostasis, and memory. The extensive areas of overlap between the rhinencephalon and the limbic system in the human nervous system are important for the affective and emotional dimensions of olfactory perception. These areas of overlap are summarized in Table 22–1.

Two other cortical areas add some confusion to the definition of the limbic lobe: the *piriform cortex* (*olfactory cortex*) and the *entorhinal cortex*. Many species differences in these cortical areas exist. Often, different criteria are employed for their definition. Both cortical areas are components of the limbic lobe and of the rhinencephalon. The following definitions, although simplistic, are sufficient for the purpose of this discussion.

Together, the entorhinal cortex and the piriform cortex occupy most of the *parahippocampal gyrus*. The parahippocampal gyrus lies on the medial surface of the temporal lobe, parallel to the hippocampal formation. The *hippocampal sulcus* separates the parahippocampal gyrus from the hippocampus: the *rhinal* and *collateral sulci* separate the parahippocampal gyrus from the adjacent neocortical temporal lobe association areas (see Figs. 22–1, 22–4, and 22–5). The most anterior portion of the parahippocampal gyrus folds back on itself to form a "hook" or fist-shaped area of cortex called the *uncus*. The amygdaloid nuclei lie deep to the uncus in the rostral part of the temporal lobe.

The *piriform cortex* is the anterior part of the parahippocampal gyrus, including the uncus. Included in the definition of piriform cortex, but *not* a component of the limbic lobe, is the lateral olfactory gyrus (see Chapter 13). The term piriform means pear-shaped, and this cortical area is roughly shaped like a pear (see Fig. 22–4). The entire piriform cortex is paleocortex and contains from three to five layers.

The remainder of the parahippocampal gyrus, principally Brodmann's area 28, is the *entorhinal*

cortex. The rostral boundary of the entorhinal cortex is the piriform cortex. The posterior boundary is the isthmus of the cingulate gyrus (see Fig. 22–4). Areas of the entorhinal cortex that are anterior and superior (i.e., adjacent to the subiculum) are paleocortical and contain up to five layers. Areas that are more inferior (i.e., adjacent to the temporal association cortex) and posterior are neocortical and contain six layers.

Some workers include the subiculum in the definitions of the entorhinal cortex and the parahippocampal gyrus. In this text, the subiculum is considered a part of the hippocampal formation, creating a transitional zone between the hippocampus and the adjacent entorhinal cortex.

ISTHMUS AND THE CINGULATE GYRUS

The *isthmus of the cingulate gyrus* (*isthmus gyrus cinguli*) lies adjacent to the splenium of the corpus callosum, on the medial surface of the cerebral hemisphere. The isthmus forms a constricted segment of neocortex interconnecting the *cingulate* and *parahippocampal gyri*. The *cingulate gyrus* is an arch-shaped convolution of neocortex, also on the medial surface of the cerebral hemisphere. The cingulate gyrus lies dorsal to the corpus callosum, separated from it by the *callosal sulcus* (see Figs. 22–1 and 22–3). Deep to the surface of the cingulate gyrus, and running parallel to it, is the *cingulum*, a large cortical association bundle.

SUBCALLOSAL GYRUS AND PAROLFACTORY AREA

As the cingulate gyrus curves forward and then inferiorly, around the genu and rostrum of the corpus callosum in the frontal lobe, it becomes continuous with the *subcallosal gyrus* (*paraterminal gyrus*). The subcallosal gyrus forms a thin sheet of cortex ventral to the rostrum of the corpus callosum and anterior to the lamina terminalis (see Figs. 22–1 and 22–3). The *parolfactory area* (*subcallosal area*) is a small area of cortex on the medial surface of the frontal lobe, immediately in front of and below the subcallosal gyrus.

RELATED NEOCORTICAL ASSOCIATION AREAS

Extensive connections exist between the limbic system and many of the cortical association areas in the frontal and temporal lobes. Generally, these association areas are not considered limbic structures. These neocortical areas include the *orbitofrontal* and *dorsolateral prefrontal association areas*, along with the *inferior* and *anteromedial temporal association areas* (see Chapter 21). These same neocortical areas also have strong connections with the ventral striatum, as do all areas of the limbic lobe.

The *anteromedial temporal association area* does contain a portion of the limbic lobe (the piriform and entorhinal areas), in addition to the adjacent neocortex on the inferomedial surface of the temporal lobe. Both the anteromedial and inferior temporal association areas are involved in memory mechanisms (see subsequent discussion).

The *orbitofrontal areas* are also the neocortical representation areas for olfaction. Cortical projections of the olfactory system from the mediodorsal nucleus of the thalamus terminate principally in the *orbital gyri*. Patients with lesions in this area are unable to discriminate between odorants. This area is also important in the affective and emotional dimensions of olfaction.

Damage to the *dorsolateral* or *orbitofrontal association areas* can lead to emotional disturbances. Electrical stimulation of these areas —especially the orbitofrontal area—leads to autonomic nervous system responses and emotional reactions. Both areas have extensive interconnections with limbic areas. These include the reciprocal thalamic connections, principally with the mediodorsal nucleus; cortical association pathways, including the cingulum; strong reciprocal connections with the ventral striatum; and *direct* projections to the hypothalamus. These are the only neocortical areas with direct projections to the hypothalamus. Interconnections of the *orbitofrontal area* are almost exclusively *limbic* in nature. The *dorsolateral area* has more interconnections with *other areas of the neocortex*, in addition to those with the *limbic system*.

Septum and Forebrain Structures

COMPONENTS OF THE SEPTAL COMPLEX

In the human brain, most of the nuclei of the septal complex are ventral to the *septum pellucidum*. These nuclei extend into the forebrain, toward the subcallosal gyrus, and form the "true septum" or *septum verum*. Only a few scattered neurons extend into the septum pellucidum. The most prominent nuclei of the septum verum are

the *medial, lateral,* and *dorsal septal nuclei*. Associated with these nuclei, and part of the *septal complex*, are the *nucleus of the diagonal band*, the *bed nuclei of the stria terminalis*, and the *bed nuclei of the anterior commissure*. The *nucleus accumbens* is also continuous with the posterior portion of the septal complex, but this nucleus is functionally more a part of the ventral striatum (see subsequent discussion).

The *diagonal band of Broca* runs along the ventral surface of the forebrain. Originating in the parolfactory area and the medial portion of the septum, this band extends along the posterior margin of the anterior perforated substance. Closely associated with the band is the *nucleus of the diagonal band*. The nucleus of the diagonal band is continuous with the *medial septal nuclei*. Together, they represent a single nuclear complex.

The *stria terminalis* runs along the inner curvature of the caudate nucleus, extending from the septal complex in the basal forebrain area to the amygdala in the temporal lobe. In the basal forebrain area and in close association with the stria terminalis is the *bed nucleus of the stria terminalis*. This nucleus is continuous with the *lateral septal nucleus*. Together, they function as a single nuclear complex.

SEPTAL PATHWAYS

The *septal complex* has extensive reciprocal connections with the *hippocampus*, the *hypothalamus*, and the *habenula*. In the circuitry of the limbic system, the septal complex lies in the middle of a principal pathway for the flow of information from the limbic lobe structures in the temporal lobe to the hypothalamus and the midbrain reticular formation. The septal complex receives extensive afferent projections from many cortical areas, as well as nuclei in the basal forebrain, hypothalamus, and brain stem. Among these afferents are brain stem monoamine projections, similar to the *extrathalamic cortical modulatory systems* discussed in Chapter 21. These include *adrenergic projections* from the locus ceruleus, *serotoninergic projections* from the dorsal raphe, and *dopaminergic projections* from the ventral tegmental area along with *histaminergic projections* from the posterior hypothalamus.

The septal complex occupies a strategic location for the modulation and relay of information passing from the hippocampal formation to the lower centers. Through modulation of this pathway, the septal complex can alter autonomic responses controlled by hypothalamic and brain stem centers (see Chapter 18). The relative roles of the *hippocampal-septal-hypothalamic pathway* of the *precommissural fornix* and the more direct *hippocampal-hypothalamic pathway* of the *postcommissural fornix* in the control of autonomic function are unknown.

Fibers from the *medial septal nuclei* and the *nuclei of the diagonal band* have strong projections to the *hippocampal formation* via the *septohippocampal tract*. Traveling in the fornix, these *cholinergic* and *GABAergic* fibers terminate in the dentate gyrus, the hippocampus, the subiculum, and the adjacent entorhinal cortex.

Glutaminergic projections from the *hippocampal pyramidal cells* reach the *lateral septal nuclei* via the fibers of the *precommissural fornix*. Many of these fibers originate in the contralateral hippocampal formation and decussate in the hippocampal commissure. Other fibers of the precommissural fornix originate in the *subiculum* and the adjacent *entorhinal cortex*. The last projections are not as specific and terminate in many nuclei in the septal complex.

Neurons from the septal nuclei project to many areas of the hypothalamus via the *medial forebrain bundle*. These targets include the *medial preoptic area*, the *lateral hypothalamus*, nuclei of the *medial hypothalamus*, and the *mammillary complex*. Some of these septal projections continue in the medial forebrain bundle to midbrain levels, terminating in the *ventral tegmental area*, the *locus ceruleus*, and the *dorsal raphe nucleus*.

Septal fibers, principally from the posterior and medial areas, project to the *habenula* via the *stria medullaris thalami*. This information, in turn, is relayed to the *interpeduncular nucleus* of the midbrain by neurons from the medial habenular nucleus. These fibers form the *habenulointerpeduncular tract*. This route to the midbrain provides feedback to the locus ceruleus and the dorsal raphe nuclei and carries information to other nuclei of the brain stem reticular formation.

OTHER FOREBRAIN STRUCTURES

The *basal ganglia* have a significant role in the modulating and processing of information related to the limbic lobe and to the neocortical associational areas of the prefrontal and temporal areas. The information processing that occurs through the basal ganglia involves an extensive series of loop circuits that interconnect the specific cortical areas, basal ganglia, and selected relay nuclei of the dorsal thalamus (see Chapter 16).

Although the caudate and putamen receive input from large areas of the cerebral cortex, the *ventral striatum* receives most of its projections from cortical areas related to the limbic system. This includes the components of the *limbic lobe*, the *prefrontal association areas*, and the *temporal association areas*.

The *ventral striatum* contains the *nucleus accumbens* and the *substantia innominata* (*nucleus basalis*) as well as the ventral divisions of both the *caudate nucleus* and the *putamen*. The *ventral pallidum* contains the ventral division of the globus pallidus (see Table 22-1).

Because both the *nucleus accumbens* and the *substantia innominata* functionally link the limbic system with the basal ganglia, they are part of the *ventral striatum*. The *nucleus accumbens* extends from the base of the septal complex laterally to the junction of the caudate and putamen, where it becomes continuous with the ventral divisions of these striatal nuclei. The *substantia innominata* is situated beneath, and is continuous with, the ventral divisions of the putamen and the globus pallidus. Anteriorly, the substantia innominata extends toward the nucleus accumbens and the amygdala, with its rostral end deep to the anterior perforated substance.

Three of the *basal ganglia-thalamocortical loop circuits* involve the limbic lobe and related prefrontal cortical association areas. These are the *limbic circuit*, the *association-1 circuit*, and the *association-2 circuit* (see Chapter 16 for details).

The *limbic circuit* projects principally to the *anterior cingulate area* (Brodmann's areas 24 and 33) and the *medial orbitofrontal area* (Brodmann's areas 10, 11, 12, 25, and 32). The *corticostriate* fibers originate from the same anterior cingulate and medial orbitofrontal areas as well as the remainder of the *limbic lobe* and the *temporal association areas*, including the temporal pole. All of these corticostriate fibers project to the *ventral striatum*. The *ventral striatum*, in turn, projects to the *ventral pallidum* and to the *pars reticulata* of the *substantia nigra* (*SNr*). The thalamocortical projections complete this loop circuit. These arise from the *mediodorsal nucleus* and terminate in the *anterior cingulate* and *medial orbitofrontal areas* (see Fig. 16-2).

The *association-1 circuit* projects principally to the *dorsolateral prefrontal area* (Brodmann's areas 8, 9, 10, and 46). These corticostriate fibers originate from the *posterior parietal association cortex* and the *premotor cortex*, in addition to the *dorsolateral prefrontal area*. These corticostriate fibers terminate in the *head* of the *caudate*. The pallidal connections are with both the *external* and *internal* divisions of the *globus pallidus* (*GPe* and *GPi*). The thalamocortical projections that complete the loop originate in both the *ventral anterior* and *mediodorsal nuclei* of the thalamus and terminate in the *dorsolateral prefrontal area* (see Fig. 16–2).

The *association-2 circuit* projects principally to the *lateral orbitofrontal area* (Brodmann's areas 10, 11, 44, 45, 46, and 47). The corticostriate projections for this circuit arise from the *auditory* and *visual association areas* of the temporal lobe; from the *superior, middle,* and *inferior temporal gyri*; from the *anterior cingulate area*; and from the *lateral orbitofrontal area*. These corticostriate fibers also terminate in the *head* of the *caudate*. The pallidal and thalamic connections are similar to those in the association-1 circuit, except that the thalamocortical fibers project selectively to the *lateral orbitofrontal area* (see Fig. 16–2).

It is difficult to distinguish between *direct* and *indirect* loops for those circuits that use the ventral pallidum. The ventral pallidum does not contain subdivisions comparable to GPe and GPi. The direct loop facilitates the flow of information from the thalamus to the cortex, whereas the indirect loop inhibits the flow of information from the thalamus to the cortex (see Chapter 16). Physiological studies, however, indicate the presence of both direct and indirect loops in the limbic circuits. Further resolution of the neuroanatomy is needed to identify both types of limbic loop.

The precise roles for these loops in the processing of limbic system information are unknown. In somatic motor systems, in which measurements of function and deficit are more precise, the loop circuits are involved in the *planning, programming,* and *execution* of complex motor tasks. Functional correlates of the prefrontal and anterior cingulate areas include *emotion, affect,* and *complex problem solving* (see Chapter 21). It is likely that these limbic-related loops have a role in the planning, programming, and execution of responses (behavioral, autonomic, and somatic motor) that are related to emotion, affect, and problem solving. Definitive information, however, awaits the development of tests that can reliably differentiate between and measure these dimensions of behavior.

The behavioral and emotional changes that often accompany disorders of the basal ganglia (e.g., Parkinson's disease and Huntington's disease) may involve areas of the caudate nucleus; the ventral striatum; or, more specifically, the

limbic loops. A role for these loops in cognition is supported by the results of positron emission tomographic studies. These findings indicate a correlation between the dementia associated with Huntington's disease and hypometabolism in the caudate nucleus. The cerebral cortex appears normal.

Amygdala

The *amygdala* or the *amygdaloid nuclear complex* is a group of nuclei in the rostral end of the temporal lobe, deep to the piriform cortex of the uncus. Developmentally, the *amygdala* differentiates from the same basal telencephalic mass as the other nuclei of the basal ganglia: the caudate, putamen, globus pallidus, ventral striatum, and ventral pallidum (see Fig. 1–19). The afferents and efferents of the amygdala, however, are unlike any of the other basal ganglia. These connections, and the *absence* of loop circuits, set the amygdala apart from the other basal ganglia and make it a functional component of the *limbic system*.

The *amygdala* is divisible into many nuclei, each with different connections and different functions. For discussion, these nuclei are grouped into three divisions, with the nuclei of each division sharing common features of connectivity and function. The three divisions are the *corticomedial*, the *basolateral*, and the *central divisions*. None of these nuclei or divisions, however, operate in isolation. Extensive interconnections exist between most of the nuclei along with commissural connections with the amygdaloid complex of the opposite side. These *interamygdaloid commissural fibers* enter the *stria terminalis* and project forward to the *lamina terminalis*, where they cross the midline in the *anterior commissure*. The crossed fibers then reach the contralateral amygdaloid nuclei by traveling in the reverse direction in the contralateral *stria terminalis*.

CORTICOMEDIAL DIVISION

The *corticomedial division* has extensive *olfactory connections* and strong reciprocal *hypothalamic connections*. Most of the fibers in the *lateral olfactory stria* terminate in the corticomedial division of the amygdaloid complex or in the overlying *piriform cortex*. Secondary projections from the piriform cortex also terminate in the corticomedial division of the amygdala or in the adjacent *entorhinal cortex.* The *ventral amygdalohypothalamic tract* is a direct pathway of reciprocal connections between the amygdala and the hypothalamus. This pathway passes from the amygdala, through the sublenticular part of the internal capsule, and directly into the hypothalamus. A less direct route is taken by other amygdalohypothalamic fibers. These fibers reach the nuclei of the anterior hypothalamus via the *stria terminalis.*

BASOLATERAL DIVISION

The corticomedial division is the oldest phylogenetically, whereas *basolateral division* is the newest. The basolateral division has extensive *reciprocal connections with the neocortical sensory association areas,* principally from the parietal and temporal lobes. This amygdaloid division also projects to both the basal ganglia and the dorsal thalamus. The size of this division correlates well with the size of the neocortex. Therefore, this division is larger in the human brain than in the brains of other mammals. Except for olfactory information, the amygdaloid complex receives only "processed" sensory information from sensory association areas. The amygdala does not receive information, either from thalamic sensory relay nuclei or from primary sensory cortices. In addition to the cortical association areas, extensive connections exist between nuclei of the *amygdala* and areas of the limbic lobe, such as the *entorhinal cortex, cingulate gyrus,* and *parolfactory area.*

CENTRAL DIVISION

Neurons in the *central division* form the principal descending pathways from the amygdala to the autonomic nervous system centers in the brain stem. These centers include the dorsal motor nucleus of the vagus, brain stem respiratory centers, and cardiovascular pressor and depressor centers (see Chapter 18). One neurochemical characteristic of the central division is a high concentration of *peptidergic neurons.* Many of the interneurons of the central division contain enkephalins; many of the projection neurons contain a variety of other peptides, including somatostatin, neurotensin, CRH, and cholecystokinin. Axon terminals from central division neurons also terminate near brain stem monoaminergic nuclei, such as the locus ceruleus, the dorsal raphe nucleus, and the ventral tegmental nucleus of the midbrain. The degree of descending amygdaloid influence on these ascending extrathalamic cortical modulatory systems is not clear.

Descending peptidergic fibers from the amygdala reach the hypothalamus and basal forebrain area by either the direct *ventral amygdalohypothalamic tract* or the *stria terminalis.* Once in the forebrain or diencephalon, many of these fibers descend through the brain stem in the *medial forebrain bundle* or the *dorsal longitudinal fasciculus (of Schütz).* A number of the projections to the midbrain reticular formation that travel in the stria terminalis respond to olfactory stimuli.

FUNCTIONS

The *amygdala* is involved in many limbic system functions. Most of these also involve other limbic structures. These limbic system functions are discussed further in this chapter. The *modulation of autonomic responses* is one direct function of the amygdala. These modulations of autonomic activity occur in two ways. The first is by modulating hypothalamic activity through the extensive reciprocal connections between the amygdala and the hypothalamus. The second is through the direct projections from the amygdala to autonomic centers in the brain stem. The first pathway acts on the autonomic nervous system's "upper motor neurons" and the second acts directly on the equivalent of the autonomic nervous system's "lower motor neurons."

Regulation of autonomic function by the amygdala is different from that of the hypothalamus (independent of amygdaloid influence). *Hypothalamic regulation* of autonomic function is *reflexive,* altering functions millisecond by millisecond according to changes in the body's *physiological condition* (see Chapter 18).

In contrast, *modulation by the amygdala is instinctive. The amygdala alters autonomic function based on learning and past experience.* The basolateral division, with its extensive neocortical connections, is the receiving station for the instinctive or learned experience. The central and corticomedial divisions are the source of the efferents with their projections to the brain stem and hypothalamus, respectively.

An individual can, for example, develop a generalized fear of dogs from a previous experience in which he or she was attacked by a vicious dog. Following such an experience, the sound or sight of any dog, violent or not, can trigger autonomic responses, such as increases in heart rate, sweating, and respiration. Under these circumstances, the autonomic changes are not in response to alterations in the body's internal physiology but in response to past experience. This example is a learned response. The amygdala is the center responsible for the final integration of these learned or conditioned responses. The hypothalamus, in the absence of amygdaloid input, does not respond instinctively, only reflexively.

The nature of the response modulated by the amygdala is not limited to instinctive fear. All types of past conditioning experiences can lead to amygdaloid modulation of functions controlled by the autonomic nervous system. These can be associated with the gastrointestinal system, sexual arousal, or any other visceromotor activity.

Olfaction

The olfactory system is the only sensory system to project directly to the limbic system (see Chapter 13). All other sensory information that reaches the limbic system is first processed in secondary cortical association areas. How the processing of primary olfactory information relates to other limbic system functions is not clear. The anatomical overlap between the *rhinencephalon* and the *limbic system* is more readily understood in lower forms, in which olfaction is an integral part of the behavioral patterns. In other mammals, for example, the autonomic responses associated with sexual drives and emotions such as fright and rage are often driven by olfactory stimuli. In the human, however, a total loss of olfactory sensation, *anosmia*, has little detectable effect on these behaviors or other limbic system functions. It is likely, however, that intact olfactory projections to limbic system structures in the human brain are important in the affective and emotional dimensions of olfactory perception.

Homeostatic Mechanisms

Homeostatic mechanisms are the control systems that stabilize the body's internal environment. When the external environment is in a constant state of flux, homeostatic mechanisms are necessary for survival. These autonomic nervous system mechanisms normally operate through a series of feedback controls that are coordinated in the hypothalamus (see Chapter 18). The limbic system, through its extensive connections with the hypothalamus, is able to modulate many of these mechanisms.

CONDITIONED RESPONSES

The *amygdala*, as noted, is the center in the limbic system that coordinates the modulation of

autonomic activities in response to past experiences. Most of these activities are in the area of *conditioned responses*. The human brain, however, also has the capacity to "voluntarily" override many visceromotor functions. This "mind-over-body" control of visceromotor functions, such as heart rate, blood pressure, and gastrointestinal motility, involves the neocortex. In this context, higher thought processes produce a type of conditioned response, if one expands the definition of a conditioned stimulus to include a cognitive or thought process.

The limbic system forms the link between cognitive activity and visceromotor response. Both the *amygdala* and the *hippocampus* provide the principal connections between the *limbic system* and the *autonomic nervous system*. The *hippocampus* modulates these mechanisms through its connections with the subiculum and the septal complex. Hippocampal modulation, however, is small in comparison to that of the amygdala. The amygdala, as we have discussed, is the primary autonomic effector of the limbic system.

THIRST DRIVE AND BODY FLUID REGULATION

The hypothalamus controls homeostatic mechanisms that regulate body fluids. Most of these mechanisms are reflexive and operate in response to specific sensors, the baroreceptors and the osmoreceptors. The *behavioral drive* to seek and consume water, however, originates in the cerebral cortex and is more complex. The *subfornical organ* contains osmoreceptors and is sensitive to circulating levels of angiotensin II (see Chapter 18). In addition to its hypothalamic connections, the subfornical organ has extensive connections with the *limbic lobe*. These connections are essential for the initiation of the behavioral drives to seek and consume water. Therefore, through the subfornical organ, many of the same thirst stimuli that drive the hypothalamus also reach behavioral and somatomotor areas of the cerebral cortex.

EATING BEHAVIOR

The hypothalamus is an important center for feeding behavior, and its pathology is often accompanied by a variety of eating disorders (see Chapter 18). Because the limbic system has extensive connections with the hypothalamus, pathology of the limbic system also can lead to eating disorders. In the absence of hypothalamic or limbic neuropathology, eating disorders may be psychogenic in origin. In these cases, the limbic system provides the link between neocortical areas and the hypothalamus.

Many eating disorders, from *anorexia nervosa* to *bulimia*, may be psychogenic or may involve limbic system pathology. Anorexia nervosa is characterized by a lack of interest in food and by an intense fear of becoming obese. When patients do eat, it often is followed by self-induced vomiting. Bulimia is characterized by an insatiable appetite for food. Patients with bulimia frequently go on eating binges that may be followed by self-induced vomiting. Unlike patients with anorexia nervosa, bulimic patients do not show extreme weight losses.

Eating disorders of psychogenic origin or of limbic lobe pathology are ultimately expressed through hypothalamic centers. The paraventricular nucleus is very important in this expression, but the mechanisms are unknown. Some evidence exists that noradrenergic projections from the locus ceruleus have a role in eating behavior. These projections, however, end in the neocortex, the limbic lobe, many basal forebrain centers, and the hypothalamus. Therefore, the noradrenergic system could be affecting eating behavior at any of these levels.

ADRENOCORTICOSTEROIDS

The *hippocampus* contains receptors that are sensitive to circulating levels of both *adrenocorticosteroids* and *ACTH*. In stressed animals, stimulation of the hippocampus decreases the secretion of adrenocorticosteroids. In resting animals, however, the same stimulation increases the rate of steroid secretion. Although these observations are from laboratory studies, a similar role has been postulated for the hippocampus in the human brain. The regulatory mechanism is presumed to act through hippocampal connections with the parvocellular neurosecretory cells of the hypothalamus.

The sensitivity of the hippocampal pyramidal cells to the circulating levels of corticosteroids may account for steroid-induced behaviors. Emotional lability and various forms of psychosis can accompany the administration of high levels of corticosteroids. These same symptoms can also accompany hyperfunction of the adrenal gland.

Emotions

Emotions are psychic states characterized by strong, generalized feelings. Love, joy, happiness, hate, anger, rage, fear, grief, sadness, and excitement are some of the more familiar emotional states. The development of these feelings is complex and draws on many neocortical processes and functions. These range from the recall of past experience, to sensory information processing, to cognitive processes.

Clinically, patients with damage to the prefrontal cortex often have very labile and unpredictable patterns of emotional behavior (see Chapter 21). These disturbances correlate well with the neuropathology. All of the factors contributing to a given emotional state, however, are not in the prefrontal lobe. This area, nevertheless, is important for the development and expression of these emotional feelings. Of the prefrontal areas, the *medial* and *lateral orbitofrontal areas* are most directly associated with emotions (see Fig. 16–2). In humans, stimulation of these cortical areas produces strong emotional feelings along with the associated visceromotor responses.

Although the *prefrontal areas* are needed for the cortical *perception of an emotion*, the *amygdala* is needed for the *expression of an emotion*. This concept is supported by the neuroanatomy and by clinical and laboratory studies. The prefrontal areas have extensive connections with the limbic system, including direct projections to the amygdala and to the hypothalamus.

Stimulation of the human amygdala also evokes both changes in emotional feeling and changes in the appropriate autonomic responses. The changes elicited cover a broad range of emotions from feelings of aggressiveness to those of generalized pleasure. The type of emotional feeling reflects the particular subnucleus of the amygdala stimulated.

The observation that amygdalectomies produced docile and tame monkeys prompted the use of amygdalectomies to alter the behavior of individuals with extremely aggressive and socially unacceptable behavior. These ablations were successful in eliminating aggressive behavior, but they also eliminated more positive emotional responses as well. The patients were described as emotionally "flat." These general observations are consistent with the findings of a large number of studies performed on laboratory animals, including primates.

Much of the available neuroanatomical and behavioral information about emotions concerns the amygdala and the prefrontal cortical association areas. Other areas of the limbic system also have important roles in the development and expression of emotions, although the details are not yet clear. The septal complex, for example, can have an important role in modulating the expression of emotions. Following an amygdalectomy, a monkey generally becomes tame and docile. If a lesion is placed in the septal complex of the same monkey at a later date, however, he becomes hyperactive and displays periods of rage. These studies illustrate the problems in ascribing specific functions to the components of an elaborately interconnected system.

Learning and Memory

Learning and memory are complex processes that involve many areas of the CNS, including the limbic system. The hippocampal formation is essential for the storage of newly acquired information, and this chapter is the appropriate place to discuss this subject.

There are many definitions of learning and memory and nearly as many theories about the neurobiological mechanisms involved in these processes. Few subjects in neurobiology are as hotly debated and discussed as those concerning learning and memory. The study of memory and learning has utilized a broad spectrum of behavioral and molecular techniques. Even with the advances gained from these interdisciplinary studies, we still lack a unified theory of learning and memory.

DEFINITION

Many definitions of learning and memory exist, each with subtle differences—differences that often reflect the orientation of the investigator. The following definitions, although oversimplifications, should serve as working guides and as useful starting points.

In this text, *learning* simply refers to the acquisition of new knowledge or information. We intentionally avoid the more elaborate definitions that relate learning to behavioral changes that occur because of past experience. Implicit in the definition of memory is the transient nature of learning, unless what is learned is stored in a retrievable form.

Memory refers to the process whereby newly acquired information is stored and retrieved for future use. Recall is part of this definition, because the only way to decide whether or not an individual remembers something is through the ability to recall it.

Memory, by most definitions, contains two components: *short-term memory* and *long-term memory*. *Short-term memory* refers to newly ac-

quired information that is lost after a brief period (seconds, minutes, or longer) unless reinforced. *Long-term memory* refers to the retention of the acquired information for extended periods of time, potentially for the life of the individual. For our definitions, *learning* is comparable to *short-term memory*.

PHYSIOLOGICAL THEORIES

If we assume that learning and memory occur within the neuronal network of the CNS, the alterations of synaptic mechanisms become likely candidates. *Short-term memory* or *learning* occurs rapidly, within milliseconds, and normally lasts for periods of a few minutes to an hour. These rapid changes, therefore, must involve mechanisms already in place at the synapse. These most likely would involve alterations in the properties of the synapses through second messenger systems, i.e., presynaptic or postsynaptic modulation of the activity of ion channels or receptors.

Synapses have a broad range of plasticity. Membrane conductance changes in the presynaptic membrane can alter both the amplitude and the duration of the presynaptic potential. If these result in an increase in the calcium influx, there will be a corresponding increase in the release of neurotransmitter, thereby amplifying the magnitude of the signal to the postsynaptic neuron. In comparison, a decrease in these parameters reduces the signal. Possible changes include postsynaptic conductance changes and altered sensitivity of receptors.

Many of these properties have been identified and studied in simple, invertebrate systems. The habituation of a simple reflex arc was shown to involve a decrease in the amount of neurotransmitter released at the synapse. This effect resulted from a cumulative inactivation of voltage-sensitive calcium channels. Another situation involved the facilitation of a synapse following prolonged stimulation. In this situation, presynaptic receptors, coupled to adenyl cyclase, activated a specific protein kinase. The kinase, in turn, phosphorylated potassium channels in the presynaptic terminal, rendering them inactive. This net reduction in potassium conductance extended the duration of the presynaptic potential. This extension, in turn, increased the calcium influx and the associated release of more neurotransmitter. The stimulation properties and the duration of responses in both examples are considered within the physiological ranges for short-term memory mechanisms.

High frequency stimulation of certain CNS synapses can produce a pronounced and prolonged potentiation of the excitatory postsynaptic potential (EPSP) and increases the probability that the postsynaptic neuron will fire with subsequent stimulation. This example of "functional modulation" is called *long-term potentiation*. Although many investigators consider this phenomenon a possible basis for short-term memory, a direct association has yet to be made. Under precise conditions of stimulation of perforant path neurons, postsynaptic granule cells of the dentate gyrus can maintain the potentiated state for as long as 2 to 3 weeks. This mechanism may involve both presynaptic and postsynaptic mechanisms. Presynaptically, an increase occurs in the amount of glutamate released—the reason is unknown. The postsynaptic events implicate the NMDA glutamate receptors, along with an increase in the calcium influx in the postsynaptic terminal (see Chapter 5). One explanation suggests that one or more of the calcium-dependent protein kinases are responsible for a modification of postsynaptic ion channels, rendering the synapse more responsive to subsequent stimuli. A large gap still exists between all these mechanisms and the actual acquisition of short-term memory in the vertebrate CNS.

Most current theories of *long-term memory* include the requirement for *de novo* protein synthesis. This, in turn, requires communication with the nucleus of the neuron and activation of the mechanisms for DNA transcription. This activation of transcription is probably linked to one or more of the second messenger systems. However, other than the knowledge that long-term memory requires the synthesis of new protein, we know little else.

DEFICITS AND DAMAGE

A review of clinical studies indicates that some regions of the CNS are more important than others in memory processes. The *inferior temporal association area* is important in short-term memory. However, the nature of the memory loss is different for each hemisphere. Damage to the right inferior temporal area leads to severe deficits in short-term visual memory. Following lesions to the left area, however, visual loss is not as severe, but deficits in short-term verbal memory occur. This lateralization of memory processing reflects the lateralization of language skills (see Chapter 21).

Some patients suffering from severe forms of temporal lobe epilepsy have undergone removal of the anterior portion of the temporal lobe, bilaterally. Neural tissue removed included the hippocampus, the amygdala, and the cortex of the anterior temporal lobe. These patients were able to *learn* at a normal pace, but the information was soon forgotten. The *short-term memory* mechanisms were intact, but the ability to consolidate information as *long-term memory* was lacking.

Other patients with damage to the dorsal thalamus, especially the mediodorsal nucleus, had problems with the initial learning of new information. Once learned, however, the information was remembered. In these patients, the mechanism for the transfer of information to *long-term memory* remained intact, although the acquisition of new information appeared impaired.

In the early stages of Alzheimer's disease, a progressive loss of the ability to consolidate short-term memory to long-term memory occurs. Neuroanatomically, the first area to show damage is the limbic system. Within the limbic system, the structure affected first and most severely is the hippocampus. This finding is further evidence that the hippocampus is essential for the consolidation of short-term memory to long-term memory. Although a coincident loss of cholinergic neurons in the nucleus basalis occurs, this appears to be secondary (see Chapter 21).

LOCALIZATION OF MEMORY

At this stage in our understanding of the memory processes, little is definitely known, but much is speculated. One area that is known to be essential to the human nervous system, however, for the consolidation of short-term memory to long-term memory is the hippocampal formation. Where long-term memory is stored along with how this memory is accessed is still a matter of speculation. The more conservative points of view favor widespread storage, involving extensive areas of the neocortex.

SUGGESTED READING

Isaacson, R. L. and K. H. Pribram (Editors) (1975). *The Hippocampus. (Volume 1, Structure and Development; Volume 2, Neurophysiology and Behavior.)* Plenum Press, New York.

This two-volume series remains today one of the most comprehensive compilations of information on the hippocampal formation. Topics include structure, neurochemistry, electrophysiology, behavior, and endocrinology. With chapters covering the interconnections of the hippocampus, most other limbic system structures, from the hypothalamus to the septal area, are discussed. This is an excellent source for the student desiring more information about the limbic system.

Isaacson, R. L. (1982). *The Limbic System*, 2nd Edition. Plenum Press, New York.

This short monograph provides the student with an introduction to the neurobehavioral study of the limbic system. Although 10 years old, this monograph is an excellent starting point and gives the student an understanding of the various components of this complex system and an appreciation of the manner in which the components are integrated.

Willner, P. and J. Scheel-Krüger (Editors) (1991). *The Mesolimbic Dopamine System: From Motivation to Action.* John Wiley & Sons, New York.

The mesolimbic dopaminergic system is involved in a variety of behavioral functions related to motivation and reward, whereas the nigrostriatal system is related more to motor and cognitive functions. This volume contains an extensive array of studies that summarizes the current status of the mesolimbic dopaminergic functions, the morphological and biochemical substrates, and their clinical implications.

Index

Note: Page numbers in *italics* refer to illustrations; page numbers followed by t refer to tables.

503

Resting potential, 61–74. See also *Membrane potential(s).*
calculation of, 68–71
current flow and, 70–72, *71*
equivalent circuit model and, *71*, 71–72
ion channels and, *63*, 63–68, *65*, *67*, *68*
ion concentration gradients and, 68t, 68–72
ion flow and, 69–70
maintenance of, *63*, 63–74, *65*, *67*, *68*
measurement of, 62, *62*
postsynaptic potential and, 61–62, 72–74, *73*
properties of, *63*, 63–68
sodium-potassium pump and, 66–68, *68*
Reticular activating system, 148, 459–460. See also *Extrathalamic cortical modulatory systems.*
Reticular formation, 149
cerebral activation by, 459–460
dorsolateral pontine, *220*, 220–221
motor system role of, 316–317, 319, 332
nucleus gigantocellularis, 220–221, 276
nucleus pontis caudalis, 276
nucleus raphe magnus, *220*, 220–221
rostral ventrolateral medullary, 395
thalamic relay and, 445
vestibular pathways and, 276
Reticulospinal tract, *125*, 126, 317, *318*, 319, *353*
lateral, *125*, 126, *318*, 319, 332
medial, *125*, 126, *318*, 319, 332
motor system role of, 319, 331–332
Retina, 224–237. See also *Visual system.*
anatomy of, 224–225, *225*, *226*, *228*
cell layers of, 225–237, *228*, *229*
cells of, 226–237, *229*
center-surround antagonism in, *234*, 234–235
fields and, 226, *227*
fovea and, *226*, *227*, *230*, 230–231
information processing in, 233–237
macula of, *230*, 230–231
membranes of, 228, *228*, *229*
neurons of, 226–237, *228*, *229*, *234*
photoreceptors of, *229–232*, 231–233
Retinal, 232–233
Retinogeniculocalcarine tract, *225*, 237–240, *238*, *239*, 248. See also *Visual system.*
Retinosuprachiasmic tract, 386t, 389
Retroflexus fasciculus (of Meynert), *147*, 149, *153*, *154*, *486*, 487, 494
Retrograde degeneration, 56, 58–59, *60*
Retroinsular area, 215, *215*, 217
Retrorubral nucleus, 341–342, 462
basal ganglia and, *341*, 341–342
Rexed's laminae, *127*, 128, *128*
Rhinencephalon. See also *Limbic system.*

Rhinencephalon *(Continued)*
components of, 163t, 163–164, 479, *481*, 491–492
smell sense and, 163t, 163–164, 296, 491–492
Rhodopsin, 231–232, *233*
biochemistry of, *233*
Rhombencephalon, 12–16, *13*, 13t, *14*
Rhombic lip, cerebellar development and, 15, *15*, 350
Rhomboid fossa, development of, 14
Ribosomes, *32*, *37*
Right-handedness, 468–472, *471*
Rigidity, basal ganglia disorders and, 346
decerebration and, 320
muscular, 320, 321, 346
spinal cord trauma and, 321
Riley-Day syndrome, 397–398
Rods of retina, *228–232*, 231–233
absorption spectrum of, *230*, 231
signal transduction in, *232–233*, 232–233
structure of, *231*, 231–232
Rolandic artery, *180*, 333
Roof plate, 13–14, *14*
Roots, dorsal, *119*, *124*, 126–127, *201*, 201–202, *202*
injury to, 220–221
spinal, 117, *118*, *119*, 120–123, *121*, *124*
ventral, 6–11, *8*, 117, *119*, 120–123, *121*, *124*, 304
Rostrum, corpus callosum, *159*, 162
Round window, 255, *257*. See also *Auditory system, ear and, inner.*
Rubrospinal tract, *125*, 126, *143*, *353*
motor system role of, 317–318, *318*
Ruffini's end organs, 200, *200*

S

Saccades, 410–411
Saccule, *268*, 268–269, *269*
Sagittal sinuses, *187*, 187–188. See also *Sinus(es) (dural).*
Salivary glands, *371*, *375*, 376, *379*, 380
autonomic innervation of, *375*, 378t, 380
diminished function in, 416, 420
innervation of, *375*, 378t, 380, 414, 419
secretions of, 380
Salivatory nucleus, inferior, 147, 376, 404t, *406*, *421*, 422
superior, 147, 376, 404t, *406*, 417–419, *418*
Saltatory conduction, 48, 77, *77*
Salty taste, 285–286
Satellite cells, 9, 55–56
Satiety center, 394
Scala media, 254, *256*, *257*
Scala tympani, 254, *256*, *257*
Scala vestibuli, 254, *256*, *257*
Scarpa's (vestibular) ganglion, 251, *268*, 271, 273–274, *274*
Schaffer collaterals, 489, *489*

Schütz, dorsal longitudinal fasciculus of, *140*, *142*, *152*, 388, 462, 487, 496
Schwann cells, capsular, 55–56
ganglia and, 55–56
morphology of, *50*, 52, *54*
myelination and, *50*, 52, *54*
origin of, 9
regeneration and, *57*, 58–59
unmyelinated axon and, 52, *55*
Sclerosis, amyotrophic lateral, 320–321
Scotoma, 247
Second messengers, cerebral receptors and, 459
G-proteins and, 93–94, *94*, 292–293
neurotransmitter systems and, 93–97, *94*, *96*, 459
olfaction and, 292–293
receptor coupled to, *81*, 84–85, 93–97, *94*, *96*, 459
Sections of brain stem, keys to, *138*, *151*
Seizures, brain waves and, *474*
Sella turcica, 188
Semicircular canals, 251, *251*, *268–272*, 268–273. See also *Vestibular system.*
ampulla of, 269, *269*, *271*
crista ampullaris of, *271*, *272*, 272–273
lateral, 268–269, *268–270*
motion effects in, *270*, 271–273, *272*
posterior, 268–270, *268–270*
superior, 268–270, *268–270*
Seminal vesicle, innervation of, 378t, 381–382
Sensory nerve fiber classification, *197*, 197–198
Sensory systems, 195–299. See also *Auditory system; Olfactory system; Somatosensory system; Taste; Touch; Vestibular system; Visual system.*
Septal area. See *Septum.*
Septomarginal fasciculus, *125*, 125–126
Septum. See also *Limbic system.*
anatomy of, *150*, *158–160*, 165, 167
fiber pathways of, 493–494
hippocampus and, 493–494
limbic system and, 480t, 484, 487, 490–491, 493–494, 497–499
nuclei of, 484
olfaction and, *297*, 297–298, *298*
pellucidum, 21, *152*, *158*, *160*, *165*, 167, 484
verum, 167, 484
Serotonin (5-hydroxytryptamine), *104*, 104–105. See also *Neurotransmitters.*
action of, 105
behavior affected by, 105
cerebral function and, 460, *460*, 461–464
degradation of, *104*, 104–105
neurons containing, 201, 236, 458, *460*, 460–462, 463–464, 491, 493
receptors for, 105
second messengers and, 105
sleep regulation and, 477